Foundations of Sensory Science

By

H. Autrum · L. M. Beidler · H. Davis · H. Engström
G. A. Fry · R. Granit · W. D. Keidel · D. R. Kenshalo
O. Lowenstein · C. Pfaffmann · L. A. Riggs · D. Schneider
T. Tomita · W. D. Wright · J. J. Zwislocki

Edited by

W. W. Dawson and J. M. Enoch

With 190 Figures

Springer-Verlag
Berlin Heidelberg New York Tokyo 1984

WILLIAM W. DAWSON

Department of Ophthalmology
College of Medicine
University of Florida
J. Hillis Miller Health Center
Gainesville, Florida 32610
USA

JAY M. ENOCH

School of Optometry
University of California
Berkeley, California 94720
USA

OPTO

ISBN 3-540-12967-7 Springer-Verlag Berlin Heidelberg New York Tokyo
ISBN 0-387-12967-7 Springer-Verlag New York Heidelberg Berlin Tokyo

Library of Congress Cataloging in Publication Data. Main entry under title: Foundations of sensory science. (Handbook of sensory physiology. Supplement) Bibliography: p. Includes index. 1. Senses and sensation–Addresses, essays, lectures. 2. Sense-organs–Addresses, essays, lectures. I. Autrum, Hansjochem. II. Dawson, William W., 1933–. III. Enoch, Jay M. IV. Series. 2P431.F68 1984 591.1'82'09 83-20107 ISBN 0-387-12967-7 (U.S.)

Typesetting, printing and bookbinding: Brühlsche Universitätsdruckerei, Giessen
2122/3130-543210

List of Contributors

AUTRUM, H., Zoologisches Institut der Universität München, Luisenstraße 14, 8000 München 2, FRG

BEIDLER, L. M., Department of Biological Science, The Florida State University, Tallahassee, Florida 32306, USA

DAVIS, H., Central Institute for the Deaf, 818 South Euclid, St. Louis, Missouri 63110, USA

ENGSTRÖM, H., Department of Oto-Rhino-Laryngology, University Hospital, 75014 Uppsala 14, Sweden

FRY, G. A., College of Optometry, The Ohio State University, 338 West 10th Avenue, Columbus, Ohio 43210, USA

GRANIT, R., The Nobel Institute for Neurophysiology, Karolinska Institutet, 10401 Stockholm 60, Sweden

KEIDEL, W. D., Institut für Physiologie und Biokybernetik der Universität Erlangen-Nürnberg, Universitätsstraße 17, 8520 Erlangen, FRG

KENSHALO, D. R., Department of Psychology, The Florida State University, Tallahassee, Florida 32306, USA

LOWENSTEIN, O., Neurocommunications Research Unit, The Medical School, The University of Birmingham, 22 Estria Road, Birmingham B15 2TJ, Great Britain

PFAFFMANN, C., The Rockefeller University, 1230 York Avenue, New York, New York 10021, USA

RIGGS, L. A., Walter S. Hunter Laboratory of Psychology, Brown University, Providence, Rhode Islands 02912, USA

SCHNEIDER, D., Max-Planck-Institut für Verhaltensphysiologie Seewiesen, 8131 Seewiesen, FRG

Tomita, T., Department of Physiology, Keio University School of Medicine, 35 Shinanomachi, Shinjuku-ku, Tokyo 160, Japan

Wright, W. D., 68 Newberries Avenue, Radlett, Herts WD7 7EP, Great Britain

Zwislocki, J. J., Institute for Sensory Research, Syracuse University, Merrill Lane, Syracuse, New York 13210, USA

Preface

When seen from an outsider's vantage point, the development of knowledge in the sensory sciences must appear massive and the result of some carefully followed master plan. In reality, it is the result of numerous relatively independent human endeavors shaped by application of the scientific method. The comprehensive construction of quantitative theories of sense organ function has occurred only recently – but at an explosive rate prefaced by centuries of expansion in the physical sciences. Predicated on this growth, the twentieth century may become known as the age of the biological sciences. With the exception of a modest number of intellectual giants, there were few contributors to the foundations of the sensory sciences before the dawn of this century. At least 90% of existing knowledge has been produced by scientists working in laboratories founded since 1920.

If any single scientist and his laboratory may be identified with the growth in the sensory sciences, it is EDGAR DOUGLAS ADRIAN, First Baron of Cambridge and leader of the Physiological Laboratory at Cambridge University, England. Lord ADRIAN's influence upon the sensory sciences was great, not only in terms of his contribution to knowledge itself but also through the influence which he exerted upon numerous young scientists who spent weeks or years at the Cambridge laboratory and who later returned to their homelands and colleagues with the seeds of vigorous research and quantitative inquiry firmly implanted. These scientists and many like them have built modern sensory science, brick by brick, laboratory by laboratory. Many of these men and women are alive today, and they have framed the research questions which will be pursued for generations. However, the death of Lord ADRIAN in 1977 marked the end of the early formative period.

The chapters in this book have been written by scientists who contributed to the forming of the foundations of the sensory sciences during the first half of the twentieth century. A diverse geographic background and a broad range of specialties are represented. The volume seeks to examine, from the viewpoint of the specialist, the numerous human factors which inadvertently affect the direction of scientific development: the influence of war, the surges of effort which follow new technical advances, the influence of colleagues and the adaption to economic necessities. The volume also seeks to look at the science which was available to these builders and at the research additions which each of them considers important to his or her speciality. The editors hope that the volume will give a glimpse of the currents which have shaped the foundations of the sensory sciences to those who will make their contributions in the future.

WILLIAM W. DAWSON
JAY M. ENOCH

Contents

CHAPTER 1

Comparative Physiology of Invertebrates: Hearing and Vision

Hansjochem Autrum

A. Introduction

When my interest in biology began, the discipline was not defined (as it usually is in our excellent modern textbooks) as the science of "the natural bodies which possess nucleic acids and proteins, and which are capable of synthesizing such molecules by themselves." In the Berlin vernacular – quick-tongued as a Berliner is – the plain retort would have been, "Right you are, but all the same it's just boloney." And later, I never asked myself whether the living processes which interested me took place in "natural bodies of proteins and nucleic acids." When I was a student, it was the Protista which fascinated me, and I built my own microscope to study them. In 1923, I also assembled a radio which had a crystal as the rectifier. At that time, it was still forbidden to build a radio, but one could buy a book, written anonymously and entitled *How the American Hobbyist Builds a Radio by Himself*. Here were the roots of my two later interests; delight in studying living animals and delight in building instruments.

To be sure, to pull these two interests together years ago was not easy. Zoological institutes had neither the equipment nor the money to provide physical apparatus. Institutes of physics – at least in Berlin – had no interest in physiological questions. Help with my interests appeared by coincidence.

My professor, Richard Hesse (1868–1944), was asked by Karl Willi Wagner (1883–1953) whether he knew someone who would like to work on the hearing of lower animals in his newly founded institute. Wagner was the Director of Heinrich Hertz Institut für Schwingungsforschung, a modern institute set up in connection with the flourishing development of radio technology and supported by the radio industry itself. To busy someone with the physiology of hearing in lower animals was a hobby of Wagner, for he had the ambition to see represented in his institute investigations of the entire spectrum of oscillatory processes – all the way from high-frequency electric to those of acoustics and music. He told me: "When you want apparatus, just let me know, for our workshop can assemble anything you need. Your concern is to find a research topic."

Of course, the post carried neither stipend nor salary. What I needed to live I had to earn by tutoring failing students, privately. And I understood nothing about acoustics. But I had every bit of help I needed from my co-workers in the Institute, even though most of them laughed at me, the "useless" outsider. What could ever come from investigations of ants and grasshoppers?

B. Hearing in Insects

I. The Theory

Opinions about hearing capacities of insects were contradictory. GRABER (1875), who was the first to examine the tympanic organs of orthopterans, stated: "I can demonstrate that the tympanic organs are not the essential hearing organs of these animals; there must be other acoustical apparatus with the same function." REGEN (1914, p. 892) reached the same conclusion for males of the genus *Thamnotrizon*, as did EGGERS (1928) for insects of the genera *Agrotis* and *Catocala*. Therefore, insects that do not have tympanic membranes were studied first of all. As examples, I chose ants (*Myrmica, Lasius,* and *Formica*). Opinions about their hearing capacities were also controversial (for the older literature, see AUTRUM 1936 a, b).

The conclusions from my investigations (AUTRUM 1936 a, b) were that there are two types of sound receiver, physically as well as biologically speaking. Sound waves can be described in terms of two characteristics. First, the oscillating particles move back and forth, and they oscillate around an average position. The movements of particles of pure tones are sinusoidal. Through friction the oscillating particles can easily set other particles into oscillation with them, just as thin ribbons or moveable hairs are set into movement by oscillations. Receivers of the types which are stimulated by the movements of sound waves are called "velocity" or "movement" receivers. Second, a sound wave also involves pressure oscillations. The particles, which move back and forth periodically, produce pressure waves.

Those two components of sound waves can be separated physically. The physicist August Adolph KUNDT (1839–1894) did this in an elegant manner. He produced standing sound waves in a tube (Fig. 1) on the bottom of which he had sprinkled very light powder – actually cork dust. By the movements of air particles, the cork particles were flung forward to positions where velocity was great. The cork dust then collected in the places where pressure oscillations were maximal and where, in comparison, the air particles' movements were minimal.

That method was also used in my investigations with the ants (AUTRUM 1936 a, b). It was found that the ants responded only to maximal movements of particles, not to the pressure maximum of the standing waves.

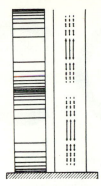

Fig. 1. Stationary airborne waves in Kundt's tube (1870). *Left,* pressure maxima and minima; *right,* velocity maxima and minima. Length of the tube: 2 λ. Phase angle between pressure and velocity: $\lambda/2$ ($= 180°$)

Thus, there are two types of sound receivers. One type responds to the periodic *movement* of particles. Examples of that type are hair sensilla and antennae. The second type responds to periodic *pressure* waves. The tympanic membranes of most vertebrates are examples of that type. As was shown later, those examples are extreme cases, for there are many hearing organs the physical characteristics of which lie between pure movement receivers and pure pressure receivers (for review see MICHELSEN and NOCKE 1974; MICHELSEN 1979).

Another parameter of a sound field is its pressure gradient. That is the difference in sound pressure between the two sides of a tympanic membrane (AUTRUM 1940). Movement, acceleration, and pressure gradient (pressure difference) are vectorial quantities. Consequently, receivers which respond to those factors have a directionality. Pure pressure receivers do not possess directionality, since sound pressure is a scalar quantity (Fig. 2).

A further characteristic of sound fields exists in close proximity to the source of the sound. There the wave fronts are not plane, but are more or less spherical, and the pressure gradient is not a simple function of the sound pressure. There, since animal sound receivers are often mixed pressure and pressure gradient receivers, measurements in the neighborhood of the source of sound are often incalculable (see MICHELSEN and NOCKE 1974). Also, in the neighborhood of oscillating bodies, under certain conditions there advance rhythmically changing medium currents the velocities of which are directly proportional to the surface of the vibrating bodies and which decrease with the square of the distance from the source. Therefore, in the far field, those currents play no roles. In some cases, the sound produced by other animals is "heard" only in the extreme near field of the sound source. Thus, a high threshold for sound under far-field conditions does not exclude a good sense of hearing in situations which are biologically important for the animals. The physical characteristics of sound fields have been presented in detail by MARKL (1973) and MICHELSEN and NOCKE (1974).

At the beginning, my conclusions about types of sound receivers in insects were a result of bad luck. In 1936, I presented a short report on the theory of velocity receivers of insects to the Zoological Congress in Freiburg. Hans Spemann, who, in

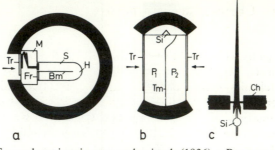

Fig. 2 a–c. Types of sound receiver in man and animals (1936). **a** Pressure receiver: the mammalian ear. The tympanum (*Tr*) is accessible to sound waves on only one side. The head acts as a firm casing. The apparatus of the middle ear (hammer, anvil, stirrup) inserts on the tympanum, and conducts movements of the tympanum to the inner ear (cochlea; organ of Corti); *Bm*, basilar membrane; *Fr*, round window; *H*, helicotrema; *M*, middle ear; *S*, cochlea. **b** Pressure gradient receiver. Sound pressure affects the two opposing sites of the tympanal membrane(*Tm*). *Si*, sensory cells of the crista acustica; Tr_1, Tr_2, tympana; P_1, P_2, tracheal air cavities. **c** Movement receiver: mobile hair of arthropods. *Si*, sensory cell(s) with a distal dendrite; *Ch*, chitin armor. Autrum (1942)

1935 had won a Nobel Prize for his work in developmental physiology, was the host and Chairman of the meetings. After my short paper, which was probably *too* short, and therefore not readily understood by a nonphysicist, Spemann made only one remark: that it was difficult to comprehend why insects could hear better when they were moving than when they were sitting still! Further discussion of my theory did not occur; the theory and the speaker were dismissed. Only von Frisch came after my presentation to hear more. He had already received the manuscript of my complete paper for publication in the *Zeitschrift für Vergleichende Physiologie* (Autrum 1936 b).

Without doubt, the work had a weakness. My theory was correct and was, in general, valid. However, for the ants which had been studied, the theory seemed to have no biological significance. Only in 1975 did Markl and Tautz renew investigations of hair sensilla of caterpillars, some of which had been started by Minnich (1925). They studied the reactions of larvae of *Barathra brassicae* (syn. *Mamestra brassicae,* commonly the cabbage dot moth) to airborne sound. Tautz (1977, 1978) described the physical basis of movement reception by hair sensilla as follows: It would be either the frictional forces or the acceleration forces of the oscillating air particles which set the receptor hairs into vibration. Markl and Tautz (1975) also explained the biological significance of the phenomenon: The filiform hairs on the thorax of the caterpillar respond to the dominant frequency (150 Hz) in the near field out to a distance of 70 cm. There the amplitude of particle displacement (peak to peak) amounts to 2.0 µm. Fletcher (1978), applying one of Stokes' (1851) laws, showed that it is the frictional forces which set the hair sensilla into vibration; those hair-like transducers react optimally to a specific frequency when their length is roughly in inverse proportion to the square root of the frequency. Such differentiation of the scalar components (e.g., pressure) from the vectorial characteristics (e.g., velocity, acceleration) of sound waves plays a role not only in the hearing of arthropods, but also in the hearing of vertebrates, e.g., fishes (for reviews see Popper and Fay 1980).

II. The Tympanic Organs of the Tettigoniidae

1. Methods

The tympanic organs, which lie below the "knee" in the proximal portion of the tibia of bush crickets, were first described by VON SIEBOLD (1844). He proved even then that the tracheal system, which runs through the tympanic organs, leaves through a bladder-like opening in the prothorax, the "hearing trumpet." The classic study of the anatomy of tympanic organs is that of SCHWABE (1906). Further anatomical studies were published by SCHUMACHER (1973) and LEWIS (1974a). REGEN (1914, 1926) demonstrated for *Thamnotrizon* that the tympanic organ is the essential, but not the sole, organ of hearing.

A new approach to the physiological investigation of such organs was described by WEVER and BRAY (1933). They recorded the summated action potentials from the femoral nerves of crickets, mole crickets, and katydids. In doing so, they used the first electrophysiological methods for investigating hearing in insects. EGGERS (1928) reviewed some of the earlier studies of hearing in these animals.

For us, bush crickets were easy to get – at least in the summer and autumn. It was much more difficult to procure amplifiers with which to record the action potentials from the crickets' hearing organs. Again my co-workers at the Heinrich Hertz Institute helped. We built ourselves a suitable ac amplifier. It was a tube amplifier with AF7 tubes approximately 7 cm in length. It was extremely sensitive to sound and tended to respond to many disturbances, above all to electric fields and acoustical feedback. A huge Faraday cage and cotton wool packing about 10 cm thick made up the circuit to the battery-operated amplifier. The apparatus was not really a pleasure.

2. The Subgenual Organs

Further difficulties accompanied our investigation. The action potentials were led from the femoral nerves of the forelegs. A needle in the femur was the reference electrode; a small silver plate lying under the tarsi was the indifferent electrode. A preparation with a tympanic organ responded well to high tones, e.g., hissing or the ultrasound of a Galton whistle (25 kHz). But – and here lay the difficulties – the slightest shaking, every footstep in the room, even light taps on the laboratory bench caused electric responses. The physicists suspected that the problem was the shaking of the electrodes. Even though careful anesthetizing of the preparation with ether disproved that idea, the physicists were not convinced.

How great did the vibrations have to be to release the response? And with which receptor organ were they received? Those were the questions to be answered next.

To produce and to measure the vibration waves, a permanent dynamic loudspeaker was used (Fig. 3). Its membrane was removed and a short rod was glued to its coil. A small silver plate was fastened to the free end of the rod, and on it rested the tarsi of the foreleg. Again, action potentials were recorded with a needle from the femoral nerves.

The system could be calibrated by measuring the sinusoidal oscillations under the microscope, for the amplitudes of vibrations are proportional to the intensity of current in permanent dynamic loudspeakers. (This type of loudspeaker was in-

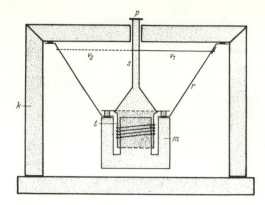

Fig. 3. The apparatus for producing vibrations (1941): k, wooden box; m, permanent magnet with a circular, ring-like fissure (in this fissure was a pasteboard cylinder holding a low-resistance coil); s, rod and funnel glued on to the pasteboard cylinder; p, vibrating silver plate; v_1, v_2, adjustment wires; r, metal frame of the loudspeaker; the vibrating loudspeaker membrane (inserting on the pasteboard cylinder) was removed. AUTRUM (1941)

vented by Werner von Siemens in 1878 in collaboration with von Helmholtz.) That linear relationship was checked under the microscope. The measurements made under magnification ($d = k \times I$; in which d = amplitude of the rod, I = effective current intensity in the coil, and k = a constant) could be extrapolated to the smallest amplitude, since the extrapolated measurements went through the zero point of the coordinates. However, even with this system, the technical difficulties were not overcome. Shaking of the apparatus had been eliminated to a great degree by placing the entire setup on a heavy plate which rested on four tennis balls. Nevertheless, its was impossible to make measurements during the daytime because vibrations in the building and those from traffic in the street could not be entirely eliminated. Consequently, measurements were made at night. For me that meant tutoring by day and doing research by night.

Then, in 1935, after an offer from Hesse, I finally received a salaried position in the Institute of Zoology of the University of Berlin. Hesse retired in that same year – early, and probably on political grounds, although he never discussed that with me. K. W. Wagner did have to relinquish the directorship of the Heinrich Hertz Institute for political reasons.

The consequence of my appointment was that I no longer had the apparatus which had been available to me in Wagner's Institute. So I had to build by myself all the equipment necessary for my research. To make the situation even more difficult, there was no workshop in the Institute of Zoology! A great help was Ferdinand Trendelenburg (1896–1973), the author of one of the first textbooks in physical acoustics, and in the 1930', the Director of the research laboratories of Siemens and Halske in Berlin; he gave me a low-frequency oscillator (20–20,000 Hz) and a power amplifier as a gift from his company. Today, after 50 years, that equipment is still fully intact.

I found that the amplitudes of vibration of the receptor organs in the tibia of the insects were surprisingly low. In *Decticus* and *Tettigonia*, the threshold amplitudes of the vibration lay in the frequency range 200–3,000 Hz and were in the

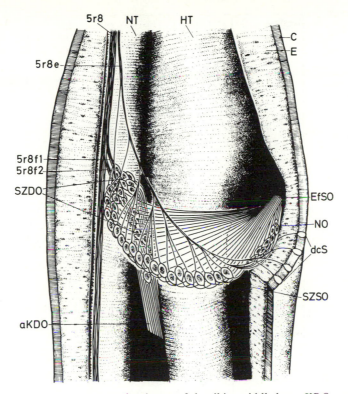

Fig. 4. *Periplaneta americana:* proximal part of the tibia, middle leg. *aKDO,* accessory cap cells of the distal organ; *C,* cuticula; *dcS,* distal campaniform sensilla; *E,* epidermis; *EfSO,* end fibers of the subgenual organ; *HT,* posterior principal trachea; *NO,* accessory organ; *NT,* anterior trachea; *SZDO,* receptor cells of the distal organ; *SZSO,* receptor cells of the subgenual organ; *5r8,* nerve innervating the sensory organs (except the proximal campaniform sensilla), with the branches *5r8e* coming from the distal campaniform sensilla, the subgenual organ and the accessory organ, and *5r8f1* and *5r8f2* from the distal organ. × 500 Schnorbus (1971)

magnitude of 10^{-8} cm (peak to peak) (Autrum 1941); and in the cockroach, *Periplaneta americana,* they were found to be even less than 10^{-9} cm at 1,500 Hz (Autrum 1943).

Those vibrations lie within atomic dimensions, about 1/25 of the diameter of the first electron ring of hydrogen atoms. We asked whether that was physically possible. We did not believe it ourselves and sought for experimental errors – in vain. First, a discussion with the physicist Karl Friedrich von Weizsäcker reassured us. (Von Weizsäcker worked at the Kaiser Wilhelm Institute of Physics in Berlin-Dahlem with Werner Heisenberg.) He pointed out that vibrations with magnitudes of 10^{-10} cm were physically conceivable, but that such sizes were the lowest possible, and vibrations with smaller amplitudes were not allowable. Von Békésy (1941) also came to those conclusions after calculating that the amplitudes of vibrations of the human tympanic membrane, and especially those of the stapes, fall in the same size range.

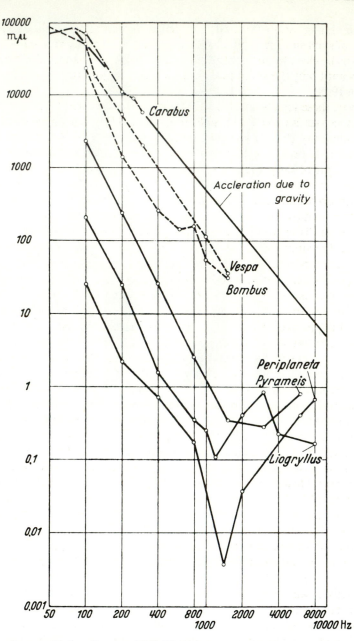

Fig. 5. Vibration sensitivity of insects (1941 ff.) *Abscissa,* vibration frequency (Hz). *Ordinate,* amplitudes (peak-to-peak) in mμ ($=10^{-7}$ cm). Autrum and Schneider (1948)

Only recently, with the modern methods of laser technology, has it been possible to measure movements smaller than 0.1 nm ($=10^{-10}$ m) (Dragsten et al. 1974). Michelsen and Larsen (1978) converted a slightly less sensitive method than Dragsten's to measure the movements and phase relationships of the tympanic membranes of insects.

For me, this question came next: Which receptor organs in insects respond to vibrations of such small magnitudes? In the tympanic region of bush crickets many sense organs lie close to one another. We successively disconnected all these receptor organs until only the subgenual organ was intact (AUTRUM 1941; AUTRUM and SCHNEIDER 1948).

However, these results (AUTRUM 1941) were also doubted (LITTLE 1962; WALCOTT and VAN DER KLOOT 1959), so SCHNORBUS (1971), at my suggestion, investigated the anatomy (Fig. 4) and the vibratory sensitivity of *Periplaneta* using the modern methods now available. She also studied the campaniform sensilla and found that some of those organs, specifically those of the distal group, responded in synchrony with sinusoidal stimuli up to approximately 40 Hz. Those of the proximal group responded to stimuli of about 70 Hz. At higher frequencies the responses alternated (there is one response for every two stimuli). We know that the subgenual organ is maximally sensitive to stimuli lying between 1,000 and 5,000 Hz, and that the vibration threshold at 2,000 Hz lies near 10^{-10} cm. The adequate stimulus is acceleration. These facts are based not only on measurements made in the subgenual organ, but also on responses recorded from interneurons in neck connectives of crickets, *Gryllus campestris* (DAMBACH and HUBER 1974).

In *Gryllus,* the frequency of impulses is linearly proportional to acceleration in the range of 0.5 to 100 cm $\times$ s^{-2}. Comparative measurements of activity in many other insects (AUTRUM and SCHNEIDER 1948; SCHNEIDER 1950) showed that vibration sensitivity, measured in terms of amplitude threshold, varies in different species (Fig. 5). In addition, when acceleration is measured at threshold, there are even greater differences between insect types. For example, for *Eristalis* the figure is 246 cm $\times$ s^{-2} at 80 Hz, and for *Periplaneta,* it is 1.6×10^{-2} cm $\times$ s^{-2} at 1,400 Hz (AUTRUM and SCHNEIDER 1948). They attributed these differences to the varying structures of the chordotonal organs in the insect legs. This assumption is still not completely compelling. Undoubtedly, the subgenual organs and the accessory organ (for discussion of that point, see SCHNORBUS 1971) are the most sensitive vibration receptor organs. However, when the earlier measurements were made, it was not considered possible that the campaniform sensilla could function as vibration receptors by summing the impulses from the femur (MARKL 1970, leaf-cutting ants; SCHNORBUS 1971, cockroaches).

The question of whether insects are also sensitive and respond to vibration of such amplitudes under natural conditions remained open. Then, in 1974, DAMBACH and HUBER showed this to be true for *Gryllus bimaculatus* and *Gryllus campestris;* electrical activity was recorded in nerves from the legs near the thoracic ganglia and from interneurons of the connective between the subesophageal and prothoracic ganglia. They not only confirmed our results (AUTRUM and SCHNEIDER 1948), but they also found a somewhat greater sensitivity in the range of 1,000 Hz. The most sensitive are the receptors of hind legs. Their threshold lies at 0.11 cm $\times$ s^{-2}, which corresponds to a peak-to-peak amplitude of 2.2×10^{-8} cm. In *Gryllus* vibratory stimuli are warning signals. In numerous other cases, the vibrations function in intraspecific communication (for reviews see MARKL 1973; SCHWARTZKOPFF 1974).

3. The Tympanic Organs: The Tympana and the Crista Acustica

WEVER and BRAY (1933), using electrophysiological measurements, had found for *Amblycorypha* and *Pterophylla* a high-frequency boundary at 45 kHz. In *Decticus* and *Tettigonia* responses to even 90 kHz were observed (AUTRUM 1940). However, at that time and for a long time afterward, sources of ultrasound were unavailable, and above all there were no properly sensitive instruments with which to make the necessary measurements. With a Galton whistle one could approach approximately 25 kHz, and in the Heinrich Hertz Institute there was a magnetostrictive device emitting ultrasound at my disposal. Actually, the transmitter was made up of short iron rods surrounded by coils of wire, which emitted – more or less directed – ultrasound of one specific frequency, when activated, at their resonance frequency, on their end surfaces.

Again both we and our physicist colleagues were amazed that the tympanic organs of the bush crickets were far more sensitive to ultrasound than were any available physical instruments. At that time, quantitative measurements in the ultrasound range were impossible. Instruments with which to measure sound pressure had been developed about that same time in the Heinrich Hertz Institute, but their sensitivity reached only to roughly 0.04 µbar, and in *Tettigonia* this threshold was already attained at 6 kHz. However, the extension of the curve showed that the sensitivity maximum must lie at an even higher frequency.

The most important results of our measurements were the findings that:
1. The tympanic organs of *Decticus* and *Tettigonia* are pressure gradient receivers;
2. In bush crickets, frequency discrimination is not possible.

Those studies were still going on in part in the Heinrich Hertz Institute, but they were being conducted predominantly in the Institute of Zoology. My association with the Heinrich Hertz Institute was broken off after 1936. Wagner's successor had no interest in the physiology of hearing in insects. Such studies served no scientific usefulness, were militarily without value, and – as I was told by the politically coordinated *Deutsche Notgemeinschaft* (Emergency Association of German Science) – were without meaning for the German people. Consequently, further support of my studies from those sources was no longer conceivable. Help came from another source, one which I hardly expected, but my research turned in a completely different direction.

But first, a few remarks about the development of our theories regarding hearing in the Tettigoniidae. LEWIS (1974 a–d) and NOCKE (1975) employed electrophysiological methods, and also investigated primarily the influence of the prothoracic hearing trumpet. MICHELSEN and LARSEN (1978) directly determined the vibration of the tympanic membrane, with the aid of a laser beam reflected from the membrane. With that method, not only the velocity, but also the phase difference of the velocity compared to the oscillating sound pressure, could be measured. At low frequencies, it was found that the hearing trumpet plays the most important role. In contrast to my earlier assumption (AUTRUM 1940), the sound waves in the low-frequency range reach the inner side of the tympanum through the hearing trumpet; only with increasing frequency do they move through the tympanic membrane itself. Thus, with low-frequency sounds, i.e., between 1 and about 10 kHz, the hearing organ is a pressure gradient receiver; with higher frequencies, it is a pressure receiver. That shows how complicated acoustical situations often are. The theory of the functioning of these hearing organs is still not completely clear, since the different types operate on the basis of various mechanisms.

C. The Eyes of Insects

I. The Eyes of Flies – At First Help in Emergency

In the years 1942–1943, work in the Institute of Zoology became increasingly endangered as a result of the bombing attacks on Berlin. And for me there was the constant threat of being drafted for military service. One day, H. Strughold asked me whether I would be inclined to work with him on an assignment from the Air Force Medical Research Institute, of which he was then the Director. Strughold was a physiologist, a student of von Frey (1852–1932). Of course, the physiology of hearing did not interest him. The physiology of vision, especially the measurement of the course of adaptation in human eyes by means of objective (i.e., electrophysiological) methods was his interest. That research problem excited me, and other important advantages would accompany my working with him, for I could procure apparatus from Strughold and he could put assistants at my disposal. Strughold was an excellent organizer, and – even more important – he had the best connections with the German Air Force. In confidential discussions, Strughold left no doubt that he believed Hitler's war to be hopeless, so he protected young scientists from military service. Because the Institute qualified as being militarily important, as a researcher there one was shielded from military service.

In 1943, I began my investigation of the human electroretinogram (ERG). With the apparatus available, it was not possible to record ERGs. The ERG had slow components; amplifiers which I built myself, with condenser-connected input, did not respond. Next a string galvanometer was used. Its deflections were enlarged with a microscope and drawn on film. Now string galvanometers are indeed extraordinarily sensitive, but unfortunately, they are not only sensitive to what is to be measured, but also to circuits connected to them. In addition, dc amplifiers were not available.

Once again a patron came to my aid. The German Postal Service had a research institute, and one of the staff, named Schöps, explained that he would be happy to develop the apparatus that I needed. For nine months he drove himself until the amplifier finally had a somewhat reliable "foolproof" construction and possessed the required amplification (Fig. 6). Contact lenses with holes bored in their sides served as the electrodes. A wool thread, moistened with saline, led through the hole to the outer surface of the eyeball. Since I had built the entire apparatus myself there was always some breakdown. That study did not lead to any substantial results. However, the work was the starting point of almost all the investigations undertaken since then on the electrophysiology of insect eyes. The way that came about follows.

In 1943 the bombing attacks on Berlin increased. Several parts of the city were destroyed, including the Air Force Medical Research Institute. On orders from Strughold, our Institute was moved to Silesia. In January 1944 we moved into a small medieval castle in Welkersdorf, in the neighborhood of Görlitz, with the apparatus we had been able to rescue. There was not a single electrical installation in the castle. With tremendous effort we laid electric cables in the cellar and first floor, having to bore through medieval walls two meters thick. I think back thankfully to the continuous cooperation of all the personnel of the Institute. I also remember with thanks a small group of Russian prisoners of war. They were me-

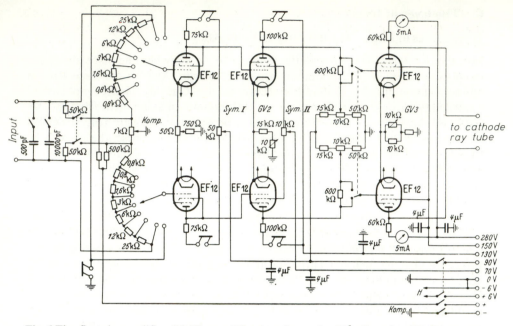

Fig. 6. The first dc amplifier (1943); amplification factor 3×10^5. Six tubes EF12. *Komp.,*
Sym. I, II, potentiometers to balance the amplifier and to compensate disturbing input dc
voltages. Autrum (1950)

chanics and locksmiths from Baku with whom we quickly established a comrade-
like working relationship. One day, when an order from their own prison camp was
announced, they even repaired the weapons of their pro forma guards. We lived
there on a peaceful island surrounded by the war, but this was coming closer and
closer.

Our attempts to record the ERG from our own eyes or from those of our associates continued to founder because of inadequacies of the apparatus. Above all,
it was always irksome to adjust the contact lenses and then to find that the apparatus did not function as it should have. Therefore, we looked for substitutes for
our own eyes, and we found them in the stalls of the farm near the castle – *Calli-*
phora, blowflies, which lived in the barn in most agreeable numbers!

In our work with *Calliphora,* one insect pin was stuck through a carefully am-
putated head and a second pin was inserted carefully in the retinula. The eye was
stimulated with flickering light, produced with a rotating sectional disk.

The results amazed us, for the fusion frequency of the flickering light we used
lay considerably higher than the fusion frequency judged subjectively with our own
eyes. At the intensities tested, we saw no flicker above about 40 Hz, but the flies'
eyes produced flicker ERGs which were distinguished from the noise of the oscilloscope even above 250 Hz.

Unfortunately, our work in Welkersdorf had to be discontinued shortly after
we recorded the ERGs from the flies, for Russian troops were standing near Breslau. In January 1945, we packed the most important apparatus in chests and sent

them to acquaintances in Thüringen, one of whom had been my technical assistant since 1940. The apparatus was buried there without packing cases, a meter deep in the ground, just a day before the American troops neared the city. With the approval of the English commander of the garrison at Göttingen, we were able to recover our equipment only a day before the American troops evacuated Thüringen and turned the zone over to the Russians.

We had sent some of our apparatus to Göttingen. Then, air attacks on the city were feared – with good reason, as the examples of Hildesheim and Würzburg showed. My wife and six-year-old daughter had accompanied me, so because of the danger in Göttingen we were sent to stay with farmers in the village of Niedernjesa, which is close to Göttingen. When the American troops finally occupied the city, they discovered our apparatus and confiscated it, for they assumed that our equipment included forbidden radio transmitters.

I drove to the American headquarters and explained to Sergant I. Schevis, A Battery, 275th. A.F.A. Battalion, that I studied the vision of insects, and that our apparatus served no military purpose. I also had a reprint of WEVER and BRAY's (1933) paper, inscribed "With Best Regards," which I showed to Sergeant Schevis. That convinced him of the truth of my statements. Since Sergeant Schevis was not to remain in the neighborhood of Göttingen, I asked him for a written statement permitting me to retain my equipment. He wrote one that protected me from renewed harassment by all American, English, and French troops. To my question "And what about the Russian troops?" he shrugged his shoulders. Fortunately, the Russians did not move in to Göttingen.

In 1946, the investigations of the flicker fusion frequency in *Calliphora* were resumed in the Institute of Zoology of the University of Göttingen. Part of the apparatus had been rescued. Other parts we built ourselves with military materials which had been strewn in the fields. We had no proper workshop, for the Zoological Institute had been destroyed, and when the University began to function again the Institute of Zoology was housed in a small, makeshift building. The space was limited: four small attic rooms had to suffice for my predoctoral students and myself.

My students were (in alphabetical order):

Dietrich Burkhardt, now professor at the University of Regensburg. He studied oscillations in the optic ganglia of insects.
Friedrich Diecke, now professor at the New Jersey Medical School in Newark. He worked on accommodation in nerve trunks and isolated nodes of Ranvier.
Ursula Gallwitz, who investigated the influence of optical ganglia on the ERG.
H.C. Lüttgau, now professor at the University of Bochum. His work focused on the dependence of stimulatory waves of isolated nodes of Ranvier on ion concentrations.
Dietrich Poggendorf. He studied absolute auditory thresholds in the catfish, *Amiurus*.
Friedrich Schlote, now professor at the University of Aachen. He recorded activity in the nerves of gastropods.
Dietrich Schneider, now professor at the University of Munich and Director of the Max Planck Institute in Seewiesen. He worked on conduction in single nerve fibers.
Günther Schneider, now professor at the University of Düsseldorf. His studies focused on the halteres of *Calliphora,* both as receptor organs and as flight stabilizers.
Wilfriede Schneider, who investigated vibration receptors in insects.
Marieluise Stöcker, who worked on vision in bees.
Hildegard Stumpf, whose research included the electrophysiology of color vision in *Calliphora* and the sensitivity of insects to polarized light.

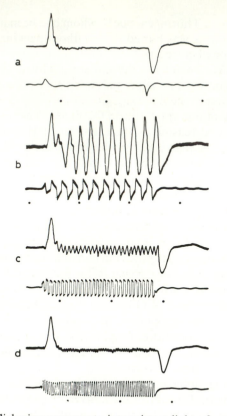

Fig. 7 a–d. *Calliphora:* flickering response to intermittent light of various flash frequencies (1944). *Upper traces,* electroretinogram; *lower traces,* light stimuli. *Time marks (points),* 0.1 s. **a** Constant stimulus of about 0.2 s; **b** 47/s; **c** 133/s; **d** 246/s. Autrum (1950)

Johann Schwartzkopff, now professor at the University of Bochum. He studied vibration receptors in birds.

So there we were – my 12 young associates and I – in four tiny rooms in an attic. Many of their research problems and results continue to be valid, and remain as important contributions to receptor and nerve physiology.

As far as my own work on the electrophysiology of insect vision was concerned, the following information came from the studies in Göttingen:

1. There are insects, e.g., *Calliphora* and *Apis,* that respond to white (as perceived by human beings) flickering light with very high flicker fusion frequencies (Autrum 1948 a, b, 1950; Fig. 7). They have a rather high temporal resolution. By measurements of responses in single photoreceptor cells, recorded with intracellular microelectrodes, Zettler (1969), using sinusoidal modulated light, confirmed this high temporal resolution. He showed also that the photoreceptor cell represents a nonlinear system.
2. There are other insects, e.g., *Dixippus* and *Tachycines,* in which flicker fusion frequencies are very much lower (Fig. 8).

Further studies (Müller 1966) showed that among insects there are many intergradations between those two extremes.

The high fusion frequency in dipterans and in many other rapidly flying insects is primarily an experimentally derived fact. That fact raised these questions:

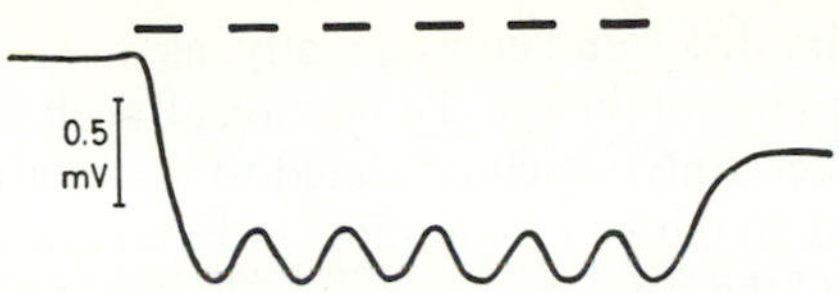

Fig. 8. *Tachycines* (Tettigoniidae): flickering response (1947). Stimulus: six flashes/s, *upper trace;* electroretinogram, *lower trace*. Fusion frequency about 20/s. AUTRUM (1950)

1. Which mechanisms are responsible for the high temporal resolution of "fast" eyes?
2. What are the differences between the mechanisms of fast eyes and "slow" eyes?
3. Of what biological significance is high temporal resolving power?

The following are some of our answers to these questions. High temporal resolution means rapid adaptation. Indeed, mechanisms which exist in bees, wasps, flies, and butterflies function quickly, and influence the pathway of light to the light-sensitive structures. In light adaptation, pigment granules move in the photoreceptive cells to the wall of the rhabdom or the rhabdomeres, and change the refractive index. These longitudinal pupil mechanisms were discovered by KIRSCH-FELD and FRANCESCHINI in 1969. The change in sensitivity occurs in only a few seconds, i.e., 1–2 log units in 10–60 s. (For reviews see MILLER 1979; STAVENGA 1979; AUTRUM 1981.).

In addition, there is a second important characteristic of the fast eyes. When the eyes of the species examined so far are stimulated with white light, the amount of unbleached photopigment remains almost constant, since light of long wavelengths reisomerizes metarhodopsin to rhodopsin (reviewed by HAMDORF 1979). Consequently, in the insects studied, under open air light conditions, the bleaching of the light-sensitive pigments is less than in vertebrates and in many other invertebrates. Whether such mechanisms exist in insects with slow eyes, e.g., *Dixippus,* is not known.

The first hypothesis regarding the significance of the extremely high temporal resolving power was that compared to eyes with only one lens (e.g., camera-type eyes) the compound eyes of insects have low spatial resolution. This is compensated for in flying insects by great temporal resolution. This hypothesis is often misunderstood, and has been refuted. First of all, it cannot be maintained that in a resting, static condition spatial resolution can be improved by temporal acuity. What is important is movement, either movement of the object or movement of the insect. Without doubt, high temporal acuity increases information capacity according to the Shannon formula given as

$$C = F \times \log_2 (1 + \sigma_s^2/\sigma_n^2) \tag{1}$$

in which C = information capacity in bits; F = upper cutoff frequency of the fastest response in Hz; σ_s^2 = variance of signals; and σ_n^2 = variance of noise (see SMOLA and GEMPERLEIN 1973; LAUGHLIN 1981, p. 219). A high-frequency response improves the channel capacity (AUTRUM 1958), but the spatial acuity is not thus improved.

Now, since in compound eyes the cutoff frequency compared to moving objects is limited by the receptor angular sensitivity function (KIRSCHFELD 1976; SNYDER 1979), the optical characteristics of the dioptric apparatus limit the resolution by such eyes. Fraunhofer's diffraction and the diameter of the pupil define the size of the diffraction disk (Airy disk), and consequently, as in all optic systems, they determine the resolution power of the eye. To be sure, all such theoretical calculations include a particular uncertainty which is related to the establishment of the diameter of the first Airy disk to the first minimum, and that question is correlated with the contrast sensitivity of the eye.

Excellent reviews of the comparisons among various types of compound eyes and the camera-type eyes of vertebrates, including that of the human, have been published by KIRSCHFELD (1976), LAUGHLIN (1981), and LAND (1981). One must be especially careful to remember that compound eyes are not only differently constructed, but also have different functions than eyes with only one lens.

The advantages of great temporal resolution have been summarized by LAUGHLIN (1981, p. 226):

> The principal advantage of a fast response is that it helps resolve moving objects (SRINIVASAN and BERNARD 1975). The sluggish responses of receptors smear a moving image across the retina. This type of effect is vividly seen when a small point source, such as flashlight, is waved around in the dark and appears to draw figures in the air with a luminous line. The point source may only be in front of a single receptor for two or three milliseconds, yet the response lasts several times longer and at any instant, the image of the point source is represented in several consecutive points in the retina. This temporal smearing is similar to the blurring of objects by the optics, but it is the receptor potential which is spread across the retina and not light intensity. The effects of temporal smearing can be analysed by considering the resolution of point sources (SRINIVASAN and BERNARD 1975), or by considering sinusoidal stimuli and converting every spatial sinusoid via velocity into a temporal intensity modulation and then passing this through the photoreceptor's frequency response. Alternatively one can use a simple and elegant approximation (conceptual method). The angular sensitivity of the photoreceptor is widened by an amount equal to the product of angular velocity and the half-time of the Gaussian approximation of the receptor's impulse response (SNYDER 1977). Whichever method one uses, a receptor's sluggish response blurs out the spatial detail from moving objects. This goes a long way towards explaining Autrum's original observation that the ERG of the fast flying insects had a better flicker fusion frequency than the slower ones (e.g., fly, cf. locust).

II. Spectral Sensitivity of Single Receptor Cells

In 1952 our time in Göttingen came to an end, for I was offered a post in Würzburg. The Zoological Institute there had also been extensively damaged. However, a small workshop was built during reconstruction. That expedited our studies, which was certainly to my advantage, because from 1953 to 1957 I was Chancellor of the University. That, too, had an advantage: I came to learn the entire spectrum of worries of a university – from those of clinical medicine on the one hand to those of theology on the other.

Then, in 1958, I became the successor to Karl von Frisch in Munich. Of the Zoological Institute, actually built for von Frisch by the Rockefeller Foundation, only the building and the extensive library remained. The rooms were completely empty and unusable. That was certainly an advantage, since everything could be newly arranged.

Dietrich Burkhardt accompanied me to Munich. We were grateful for his initiative, which allowed us to attack the problems of the physiology of vision with

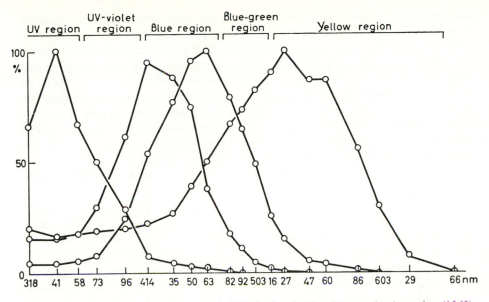

Fig. 9. Relative spectral sensitivity curves of single visual cells of the worker honeybee (1962) (AUTRUM and VON ZWEHL 1964). Regions of color discrimination after the training experiments of KÜHN (1927)

modern methods. In our workshop was built the apparatus for producing microelectrodes, and Burkhardt himself investigated single photoreceptor cells, chiefly those of flies.

The tradition of the Zoological Institute in Munich also defined our work. Von Frisch had studied color vision of honeybees in detail (for review see VON FRISCH 1965), and Karl DAUMER (1956), while a student of von Frisch, had shown by using behavioral methods that the color vision of bees has basic principles similar to those of the color vision of human beings. The bee's visible spectrum extends into the ultraviolet, and is consequently shorter at the long-wave end than that of man. The color circle is also closed in bees, and mixing of the two ends of the visible spectrum, i.e., the ultraviolet and the yellow, produces a unique color, called "bee-purple" by Daumer. Bee-purple is analogous to the purple quality seen by human beings when the red and violet ends of their spectrum are mixed. In addition, to achieve a "bee-white" the mixing of three spectral colors is necessary and sufficient.

Daumer's findings were in accord with the Young–Helmholtz hypothesis, which holds that color vision is based on the working together of three types of photoreceptors with different spectral sensitivities. But that hypothesis, even though it was almost 300 years old (for the history of theories of color vision see WEALE 1957; MARRIOTT 1962), had never been proved by direct measurements of the spectral sensitivities of single photoreceptors.

Finally, BURKHARDT (1962, 1964) determined electrophysiologically, using microelectrodes, the spectral sensitivities of single photoreceptor cells in *Calliphora*. That success encouraged us to use the same methods with honeybees. To our amazement, they proved to be extremely convenient subjects for the implantation of microelectrodes in single cells. Consequently, the spectral sensitivity of bees' single photoreceptor cells was measured directly (Fig. 9) (AUTRUM and VON ZWEHL 1962–1964; AUTRUM 1968; for reviews see AUTRUM and THOMAS 1973; MENZEL 1979). About the same time that we made those measurements in bees, others, using microspectrophotometric measurements, demonstrated that there are three different types of cone in the retinas of fish (MARKS 1963, 1965; MACNICHOL 1964), as well as in *Macaca* and *Homo* (MARKS et al. 1964; BROWN and WALD 1963, 1964; for review see GOURAS and ZRENNER 1981). Then, in 1967, TOMITA et al. established the spectral sensitivities of individual cones in fish once again by making electrophysiological, intracellular measurements. So, with these results, the three-component theory of color vision in animals was finally proved. Until that time, we had evidence only from behavioral studies that animals do see colors.

Color vision in invertebrates continues to present many problems. Very recently, we learned that there are also four-color systems, e.g., in the jumping spider, *Menemerus* (YAMASHITA and TATEDA 1976); in the moth, *Spodoptera* (LANGER et al. 1979); and in the ant, *Cataglyphis* (KRETZ 1979). In addition, the capacity to respond to polarized light and its peripheral and central analyses pose numerous questions (for reviews see WATERMAN 1981; WEHNER 1981).

One problem which has occupied me since my time in Göttingen is this: Optically speaking, to what extent is a single ommatidium a unit? I suggested even before it was proved experimentally that the single cells of an ommatidium are different, at least in terms of their spectral characteristics. Further, we (AUTRUM and STUMPF 1950) hypothesized that the individual photoreceptor cells of one ommatidium have various "preferred" directions for the analysis of the e-vector of polarized light. The further development of the analysis of polarization patterns has been discussed in detail by WATERMAN (1981).

However, whether each ommatidium actually receives light from only one field, as determined by its morphology, was not clear. And that is really the question of the correlation between the anatomical divergence angle and the field of vision of an ommatidium. That question was investigated by Ingrid Wiedemann (AUTRUM and WIEDEMANN 1962; WIEDEMANN 1965). She showed that in the open rhabdoms of *Calliphora,* the single receptor cells, i.e., the rhabdomeres of one ommatidium, have different optical axes. However, the optical axes of the various photoreceptor cells agree with those of neighboring ommatidia, in each case. These results were not pursued further by us. In the same year, KUIPER (1962) obtained the same results independently. Greater understanding of the characteristic morphology of these compound eyes was possible only after TRUJILLO-CENÓZ and MELAMED (1966), BRAITENBERG (1967), KIRSCHFELD (1967, 1969), and HORRIDGE and MEINERTZHAGEN (1970) described the pathways of axons of the photoreceptor cells to the optical ganglia. That led to the discovery of the characteristic convergence of six peripheral receptor cells from different ommatidia to one optic cartridge, typical of the neural superposition eye.

The variety of researches which followed these discoveries cannot be discussed here. The interested reader can find such discussions in the excellent reviews by HORRIDGE (1975) and ZETTLER and WEILER (1976). Further summaries have been published in the *Handbook of Sensory Physiology* (AUTRUM 1979–1981).

D. Conclusions

The beginnings of the comparative physiology of hearing and vision in inverte-brates go back a long time. After the great discoveries of Johannes MÜLLER (1826), GRABER (1875), EXNER (1891), HESSE (1896, 1897a, b, 1899), VON FRISCH (1965), and REGEN (1914), there followed, for the most part, a long pause. With only a few exceptions, new techniques, e.g., improvements in microscopy, were not decisive for the new discoveries which came later. Much more fruitful were new ideas which, often with simple technical equipment, led to unsuspected fields of research. The classic example is that of the studies by VON FRISCH (1914, 1914–1915) on the color vision of bees and on the orientation of bees to the polarization pattern of the blue sky (VON FRISCH 1949). Von Frisch used no new apparatus, but a new method, i.e., the analysis of bees' behavior in response to color and to orientational cues. Then further steps and deeper analyses demanded the use of physical and mathematical methods, once again focused at first on behavior (REGEN 1914).

Certainly, the development of physical measuring techniques stimulated con-siderable progress, and also led to new theoretical concepts. However, the physical aspects of the field required new ideas. For example, the dimensions of the acoustic and optic receptors in arthropods are often very small relative to the physical pa-rameters to which they respond. That has been appreciated only since about 1970, and has necessitated unique, detailed mathematical and physical analyses for the-oretical as well as experimental considerations of the problem.

Since the history of the modern development of these fields cannot be included here, the interested reader is referred to the comprehensive reviews by HORRIDGE (1975), SNYDER (1979), LAUGHLIN (1981), LAND (1981), and WEHNER (1981) for the arthropod eye; by MICHELSEN (1973, 1978, 1979), and MICHELSEN and NOCKE (1974) for the physiology of hearing; by MARKL (1973) for vibration receptors; and by MENZEL (1979) for the physiology of color vision in insects.

Acknowledgement. I wish to thank Professor MIRIAM F. BENNETT, Colby College, Waterville, Maine, for the English translation, and HERTA TSCHARNTKE (since 1941) and IN-GE THOMAS (since 1958) for their assistance in experiments and accurate help in the prepa-ration of my manuscripts.

References

Names containing *von* are alphabetized in this list under *v*

Autrum H (1936a) Eine Theorie der Schallwahrnehmung für Luftarthropoden. Verh Dtsch Zool Ges 1936:125–134
Autrum H (1936b) Über Lautäußerungen und Schallwahrnehmung bei Arthropoden. I. Untersuchungen bei Ameisen. Eine allgemeine Theorie der Schallwahrnehmung bei Ar-thropoden. Z Vgl Physiol 23:332–373
Autrum H (1940) Über Lautäußerungen und Schallwahrnehmung bei Arthropoden. II. Das Richtungshören von *Locusta* und Versuch einer Hörtheorie für Tympanalorgane vom Locustidentyp. Z Vgl Physiol 28:326–352
Autrum H (1941) Über Gehör und Erschütterungssinn bei Locustiden. Z Vgl Physiol 28:580–637
Autrum H (1942) Schallempfang bei Tier und Mensch. Naturwissenschaften 30:69–85
Autrum H (1943) Über kleinste Reize bei Sinnesorganen. Biol Zentralbl 63:209–236

Autrum H (1948 a) Über das zeitliche Auflösungsvermögen des Insektenauges. Nachr Akad Wiss Göttingen Math-Phys Kl 2:8–12

Autrum H (1948 b) Zur Analyse des zeitlichen Auflösungsvermögens des Insektenauges. Nachr Akad Wiss Göttingen Math-Phys Kl 2:13–18

Autrum H (1950) Die Belichtungspotentiale und das Sehen der Insekten (Untersuchungen an *Calliphora* und *Dixippus*). Z Vgl Physiol 32:176–227

Autrum H (1958) Electrophysiological analysis of the visual system in insects. Exp Cell Res [Suppl] 5:426–439

Autrum H (1968) Colour vision in man and animals. Naturwissenschaften 55:10–18

Autrum H (ed) (1979–1981) Vision in invertebrates. Springer, Berlin Heidelberg New York (Handbook of sensory physiology, vols VII/6A, B, and C)

Autrum H (1981) Light and dark adaptation in invertebrates. In: Autrum H (ed) Invertebrate visual centers and behavior II. Springer, Berlin Heidelberg New York, pp 1–91 (Handbook of sensory physiology, vol VII/6C)

Autrum H, Schneider W (1948) Vergleichende Untersuchungen über den Erschütterungssinn der Insekten. Z Vgl Physiol 31:77–88

Autrum H, Stumpf H (1950) Das Bienenauge als Analysator für polarisiertes Licht. Z Naturforsch [B] 5:116–122

Autrum H, Thomas I (1973) Comparative physiology of colour vision in animals. In: R. Jung (ed) Integrative functions and comparative data. Springer, Berlin Heidelberg New York, pp 661–692 (Handbook of sensory physiology, vol VII/3A)

Autrum H, von Zwehl V (1962) Zur spektralen Empfindlichkeit einzelner Sehzellen der Drohne (*Apis mellifica♂*). Z Vgl Physiol 46:8–12

Autrum H, von Zwehl V (1963) Ein Grünrezeptor im Drohnenauge (*Apis mellifica♂*). Naturwissenschaften 50:698

Autrum H, von Zwehl V (1964) Die spektrale Empfindlichkeit einzelner Sehzellen des Bienenauges. Z Vgl Physiol 48:357–384

Autrum H, Wiedemann I (1962) Versuche über den Strahlengang im Insektenauge (Appositionsauge). Z Naturforsch [B] 17:480–482

Braitenberg V (1967) Patterns of projection in the visual system of the fly. I. Retina-lamina projections. Exp Brain Res 3:271–298

Brown PK, Wald G (1963) Visual pigments in human and monkey retinas. Nature 200:37–43

Brown PK, Wald G (1964) Visual pigments in single rods and cones of the human retina. Science 144:45–52

Burkhardt D (1962) Spectral sensitivity and other response characteristics of single visual cells in the arthropod eye. Symp Soc Exp Biol 16:86–108

Burkhardt D (1964) Colour discrimination in insects. Adv Insect Physiol 2:131–203

Dambach M, Huber F (1974) Perception of substrate vibration in crickets. In: Schwartzkopff J (ed) Symposium mechanoreception. Abh Rheinisch-Westfäl Akad Wiss 53:263–280

Daumer K (1956) Reizmetrische Untersuchung des Farbensehens der Biene. Z Vgl Physiol 38:413–478

Dragsten PR, Webb WW, Paton JA, Capranica RR (1974) Auditory membrane vibrations: measurements at sub-angstrom levels by optical heterodyne spectroscopy. Science 185:55–57

Eggers F (1928) Die stiftführenden Sinnesorgane. Zoologische Bausteine, vol 2/1. Gebr. Bornträger, Berlin

Exner S (1891) Die Physiologie der facettirten Augen von Krebsen und Insecten. Deuticke, Leipzig

Fletcher WH (1978) Acoustic response of hair receptors in insects. J Comp Physiol 127:185–189

Gouras P, Zrenner E (1981) Color vision: a review from a neurophysiological perspective. Prog Sensory Physiol 1:139–179

Graber V (1875) Die tympanalen Sinnesapparate der Orthopteren. Denkschr Wiss Akad Wien 36:1–140

Hamdorf K (1979) The physiology of invertebrate visual pigments. In: Autrum H (ed) Invertebrate photoreceptors. Springer, Berlin Heidelberg New York, pp 145–224 (Handbook of sensory physiology, vol VII/6A)

Hesse R (1896) Untersuchungen über die Organe der Lichtempfindung bei niederen Thieren. I. Die Organe der Lichtempfindung bei den Lumbriciden. Z Wiss Zool 61:393–419

Hesse R (1897a) Untersuchungen über die Organe der Lichtempfindung bei niederen Thieren. II. Die Augen der Plathelminthen. Z Wiss Zool 62:527–582

Hesse R (1897b) Untersuchungen über die Organe der Lichtempfindung bei niederen Thieren. III. Die Sehorgane der Hirudineen. Z Wiss Zool 62:671–707

Hesse R (1899) Untersuchungen über die Organe der Lichtempfindung bei niederen Thieren. V. Die Augen der polychaeten Anneliden. Z Wiss Zool 65:446–516

Horridge GA (ed) (1975) The compound eye and vision of insects. Clarendon, Oxford

Horridge GA, Meinertzhagen IA (1970) The exact neural projections of the visual fields upon the first and second ganglia of the insect eye. Z Vgl Physiol 66:369–378

Kirschfeld K (1967) Die Projektion der optischen Umwelt auf das Raster der Rhabdomere im Komplexauge von *Musca*. Exp Brain Res 3:248–270

Kirschfeld K (1969) Optics of the compound eye. In: Reichardt W (ed) Processing of optical data by organisms and by machines. Academic, New York, pp 144–166

Kirschfeld K (1976) The resolution of lens and compound eyes. In: Zettler F, Weiler R (eds) Neural principles in vision. Springer, Berlin Heidelberg New York, pp 355–370

Kirschfeld K, Franceschini N (1969) Ein Mechanismus zur Steuerung des Lichtflusses in den Rhabdomeren des Komplexauges von *Musca*. Kybernetik 6:13–22

Kretz R (1979) A behavioural analysis of colour vision in the ant *Cataglyphis bicolor* (Formicidae, Hymenoptera). J Comp Physiol 131:217–233

Kühn A (1927) Über den Farbensinn der Bienen. Z Vgl Physiol 5:762–800

Kuiper JW (1962) The optics of the compound eye. Symp Soc Exp Biol 16:58–71

Land MF (1981) Optics and vision in invertebrates. In: Autrum H (ed) Invertebrate visual centers and behavior I. Springer, Berlin Heidelberg New York, pp 471–592 (Handbook of sensory physiology, vol VII/6B)

Langer H, Hamann B, Meinecke CC (1979) Tetrachromatic visual system in the moth *Spodoptera exempta* (Insecta: Noctuidae). J Comp Physiol 129:235–239

Laughlin SB (1981) Neural principles in the peripheral visual systems of invertebrates. In: Autrum H (ed) Invertebrate visual centers and behavior I. Springer, Berlin Heidelberg New York, pp 133–280 (Handbook of sensory physiology, vol VII/6B)

Lewis DB (1974a) The physiology of the tettigoniid ear. I. The implications of the anatomy of the ear to its function in sound reception. J Exp Biol 60:821–837

Lewis DB (1974b) The physiology of the tettigoniid ear. II. The response characteristics of the ear to differential inputs: lesion and blocking experiments. J Exp Biol 60:839–851

Lewis DB (1974c) The physiology of the tettigoniid ear. III. The response characteristics of the intact ear and some biophysical considerations. J Exp Biol 60:853–859

Lewis DB (1974d) The physiology of the tettigoniid ear. IV. A new hypothesis for acoustic orientation behavior. J Exp Biol 60:861–869

Little HF (1962) Reactions of the honeybee *Apis mellifera* L. to artificial sounds and vibrations of known frequencies. Ann Entomol Soc Am 55:82–89

MacNichol EF Jr (1964) Retinal mechanisms of colour vision. Vision Res 4:119–133

Markl H (1970) Die Verständigung durch Stridulationssignale bei Blattschneiderameisen. III. Die Empfindlichkeit für Substratvibrationen. Z Vgl Physiol 69:6–37

Markl H (1973) Leistungen des Vibrationssinnes bei wirbellosen Tieren. Fortschr Zool 21:100–120

Markl H, Tautz J (1975) The sensitivity of hair receptors in caterpillars of *Barathra brassicae* L. (Lepidoptera, Noctuidae) to particle movements in a sound field. J Comp Physiol 99:79–87

Marks WB (1963) Difference spectra of the visual pigment in single goldfish cones. PhD dissertation, Johns Hopkins University, Baltimore

Marks WB (1965) Visual pigments of single goldfish cones. J Physiol 178:14–32

Marks WB, Dobelle WH, MacNichol FF Jr (1964) Visual pigments of single primate cones. Science 143:1181–1183

22 H. Autrum

Marriott FHC (1962) Colour vision: theories. In: Davson H (ed) The eye, vol 2. Academic, New York, pp 299–320
Menzel R (1979) Spectral sensitivity and colour vision in invertebrates. In: Autrum H (ed) Invertebrate photoreceptors. Springer, Berlin Heidelberg New York, pp 503–580 (Handbook of sensory physiology, vol VII/6A)
Michelsen A (1973) The mechanics of the locust ear: an invertebrate frequency analyzer. In: Møller AR (ed) Basic mechanisms in hearing. Academic, New York, pp 911–931
Michelsen A (1978) Sound reception in different environments. In: Ali MA (ed) Sensory ecology. Plenum, New York, pp 345–373
Michelsen A (1979) Insect ears as mechanical systems. Am Sci 67:696–706
Michelsen A, Larsen ON (1978) Biophysics of the ensiferan ear. I. Tympanal vibrations in bushcrickets (Tettigoniidae) studied with laser vibrometry. J Comp Physiol 123:193–203
Michelsen A, Nocke H (1974) Biophysical aspects of sound communication in insects. Adv Insect Physiol 10:247–296
Miller WH (1979) Ocular optical filtering. In: Autrum H (ed) Invertebrate photoreceptors. Springer, Berlin Heidelberg New York, pp 69–143 (Handbook of sensory physiology, vol VII/6A)
Minnich DE (1925) The reactions of the larvae of *Vanessa antiopa* Linn. to sounds. J Exp Zool 42:443–469
Müller A (1966) Über die Abhängigkeit von Retinogrammform und Verschmelzungsfrequenz bei Insekten. Dissertation, University of Würzburg
Müller J (1826) Zur vergleichenden Physiologie des Gesichtssinnes des Menschen und der Thiere nebst einem Versuch über die Bewegungen der Augen und über den menschlichen Blick. Cnobloch, Leipzig
Nocke H (1975) Physical and physiological properties of the tettigoniid ("grasshopper") ear. J Comp Physiol 100:25–57
Popper AN, Fay RR (eds) (1980) Comparative studies of hearing in vertebrates. Springer, New York Heidelberg Berlin
Regen J (1914) Untersuchungen über die Stridulation und das Gehör von *Thamnotrizon apterus* Fab. Sitzgsber Akad Wiss Wien Math Naturwiss Kl Abt I 123:853–892
Regen J (1926) Über die Beeinflussung des Stridulierens von *Thamnotrizon apterus* Fab. ♂ durch künstlich erzeugte Töne und verschiedenartige Geräusche. Sitzgsber Akad Wiss Wien Math Naturwiss Kl Abt I 135:329–368
Schneider W (1950) Über den Erschütterungssinn von Käfern und Fliegen. Z Vgl Physiol 32:287–302
Schnorbus H (1971) Die subgenualen Sinnesorgane von *Periplaneta americana:* Histologie und Vibrationsschwellen. Z Vgl Physiol 71:14–48
Schumacher R (1973) Beitrag zur Kenntnis des tibialen Tympanalorgans von *Tettigonia viridissima* L. (Orthoptera: Tettigoniidae). Mikroskopie 29:8–19
Schwabe J (1906) Beiträge zur Morphologie und Histologie der tympanalen Sinnesapparate der Orthopteren. Zoologica Heft 50
Schwartzkopff J (1974) Mechanoreception. In: Rockstein M (ed) The physiology of insecta. Academic, New York, pp 273–352
Smola U, Gemperlein R (1973) Rezeptorrauschen und Informationskapazität der Sehzellen von *Calliphora erythrocephala* und *Periplaneta americana*. J Comp Physiol 87:393–404
Snyder AW (1977) Acuity of compound eyes: physical limitations and design. J Comp Physiol 116:161–182
Snyder AW (1979) Physics of vision in compound eyes. In: Autrum H (ed) Invertebrate photoreceptors. Springer, Berlin Heidelberg New York, pp 225–313 (Handbook of sensory physiology, vol VII/6A)
Srinivasan MV, Bernard GD (1975) The effect of motion on visual acuity of the compound eye: a theoretical analysis. Vision Res 15:515–525
Stavenga DG (1979) Pseudopupils of compound eyes. In: Autrum H (ed) Invertebrate photoreceptors. Springer, Berlin Heidelberg New York, pp 357–439 (Handbook of sensory physiology, vol VII/6A)
Stokes GG (1851) On the effect of the internal friction of fluids on the motion of pendulums. Trans Cambridge Philos Soc 9:8 ff

Tautz J (1977) Reception of medium vibration by thoracal hairs of caterpillars of *Barathra brassicae* L. (Lepidoptera, Noctuidae). I. Mechanical properties of the receptor hairs. J Comp Physiol 118:13–31

Tautz J (1978) Reception of medium vibration by thoracal hairs of caterpillars of *Barathra brassicae* L. II. Response characteristics of the sensory cell. J Comp Physiol 125:67–77

Tomita T, Kaneko A, Murakami M, Pautler EL (1967) Spectral response curves of single cones in the carp. Vision Res 7:519–531

Trendelenburg F (1939) Einführung in die Akustik. Springer, Berlin

Trujillo-Cenóz O, Melamed J (1966) Compound eye of dipterans: anatomical basis for integration, an electron microscope study. J Ultrastr Res 16:395–398

von Békésy G (1941) Über die Messung der Schwingungsamplitude der Gehörknöchelchen mittels einer kapazitiven Sonde. Akust Z 6:1–15

von Frisch K (1914) Demonstration von Versuchen zum Nachweis des Farbensinnes bei angeblich total farbenblinden Tieren. Verh Dtsch Zool Ges 1914:50–58

von Frisch K (1914–1915) Der Farbensinn und Formensinn der Bienen. Zool Jahrb Abt Allg Zool Physiol Tiere 35:1–188

von Frisch K (1949) Die Polarisation des Himmelslichts als orientierender Faktor bei den Tänzen der Bienen. Experientia 5:142–148

von Frisch K (1965) Tanzsprache und Orientierung der Bienen. Springer, Berlin Heidelberg New York

von Siebold CTF (1844) Über das Stimm- und Gehörorgan der Orthopteren. Arch Naturgesch 10:71–86

Walcott C, van der Kloot WG (1959) The physiology of the spider vibration receptor. J Exp Zool 141:191–244

Waterman TH (1981) Polarization sensitivity. In: Autrum H (ed) Invertebrate visual centers and behavior I. Springer, Berlin Heidelberg New York, pp 281–469 (Handbook of sensory physiology, vol VII/6B)

Weale RA (1957) Trichromatic ideas in the seventeenth and eighteenth centuries. Nature 179:648–651

Wehner R (1981) Spatial vision in arthropods. In: Autrum H (ed) Invertebrate visual centers and behavior II. Springer, Berlin Heidelberg New York, pp 287–616 (Handbook of sensory physiology, vol VII/6C)

Wever EG, Bray CW (1933) A new method for the study of hearing in insects. J Cell Comp Physiol 4:79–93

Wiedemann I (1965) Versuche über den Strahlengang im Insektenauge (Appositionsauge). Z Vgl Physiol 49:526–542

Yamashita S, Tateda H (1976) Spectral sensitivities of jumping spider eyes. J Comp Physiol 105:29–41

Zettler F (1969) Die Abhängigkeit des Übertragungsverhaltens von Frequenz und Adaptationszustand, gemessen am einzelnen Lichtrezeptor von *Calliphora erythrocephala*. Z Vgl Physiol 64:432–449

Zettler F, Weiler R (eds) (1976) Neural principles in vision. Springer, Berlin Heidelberg New York

CHAPTER 2

The Development of Auditory Neurophysiology*

Hallowell Davis

* The preparation of this chapter was supported by U.S. Public Health Service Department
of Health, Education, and Welfare research grant NSO3856 from the National Institute
of Neurological and Communicative Disorders and Stroke to Central Institute for the
Deaf

A. Background

This chapter will be strongly autobiographical, which I understand is the intent of the editors of this volume. I shall emphasize the context and the thinking that influenced my own choices of problems and projects in auditory neurophysiology. Two secondary themes will be the gradual refinement of "auditory theory" and the importance of technical advances in other fields, notably electronics.

I. My Start in Neurophysiology

I became a neurophysiologist immediately after graduation from medical school in 1922. I spent a postdoctoral year in Cambridge, England, in the laboratory of Edgar D. Adrian, and continued at Harvard Medical School under Alexander Forbes. These fortunate choices placed me in the mainstream of the technical developments that followed the first application of a vacuum tube amplifier to neurophysiology by FORBES and THATCHER (1920), the development of the Matthews oscillograph and its use by Adrian, and the introduction by GASSER and ERLANGER (1922) of the Braun tube, the prototype of the cathode ray oscilloscope. Our central concern at that time was the nerve impulse and how with its rigid all-or-none limitations it controls motor performance and conveys sensory information. This interest is well illustrated by FORBES's (1922) classic review, "The Interpretation of Spinal Reflexes in Terms of Present Knowledge of Nerve Conduction," which united the Lucas–Adrian school of electrophysiology at Cambridge with the central nervous system physiology at Oxford. Forbes was wrong in many details of his theoretical mechanisms, but he did show that mechanisms could be conceived that would do the job.

II. The All-or-None Law

A central idea in Forbes's interpretations was the all-or-none law for the nerve impulse in normal nerve fibers. The strength of the nerve impulse is independent of the strength of the stimulus; also each impulse is limited in duration and is followed by a refractory period. A second idea was "conduction with a decrement," thought to occur in a region of nerve exposed to a narcotic such as alcohol. Here the impulse was thought to become progressively weaker, i.e., to be conducted with a decrement and perhaps extinguished. Forbes in his review hypothetically applied this idea to synaptic connections. Forbes was unhappy about the contradiction between all-or-none behavior and conduction with a decrement, and he formulated an experiment in which we would measure the action current of a nerve at several points in and beyond a region of narcosis in the long uniform peroneal nerve of cat.

The experiment gave a decisive result (DAVIS et al. 1926). It disproved the idea of conduction with a decrement and completely validated the all-or-none law. It supported the participation of the action current in the conduction of the impulse.

Our complete paper (DAVIS et al. 1926), "Studies of the Nerve Impulse: II The Question of Decrement," was published in the *American Journal of Physiology* in April 1926, but while the manuscript was in preparation a monograph by Genichi Kato, with many collaborators, was published in Tokyo (KATO 1924). Its title was *The Theory of Decrementless Conduction in Narcotized Region of Nerve*. It antedated our preliminary report of March 1925 by a year. It contained a variety of different experiments, including one that was a simplified version of our own – but they all pointed to the same conclusion. The nerve impulse is conducted without decrement in a region of narcosis. Like Forbes, Kato had found a long uniform nerve – in the gigantic Japanese bullfrog. The convergence of our work with that of Kato's group led to the general acceptance of the principle of decrementless conduction by nearly all neurophysiologists (with the notable exception of Raphael Lorente de Nó).

Studies in other laboratories also made it clear that the nerve impulse involved metabolic work and was not a passive physical process. It was my good fortune to be invited to assemble these and other related experimental findings in an article in *Physiological Reviews* entitled "The Conduction of the Nerve Impulse" (DAVIS 1926). This article, with Kato's monographs, closed a chapter in electrophysiology.

III. Sensory Physiology 1924–1929

Gasser and Erlanger, joined by Bishop, were analyzing the compound action potentials of isolated nerve trunks. Adrian and his series of distinguished collaborators at Cambridge (Zotterman, Bronk, Hoagland, Cattell, Matthews, and others), with amplifiers and improved oscillographs, analyzed the behavior of single motor units and also extended their analysis to sensory units, notably to muscle proprioceptors. To obtain responses of single units in motor nerves it was necessary to cut the other fibers, by laborious dissection, until only one or two remained intact. The single impulses were, of course, all-or-none in amplitude, but the frequency of discharge varied with the intensity of the stimulus, fatigue, adaptation, and other factors. Thus the "neural code" for sensory action was established, and was clearly stated by ADRIAN (1928) in his famous little volume *The Basis of Sensation: the Action of Sense Organs* for several mechanical stimuli, including muscle stretch, cutaneous touch, pressure, and bending of hairs. The volume contains preliminary experiments on vision and on noxious stimuli. Adrian's experiments, however, did not include the ear until 1930. The code seemed to be the same for all modalities studied, and is summarized in Fig. 1, which is taken from Adrian's monograph.

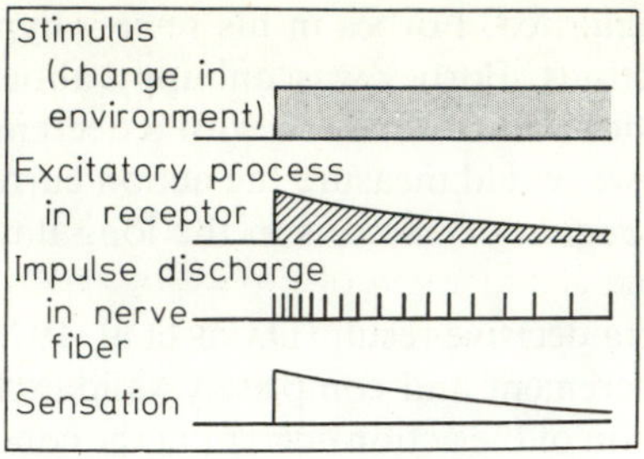

Fig. 1. The relation between stimulus, sensory message, and sensation. ADRIAN (1928)

IV. Auditory Neurophysiology Begins

Mammalian auditory action potentials were first reported by FORBES et al. (1927) in decerebrate cats. They applied wick electrodes to the dorsal surface of the medulla and the posterior colliculus, and obtained clear repetitive volleys of impulses in response to clicks at various frequencies, as produced by a "watchman's rattle" or by a visiting card held against the edge of a hand-turned cogwheel. They noted that the frequency following was excellent at low frequencies but could not be detected (with their string galvanometer) above about 200 Hz.

In this paper (FORBES et al. 1927) Forbes discussed the two major rival theories of audition. The so-called frequency or telephone theory, proposed originally by RUTHERFORD (1886), assumed that the waveforms of sound waves were carried by nerve impulses to the brain, where they were analyzed and "heard" by some unspecified central mechanism. Intensity was originally thought to be coded as differences in the magnitude of nerve impulses. Of course, the all-or-none law made this type of coding impossible, and waveforms could not be carried as such, so the revised frequency theory assumed that the frequencies of sound waves were coded as frequencies of nerve impulses and intensity as the number of nerve fibers activated. Forbes favored the "resonance" or "place" theory, as propounded by VON HELMHOLTZ (1863). The organ of Corti was assumed to contain a series of resonators, so that the nerve fibers were excited selectively according to the tuning of the resonators that they innervated. Thus the frequencies of the sound waves determined which fibers were stimulated. The frequency of nerve impulses would, of course, follow that of the sound waves at low frequencies but would be limited by the refractory period at higher frequencies. This interpretation required that intensity be coded simply in terms of the number of fibers stimulated, and not, as for the mechanoreceptors studied by Adrian, by frequency of impulses.

By a curious coincidence another member of the Harvard faculty, E. G. Boring, Professor of Psychology, had published a very different theory of audition just a year earlier (BORING 1926). This was "Auditory Theory with Special Reference to Intensity, Volume, and Localization." Boring's theory is self-consistent and explains several puzzling aspects of audition, but is elaborate and not easy to understand. He espoused the frequency theory for the coding that leads to pitch perception. He recognized two major objections to this. One was the absolute refractory period of nerve, which he disposed of by an ad hoc hypothesis. The other was

Ohm's (acoustic) law, which states that the ear can analyze a complex sound into its component frequencies and hear their pitches separately. This ability is easily explained by the resonator (place) theory, but not by the frequency theory. Boring simply left it unexplained.

In 1928 Forbes and Boring engaged in a friendly informal debate on auditory theory in a seminar in the Department of Physiology at Harvard Medical School. I attended, and was strongly influenced by it. Forbes and Boring agreed that more experimental evidence was necessary for a decision between them. The experiments cited were completely different – experimental psychology versus electrophysiology – and there was quite an aura of "east is east and west is west" about it all. Boring postulated that the auditory nerve, although its impulses were all or none, differed quantitatively from other mammalian nerves and had a refractory (recovery) period that was more than an order of magnitude shorter. This, he suggested, was an ad hoc evolutionary development. I was impressed by the completeness of Boring's theory, but I stayed with Forbes and the von Helmholtz place theory.

V. The Year 1929

Several notable events occurred in 1929 which influenced the development of sensory physiology in later years, although many of us were not aware of them at the time.

In 1928 and 1929 the classic papers by VON BÉKÉSY on the biophysics of the inner ear and the traveling wave on the basilar membrane appeared in German in the *Physikalische Zeitschrift* (VON BÉKÉSY 1960). The circulation of this journal was restricted, but by 1934 von Békésy's papers had been read by my associate S. S. Stevens, among others. The impact of von Békésy's observations was tremendous. They are well summarized and evaluated in another chapter of this volume.

In 1929 another obscure publication in Germany was destined to be as great a stimulus to cortical electrophysiology as von Békésy's contributions were to bioacoustics. This was Hans BERGER's (1929) first paper on the human electroencephalogram, „Über das Elektrenkephalogramm des Menschen I. Mitteilung." He was a psychiatrist in Jena and published in a psychiatric journal. It could hardly have been better hidden from English-speaking physiologists, but somehow, indirectly it came to the attention of Adrian in England and of my group in the United States by about 1933. Berger's observations on the spontaneous electrical activity of the brain were then promptly confirmed and publicized.

In 1929 the Acoustical Society of America was organized, chiefly by electronic and acoustic engineers of the Bell Telephone Laboratories. The work of this group had previously been published in the *Bell System Technical Journal,* but from 1929 onward information flowed more widely and quickly. And very appropriately, Harvey FLETCHER's (1929) monograph *Speech and Hearing* was first published in the same year. It summarized the studies in the Bell Telephone Laboratories of the human voice and hearing, using the new instrumentation of electroacoustics. The phonograph was a major new tool, and better generation and measurement of sound were possible.

Speech and Hearing was a landmark publication. Its first section deals with speech, including its production, the characteristics of speech sounds, and the phonographic method of recording. Much attention is given to the form of typical speech waves, and to the theory of vowel production and to the power of speech sounds. In the second section music and then noise are given similar treatment. The next section, on hearing, begins with an anatomical description of the ear and then an unqualified acceptance of "an extension of [the theory] orginally proposed by Helmholtz." Fletcher gives three pages of quotations from *Sensations of Tone* (1948) to explain it, and merely footnote references to "other theories." The all-or-none law and the refractory period are, of course, included in his extension of the theory.

Fletcher then turns to psychoacoustics and gives the limits of audition in terms of intensity and frequency. Next come the minimum perceptible differences of intensity and frequency and his well-known description of the "auditory area." Another section deals with masking effects, subjective tones, binaural beats, and other phenomena. Repeatedly, the question is considered as to how the various effects are related to position and extent of activity of the basilar membrane. The measurement of hearing and an analysis of familiar tests of hearing such as watch tick and tuning forks leads up to a description of the first four models of the electric audiometer that were developed by the Bell Telephone Laboratories.

The final section, devoted to the perception of speech and music, includes an important chapter on the loudness of sounds. Fletcher indulges in some theoretical calculations of the numbers of nerve impulses (per second) that are involved. In his "code" loudness is proportional to the total number of impulses per second reaching the brain. The loudness of a sound heard binaurally is (assumed to be) twice that of the same sound heard monaurally, and the number of impulses is obviously twice as great.

A final item in the last section is the use of speech sounds, words, and sentences to measure the "articulation" of the sounds and the "intelligibility" of sentences. The method and the various lists of test items were to become even more powerful tools in later years.

The philosophy both of the Bell Telephone Laboratories and of the physicist Georg von Békésy was the engineering approach. Both applied precise physical measurements and concepts to the problem of hearing. Von Békésy added the direct anatomical approach. I once heard him explain in a lecture why he undertook his study of the ear. He said, in effect:

I was put in charge of the telephone laboratory of the Hungarian Post Office Department. The telephone system was government-owned and -operated. The job of my laboratory was to improve the telephone, but the first thing I needed to know was whether the telephone was already as good an acoustic instrument as the ear. If it was, then no further improvement of the telephone would be necessary, so I set out to examine the ear as an acoustical instrument. I soon found out that it was much better than the telephone, but I had become interested in it.

And in 1929 Wever and Bray performed the famous experiment that initiated a new era in auditory neurophysiology.

B. The Wever and Bray Experiment and Its Repercussions

The new era in auditory physiology really began in 1930 with the publication by E. G. Wever and C. W. Bray of "Auditory Nerve Impulses" (WEVER and BRAY

1930 a). Wever, a professor of psychology at Princeton University, had taken his PhD degree at Harvard under Boring in 1926. In 1929, with the assistance of Bray and with sound critical advice from E. Newton Harvey, Professor of Biology, he undertook to determine the frequency of impulses in the cat's auditory nerve with an instrument capable of dealing with high audio frequencies. The instruments chosen were the telephone and the ear (not the eye) of an observer. A rather large electrode was placed on the auditory nerve in the internal auditory meatus of a decerebrate cat in a quiet experimental room, and another member of the team listened to the signals in a telephone in a distant quiet room. Voices of the experimenters could not be heard directly, but in the telephone receiver the listener could hear clearly any words spoken near the cat. He could not only understand the words, he could recognize the talker's voice. Transmission ceased with the death of the animal.

Forbes and I shared a mixture of disbelief and puzzlement, but within two months we witnessed a perfect demonstration in Wever's laboratory. Harvey had been meticulous in requiring both biological and electrical controls. We were completely convinced that the "Wever and Bray effect" was real, and that Boring's frequency theory of coding for pitch was strongly supported. The high frequencies of our voices were definitely present in the action potentials of the auditory nerve.

And Wever had an answer for our concern about refractory periods of a millisecond in duration. It is not necessary to suppose, Wever argued, that any one fiber carries a frequency higher than about 500/s, but the impulses in every fiber will be initiated in the same phase relation to the sound waves. Each fiber will respond, according to its refractory period, to every second, third, fourth, or nth wave, and there is no reason why the fibers should all respond to the *same* waves. *Some* fibers will thus respond to *every* wave, and the frequency of the sound waves will thus be carried by the nerve as a whole to the brain and give rise there to the corresponding pitch sensation. This idea he termed his "volley theory," and it still stands today as a valid concept. Wever was "one up." He summarized his case in an article in *Psychological Reviews* entitled "Present Possibilities for Auditory Theory" (WEVER and BRAY 1930 b).

The Wever and Bray experiment turned my personal attention strongly to the auditory system. In 1931 Forbes took time away from his laboratory to carry out a survey of the coast of northern Labrador by means of aerial photography. He practically turned the laboratory over to me. I had decided in 1930 to concentrate on the electrophysiology of the auditory system, both peripheral and central, and in 1931 began to acquire up-to-date amplifiers, a cathode ray oscilloscope, and appropriate electroacoustic equipment. It took nearly three years to assemble resources and for my engineer, E. L. Garceau, to design and construct the overall assembly. In the meantime, with L. J. Saul as my chief collaborator, I began our attack on the auditory system with Forbes's original amplifier, expanded to two stages, and a string galvanometer. This was supplemented with a six-stage resistance-coupled amplifier that activated a pair of earphones.

Our first objective was to map the auditory tracts physiologically from the auditory nerve to the cortex. Our best tool for localized detection of action potentials in nerve tracts was the concentric needle electrode pair that had been developed by ADRIAN and BRONK (1929) for isolation of the electrical output of single motor units in their own muscles. A fine insulated silver wire is inserted in the bore of an ordinary hypodermic needle and is ground off flush with the bevel of the needle. The outer needle and the subject are grounded. A less selective input is obtained with a fine needle, insulated except for the very tip, and a diffuse ground electrode. With such electrodes in decerebrate cats we detected, as expected, activity in somato-sensory pathways following electrical stimulation of the popliteal nerve. In the auditory system, under tribromoethanol anesthesia, we traced activity through the medulla to the inferior colliculus, the brachium, the medial geniculate body, and the auditory radiations.

With a needle electrode on the auditory nerve we confirmed the Wever and Bray experiment, but with the concentric electrodes we (Saul and Davis 1932a) were able to distinguish "at least two effects: 1) true nerve action currents (nerve impulses) which travel only up the auditory tracts; and 2) a diffuse electrical "spread," which seems to originate in the cochlea and which broadcasts through all the tissues of the head." The point of maximum response of the spread was the subarcuate fossa of the petrous bone. (We did not open the bulla and try the round window in our first experiments.) And the action currents were depressed much more rapidly than the spread by anesthetics and by anoxia.

As for speech, "when heard in the loudspeaker the action currents reproduce poorly the sounds applied to the ear. The general form of speech is retained but the actual words are unrecognizable." We concluded that frequencies over 1,000 Hz were not transmitted by individual nerve fibers. The best we could find was that "a considerable degree of the original pattern and frequency of auditory stimuli is still maintained in the action current from regions that are separated from the ear by at least one and perhaps as many as three or four synapses" (Saul and Davis 1932b).

We were not the only investigators to confirm the Wever and Bray experiment. At least six groups had so reported by 1933. Particularly notable was the brief communication by Adrian (1931). He led off from the round window (of cat), and he interpreted his responses as due to a "microphonic action of the cochlea," and gave considerable experimental evidence in support of this view, which was ultimately established as correct. This "microphonic action" was of course our (Saul and Davis's) "spread" and the "cochlear response" of most other investigators; but, still in 1931, in collaboration with Bronk and Phillips, Adrian apparently reversed his judgment, tacitly assuming that only one type of response, true action potentials, was present (Adrian et al. 1931). He evidently did not yet feel the necessity of multiplying his hypotheses. In *The Mechanism of Nervous Action,* Adrian (1932) quotes our (Saul and Davis's) demonstration of frequencies up to 1,000 Hz in the auditory tracts, mentions "the large cochlear effect," and explicitly accepts Wever's volley theory as the basis of the intelligibility of speech in the Wever and Bray experiment. His final pronouncement is in favor of Wever's modification of the frequency theory. Here are excerpts from the two final paragraphs of his section on the action of the sense organs.

It is, I think, an open question whether there will be much left of the resonance hypothesis of the cochlea when Wever and Bray have finished their investigations; the structure of the cochlea is the main argument for the resonance hypothesis, but it is clear that we might expect to obtain something like the Wever and Bray effect in any preparation of tactile receptors thrown into rapid vibration . . .

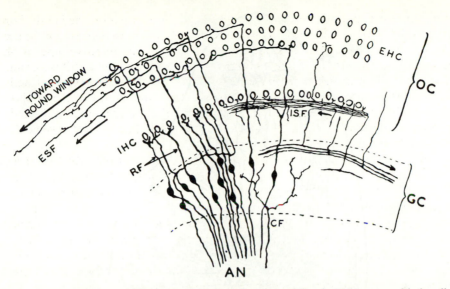

Fig. 2. The innervation of the organ of Corti. *OC*, organ of Corti; *EHC*, external hair cells; *ESF*, external spiral fibers, each innervating many external hair cells; *ISF*, internal spiral fibers, of unknown function; *IHC*, internal hair cells; *RF*, radial fibers, innervating the internal hair cells; *GC*, ganglion of Corti. *Arrows* show the direction of the fibers away from their cell bodies. *CF*, centrifugal fibers, of unknown function; *AN*, auditory nerve. STEVENS and DAVIS (1938), after LORENTE DE NÓ (1933)

The conclusion seems to be that with the auditory as with the tactile nerve fibres we judge the intensity of the stimulus by the number of impulses making up each volley, and that we judge the pitch of a note by the frequency of the volleys without regard to the frequency in each nerve fibre ... It will be time to discuss the knotty problems of central activity when we are more certain of the peripheral events.

C. A Decade of Expansion: 1931–1941

I. Books and People

In 1933, soon after our new amplifier and oscilloscope came into action, Moses H. Lurie joined our team. He was a member of the Department of Otolaryngology, and for the next 15 years he provided us with invaluable assistance in the form of anatomical examinations of our experimental specimens. And as a practicing otolaryngologist, Lurie was an important link in our association with the American Otological Society. In the 1930s our association with otology was much closer than with psychology.

Several books, papers, and individuals strongly influenced my thinking during this decade. In psychology, *Sensation*, vol. II of L. TROLAND's (1930) *Psychophysiology*, and E. G. BORING's (1933) *The Physical Dimensions of Consciousness* taught me about sensory qualities and magnitude. A landmark article was published by R. LORENTE DE NÓ (1933), entitled "Anatomy of the Eighth Nerve. The Central Projection of the Nerve Endings of the Internal Ear." Lorente really made

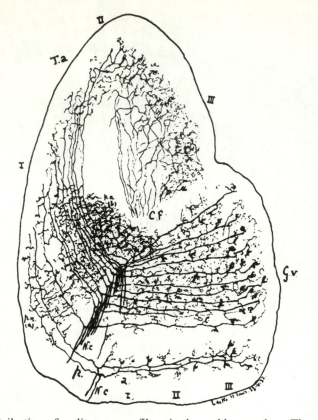

Fig. 3. The distribution of auditory nerve fibers in the cochlear nucleus. The primary bifurcation of the incoming fibers is in the lower left quadrant. Three major subdivisions of the nucleus are obvious; *Gv*, ganglion ventrale of the cochlear nucleus; *pn*, posterior nucleus; *Ta*, tuberculum acusticum; *I*, *II*, and *III* indicate regions of specific structure within the tuberculum acusticum and the ganglion ventrale; *Cf*, centrifugal fibers from higher auditory nuclei; *Nc*, fibers of the cochlear auditory nerve, with anterior branches (*a*) for the ganglion ventrale and posterior branches (*p*) for the tuberculum acusticum and posterior nucleus. LORENTE DE NÓ (1933)

me aware of microscopic neuroanatomy. Two of his illustrations, based on the Golgi method, are recognized classics (Figs. 2 and 3). The former was our guide for innervation until, in the 1950s, Rasmussen (1953) described the efferent olivocochlear system, and then in the 1970s Spoendlin completely revised our notions about afferent innervation.

Very important for me also was H. FLETCHER's (1930) paper entitled "A Space–Time Pattern Theory of Hearing." His thinking about nerve impulses and the place theory were very congenial to me, but not until 1935 did I begin to understand Fletcher's arguments based on masking or his "critical band." It was S. S. Stevens who made me appreciate psychoacoustics. In 1935 Stevens had just received his PhD degree from Harvard under the tutelage of E. G. Boring. He joined my team to gain some firsthand contact with experimental physiological psychology.

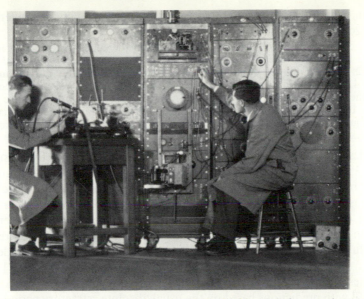

Fig. 4. Equipment used by myself (*right*) and A. J. Derbyshire (*left*) for experiments on auditory electrophysiology. Photograph taken in the corridor of Building C of Harvard Medical School on 5 December 1934. In actual use the animal table (*left center*) was in a separate sound-treated and electrically shielded booth. Center rack carries cathode ray oscilloscope (CRO) (*middle*), a camera for still or moving film (*bottom*) which can be swung up in front of CRO, and our first ink-writing electroencephalograph (*top*)

A more remote influence in the 1930s was the development of microdissection as a method for the direct study of the physiology of single nerve fibers and even single nodes of Ranvier by G. Kato and his pupils. His book *The Microphysiology of Nerve* appeared in 1934 (KATO 1934). The development was part of the trend, initiated by Adrian, toward isolation and study of single functioning units in both motor and sensory systems. My own personal contact with Kato developed through the triennial International Congresses of Physiology. It was in 1935 in Moscow that I first met I. Tasaki, the youngest member of Kato's retinue of that year. Tasaki joined me in St. Louis in 1951 for a very fruitful collaboration in auditory physiology, and later became an American citizen.

II. Electric Response of the Cochlea and Nerve Impulses

In 1934 our electronic equipment, designed and constructed by E. L. Garceau, represented a new level of sophistication, but it is amusing to look back at the bulky installation (Fig. 4) on five relay racks and containing 47 vacuum tubes. However, this equipment served us well until I moved from Harvard to St. Louis in 1946. Our favorite form of recording was by the standing-wave technique, synchronizing our oscilloscope with the stimulating tone or clicks. This is, of course, a simple form of response averaging.

In 1933 we (DAVIS et al. 1934a) submitted for publication in the *American Journal of Physiology* our definitive study of the electric response of the cochlea, based chiefly on recordings from the round window of cat. The major characteristics we summarized in 1934 (DAVIS et al. 1934 b) as follows:

The cochlear response differs fundamentally from the action potentials of nerve and muscle: 1. It shows no characteristic wave form of its own, but reproduces that of the stimulus. 2. It is not followed by a refractory period. 3. It is immune to fatigue, anaesthesia and cold. 4. It may begin by either a positive or a negative electrical change depending on whether the initial stimulating (sound) pressure is positive or negative. We have also confirmed the observation of Howe and Guild that this response is absent in albinic cats which on histologic examination are found to lack the organ of Corti. We have ventured the hypothesis that the sensory cells of this organ are responsible for the electrical change ...

The description of the action potentials of the auditory nerve (DERBYSHIRE and DAVIS 1935) followed very soon. It included identification of the delay of the action potential relative to the cochlear response by "at least 0.6 msec." The cochlear response was thus established conclusively as nonneural in character. Neural on-effects and off-effects were identified, but particular attention was given to the changes in amplitude of the neural response related to the intensity, the frequency, and the duration of a stimulating tone. [The cochlear response was excluded by recording from the auditory nerve with coaxial (concentric) electrodes.] Critical frequencies at which rather abrupt changes in amplitude were found corresponded rather well with predictions based on the usual absolute refractory period of other nerves. The first critical frequency was at about 900 Hz, which was interpreted as the frequency at which systematic alternation of response in the auditory nerve fibers began.

Our strong interest in the question of frequency in individual fibers was due to our desire to construct an "auditory theory" for the coding of the frequency and the intensity of sound and to relate the auditory code to Adrian's general rules. Data derived from single auditory units were not yet available, and we were forced to rely on indirect methods. One of our more direct observations was to use our auditory monitor to listen for synchronized neural activity in the medial geniculate body, in the cortex, and elsewhere. The highest frequency from the cortex was heard in response to clicks delivered at 100/s.

III. Localization of Pitch Perception

During 1933 and 1934 Lurie, Derbyshire, and I gave considerable attention to abnormal ears of cats and guinea pigs that we encountered, and so did several investigators in other laboratories, including H. A. Howe, S. R. Guild, and W. Hughson in Baltimore. With the help of E. H. Kemp and M. Upton we produced cochlear injuries in guinea pigs by prolonged exposure to loud sound, following the model of early experiments by WITTMAACK (1907) and by YOSHIE (1909).

In 1935 we (STEVENS et al. 1935) employed the cochlear response recorded from the round window of anesthetized guinea pigs to "localize pitch perception on the basilar membrane." We determined the threshold of detectability of the response at 26 frequencies (60–12,000 Hz), then drilled a small hole into the cochlea to produce a local injury and immediately determined the same set of thresholds, and finally removed the temporal bone and fixed the specimen for subsequent sectioning and microscopic examination (by M. H. Lurie). We noted immediately that

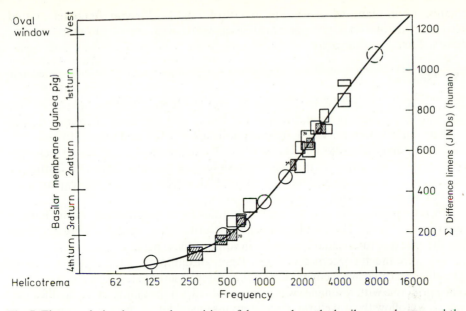

Fig. 5. The correlation between the position of damage along the basilar membrane and the associated changes in the audiogram. The *width of each rectangle* represents the frequency range within which the deviation from normal sensitivity occurs, and its height represents the zone on the basilar membrane separating definitely normal from definitely abnormal hair cells. The *centers of the circles* indicate the centers of peaks or depressions in the audiograms and the centers of isolated normal regions or zones of damage of the organ of Corti. The *solid line* represents the integration of SHOWER and BIDDULPH's (1931) data for human pitch discrimination. *VEST,* vestibular portion of basilar membrane; *JND,* just noticable differences. STEVENS et al. (1935)

complete destruction of the organ of Corti produces no more than about a 30-dB loss of response ... even when more than half of the organ of Corti is destroyed ... [This] suggests that when a tone is raised to about 30 dB above threshold intensity, parts of the mechanism far removed from the place tuned to the frequency of the tone are sufficiently agitated to produce a response. The spread of excitation is apparently greater for low tones than for high.

We therefore looked for, and found, *small* abrupt drops of the order of 10 dB in the audiograms made after injury. The locations of the operative lesions were determined by a careful examination of the serial sections of each cochlea. The basilar membrane was divided longitudinally into nine, two divisions for each full turn, and the beginning and end of the damaged region was located in the upper, middle, or lower third of a division.

The correlation between the frequencies at which there were deviations of sensitivity in the audiograms and the zones separating normal from abnormal hair cells is shown in Fig. 5. I well remember an evening at Lurie's home. He, looking through his microscope, identified the positions and Stevens then read off the predetermined breaks in the audiograms and I plotted the rectangles and circles on a large sheet of coordinate paper. Stevens had already plotted the heavy curve that represents the integration of SHOWER and BIDDULPH's (1931) data for human pitch discrimination, with scale adjusted to correct for the different length of the basilar membrane in man and guinea pig. Every one of the 25 symbols that I plotted touched this psychoacoustically derived curve! It was one of the most exciting hours of my scientific career.

IV. Hearing

With the data concerning localization of pitch perception and the inferences that followed from them in hand, Stevens and I prepared our book *Hearing: Its Psychology and Physiology*. The book was published in 1938, and proved to be a very timely summary (STEVENS and DAVIS 1938). We dedicated it "To the two men who first excited our interest in the psychophysiology of hearing: Edwin G. Boring by his constant concern for auditory theory, and Alexander Forbes by his experiments on the electrophysiology of the auditory pathways."

In retrospect I note that we quoted 25 titles by G. von Békésy, 24 in German and one in French. The traveling wave we described, but we did not greatly stress the sharpness of tuning that is revealed in some of these papers.

We were much concerned with the degree of damping of the auditory system. The dilemma that we recognized was that pitch discrimination on the basis of a place principle with resonance was incompatible with the ability of the cochlear response to follow the waveform of the stimulus in sudden changes such as an abrupt reversal of phase. Implicitly, the cues for auditory lateralization showed that an interaural time difference of 0.1 ms was significant. Such excellent time resolution implies heavy damping, but good frequency resolution requires light damping. (Parenthetically, we may note that in 1983 the dilemma is still with us.) The ear can resolve small differences in *both* time and frequency. And the volley theory as an alternative is at best only a partial solution.

We (STEVENS and DAVIS 1938) took refuge in a place theory based on the concept of the transmission of pressure waves in tubes with elastic walls, and quoted hopefully von Békésy's law of contrast based on an experiment by Mach.

When a sensitive surface of the body, either in the eye or on the skin, is subjected to a stimulus in which there is a change of gradient from place to place, the change of gradient stands out prominently in sensation. If we regard the basilar membrane as such a sensitive surface of the body, we might expect to find a similar effect – an effect which would make the relatively sharp change of gradient in excitation at the maximum of a basilar disturbance stand out in sharp contrast to the rest of the disturbance.

It was not until 1956 that Hartline and his associates gave direct experimental support to this idea by demonstrating "lateral inhibition" in the compound eye of *Limulus* (HARTLINE et al. 1956). The general idea has now become basic in sensory physiology, and the neural inhibitory effects that are involved were the stimulus for von Békésy's experimental work after 1957.

The discussions in *Hearing* of both loudness and pitch involve the work with which Stevens was already deeply concerned of establishing sensory scales, both intensive and numerical. The method of fractionation was his favorite. We employed the concepts of the *mel* as the unit for the pitch scale and of the *sone* for the loudness scale. The relation of the sone to the difference limen (DL) for intensity is discussed and the DLs are shown to be unequal in size. Therefore, "the integration of DLs for the purpose of obtaining a numerical scale of loudness is not permissible."

We (STEVENS and DAVIS 1938) treated loudness a little more firmly than pitch. Its physiological basis was inferred to be the number of active fibers rather than the rate of incoming nerve impulses or the frequency in particular fibers. Here, as elsewhere, Stevens and I had begun to perceive the vast complexity of the nervous system and the improbability of establishing a theory of hearing in terms of the flow of nerve impulses.

With respect to the "cochlear microphonic" (CM), as we now called the cochlear response, I explicitly supported the theory that CM arises as a piezoelectric effect in the hair cells of the organ of Corti. I was right about the hair cells as the source but wrong about the mechanism.

D. Distractions: Scientific and Military

I. The Revolution in Neurophysiology

In 1939 what BULLOCK (1959) later called "the revolution in neurophysiology" was already in progress, but it was accelerated by the advent of electroencephalography. In my opinion the foundation of the revolution was the general acceptance of the principle of chemical mediation at synapses. It was not difficult to extend the idea of chemical excitability to include persistent graded excitatory processes capable of spatial and temporal summation, and then to inhibitory processes and multiple chemical mediators as well. SHERRINGTON'S (1925) postulated central excitatory state and central inhibitory state were transformed into specific neurophysiological models with (ultimately) very direct experimental support. Most important of all, neurophysiology was freed from the straitjacket of the all-or-none nerve impulse as the only means of communication within the central nervous system. This parsimonious hypothesis, originating with Keith Lucas and ably promoted later by Alexander Forbes and Herbert Gasser, was recognized as totally inadequate. The slow potential changes of the electroencephalogram were seen as true physiological phenomena and not merely as volleys of nerve impulses in axons.

A productive study of cortical activity was carried out at Johns Hopkins University by E. M. Walzl and C. Woolsey. The results (WALZL and WOOLSEY 1942, 1946) are a landmark in auditory neurophysiology. They established the tonotopic organization of the auditory cortex in cat. Walzl and Woolsey simplified the sensory input by opening the cochlea and injuring locally the organ of Corti. Later they stimulated electrically the nerve fibers in a restricted segment of the habenula perforata. They simplified the background electroencephalogram by deep barbiturate anesthesia. Under these conditions the auditory evoked potential could be mapped clearly and the projection of the sensory surface of the organ of Corti on the cortex was evident. This had, of course, been expected in the anatomical primary projection area, but, as always seems to be the case, the central nervous system is more complicated than we have any right to anticipate. The organ of Corti was mapped twice, in opposite directions. Later studies with lighter anesthesia showed that there are not only two but half a dozen auditory areas, each with something of a tonotopic organization.

Another activity in auditory physiology was the use of the CM as a tool for studying the transmission of sound across the middle ear. The CM of the basal turn

is easily recorded from the round window. It follows the waveform of the movement of the foot plate of the stapes with no appreciable latency and, at moderate
intensities, no significant nonlinear distortions. These advantages were exploited
in several laboratories, and the intraaural or stapedial reflexes began to receive
well-deserved attention. The volume entitled *Physiological Acoustics* by WEVER
and LAWRENCE (1954) later summarized much of this work.

II. Military Distractions

World War II disrupted the progress of sensory science and the lives and careers
of many individual scientists. Our concerns, our anxieties, our ambitions, our daily
activities were centered on the military effort and our participation in it. Teaching
remained as a familiar routine for those of us in academic positions, but our research was abruptly reoriented to intensely practical applications of military significance.

From a five-year excursion into electroencephalography I was recalled very
abruptly to acoustics. In 1942 I was appointed as one of the original members of
the National Defense Research Committee. Harvey Fletcher was also a member,
and it was he who explained to me that a highly classified mission for us was the
possible use of sound as an offensive military weapon and means of defending
against it. Fletcher, at the Bell Telephone Laboratories, was to design and construct sound sources. I, at Harvard, was to find out how much and what kind of
sound it took to injure or temporarily incapacitate a man. Vern Knudsen, at the
University of California, Los Angeles, was to develop ear defenders and to consider problems of outdoor acoustic transmission. No limits were set on our
budgets, the entire project was secret, and in an outrageous conflict-of-interests situation we were scientifically responsible only to our own subcommittee of three
and to an unspecified military board, probably the Chiefs of Staff.

I enlisted my junior teaching staff at the Department of Physiology, Joseph E.
Hawkins Jr., Robert Galambos, and Horace O. Parrack, my laboratory technician,
Franklin Smith, and a psychology postdoctoral student, Clifford Morgan. We located a secluded suite of rooms in the basement of the biological laboratories in
Cambridge. The Navy provided a tremendous loudspeaker, a "bullhorn," used to
address the deck crew on an aircraft carrier. The Bell Laboratories built us special
amplifiers to drive the bullhorn to its limit, and provided measuring instruments.
At the nodes of standing waves in our reverberant chamber we easily reached a
sound pressure level (SPL) of 150 dB at favorable frequencies.

I also read avidly all that I could find about the observed effects of loud noise
on man, including psychological effects, and separated them from popular super-
stitions and literary fantasies, such as that in *The Nine Tailors* by Dorothy Sayers
(1962). I did some calculations concerning acoustic energy, sound absorption, and
sound reflection, and of course we exposed ourselves to the sound of our bullhorn.

Very soon I was able to give our military authorities my expert opinion:

Sound won't hurt a man except for his ears. It is not worth the effort to develop sound
as a weapon, but it might have useful psychological effects on civilian populations. Noise
can interfere seriously with communication by speech and can permanently impair hearing.
The development of ear defenders should be continued.

The bullhorn rewarded us with a fine bit of serendipity. Our experimental objective was to explore the limits of tolerance of the human ear to sustained sound, as opposed to explosions. We took turns exposing one ear at a time and measuring the recovery of sensitivity from our "temporary deafness." If recovery was complete (within 5 dB) within 24 h we considered the exposure "safe" in the military context. Our criteria of tolerance were very very different from those now invoked for control of noise pollution, and even from those for protection of hearing in industry. We raised the ceiling of tolerance a full 20 dB above our original expectations (DAVIS et al. 1950a). The serendipity was to find that when we exposed our ears to a pure tone from the bullhorn the temporary elevation of threshold was always greatest at a frequency about half an octave above that of the exposure tone. Sometimes the threshold at the exposure tone was shifted no more than 10 dB, while half an octave higher the shift 2 min after exposure might be 50 dB. There were no exceptions to the rule. We were completely baffled for an explanation. Only in 1981 did I realize that an explanation of the displaced threshold shift is to be found in terms of the "tips" and the "tails" of the tuning curves of individual auditory units.

III. The Psycho-Acoustic Laboratory

Meanwhile, at the newly organized Psycho-Acoustic Laboratory in the basement areas of Memorial Hall at Harvard, S.S. Stevens' team of experimental psychologists determined the effects of sustained noise, like the noise in the cockpit of a bomber, on a great variety of psychological and psychomotor functions. They established that there were no measurable deleterious effects, and the Psycho-Acoustics Laboratory then turned its attention to speech communication in noise. By 1943 it had become the national center for the study of speech communication under difficult conditions, for the improvement of electroacoustic equipment to deal with the difficulties, for the development of ear defenders, and for the application of acoustic methods or principles to a wide variety of other military problems of airborne sound. A project under my own direction was to determine the design objectives for hearing aids, for the benefit of hearing-impaired veterans (DAVIS et al. 1947).

The gathering together of the group at the Psycho-Acoustics Laboratory to work on common problems under effective leadership and with generous financial support had far-reaching effects on the development of psychoacoustics and physiological acoustics that are still felt. Nearly all of the untenured psychoacoustic postdoctoral investigators in the United States and many graduate students as well were enlisted and brought to Cambridge. The close personal friendships that were developed have persisted over the years. The group formed the nucleus after the war of the section on physiological and psychological acoustics of the Acoustical Society of America. One result has been that auditory physiology in the United States has remained closely associated with psychoacoustics, secondarily associated with otology, and very weakly associated with neurophysiology.

IV. Single Auditory Units

Even when we were busiest exposing our own ears to the sound of the bullhorn, R. Galambos and I continued to conduct animal experiments in pure auditory

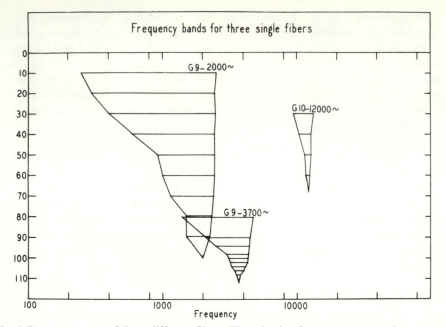

Fig. 6. Response areas of three different fibers. The criterion for response was a just-percep-tible increase in rate over the spontaneous rate, usually about 10%, as judged by listening to the audio monitor. The characteristic frequencies are 2,000, 3,700, and 12,000 Hz. The intensity scale is in decibels relative to an arbitrary high intensity level. GALAMBOS and DAVIS (1943)

physiology. Galambos undertook to isolate the output of a single auditory neural unit. We chose the cat, and Galambos finally mastered the intracranial approach and lowered his fluid-filled pipette microelectrodes into the internal auditory meatus. The electrodes were still very large by modern standards, but on cat number 9, in November 1941, *mirabile dictu,* they worked! The cat's ear was being stim-ulated by "white" noise, and in our auditory monitor we suddenly heard the ex-pected rat-tat-tat-tat-tat of nerve impulses. They nearly stopped when the noise was turned off and they were very sensitive to further movements of the electrode. Before the evening was over we had observed the spontaneous activity of units without acoustic stimulation, we had plotted the first tuning curve outlining a re-sponse area, and had found sharp tuning to different frequencies for different units (see Fig. 6). Later, GALAMBOS (1944) observed inhibition. A tone or noise outside the response area could reduce or completely inhibit the response of a unit to a tone at its characteristic frequency and comfortably above its threshold.

We proudly published our observations under the title "The Response of Single Auditory Nerve Fibers to Acoustic Stimulation" (GALAMBOS and DAVIS 1943). Our observations were all correct and subsequently confirmed. Only one thing was wrong. We had not recorded from primary auditory nerve fibers as we thought. We had actually encountered the cell bodies of second-order units in the cochlear nucleus. By a lucky anatomical accident, in cat some of these units are located far down in the internal auditory meatus. The cell bodies were large targets, suitable

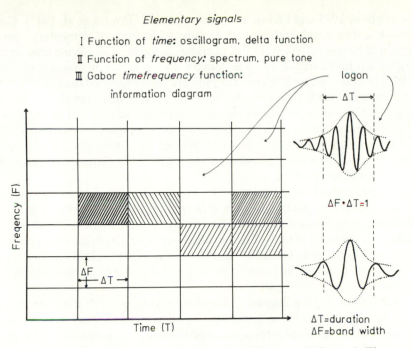

Fig. 7. The information diagram and Gaussian elementary signals (logons). The envelopes (*dotted lines*) of the wave trains are intended to be Gaussian probability functions. The intensity of the logons in the diagram is represented by the density of the *shading* as in one form of "visible speech." DAVIS (1952), after GABOR (1950)

for our crude "micropipette" electrodes. Fortunately, as Tasaki and then Kiang showed later, the pattern of traffic of nerve impulses in many second-order neurons is nearly the same as in the primary units. Our error was suspected early by H. K. Hartline, and in 1948 we finally carried out a proper anatomical control study and admitted our error (GALAMBOS and DAVIS 1948). We had not done postmortem anatomical controls in the original experiments because facilities were not available to us due to wartime conditions. In summary, we had blazed the trail for the study of single auditory units and established tuning curves and response areas. It was KIANG (1965) and his collaborators who really introduced the modern era of the study of such single units, whether primary or secondary or higher order, with computer techniques. WEVER (1949), in his book *Theory of Hearing,* and WEVER and LAWRENCE (1954), in their book *Physiological Acoustics,* gave excellent syntheses of the earlier and of our new data, and an era of controversy ended. Or at least the controversies moved on to new topics.

V. Gabor and the Logon

An interesting sequel to the Galambos study was our interaction with Denis Gabor, Nobel laureate in physics in 1971, a Hungarian-born mathematical physicist and a professor at Imperial College in London. Gabor had noticed the techniques of visual representation of speech sounds as developed at the Bell Telephone Laboratories about 1945 and known as "visible speech" (POTTER et al. 1947). Gabor undertook a theoretical analysis to determine what form of elementary acoustic signal would be most efficient for this purpose, in the sense of having least overlap among signals in the frequency–time domain. In a brief summarizing article (GABOR 1947) he described such "elementary signals" and suggested the name "logon." His mathematical methods are closely related to those of quantum theory, and lead to an uncertainty principle that expresses an inescapable trade-off between precision in time and precision in frequency. By a rather complex mathematical definition of his units of time and frequency he derived the simple equation $\Delta t \times \Delta f \geqq 1$ (GABOR 1950). This is exactly analogous to the familiar Heisenberg uncertainty principle in quantum physics.

In his 1947 paper GABOR further writes that the simplest elementary signals are harmonic oscillations modulated by a (Gaussian) probability pulse (Fig. 7). The ear, he notes, possesses a threshold area of discrimination (dimensions of time and frequency) of the order of unity. Gabor called our attention to his articles in a very friendly personal letter to Galambos in 1947. He saw that some interaction among the fibers must occur in the brain to extract different kinds of information from the ensemble.

I later (DAVIS 1952) published a simplified statement of Gabor's uncertainty principle and its application in audiology. By then I had adopted "tone pips" (filtered clicks) as my standard form of acoustic stimulus in experiments on the guinea pig cochlea. The tone pip is an approximate logon.

E. After World War II but Before Computers

I. Background Publications

We all made a fresh start about 1948 with an academic outlook once more and freedom to communicate again with one another. For auditory neurophysiology and psychoacoustics the state of knowledge and theory were summarized almost simultaneously by WEVER (1949) in his book *Theory of Hearing,* and by myself (DAVIS 1951) in a chapter entitled "Psychophysiology of Hearing and Deafness" in the *Handbook of Experimental Psychology* edited by S. S. STEVENS. Other noteworthy chapters in the *Handbook* included "Basic Correlates of the Auditory Stimulus" by J. C. R. LICKLIDER, "The Perception of Speech" by J. C. R. LICKLIDER and G. A. MILLER, and "The Mechanical Properties of the Ear" by G. VON BÉKÉSY and W. A. ROSENBLITH.

The chapter by von Békésy and Rosenblith is particularly significant because it assembled concisely the gist of von Békésy's fundamental contributions to bioacoustics, which began in 1928. His papers before 1947 had been published in German, many of them in a journal not readily available in USA. With the 1951 chapter and with the introduction of his subject-operated recording audiometer in 1947, von Békésy emerged as the dominant figure in auditory physiology, to be recognized as such in 1961 by a Nobel Prize. The publication of the book by VON BÉKÉSY (1960), ably edited by Wever, entitled *Experiments in Hearing* was another landmark event.

WEVER's (1949) *Theory of Hearing* is oriented to the history of anatomical knowledge of the ear and to some 20 theories of how it works. Nearly two-thirds of it are devoted to elaboration of the volley theory, and in WEVER and LAWRENCE's (1954) *Physiological Acoustics,* Galambos's single-unit data and their implications are fully incorporated in the volley theory.

My own chapter (DAVIS 1951) in the *Handbook of Experimental Psychology* gives prominence to the advances in cortical localization, achieved in animal experiments, by Woolsey and Walzl, Ades, Tunturi, Neff, and others. In particular, the existence of two primary cortical projection areas, each with its own tonotopic organization, emerges as a new principle. Actually, I had been personally diverted from auditory neurophysiology in 1935 to the new field of clinical electroencephalography, in which I was one of the American pioneers. I was next involved deeply in war work related to noise. In 1946 I left Harvard to found a research department at Central Institute for the Deaf in St. Louis. There, in 1948, I resumed active experimentation in cochlear electrophysiology.

II. Analysis of Cochlear Potentials

1. Differential Recording with Intracochlear Electrodes

A major experimental advance during the decade from 1950 to 1960 was the development of the intracochlear recording of cochlear potentials. Before World War II the potentials had been recorded from electrodes on the round window, in the auditory nerve, or on the bony shell of the cochlea (of guinea pigs). About 1950, in response to the demand of otologic surgeons for better visualization of the ossicles and of the delicate procedures of the fenestration operation, the optical industry produced an operating room binocular microscope with a long working distance between the objective and the operative field and magnification up to 45 diameters. These instruments, now a commonplace in neurophysiological laboratories, opened the way for electrical exploration of the cochlea.

I was probably the first to place an intracochlear electrode in an experimental animal. The guinea pig, with its exposed cochlea in the auditory bulla and its greatly enlarged basal turn, offered an excellent target, and I soon found (DAVIS et al. 1949) that from a fine wire electrode introduced through a drill hole excellent recordings could be made, and when two electrodes were introduced, one in scala tympani and the other in the smaller scala vestibuli, the power of intracochlear electrodes became apparent.

The output from scala vestibuli, referred to an electrode on the neck muscles, is a combination of the cochlear microphonic (CM) and action potentials of the auditory nerve. The output from scala tympani is similar, except that the CM is in opposite phase. Thus it is easy, by connecting the two intracochlear electrodes in parallel (and adjusting the relative amplitudes with a potentiometer if necessary), to cancel the CM and observe the uncontaminated action potentials of the nerve. The action potentials can be eliminated and the CM retained if the two inputs to the amplifier are connected to scala vestibuli and scala tympani respectively. This configuration has been designated "differential recording." The CM is a potential difference between the two scalae, generated within the organ of Corti.

A second step was the placement of pairs of electrodes in two or even three different turns of the cochlea, first accomplished by Tasaki (TASAKI et al. 1952). He, with myself and Legouix, compared the velocity and amplitude of the traveling wave of CM along the basilar membrane with von Békésy's observations of mechanical displacement, and found excellent agreement. The CM became a tool for study of mechanical movement.

I recall very vividly a day in 1950 when von Békésy visited Central Institute for the Deaf as a member of a project site visit team. The intracochlear recording of CM was demonstrated. Von Békésy was the last of the visitors to leave the laboratory. He sat a long time with chin in hand before the oscilloscope. He nodded his head slowly and I, standing behing him, heard him murmur half to himself, "and you can make measurements." And within a year von Békésy did make measurements which combined electrical with his own mechanical techniques. I believe that this is probably the only time I directly influenced von Békésy.

2. The Summating Potential

In 1950 my associates and I described the summating potential (SP) (DAVIS et al. 1950 b). This curious name resulted from a false interpretation of a new phenomenon. The new phenomenon was a dc response to acoustic stimulation of the cochlea. The ac response (the CM) was superimposed on it. The new response appeared at moderate to strong levels of stimulation. I found SP because I was looking for it. In spite of my neutral position in my chapter in the *Handbook of Experimental Psychology,* I actually favored the theory of chemical mediation at synaptic junctions between hair cells and the afferent nerve fibers. There should therefore be a postsynaptic "generator" potential (a partial depolarization) produced locally by the chemical mediator and serving to initiate the nerve impulses. The chemical mediator liberated by one phase of a sound wave would not be reabsorbed during the opposite phase, providing a rectifying action, and the excitatory effects of successive sound waves would "summate" to produce a more or less continuous excitation. I looked for a dc response and when I found it I dubbed it the "summating potential," and the name stuck. Perhaps my guess was partly correct. At least four components of SP have now been identified by DALLOS (1973) and his associates, and one of them may be the elusive generator potential of the afferent synapses. SP is complex: for one thing an unsymmetrical mechanical nonlinearity accounts for a considerable part of SP as usually recorded.

3. Von Békésy's Experiment with a Vibrating Electrode

VON BÉKÉSY (1951) combined mechanical and electrical techniques to perform one of his pivotal experiments. He demonstrated first that the critical mechanical movement for the generation of the CM is movement of the tectorial membrane in a *radial* direction, away from the modiolus; secondly, that the CM depends on the displacement and not on the velocity of the movement; and thirdly, that more (electrical) energy may be released in the CM than is imparted to the system by moving the tectorial membrane. A fine metal stylus served both as an electrode to record the electric potential at its point of contact with the tectorial membrane and as the driver to move the membrane in any desired direction. The trapezoidal maneuver showed that the resulting voltage was proportional to the displacement and not to the velocity of the movement. The effective direction was radial, away from the modiolus. If the tectorial membrane was simply held stationary after radial displacement the voltage maintained its new value for several seconds at least. Calculations of the electrical energy dissipated in this situation showed that the dissipation far exceeded the energy required to produce the movement. This result proved that the energy of the CM was supplied by the tissues of the organ of Corti, not by the sound stimulus – and it effectively disposed of the piezoelectric theory of the production of the CM.

4. The Endolymphatic Potential

In the course of his electrical explorations of the cochlea VON BÉKÉSY (1952) discovered the large positive polarization of the endolymph of the scala media. It is about 80 mV positive relative to the perilymph in scala tympani. The dc differences between other structures and positions throughout the membranous labyrinth are of the order of 5 mV or less. The technical advance that made entry into scala media possible without disruptive injury was the use of a very fine micropipette, filled with a strong solution of KCl to make it an electrical conductor. This type of electrode had been developed by electrophysiologists to explore intracellular potentials. Micropipettes a few microns in diameter at the tip became feasible when amplifiers were developed with sufficiently high input impedance to match the impedance of the pipette.

The original name of von Békésy's new potential, the "endolymphatic potential" (EP), proved later to be misleading because the endolymph within the vestibule, saccule, and semicircular canals does not share in the high positive polarization (SMITH et al. 1958). The term "endocochlear potential" is more accurate. The source was identified as the stria vascularis by exploration of the walls of scala media emptied of its endolymph (TASAKI and SPYROPOULOS 1959). It had been established much earlier that in anoxia the positive potential fell rapidly to a negative value and was restored equally rapidly by readmitting oxygen.

Tasaki, Eldredge, and I (TASAKI et al. 1954) utilized the endocochlear potential in our localization of the generator of CM in the plane of the recticular lamina. A micropipette was advanced through the organ of Corti while the guinea pig's ear was stimulated with a 500-Hz tone. The electrical output from the pipette was recorded continuously with both an ac amplifier and a dc amplifier. When the pipette entered scala media the dc potential jumped abruptly from a low or a negative value to +80 mV. The electrode now "saw" the opposite side of the dipole generator of CM, in opposite phase.

III. Impulses in Single Auditory Nerve Fibers

TASAKI succeeded at last (1954), with improved microelectrodes, in recording nerve impulses from single auditory nerve fibers. The animal was the guinea pig. The operative approach to the nerve was through a hole drilled through the petrous bone from the auditory bulla to the internal auditory canal. No possibility here of encountering second-order neurons, as Galambos and I had done in cat (GALAMBOS and DAVIS 1943). The fibers were spontaneously active. The rate of discharge increased when a test tone or noise was increased, up to a saturation rate. These units showed the same patterns of activity and relations to acoustic stimuli as had the second-order neurons of the cat's cochlear nucleus, except that no inhibition of one tone by another was seen, beyond the familiar physical two-tone interactions observable in the CM.

IV. My Theory of Cochlear Excitation

Very soon after von Békésy had discovered the dc polarization of the scala media, I (DAVIS 1953) incorporated it into a theory of the action of the hair cells that still remains the most generally accepted. The negative polarization of about 60 mV of the interior of the hair cells was well known. Von Békésy had shown that the tissues of the cochlea provide the energy for the CM, and I proposed a simple mechanism by which this might occur. A large potential difference, about 140 mV, exists across the reticular lamina between scala media and the interior of the hair cells and the cilia are located in just this region. I assumed that the dc resistance across the reticular lamina is variable, controlled by the position of the cilia. The mechanism, at the molecular level, was and still is entirely hypothetical, but the action would be that of a mechanical valve controlling electric current flow from scala media into the hair cells. The CM is simply the IR drop across the variable resistance. (The "IR drop" is a well-known corollary of Ohm's law.) This is my hypothesis for the generation of the CM. The critical event for activation of the hair cell is the current flow, which causes partial depolarization of the hair cells during the excitatory half of the acoustic cycle.

Other hypotheses are needed to complete the process of initiation of nerve impulses. The transmission of the depolarization from reticular lamina to synapse is by electrotonic spread like that along a nerve fiber in advance of a nerve impulse. At the synapse there might be direct electrical excitation of the nerve by the CM. Such synapses are rare, however, in mammalian systems. Also a rectifier action is needed to permit efficient stimulation of the nerve at high audio frequencies. With chemical mediation we merely assume that the CM half-cycle of depolarization causes liberation of the chemical mediator and that it is not reabsorbed.

In 1961 I pointed out in an article in *Physiological Reviews* (DAVIS 1961) that a common feature of all sense organs is a partial depolarization of the sensory cell. In most cases the sensory cells are independent (like the hair cells) and excite their afferent nerves through a synaptic connection. I urged that the term "receptor potential" be used to designate the initial depolarization of the sensory cell, and that "generator potential" be reserved for the potential, usually postsynaptic, that initiates nerve impulses. I identified the CM as the receptor potential of the organ of Corti. I further clarified my theory of CM at a symposium at Cold Spring Harbor in 1965 (DAVIS 1965).

V. Contributions from Morphology

During the period from 1930 onward, improved methods led to more precise knowledge of the nuclei of the central nervous system and the tracts that interconnect them. Two developments in the postwar period had a profound influence on our physiological thinking and investigation.

1. Efferent Innervation of the Cochlea

Known as the olivocochlear system or "bundle," the efferent innervation of the cochlea was described by Grant RASMUSSEN in 1946 and 1953, although in Europe it is often called the "bundle of Portmann." It arises in the superior olivary complex of the brain stem, crosses the floor of the fourth ventricle, passes close to the cochlear nucleus, and becomes part of the eighth (auditory) cranial nerve. It terminates with rich synaptic endings on the hair cells of the cochlea, chiefly on the outer hair cells. A few years later RASMUSSEN (1960) described a second, smaller bundle that arises near the origin of the larger bundle but does not cross the midline. Instead it is distributed to the homolateral cochlea. The efferent system is much smaller than the afferent system, with only about 500 fibers running to each cochlea (in cat). Each fiber branches richly within the organ of Corti and innervates a set of some 20 hair cells. The peripheral distribution of these fibers had been described many years previously, but it had been assumed that they were afferent fibers, in spite of the implausible pattern of one fiber innervating so many sensory cells. Auditory physiologists immediately sought its function. The obvious model was the muscle spindle, with its small-fiber (gamma) efferent innervation that serves to adjust the sensory structure to operate at different lengths, appropriate to the posture of the limb or body. And at about this time experimental psychologists speculated that the focusing of attention on one particular sensory input might depend on or be facilitated by partial inhibition of other competing inputs. This inhibition or "gating" might be accomplished by efferent neural action on the peripheral sense organ. The efferent olivocochlear system fitted this hypothesis exactly, and just such an effect was soon demonstrated. GALAMBOS (1956), DESMEDT (1960), and FEX (1959, 1965, 1967) all contributed to showing (in cats) that the whole-nerve action potential in response to clicks could be reduced in amplitude by stimulation of the crossed olivocochlear bundle where it crosses the midline in the floor of the fourth ventricle. At the same time the CM output of the hair cells was slightly increased. The efferent fibers were rich in acetylcholinesterase, and it was generally agreed that acetylcholine was released as a chemical transmitter to the external hair cells.

The reduction in the action potential of the auditory nerve produced by maximal stimulation of the crossed olivocochlear bundle corresponded to that produced by reducing the strength of the clicks by about 15 or 20 dB, but the stimulation had to be strong and the frequency of the stimuli had to be high, far above the rate of spontaneous discharge which was found (by Fex) to be about 10/s.

A variety of positive effects were reported, but all of the effects were minor, and interest in the efferent system gradually waned. The physiological significance of the auditory efferent system still remains a mystery in 1983.

2. Electron Microscopy

In a very few years after electron microscopes became commercially available they revolutionized our thinking about the detection of sound by the cochlea, both at the level of the bioacoustics of the organ of Corti and at the level of its nerve supply. It took us from the vague outlines of the cilia of the hair cells to the details of their internal structure and their relations to one another and to the tectorial membrane. It showed not only the presence of typical synapses at the junctions of nerves with hair cells, but also which ones were afferent and which were efferent. It revealed nerve fibers too small to be traced except by uncertain methods of impregnation. It allowed the reliable tracing of neural pathways by detecting subtle degenerative changes after nerve section. It opened a new chapter in the study of the pathology of the ear, particularly of the noxious effects of excessive noise exposure. Unfortunately, the electron microscope stops just short of revealing structure at the molecular level, and it is now clear that the secret of mechanical as well as chemical sensory action still lies out of sight.

VI. Acoustic Trauma

Since World War II auditory physiology has been influenced by the social problem of the impairment of hearing caused by noise. The problem of noise in industry emerged from a previous conspiracy of silence when, in 1948, the Court of Appeals in New York State ruled that such permanent impairment of hearing was compensable under the Workmen's Compensation Act of 1935. The condition known as "boilermakers' deafness" and the prevalence of hearing loss among weavers had been recognized for decades, but in the 1950s the problem of danger from exposure to noise of certain kinds suddenly became a matter of public concern and active investigation.

The study of the effects of noise on hearing gave auditory physiologists a new tool, namely controlled exposures of animals to various noises, for producing fairly predictable injuries to the organ of Corti. The study also provided a new question: "What is the relation of the temporary elevation of auditory thresholds produced by brief severe noise exposure to the permanent threshold shift produced by habitual noise exposure for many hours a day for a period of years?" The electron microscope has shown that the effects of moderate noise exposure are more subtle than the partial loss of hair cells. Apparently, the cilia, particularly the cilia of the outer hair cells, may be visibly injured, but many observations suggest the presence of some still more subtle form of injury from noise exposure.

F. The Computer Era Begins

I. Averaged Responses

For auditory physiology the computer era really began in 1960 with a PhD dissertation by C. D. Geisler (1960) at Massachusetts Institute of Technology, entitled *Average Responses to Clicks in Man Recorded by Scalp Electrodes*. Geisler used a large digital computer, ARC-1, owned by the Air Force, to perform what is in principle a very simple operation, namely to add together successive electric responses that are time-locked to a series of similar stimuli. The method in the context of human evoked potentials actually originated in experiments by Dawson (1947) on

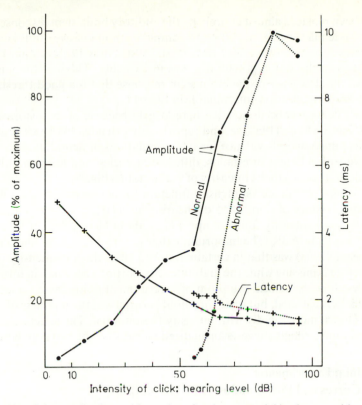

Fig. 8. Graphs of the amplitudes and latencies of action potential in electrocochleograms of a normal and an abnormal ear. Electrode on promontory. Stimulus = unfiltered click. Note that the amplitude is expressed as a percentage of the maximum response of that ear, in each case at 90 dB HL. DAVIS (1976), after ARAN (1968)

the somatosensory system, using first photographic superposition and later (DAWSON 1954) a hand-built electrical analog summing device with a mechanical commutator. Small electric responses were extracted from the background of muscle potentials and the electroencephalogram.

II. Application to Humans: Average Evoked Potentials – The Cochlea and Brain Stem

The human electrocochleogram (ECochG) can be recorded most effectively from a needle electrode that enters the external ear canal, pierces the tympanic membrane, and makes contact with the promontory of the medial wall of the middle ear (ARAN and LeBERT 1968). Other placements outside of the canal, but still close to the ear, are also possible (SOHMER and FEINMESSER 1967). YOSHIE et al. (1967) placed a needle in the wall of the canal. The most careful and extensive exploration of ECochG was described by EGGERMONT et al. (1974) in Utrecht, Netherlands.

The action potential of the auditory nerve is a very robust response. It can be detected very close indeed to the behavioral threshold, but ECochG as a clinical tool has been replaced almost entirely by the auditory brain stem responses (ABR). The electrode placements for ABR are completely noninvasive, and the information obtained from P_6 (wave V of JEWETT and WILLISTON 1971) is almost identical with that from the action potential waves in ECochG. The sensitivity is equally good, and the slow wave of the brain stem response that is a good threshold indicator for low frequencies is not available in ECochG.

The ECochG has been included here largely because of its historical importance. It was YOSHIE's (1968) second report, ably extended by ARAN et al. (1972), which gave unequivocal evidence for two populations of neural units in the auditory nerve with different thresholds, different latencies, and different relations of amplitude and latency to the intensity of the stimulus (Fig. 8).

The normal amplitude vs intensity function for action potential shows a clear break with a change of slope at 55 dB hearing level (HL). A corresponding break in the latency vs intensity function appears at about 60 dB. Similar functions are obtained for P_6 in ABR. The important extension made by Aran and also hinted at by YOSHIE (1968) was that in certain abnormal ears the low-intensity branch of each function is missing while the high-intensity portion is normal, in form at least. These ears show the clinical symptom of "recruitment of loudness." Their threshold for clicks is elevated, but once threshold is surpassed the loudness of the clicks increases much more rapidly with intensity than normal. The selective absence of one population strongly suggests an anatomical basis for the two populations.

III. Animal Experiments:
Tuning Curves and Poststimulus Time Histograms

Animal experiments permit the use of microelectrodes and the study of the nerve impulses in single neural units, and sometimes even the identification of the particular cell studied. About 1960 sensory neurophysiology became the physiology of the traffic of nerve impulses in axons, whether in peripheral nerves, the white matter (nerve tracts) of the central nervous system, or of units in the gray matter.

In addition to plotting the "response areas" or "tuning curves" of individual units, a very effective form of analysis of the activity of a unit is a latency or "poststimulus time" (PST) histogram of its nerve impulses. A long series of stimuli is presented and the latencies of the impulses detected by the microelectrode are displayed graphically. Responses that occur at random time intervals, such as the spontaneous discharge in auditory nerve fibers, show no grouping in time; there are no peaks in the histogram generated from scanning many successive samples. However, if clicks are presented as stimuli the histogram of a fiber with a characteristic frequency (CF) below about 4 kHz shows a remarkable grouping of the impulses at intervals which are the reciprocal of the CF. Evidently, the impulses are time-locked to some feature of the excitatory mechanism that seems to resonate at the CF of the neural unit.

The monograph by N.Y-S. KIANG (1965) entitled *Discharge Patterns of Single Fibers in the Cat's Auditory Nerve,* based on such methods, was a landmark event in sensory neurophysiology. It comprises the spontaneous discharges, the sharp tuning of the units at low intensities and their very broad tuning at high levels, the synchronization of impulses with the sound waves of the stimulus at frequencies below 5 kHz, the grouping in the PST histogram of impulses following a click stimulus into peaks separated by intervals that are equal to 1/CF, the adaptation in rate of discharge over time and the saturation of rate with respect to intensity, and many more.

Kiang's interpretive comments are as cautious as his observations are prolific. Perhaps this is one reason why most of them are still valid. Here are a few of them.

No criterion has been found which allows us to divide primary units into two distinct types that can be correlated either with inner and outer hair cells or with radial and spiral fibers.

We made extensive attempts to demonstrate inhibition of spontaneous activity by a single tone but did not succeed.

It seems reasonable to adopt the position that psychophysical judgments do not necessarily bear simple relationships to events at the level of the auditory nerve. Tasks such as pitch or loudness judgments may depend on an elaboration of many different aspects of auditory nerve activity.

The work of Kiang and his team did not terminate with the monograph. They have provided much additional data on the tuning curves of primary auditory units. Improved methods have allowed the study of units in sufficient numbers to begin a statistical approach to some problems. They have established a clear difference in the sharpness of tuning as a function of CF: much sharper in the high-frequency range. They and many other investigators, notably J. Rose and J. E. Hind and their collaborators at the University of Wisconsin, have extended the range of single unit analysis anatomically into the midbrain, but limitations of space prevent us from attempting to extend our present survey above the level of the auditory nerve (ROSE et al. 1967, 1971).

G. An Era of Puzzlement

I. Progress and Puzzles

By 1970 the sensory process of the cochlea had turned out to be unexpectedly complex. It is appropriate to call the decade of the 1970s not only an era of rapid progress but equally an era of puzzlement. The following summary is very personal in its choice of topics. Many features of current auditory science, such as comparative anatomy and the process of echolocation, and also advances in central neurophysiology are arbitrarily omitted.

I shall draw freely on two important symposia that I attended, one in Stockholm under the auspices of the Royal Swedish Academy of Sciences (Basic Mechanisms of Hearing, 1973), the other in Paris at the 1974 meeting of the International Society of Audiology, entitled "Cochlear Function."

II. The Sharpness of Tuning of the Basilar Membrane

In his first description of the relation of the locus of maximal amplitude to acoustic frequency, von Békésy noted that the "tuning" of the cochlear partition, although fairly sharp on the high-frequency side, is very broad toward the low frequencies

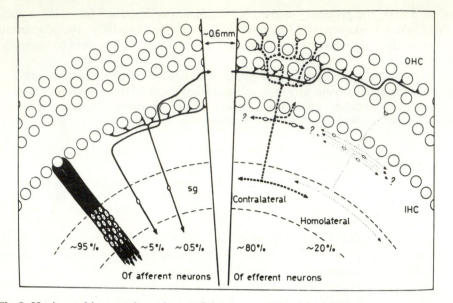

Fig. 9. Horizontal innervation schema of the organ of Corti with the different types of afferent neurons on the *left* and of efferent neurons on the *right* with their corresponding approximate percentages. *OHC,* outer hair cells; *IHC,* inner hair cells; *sg,* spiral ganglion. Spoendlin (1975)

and could hardly provide unaided the fine discrimination of pitch, related to frequency, that is shown by psychoacoustic methods. He invoked Mach's principle of contrast. Such interaction is carried out by nerve impulses and inhibitory synapses, but no neural interconnections among the hair cells or their afferent nerves have ever been demonstrated in the organ of Corti.

But is the von Békésy envelope really so rounded? Three delicate micromethods have been applied to the problem. One depends on the Mössbauer effect. It makes use of a tiny bit of radioactive material that is placed on the basilar membrane. A probe nearby detects fluctuations in the radiation received, related to movement of the source – a sort of Doppler effect. Elegant experiments by Johnstone and Boyle (1967) and by Rhode (1971) and others on guinea pigs and on squirrel monkeys show that the slope of the mechanical tuning curve of the membrane is very steep indeed on the high-frequency side and may approximate to that of the neural response areas, but on the low-frequency side the mechanical tuning is far too flat.

Another micromethod employs a laser beam (Kohllöffel 1973), and yields very similar results.

A third method, using a capacitative electrical probe, has overcome some of the criticisms raised against the Mössbauer effect (Wilson and Johnstone 1975). With it Evans and Wilson (1975) demonstrated in cats a very broad tuning of the basilar membrane, while recording concurrently a very sharp tip of the response area of a single nerve fiber. They concluded, quite reasonably, that a second filter is a necessary assumption.

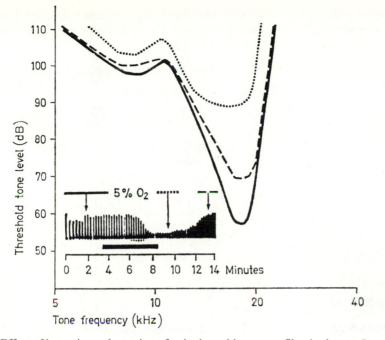

Fig. 10. Effect of hypoxia on the tuning of a single cochlear nerve fiber in the cat. *Inset* shows time course of gross cochlear action potential (AP) response amplitude to click stimuli of constant intensity. *Black bar* indicates duration of administration of 5% O_2 in N_2O. *Bars over the AP record* indicate the time during which determinations of the frequency threshold curve (FTC) for the fiber, illustrated in the main figure, were taken. The *solid curve* is the control FTC. The *upper dotted curve* is the FTC of the fiber at the height of the hypoxia, the *middle dashed curve* during partial recovery. EVANS (1975)

III. Innervation of the Organ of Corti

H. Spoendlin of Innsbruck, Austria, almost single-handedly, has since 1967 completely revised our ideas about the innervation of the organ of Corti. He has traced degeneration following nerve sections, using the electron microscope, and has counted nerve fibers and cell bodies. His favorite animal is cat, but the general pattern that he has developed is now generally accepted and extrapolated to humans (Fig. 9).

Of the afferent neurons in the auditory nerve about 95% innervate inner hair cells. Each inner hair cell receives about 20 afferent neurons. About 5% of afferent neurons make contact with outer hair cells by way of spiral bundles. Each of these neurons innervates about ten cells. In addition, about 0.5% of afferents, also in spiral bundles, each innervate a group of about ten inner hair cells.

There are about 60,000 afferent fibers from each ear, but only about 500 efferents. The larger (contralateral) olivocochlear system (80%) goes chiefly in radial bundles to the outer hair cells, particularly of the basal and middle turns. Each fiber makes synaptic contact with a cluster of about 20 hair cells. The homolateral system (20%) is distributed in spiral bundles chiefly to the afferent neurons under the inner hair cells.

The most startling feature of this pattern of innervation is the very small percentage of afferent fibers from the outer hair cells. What now is the function of the outer hair cells and their efferent nerve supply?

IV. The Dual Nature of Single-Unit Tuning Curves

E. F. EVANS (1975, 1978) summarized evidence that there are two components of the response area of a single neuron in the auditory nerve. One part that he called the "tip" is sharply tuned and very sensitive (Fig. 10). The tip centers on the CF. The remainder of the area, the "tail", consisting of the tones that stimulate only at medium or high intensity levels, is very broadly tuned. The best evidence that there are two components is that the tip is selectively vulnerable to anoxia and to certain ototoxic drugs, including kanamycin (KIANG et al. 1970). It is particularly significant that the suppression of the tip in anoxia is reversible. It is the outer hair cells that are particularly susceptible to kanamycin and other noxious influences. The outer hair cells thus become the basis, somehow, for the tips.

V. The Second Filter

I believe that the term "second filter" was first introduced in discussions of possible origins of the "cubic difference tone" $(2f_1-f_2)$, which has puzzled psychoacousticians for many years. The generation of this tone can be accounted for, according to PFEIFFER (1970; PFEIFFER and KIM 1973) by a primary filter followed by a non-linear element followed by a second filter. Everyone agrees that the basilar membrane is the mechanism for the first filter.

RUSSELL and SELLICK (1978) introduced a micropipette into an inner hair cell in a living guinea pig and measured its internal electric potentials as it was stimulated by sound. They proved the identity of the cell by introducing a marker dye through the pipette electrode. They found the expected negative resting potential, and under stimulation an ac potential and a dc shift, corresponding to CM and SP, appeared. The magnitude of these electric responses varied with the intensity and the frequency of the stimulating tone. Tuning curves were plotted, and they showed sharp sensitive tips as well as the long low-frequency tails. Thus the interior of the inner hair cells was proved to be located beyond the second filter. This experiment rules out any neural interaction between inner and outer cells as the basis for the sharp tuning, as suggested by ZWISLOCKI (1975). Excluded also is any possible "molecular tuning" at the first synapse.

A curious feature of the second filter is that its resonant frequency, which yields the tip of the tuning curve, is appreciably higher than that of the secondary peak of sensitivity that is shown by the tail of the tuning curve when the tips have been suppressed by anoxia or ototoxic drugs (Fig. 10). Apparently, the tail represents the classic von Békésy envelope, i.e., the action of the first filter, and the tip is located near the extreme low-frequency (apical) end of the envelope of the traveling wave.

The displacement of the temporary threshold shift to frequencies above that of the exposure tone, noted in Sect. D. II, rests on this relation. It is the vulnerable tips of the tuning curves of auditory units that are affected by excessive amplitudes of the von Békésy traveling wave (DAVIS, 1983).

How can a microscopic structure in the organ of Corti act as a second resonant filter? The idea of electrical stimulation or a facilitation of the inner hair cells by the CM of the outer hair cells has been suggested. This idea encounters very serious difficulties, but nevertheless many investigators of the cochlea accepted RYAN and DALLOS's (1975) proposition that the outer hair cells "sensitize" the inner hair cells by some unspecified mechanism.

VI. Cochlear Latency

While conducting clinical testing of ears by auditory brain stem responses (DAVIS and HIRSH 1979), I noted the great prolongation near threshold of the latency of the neural response to 4-kHz tone pips. The prolongation cannot be accounted for by physical or neural conduction times or the traveling wave delay (DAVIS 1981, 1983). But this is exactly the way the second filter should work. The high-intensity system, corresponding to the tails of the response areas of the neurons, is excited directly by a 60-dB tone pip without the intervention of the second filter, and its latency is short, but for a stimulus near threshold the second filter must act. It is essentially a lightly damped resonator and has a high Q. It therefore requires several periods of the tone for amplitude to build up to a threshold strength for the neuron. The second filter gives the auditory unit greater sensitivity, but the price of this is a longer latency.

VII. The Cochlear Echo: Acoustic Emissions

A climax of implausibility was provided by KEMP (1978). He placed a sensitive microphone in the human external ear canal and arranged for it to "listen" for a few milliseconds just after a tone pip had been delivered to the ear. By the method of averaged responses he detected an echo. It was too early to involve any neural reflex and too late to be a physical reverberation in the canal.

Kemp's claims were confirmed and extended. In fact the cochlea seems sometimes to return more energy than can reasonably be expected as a simple echo from a passive system. For this reason we now speak of "acoustic emissions." An important symposium on the subject was held in London in 1979 under the title "Nonlinear and Active Mechanical Processes in the Cochlea." (KEMP and ANDERSON 1980.)

It is now impossible to avoid the idea of *positive feedback*, and idea put forward by GOLD in 1948, 30 years ahead of its time. Positive feedback can provide the high Q (light damping) that seems so necessary for the second filter.

The idea of positive feedback revived interest in *audible tinnitus*, tinnitus audible to a second listener. Such tinnitus is clearly tonal in character, does not pulsate, can be clearly traced to the cochlea, and interacts with external tones. Now investigators have begun to "listen", with microphone and filters, to normal human ears and to the ears of animals that have been subjected to acoustic trauma. As this

chapter was being written, Zurek (1981) and Zurek and Clark (1980) were reporting their observations on narrow-band acoustic emissions from humans and
noise-exposed chinchillas.

H. Auditory Theory Today

I. What is Auditory Theory?

What does or should the term "auditory theory" denote today? At one time it
seemed to consist of speculations as to what physical and physiological mechanisms lie between the acoustic stimulus and auditory sensation and perception.
At another time it seemed to be the narrower question of how acoustic/auditory
information is encoded in the auditory nerve. Today interest seems divided among
the most recent answers to the old questions plus a great concern with peripheral
auditory mechanisms in the realm of biophysics and neurophysiology. Another
major concern is with the "processing" of neural information within the central
nervous system in the areas of neuroanatomy, neurophysiology, and psychology.
There the gap between physiology and psychology is as wide as ever, and no appreciable progress has been made toward solving the key problem of the physiological mechanism(s) of memory.

Historically, auditory theory has been dominated by the question of how information about acoustic frequency is carried to the brain, whether by particular
nerve fibers excited selectively by a resonance (place) mechanism or directly, according to the volley theory. Both theories have been established as correct. The
upper limit of detectable synchronization of impulses is at about 5,000 Hz, and it
is agreed that the psychoacoustic phenomena of "periodicity pitch" or "residue
pitch" depend on such synchronization (Evans 1978). The synchronization cannot
be detected above the level of the inferior colliculus, and also each fiber has its own
response area, with greatest sensitivity at its CF. Each theorizer must decide for
himself what he believes to be the relative importances of the place and the volley
principles for pitch perception and the "quality" of sounds. There is a large transition range in which both principles are operating.

As the first step in peripheral frequency analysis, the tuning of the basilar membrane as described by von Békésy is unchallenged, together with its secondary feature, the traveling wave pattern on the cochlear partition.

The revised scheme of innervation of the organ of Corti as summarized by
Spoendlin has been accepted tacitly, with almost no audible dissent. This actually
involves a revolutionary modification of auditory theory because it implies that all
or nearly all of our auditory information passes through the channel of the inner
hair cells. The innervation of the inner hair cells, 20 nerve fibers to each cell, is highly redundant. There seems to be only one population of afferent nerve fibers, and
auditory theory today has difficulty in assigning any clear function to the outer hair
cells or, for that matter, to the efferent nerves in the organ of Corti (the
olivocochlear bundles). In fact, peripheral auditory theory is in such a state of dis-
array that most of us are simply waiting for more experimental facts or perhaps
the emergence of a coherent theory of the peripheral mechanism. A disputed question in auditory theory is whether a second filter must be postulated, and if so

where it is and how it works. I personally believe that the second filter is real and I include here some of my recent speculations (DAVIS 1981, 1983) to show the direction that I expect auditory theory to take.

II. My Present Auditory Theory

My present theory includes the principle of positive feedback in the organ of Corti. I accept the hypothesis of positive feedback because I think it is needed to make the second filter work, and with it the second filter solves several problems. It is a bold hypothesis: it assigns an active role to the cochlea in the detection of faint signals.

I believe intuitively that nature did not develop the second filter primarily to improve frequency discrimination but to improve sensitivity for faint but coherent acoustic signals. I believe that the second filter is fundamentally a resonator. In order for the resonator to improve sensitivity by summing energy over several cycles of the signal it must be lightly damped, and in positive feedback I see the most plausible mechanism for achieving this property in the fluid medium within the organ of Corti. A price that is paid for the sensitivity of a resonant system is its longer latency of response, particularly near threshold.

As a slight digression I note that the redundant innervation of the inner hair cells and the spontaneous discharge of impulses in each nerve fiber may serve the same purpose of increasing sensitivity. A quantal jump is necessary for the excitation of an impulse in a quiescent nerve fiber, but a very slight increase in the amount of chemical mediator being released can lead to an increase in the rate in each fiber, and if there are many fibers the probability of detection of an overall increase in the cochlear nucleus is greater. But an even more sensitive mechanism may be the synchronization of spontaneous discharges in the group of fibers that innervate a single cell, without increasing the overall rate. Just such a relation has been demonstrated very recently (JOHNSON 1980). But near the threshold the advantage of many fibers is lost unless they innervate the same cell. This is because each position along the basilar membrane has a different characteristic frequency, and the tips of the neural response areas are very sharply tuned.

I believe that the outer hair cells are involved in the positive feedback system and that this is their chief or only function. I make them responsible for the tips of the response areas. The CM of the outer hair cells is part of the feedback mechanism, but I shall not speculate further here on the possibility of direct electrical influence on the inner hair cells or on a putative piezoelectric effect that would amplify the mechanical movements of their cilia (DAVIS 1981, 1983).

I state here a favorite proposition of mine about the processing and transmission of auditory information. Mechanisms are highly refined to deal with differences in the auditory spectra of signals (frequency discrimination), with intensity (both absolute sensitivity and intensity differences), and with time differences (notably in binaural interactions). Each class of information is extracted from the ensemble of nerve impulses in the auditory nerve, and I believe that this extraction takes place at a very low level in the brain stem. The branching of the auditory nerve fibers in the cochlear nucleus is the first step. Then comes a fundamentally different process for each class of information: mutual inhibition to enhance contrast for frequency discrimination, spatial summation for overall loudness and for critical band effects, and a very secure one-to-one transmission across the first few synapses to preserve synchronization (or time differences) until binaural inter-actions have occurred. These three processes are mutually exclusive. Intensity in-formation is lost in mutual inhibition and frequency information is lost in summa-tion for intensity, and once information is lost it cannot be recovered. However, the information that *has* been extracted can be recoded and transmitted elsewhere in the very reliable basic code of all-or-none nerve impulses in particular nerve fi-bers. A conclusion is that there should be *at least three separate auditory systems* in the brain stem: one for acoustic spectrum, one for intensity, and one for time information. They must be separate physiologically, although they may be inter-mingled anatomically: and of course they interact physiologically in the gray mat-ter of the nuclei, where "feature extraction" takes place. We may need an auditory theory for each level of extraction, recording, transmission, and interaction. This implies also a supertheory: a theory of auditory theories.

Somehow frequency discrimination (pitch) historically captured center stage and held it. Perhaps the place principle and the recognition of tonotopic organiza-tion up to and including the auditory cortex gave us a (false) sense of security in thinking about how the central nervous system deals with the acoustic spectrum. But the mechanism for intensity (loudness) I find even more difficult to imagine when I consider its tremendous dynamic range.

I conclude with a sample question for future auditory theory: "What is the physiological mechanism that underlies the psychophysical power law for loudness as enunciated by S. S. Stevens (1975)?" Does this question involve the forbidden mixing of the subjective and the objective aspects of audition?

References

Names containing *von* are alphabetized in this list under *v*

Adrian ED (1928) The basis of sensation: the action of sense organs. Norton, New York
Adrian ED (1931) The microphonic action of the cochlea: an interpretation of Wever and Bray's experiments. J Physiol 71:28
Adrian ED (1932) The mechanism of nervous action. University of Pennsylvania Press, Phil-adelphia
Adrian ED, Bronk DD (1929) The discharge of impulses in motor nerve fibers. II. The frequency of discharge in reflex and voluntary contractions. J Physiol 67:119–151
Adrian ED, Bronk DD, Phillips G (1931) The nervous origin of the Wever and Bray effect. J Physiol 73:2
Aran J-M, LeBert G (1968) Human nervous cochlear responses as an image of the working of the ear and a new test of objective audiometry. (Les réponses nerveuses cochléaires chez l'homme. Image du fonctionnement de l'oreille et nouveau test d'audiometrie ob-jective.) Rev Laryngol otol Rhinol (Bord) 89:361–378
Aran J-M, Portmann C, Pelerin J (1972) Electrocochléogramme chez l'adulte et chez l'en-fant. Audiology 11:77–89
Berger H (1929) Über das Elektroenkephalogramm des Menschen: I. Arch Psychiatr Ner-venkd 87:527–570
Boring EG (1926) Auditory theory with special reference to intensity, volume, and localiz-ation. Am J Psychol 37:157–188
Boring EG (1933) The physical dimensions of consciousness. Century, New York
Bullock TH (1959) Neuron doctrine and electrophysiology. Science 129:997–1002

Dallos P (1973) The auditory periphery. Academic, New York

Davis H (1926) The conduction of the nerve impulse. Physiol Rev 6:547–595

Davis H (1951) Psychophysiology of hearing and deafness. In: Stevens SS (ed) Handbook of experimental psychology. Wiley, New York, pp 1116–1142

Davis H (1952) Information theory: 3. Applications of information theory to research in hearing. J Speech Hear Disord 17:189–197

Davis H (1953) Energy into nerve impulses. Hearing. Med Bull St. Louis University 5:43–48

Davis H (1961) Some principles of sensory receptor action. Physiol Rev 41:391–416

Davis H (1965) A model for transducer action in the cochlea. Cold Spring Harbor Symp Quant Biol 30:181–190

Davis H (1976) Principles of electric response audiometry. Ann Otol Rhinol Laryngol Suppl 28. 85:1–96

Davis H (1981) The second filter is real, but how does it work? Am J Otolaryngol 2:153–158

Davis H (1983) An active process in cochlear mechanics. Hear Res 9:79–90

Davis H, Hirsh SK (1979) A slow brainstem response for low-frequency audiometry. Audiology 18:445–461

Davis H, Forbes A, Brunswick D, Hopkins AMcH (1926) Studies of the nerve impulse. II. The question of decrement. Am J Physiol 76:448–471

Davis H, Derbyshire AJ, Lurie MH (1934a) A modification of auditory theory. Arch Otolaryngol 20:390–395

Davis H, Derbyshire AJ, Lurie MH, Saul LJ (1934b) The electric response of the cochlea. Am J Physiol 107:311–332

Davis H, Stevens SS, Nichols RH Jr, Hudgins CV, Marquis RJ, Peterson EC, Ross DA (1947) Hearing aids: a experimental study of design objectives. Harvard University Press, Cambridge, MA

Davis H, Gernandt BE, Riesco-MacClure JS, Covell WP (1949) Aural microphonics in the cochlea of the guinea pig. J Acoust Soc Am 21:502–510

Davis H, Morgan CT, Hawkins JE Jr, Galambos R, Smith FW (1950a) Temporary deafness following exposure to loud tones and noise. Acta Otolaryngol (Stockh) [Suppl] 88

Davis H, Fernandez C, McAuliffe DR (1950b) The excitatory process in the cochlea. Proc Nat Acad Sci USA 36:580–587

Dawson GD (1947) Cerebral responses to electrical stimulation of peripheral nerve in man. J Neurol Neurosurg Psychiatry 10:137–140

Dawson GD (1954) A summation technique for the detection of small evoked potentials. Electroencephalogr Clin Neurophysiol 6:65–84

Derbyshire AJ, Davis H (1935) The action potentials of the auditory nerve. Am J Physiol 113:476–504

Desmedt JE (1960) Neurophysiological mechanisms controlling acoustic input. In: Rasmussen GL, Windle W (eds) Neural mechanisms of the auditory and vestibular systems. Charles C Thomas, Springfield 11:152–164

Eggermont JJ, Odenthal DW, Schmidt PH, Spoor A (1974) Electrocochleography: basic principles and clinical application. Acta Otolaryngol (Stockh) [Suppl] 316

Evans EF (1975) The sharpening of cochlear frequency selectivity in the normal and abnormal cochlea. Audiology 14:419–442

Evans EF (1978) Place and time coding of frequency in the peripheral auditory system: some physiological pros and cons. Audiology 17:369–420

Evans EF, Wilson JP (1975) Cochlear tuning properties: concurrent basilar membrane and single nerve fiber measurements. Science 190:1218–1221

Fex J (1959) Augmentation of cochlear microphonic by stimulation of efferent fibers to the cochlea. Acta Otolaryngol 50:540–541

Fex J (1965) Auditory activity in uncrossed centrifugal cochlear fibres in cat. A study of a feedback system, II. Acta Physiol Scand 64:43–57

Fex J (1967) Efferent inhibition in the cochlea related to hair-cell dc activity: study of postsynaptic activity of the crossed olivocochlear fibers in the cat. J Acoust Soc Am 41:666–675

Fletcher H (1929) Speech and hearing. Van Nostrand, New York

Fletcher H (1930) A space-time pattern theory of hearing. J Acoust Soc Am 1:311–343

Forbes A (1922) The interpretation of spinal reflexes in terms of present knowledge of nerve conduction. Physiol Rev 2:361–414

Forbes A, Thatcher C (1920) Amplification of action currents with the electron tube in recording with the string galvanometer. Am J Physiol 52:409–471

Forbes A, Miller RH, O'Connor J (1927) Electric responses to acoustic stimuli in the decerebrate animal. Am J Physiol 80:363–380

Gabor D (1947) Acoustical quanta and the theory of hearing. Nature 159:591–594

Gabor D (1950) Communication theory and physics. Philosophical Mag 41:1161–1187

Galambos R (1944) Inhibition of activity in single auditory nerve fibers by acoustic stimulation. J Neurophysiol 7:287–303

Galambos R (1956) Suppression of auditory nerve activity by stimulation of efferent fibers to cochlea. J Neurophysiol 19:424–437

Galambos R, Davis H (1943) The response of single auditory nerve fibers to acoustic stimulation. J Neurophysiol 6:39–58

Galambos R, Davis H (1948) Action potentials from single auditory-nerve fibers? Science 108:513–514

Gasser HS, Erlanger J (1922) A study of the action currents of nerve with a cathode ray oscillograph. Am J Physiol 62:496–524

Geisler CD (1960) Average responses to clicks in man recorded by scalp electrodes. Dissertation, Massachusetts Institute of Technology, Research Laboratory of Electronics. Technical report 380. Cambridge, MA

Gold T (1948) The physical basis of the action of the cochlea. Proc R Soc Lond (Biol) 135:492–498

Hartline HK, Wagner HC, Ratliff F (1956) Inhibition in the eye of *Limulus*. J Gen Physiol 39:651–673

von Helmholtz HLF (1948) On the sensations of tone, 6th ed Smith, New York. Translation of: Die Lehre von den Tonempfindungen als physiologische Grundlage für die Theorie der Musik. Vierweg, Braunschweig, 1863

Jewett DL, Williston JS (1971) Auditory-evoked fair fields averaged from the scalp of humans. Brain 94:681–696

Johnson DH (1980) The relationship between spike rate and synchrony in responses of auditory-nerve fibers to single tones. J Acoust Soc Am 68:1115–1122

Johnston BM, Boyle AJF (1967) Basilar membrane vibration examinded with the Mössbauer technique. Science 158:389–390

Kato G (1924) The theory of decrementless conduction in narcotized region of nerve. Nankodo, Tokyo

Kato G (1934) The microphysiology of nerve. Maruzen, Tokyo

Kemp DT (1978) Stimulated acoustic emissions from within the human auditory system. J Acoust Soc Am 64:1386–1391

Kemp DT, Anderson SD (eds) (1980) Nonlinear and active mechanical processes in the cochlea (proceedings of a symposium). Hear Res 2:169–604

Kiang NY-S (1965) Discharge patterns of single fibers in the cat's auditory nerve, research monograph no 35. Massachusetts Institute of Technology Press, Cambridge

Kiang NY-S, Moxon EC, Levine RA (1970) Auditory-nerve activity in cats with normal and abnormal cochleas. Ciba Foundation symposium on sensorineural hearing loss. Churchill, London, pp 241–273

Kohllöffel LVE (1973) Observations of the mechanical disturbances along the basilar membrane with laser illumination. In: Møller AR (ed) Basic mechanisms in hearing. Academic, New York, pp 95–118

Licklider JCR (1951) Basic correlates of the auditory stimulus. In: Stevens SS (ed) Handbook of experimental psychology. John Wiley & Sons, Inc. New York 25:985–1039

Licklider JCR, Miller GA (1951) The perception of speech. In: Stevens SS (ed) Handbook of experimental psychology. John Wiley & Sons, Inc. New York 26:1040–1074

Lorente de Nó R (1933) Anatomy of the eighth nerve. The central projection of the nerve endings of the internal ear. Laryngoscope 43:1–38

Pfeiffer RR (1970) A model for two-tone inhibition of single cochlear nerve fibers. J Acoust Soc Am 48:1373–1378

Pfeiffer RR, Kim DO (1973) Considerations of nonlinear response properties of single cochlear nerve fibers. In: Møller AR (ed) Basic mechanisms in hearing. Academic, New York

Potter RK, Kopp GA, Green HC (1947) Visible speech. Van Nostrand, New York

Rasmussen GL (1946) The olivary peduncle and other fiber projections of the superior olivary complex. J Comp Neurol 84:141–200

Rasmussen GL (1953) Further observations of the efferent cochlear bundle. J Comp Neurol 99:61–74

Rasmussen GL (1960) Efferent fibers of the cochlear nerve and cochlear nucleus. In: Windle WF (ed) Neural mechanisms of the auditory and vestibular systems. Thomas Springfield, pp 105–115

Rhode WS (1971) Observations of the vibration of the basilar membrane in squirrel monkeys using the Mössbauer technique. J Acoust Soc Am 49:1218–1231

Rose JE, Brugge JF, Anderson DJ, Hind JE (1967) Phase-locked response to low-frequency tones in single auditory nerve fibers of the squirrel monkey. J Neurophysiol 30:769–793

Rose JE, Hind JE, Anderson DJ, Brugge JF (1971) Some effects of stimulus intensity on response of auditory nerve fibers in the squirrel monkey. J Neurophysiol 34:685–699

Russell IJ, Sellick PM (1978) Intracellular studies of hair cells in the mammalian cochlea. J Physiol 284:261–290

Rutherford W (1886) A new theory of hearing. J Anat Physiol 21:166–168

Ryan A, Dallos P (1975) Effect of absence of cochlear outer hair cells on behavioural auditory threshold. Nature 253:44–46

Saul LJ, Davis H (1932 a) Electrical phenomena of the auditory mechanism. Trans Am Otolaryngol Soc

Saul LJ, Davis H (1932 b) Action currents in the central nervous system: I. Action currents of the auditory tracts. Arch Neurol 28:1104–1116

Sayers DL (1962) Nine tailors. Sayers tandem. Gollancz

Sherrington CS (1925) Remarks on some aspects of reflex inhibition. Proc R Soc Lond (Biol) 97B:519–545

Shower EG, Biddulph R (1931) Differential pitch sensitivity of the ear. J Acoust Soc Am 3:275–287

Smith CA, Davis H, Deatherage DH, Gessert CF (1958) DC potentials of the membranous labyrinth. Am J Physiol 193:203–206

Sohmer H, Feinmesser M (1967) Cochlear action potentials recorded from the external ear in man. Ann Otolaryngol 76:427–435

Spoendlin H (1975) Neuroanatomical basis of cochlear coding mechanisms. Audiology 14:383–407

Stevens SS (1975) Psychophysics: introduction to its perceptual, neural, and social prospects. Wiley, New York

Stevens SS, Davis H (1938) Hearing: its psychology and physiology. Wiley, New York

Stevens SS, Davis H, Lurie MH (1935) The localization of pitch perception on the basilar membrane. J Gen Psychol 13:297–315

Tasaki I (1954) Nerve impulses in individual auditory nerve fibers of guinea pig. J Neurophysiol 17:97–122

Tasaki I, Spyropoulos CS (1959) Stria vascularis as source of endocochlear potential. J Neurophysiol 22:149–155

Tasaki I, Davis H, Legouix J-P (1952) The space-time pattern of the cochlear microphonics (guinea pig), as recorded by differential electrodes. J Acoust Soc Am 24:502–519

Tasaki I, Davis H, Eldredge DH (1954) Exploration of cochlear potentials in guinea pig with a microelectrode. J Acoust Soc Am 26:765–773

Troland LT (1930) The principles of psychophysiology. Volume II Sensation. Van Nostrand, New York

von Békésy G (1951) Microphonics produced by touching the cochlear partition with a vibrating electrode. J Acoust Soc Am 23:29–35

von Békésy G (1952) Gross localization of the place of origin of the cochlear microphonics. J Acoust Soc Am 24:399–409

von Békésy G (1960) Experiments in hearing. McGraw-Hill, New York, pp 411–414 von Helmholtz HLF (1948) On the sensations of tone, 6th edn. Smith, New York Translation of: Die Lehre von den Tonempfindungen als physiologische Grundlage für die Theorie der Musik. Vierweg, Braunschweig, 1863

Walzl EM, Woolsey CN (1942) Effects of cochlear lesions on click responses in the auditory cortex of the cat. Fed Proc 1:88

Walzl EM, Woolsey CN (1946) Effects of cochlear lesions on click responses in the auditory cortex of the cat. Bull Johns Hopkins Hosp 79:309–319

Wever EG (1949) Theory of hearing. Wiley, New York

Wever EG, Bray CW (1930a) Auditory nerve impulses. Science 71:215

Wever EG, Bray CW (1930b) Present possibilities for auditory theory. Psychol Rev 37:365–380

Wever EG, Lawrence M (1954) Physiological acoustics. Princeton University Press, Princeton

Wilson JP, Johnstone JR (1975) Basilar membrane and middle-ear vibration in guinea pig measured by capacitive probe. J Acoust Soc Am 57:705–723

Wittmaack K (1907) Über Schädigung des Gehörs durch Schalleinwirkung. Z Ohrenhk 54:37–80

Yoshie N (1968) Auditory nerve action potential responses to clicks in man. Laryngoscope 78:198–215

Yoshie N, Ohashi T, Suzuki T (1969) Non-surgical recording of auditory nerve action potentials in man. Laryngoscope 77:76–85

Yoshie U (1909) Experimentelle Untersuchungen über die Schädigung des Gehörorganes durch Schalleinwirkung. Z Ohrenhk 58:201–205

Zurek PM (1980) Spontaneous narrowband acoustic signals emitted by human ears. J Acoust Soc Am 69:514–523

Zurek PM, Clark WW (1980) Objective tonal tinnitus induced by noise exposure in chinchillas. J Acoust Soc Am [Suppl] 68:44

Zwislocki JJ (1975) Phase opposition between inner and outer hair cells and auditory sound analysis. Audiology 14:443–455

CHAPTER 3

Microstructure of the Inner Ear*

Hans Engström

A. Introduction

In morphological research, as in many other scientific areas, the development of
new techniques has often furthered our knowledge in a stepwise fashion. This
proved to be very true in the case of research concerned with inner ear morphology
when Corti (1851) published his first report on inner ear structure. Suddenly, the
interest became very intense, and in the course of a few decades, excellent publications appeared. These publications described the organ of Corti and the vestibular labyrinth and their blood vessels, as well as other related structures in the ear,
and within a short period we saw an enormous upsurge of development in this field.
Personally, I regard Retzius' publications from the 1880s as the highlight of this
period, and he developed a proprietary technique of preparation and illustration
which has hardly been surpassed since then. I shall return to this point later.

---

* This study has been supported by the Swedish Medical Research Council, grant no.
  B81-17x-03156-10

During this period, the possibilities for functional studies were considerably more limited than they are today. The development of neurophysiological technology and audiology, combined with the methods using modern electronics, suddenly increased our knowledge of the function of inner ear sensory cells and their neural pathway. At the same time, it increased the demands on morphologists and pathologists, leading to the beginning of a most rewarding collaboration whereby sometimes morphology presented new information to neurophysiologists and sometimes neurophysiological findings brought up questions for the morphologists.

Even if certain periods were especially important to the development of our knowledge of the inner ear and its normal function, important research of great clinical interest was continuously being carried out by scientists in different parts of the world. Typical examples are the standard work by RÜEDI and FURRER (1947) on acoustic trauma, the work on ototoxic substances by many authors (in the period before ototoxic antibiotics had been developed), and the basic research on otosclerosis and its surgical treatment (by Holmgren, Sourdille, Lempert, Rosen, and others). My personal contact with inner ear research started when Gunnar Holmgren, President of the Karolinska Institute in Stockholm and Professor of Otolaryngology, called me in as a histologist with a certain knowledge of bone histopathology to cooperate with him and F. R. Nager of Zürich in studies on the prevention of closure of labyrinthine fistulas made during otosclerosis operations.

This commenced in 1936 and has lead to continuous work on inner ear morphology since. For my own career, and for international research carried out by other scientists, technological innovations since then have been of extreme importance. This is especially true of the development of electron microscopy in the field of inner ear morphology. During recent years, modern methods of histochemistry, chromatography, radioimmunassay, and freeze fracturing have opened up new possibilities of combining morphology and chemistry with function. Also important have been the new tracer techniques which permit us to follow neural pathways in a most interesting way. In the following review, I shall give a description of some of the many facets of the development of inner ear morphology. It has been stipulated by the editors of this volume that this description should include a great deal about my personal contact with the research carried out from around 1950 onward. This will also mean that I shall to a great extent deal with topics which have had a special personal interest for me.

B. The Organ of Corti

I. Some Notes on the Early Studies on Inner Ear Morphology

In the internationally accepted nomenclature the acoustic portion of the inner ear has its sensory cells in the organum spirale, but the name "organ of Corti" has become so standardized that it seems very difficult to change it and I believe that more than nine papers out of ten still use this name. So fundamental and so important has Corti's 1851 discovery been considered, in spite of the fact that today's description in certain ways differs markedly from that given by Corti. It is, how-

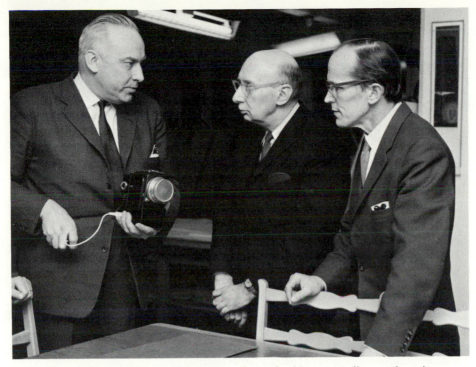

Fig. 1. G. von Békésy (*center*), Nobel prize winner for his outstanding work on inner ear function. Von Békésy and the author are here visiting the Hasselblad photofactory and receiving information concerning a new camera development

ever, interesting to see that the descriptions by SCARPA (1789) of the osseous and membranous labyrinth are considerably more in agreement with our present concept. Many scientists are certainly unaware of the fact that BRESCHET (1833), as well as TODD and BOWMAN (1845) and others, also produced descriptions of the ear, and that the time was in fact right for Corti to make his fundamental observations.

Many important observations based upon the microdissection of the inner ear appeared during the following decades. This period of microdissection culminated in the excellent results of RETZIUS (1884) described in his monumental work *Das Gehörorgan der Wirbelthiere II*. A work of art as well as of science, this is unsurpassed in its accurate descriptions of the inner ear of man and many animals. In discussions with von Békésy (Fig. 1) I found out how he often turned to this almost 100-year-old book for information. It is constantly at hand for my own needs and information, and I know that this is true for many of my colleagues working on inner ear morphology.

Retzius' skill with preparations must have been enormous, and this, combined with his illustrative competence (Fig. 2) has provided us with a reference book which is still of considerable importance. About 20 years ago, I found four of the original plates used by Retzius and engraved by Magnus Petersen. We made five prints of each plate, all of good quality. It is a pity that most of the plates now seem

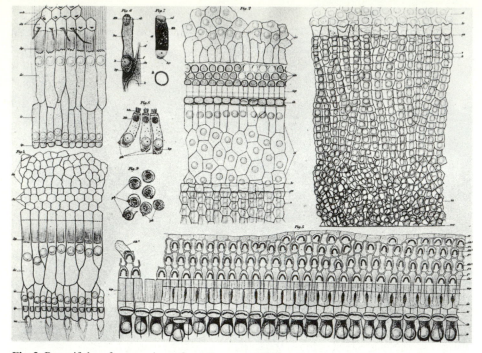

Fig. 2. Beautiful surface specimen from Retzius (1884)

to have been lost but at least some of his original drawings have been found recently.

Retzius' figures are of value in more ways than one. In his microdissections, he used techniques recently developed by several scientists (Engström 1951; Engström et al. 1966; Neubert 1952; Vinnikov and Titova 1961; Spoendlin and Brun 1974; and many others). In fact, some of his figures of the "surface specimen" type from the human cochlea (Fig. 2) compare well with those we can produce today.

It is a pity that decalcification and sectioning techniques came to dominate so much during the following years that it was not until 70–80 years later that the surface specimen technique returned to popularity as a worldwide method of cochlear investigation. As a means of understanding the supporting structures, I regard Held's (1926) paper as the most important. When interpreting scanning electron micrographs, we often return to Held's and Retzius' descriptions, which we deem very correct and informative.

The period of decalcification coincided very much with the period when histopathology entered the realm of inner ear research. In 1936 I was invited, as mentioned above, by Gunnar Holmgren and F. R. Nager (Fig. 3) to take part in a research project on otosclerosis and the prevention of healing of labyrinthine fistulas made by surgery. During the period 1936–1941, I and others in search of otosclerotic foci made hundreds of thousands of sections of human temporal bones. At the same time, many monkeys were operated upon in the attempt to find a method

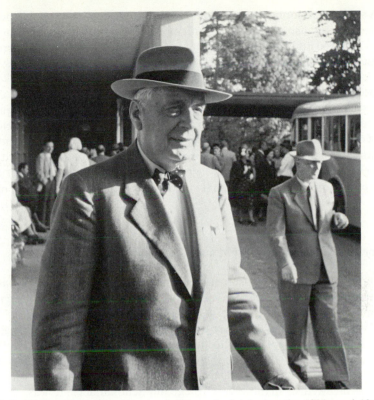

Fig. 3. F. R. Nager, leading European otolaryngologist during the 1930s and 1940s, with whom the author worked on his thesis in 1937–1938

of improving hearing. It can today be stated that the pioneer work done by Holmgren, Lempert, Sourdille, Rosen, Schuknecht, House, and many others produced a most interesting and successful solution to a severe clinical illness.

This clinical research provided inner ear studies with new tools. The new otomicroscope afforded excellent possibilities of observing middle ear structures, and even of looking into the inner ear. Surgeons could suddenly see the maculae of the saccule and utricule during operations, and in some operations of a destructive type, even the inside of the cochlea became visible to the surgeon. This contributed without doubt to a further extension of inner ear observations and microdissection under good illumination, which in turn steered the interest of morphologists toward a detailed microdissection of both cochlear and vestibular portions of the inner ear. A natural consequence was to combine microdissection with embedding and sectioning in unorthodox planes. Within a short period it became clear that transmodiolar sections through the cochlea were perhaps not the only way of visualizing the inner ear. By direct observation of the organ of Corti, prepared more or less as a whole unit, an excellent view of sensory cells under normal and pathological conditions could be obtained. This could also be done by sectioning in unconventional directions. I published some such pictures in 1951 (ENGSTRÖM

1951). A similar development came from NEUBERT (1952), who has published many interesting papers using a similar kind of surface preparation. A number of scientists followed his lines and contributed with many publications of interest. The technique of micropreparation and of surface specimens developed considerably when electron microscopy came into use. It then became necessary to make extensive microdissections, and it soon became very evident that the organ of Corti could be studied in its entirety by appropriate preparation. Several techniques were developed, and I devoted much work to a basic publication in this field (ENGSTRÖM et al. 1966). The tendency to observe the inner ear sensory epithelia by microdissection and more or less unsectioned specimens has now become standard. Excellent achievements can be mentioned, such as those of SPOENDLIN and BRUN (1974) or the preparations using the Nomarski technique. I shall return to these methods later.

II. Inner Ear Studies Using Light and Electron Microscopy

It was stated above that microsurgery and microdissection of the cochlea clearly demonstrated possibilities of studying the organ of Corti in a way different from the commonly used decalcification – mid-modiolar sectioning.

In 1950, I was forced to take over the professorship in histology during the vacation of the ordinary professor, Gösta Häggqvist. I had by then obtained much experience of middle ear surgery and stereoscopic observations of middle and inner ear structures. At this time the Department of Histology received an electron microscope of Swedish manufacture (Siegbahn-Schönander). It was, of course, most intriguing to try to study the inner ear, taste buds, and olfactory region to see if we could add new information to our knowledge. Only those who worked with the early instruments know the problems encountered when waiting for evacuation for several hours, a wait that forced us to place a bed and an alarm clock in the microscope room. Four young students helped me to form a group. Three of these have become excellent electron microscopists: Jan Wersäll in otolaryngology; Ove Nilsson in anatomy, with special reference to fertility studies; and Gunnar Bloom in studies primarily connected with blood cells. In a superb camaraderie many of the problems were overcome. It should also be stated that we had good help at this time from F. S. Sjöstrand from the Department of Anatomy, and when he got his first electron microscope, an RCA 2a, we obtained access to that instrument.

Our trials with the organ of Corti were not too successful at the beginning, and studies on tracheal cilia and the olfactory region came in when the problems seemed too difficult to overcome. The first electron microscopic picture of the ear was of a statoconium, however, and was presented at the International Audiology Meeting in Stockholm in 1950.

At this time we used steel knives and a primitive method of thermoexpansion for sectioning, and many hours were lost before Kerstin Björkroth, then Wersäll's fiancée, one day succeeded in getting some sections through the hairs of a cochlear hair cell. When the ice was broken, development was rapid, and in the years 1951–1953 we were able to present several papers on the structure of the organ of Corti.

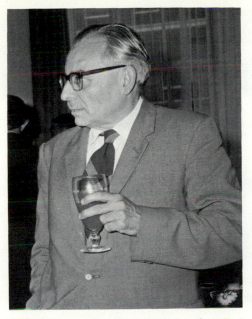

Fig. 4. Otto Lowenstein, physiologist with wide knowledge of vestibular function. His interest in morphology and function has stimulated many scientists. He received the Bárány gold medal in 1973

In the studies on the inner ear, Wersäll and I worked closely together, and the outcome can certainly be regarded as the result of excellent teamwork.

In 1953 I made the first international presentation of the electron microscopy of the inner ear at the international meeting in Amsterdam (ENGSTRÖM et al. 1953). It was with a certain amount of excitement that I entered the lecture room. At the door stood C. S. Hallpike and Simpson Hall, greeting me with the words: "Now we are going to get some real meat." It was nice to hear Hallpike's comment at the exit: "It was real meat." We became great friends in the future, and cooperated well during my time as President of the Bárány Society, the international society for vestibular research.

The great possibilities of electron microscopy soon became evident, and several approaches were made. The new openings for research were evidently also appreciated internationally, and visitors from abroad began to come. It is a pleasure to remember that Heinrich Spoendlin from Zürich was one of the first. His first paper using electron microscopy was written together with myself and Sjöstrand in Stockholm. His considerable importance with regard to our knowledge of the ultrastructure of the inner ear will be dealt with later. Today he is one of the leading scientists in this field.

In 1956 Wersäll finished his doctoral thesis on the vestibular sensory epithelia, a paper which today forms the basis for many investigations on the inner ear (WERSÄLL 1956). When I moved to Gothenburg in 1955, Wersäll soon formed his own group, and the addition of Flock, Lundqvist, Bagger-Sjöbäck, Anniko, and others to that group has proved to be of very great importance.

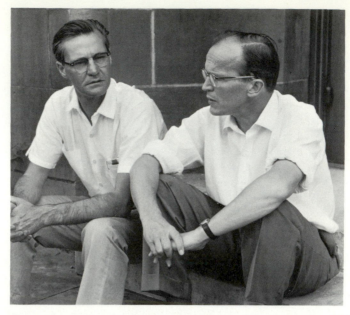

Fig. 5. Cesar Fernandez (*left*) and the author on the steps of the University of Chicago during a pause in work on the distribution of the olivocochlear efferents. Fernandez has also received the Bárány medal (1978)

Shortly after Wersäll's publication in 1956, C. Smith from St. Louis, working with Davis and others, published her paper on the vestibular maculae. She later spent a year with Sjöstrand in Stockholm, and she has in many interesting later publications enriched our knowledge of the inner ear (SMITH 1966, 1968; SMITH and RASMUSSEN 1963 a, b, 1965; SMITH and SJÖSTRAND 1961). One subsequent visitor among many others was Robert Kimura from Chicago and Boston. His knowledge of histological techniques for light microscopy was well known, and his present capacity as a specialist in the ultrastructure of the inner ear is extremely well documented (KIMURA 1966, 1975). At the beginning of the 1950s there were only a few research workers using the electron microscope. The spread of the technique was very rapid, however, and all over the world new developments appeared. The new morphological possibilities became of interest to neurophysiologists and important stimulation came from scientists like O. Lowenstein (Fig. 4), H. Davis, N. Kiang, C. Fernandez (Fig. 5), and L. Goldberg.

The preparation techniques in electron microscopy differed, but as already described, scientists also began to view the inner ear sensory epithelia in a different way from when using the light microscope. Phase contrast microscopy became at this time a much appreciated technique. Some of its possibilities were summarized by myself and my colleagues ENGSTRÖM et al. (1966) in our monograph *Structural Pattern of the Organ of Corti*. Many of the inherent problems were being studied at the same time by other scientists like VINNIKOV and TITOVA (1961) and many later authors in Russia. My contact with Vinnikov has been kept open only as a pen friend for more than 20 years, but the exchange of information has been considerable. It is not possible to name all the visitors who have played an important role in the development of inner ear research. Imre Friedmann of "Gray's Inn Road" (part of the Royal National Ear, Nose and Throat Hospital) in London understood the possibilities of electron microscopy at an early stage (FRIEDMANN and BIRD 1967; FRIEDMANN 1968, 1969), and I received repeated invitations to lecture in London. His own contributions have been considerable and his use of the "otocyst" as an experimental tool has been of special importance. Today, van de Water, another propagator of the otocyst, is a frequent and welcome guest in Stockholm, where his techniques are now in routine use.

Transmission electron microscopy has in a few decades spread all over the world, and a kind of fraternity has developed in inner ear research as a result of this technique. We have had the opportunity of cooperating with many scientists from all parts of the world, and many Japanese scientists have been our guests. A very welcome guest researcher was K. Watanuki, who spent a year in Uppsala doing research and teaching us his technique of using silver nitrate for the visualization of the pattern of sensory cells in the inner ear (WATANUKI et al. 1970). One of the micrographs he made during his stay in Sweden is to be seen in Fig. 9 b.

An important step came in 1957, when Humberto Fernandez-Morán arranged a meeting in Caracas. At this meeting many new concepts concerning sensory organs and their innervation were presented by people such as Kuffler, Bullock, Autrum, Jung, and Porter. At this time I had already formed my ideas about the double innervation of the inner ear sensory epithelia, but these were first met by much opposition because of the size of the very large efferent endings in the organ of Corti. Kuffler's ideas were especially important, as were later discussions with Eccles at various meetings.

The visit to Fernandez-Morán's lab was important to our work in yet another way. We had earlier used metal knives. When leaving Caracas I received a precious gift of two diamond knives from Morán. They opened up a new path for sectioning in our laboratory and were most welcome. A good diamond knife has since then always been a very highly valued aid.

Another meeting of importance was held in the stone house at the National Institutes of Health in Bethesda (1959). Here I met Harlow W. Ades (Fig. 6), who was especially interested in hearing and hearing loss.

Ades and I and our associates formed a Swedish-American team which collaborated until the sudden death of Ades a few years ago. This collaboration started a series of experiments on the damaging effect of noise, which were followed or paralleled by numerous similar studies on a worldwide basis. Two collaborators especially, who have contributed in an important way to the structural research of the inner ear, should be mentioned. Bredberg, who is now doing excellent scanning electron microscopy, wrote his thesis on the human cochlea (BREDBERG 1968) and Lindeman wrote his thesis on the vestibular labyrinth (LINDEMAN 1969). Both these papers have formed important foundations for further research. Bredberg in particular has over the years published many papers about cochlear structure (BREDBERG 1977; BREDBERG et al. 1972; BREDBERG and HUNTER-DUVAR 1975).

In autumn 1968, a new type of microscope was placed at the disposal of O. Nilsson, my former associate at the Department of Anatomy in Uppsala. This scanning electron microscope was soon employed by myself and my daughter Berit

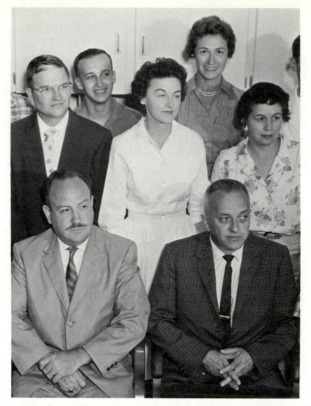

Fig. 6. For many years the author cooperated with members of this group from US Naval Air Station Pensacola, Florida. The group was formed by Harlow Ades (*front right*). *At his right side,* Gilbert Tolhurst; *behind Tolhurst,* Bobby Camp; and *in the background* Claire Ades. When Ades moved to University of Illinois, Urbana, and later to the University of Western Florida, the work continued there

Engström, who has for more than ten years been my highly valued collaborator and who has developed considerable skill in electron microscopic research. Our first scanning electron microscopic (SEM) presentation came at the beginning of 1969, and when we gave our third presentation, Jan Wersäll came back from the United States and reported that he had seen similar studies carried out by David Lim of Columbus, Ohio. I do not know who came first with SEM studies; at all events the question is of small importance. Lim and I have become great friends, and it has been enormously interesting to see how the SEM technique has rapidly conquered the world. Its beautiful pictures and three-dimensional quality are very impressive and, owing to the cytoarchitecture of the inner ear, especially the cochlea, these cells are extremely well suited to SEM observations. It is impossible to mention all the excellent publications now in print. The Uppsala group had as a visitor for two years Ivan HUNTER-DUVAR (1978), now one of the leading SEM specialists in inner ear research. Interesting studies of the statoconia have been made by a group lead by MURIEL ROSS (to be published) in Ann Arbor, with which I am now collaborating.

In a very short space of time a further technique has become of importance in inner ear research, and that is the freeze fracture technique. Important contact with this technique came through JAHNKE (1975) and through Iurato (IURATO et al. 1976), both well-known research workers in inner ear morphology. Iurato belongs to the pioneers in the field of ultrastructural inner ear research. In a series of publications, he has followed and contributed to all facets of modern inner ear research: light microscopy, transmission electron microscopy, scanning electron microscopy, histochemistry in electron microscopy, micro-X-ray technique, and freeze fracturing (IURATO 1962, 1967, 1974; IURATO et al. 1976). I shall return to some of these studies later.

One of the visitors to my group in the early 1960s was Joe E. Hawkins Jr., who spent more than two years in Sweden. His work on ototoxic antibiotics was well known, and he and members of his group have continued this work; for several years now, Hawkins, Lars Johnsson, and other members of the Kresge group in Ann Arbor have provided inner ear morphology with excellent contributions. Their information concerning the human ear, where they have worked with methods similar to that used by Bredberg and mentioned earlier, is very impressive. They have at present a very representative material of human ears (cf. JOHNSSON and HAWKINS 1976).

In inner ear morphology the interrelation of different anatomical structures is very important to the understanding of the physiology of the cochlea. The special composition of the endolymph as compared to the perilymph and the risk of mixing the two fluids during microscopy, thus disturbing the interrelation of the structures, has bothered many research workers. Several scientists have tried to overcome this problem by using artificial endolymph. This has been very difficult, but recent studies by KRONESTER-FREI (1977) and by LIM (1980) have perhaps come closest to a solution of the problem.

In recent years the close interaction between physiologists and morphologists has been very fruitful. A typical example is Nelson-Kiang and his collaborators, who combine high-quality neurophysiology with important morphological studies. New questions have been brought up and new techniques have been developed. Other typical examples are the numerous studies where physiological testing and morphology have been used in research on cochlear damage. This is true of studies on ototoxic antibiotics and on noise damage and the research on cochlear implants. The research on such implants in relation to inner ear structures is of great interest. Another important question is what kind of cochlear damage can benefit from cochlear implants. Also in this field, Spoendlin has made important contributions. From a clinical point of view, both the California groups (House group, San Francisco group) and the French group (Pialoux and Chouard), as well as other scientists, have brought up many new questions to be solved in cooperation with morphologists.

It has during recent years been most interesting to see how clinical medicine needs morphological cooperation for the solution of surgical problems. This has been especially true in the research on Meniere's disease. Light microscopy, electron microscopy, and freeze fracturing are now being used in studies of the function of the cochlear and vestibular aqueducts (Stahle's group, RASK-ANDERSEN 1979). In this work X-ray anatomy has also attained great interest (Wilbrand).

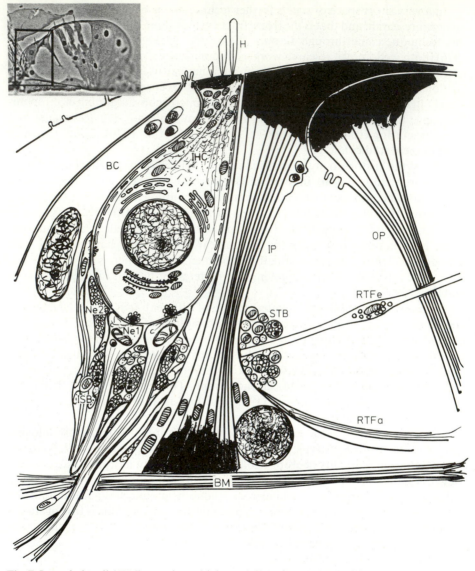

Fig. 7. Inner hair cell (*IHC*) together with inner (*IP*) and outer (*OP*) pillars. On the modiolar side of the inner hair cell is a border cell. *H*, hairs; *ISB*, inner spiral bundle with afferent (*Ne 1*) and efferent (*Ne 2*) nerve endings; *STB*, spiral tunnel bundle; *RTFa*, radiating tunnel fibers, mainly efferent; *RTFb*, mainly afferent fibers

III. Present Status of Our Knowledge Concerning the Organ of Corti

The sensory cells in the organ of Corti, the inner and outer hair cells, are today quite well known. Their form can best be seen in Figs. 7–9. They are surrounded by a complicated system of supporting and/or nutritive cells (Figs. 8, 9, 12). The organ of Corti rests on the basilar membrane, which consists of two portions: pars

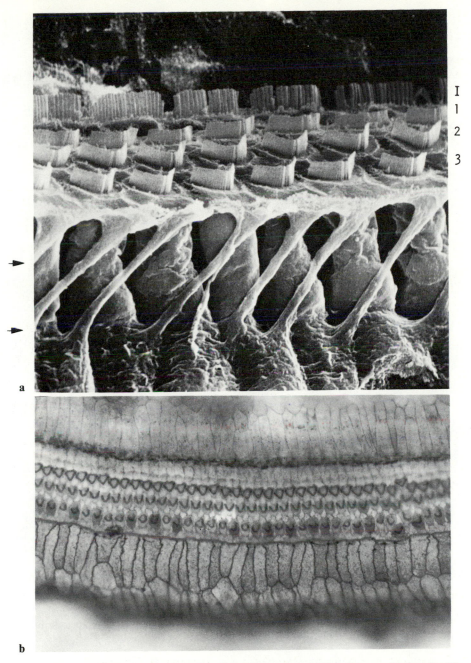

I
1
2
3

a

b

Fig. 8. a Scanning electron micrographs of inner (*I*) and outer (*1,2,3*) rows of hair cells. The phalangeal processes of the Deiters' cells are very well visible (*arrows*). **b** Silver-stained specimen from a guinea pig ear made by K. Watanuki during his work in Uppsala. With this technique excellent survey pictures can often be made

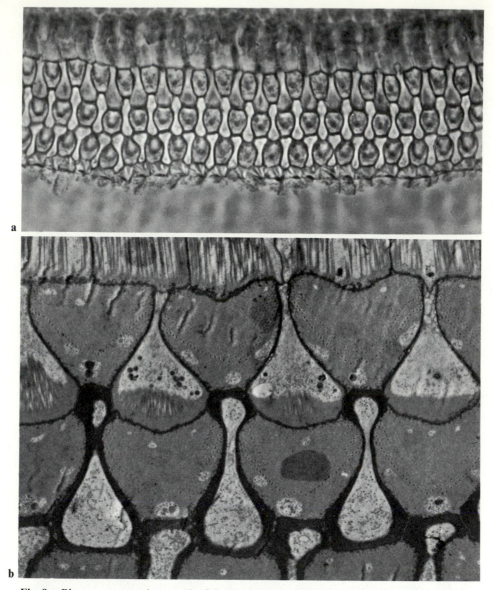

Fig. 9. a Phase contrast micrograph of the organ of Corti from a guinea pig. A typical surface specimen. **b** Corresponding area from the organ of Corti of a rabbit. Section through the cuticular plate. The rootlets of hairs are visible. The angle (just above 90°) indicates that the specimen is from the lower middle portion of the organ of Corti

tecta and pars pectinata. Over the hairs of the sensory cells there is a gelatinous, fibrous tectorial membrane, which covers the organ of Corti. Both inner and outer hair cells are regarded as highly specialized receptors for sound waves. For a very long time the more numerous outer hair cells were regarded as the most important ones. In a series of fundamental papers (cf. SPOENDLIN 1979), Spoendlin demon-

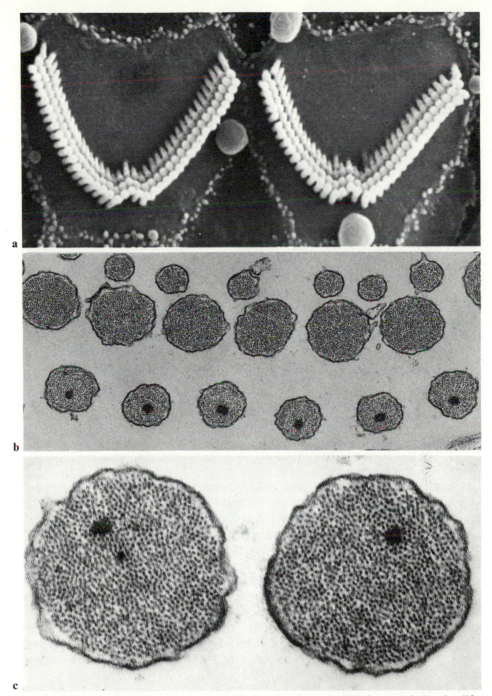

Fig. 10. a Hairs on outer hair cell from rabbit showing the typical W shape and also the different lengths in the rows of hairs. **b** Cross-sectioned hairs on outer hair cell, squirrel monkey. **c** High magnification of inner hair cell hairs, squirrel monkey. Observe the darker core, which is much more variable on inner than on outer hair cells.

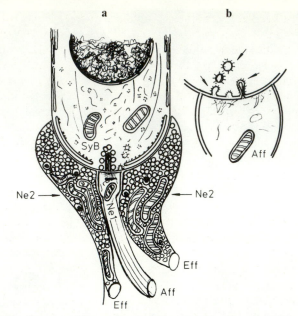

Fig. 11. a Schematic diagram of base of outer hair cell with afferent (*Aff*) and efferent (*Eff*) endings. Synaptic bar is found close to the afferent ending. **b** Invaginations, recycling? Often seen in synaptic areas

strated that only a very few inward-leading afferent nerve fibers emanate from the outer hair cells, while 90%–95% come from the inner hair cells. His observations are today generally accepted, and this has resulted in an enormously increased interest in studies of the inner hair cells.

The cochlea is innervated by at least three different neural components: afferent fibers with their ganglion cells in the spiral ganglion, and efferent fibers from the contralateral and ipsilateral superior olive complexes. The course of these fibers was well described by Rasmussen (1946), and they have recently been studied in great detail by several authors using different tracers (cf. Warr 1978, 1979; Smith and Rasmussen 1963a, b, 1965; Rossi and Cortesina 1962; Rossi et al. 1964). There is a third, adrenergic, innervation through the truncus cervicalis and the stellate ganglion. The total number of nerve fibers in the cochlear nerve varies in different species: 35,000–50,000 fibers have been found in man, 50,000–60,000 in the cat, and about 250,000 in the whale. These fibers innervate approximately 3,000 inner and 12,000 outer hair cells (more in the whale).

The sensory cells are all built according to a common principle. They are oblong cells with a free upper surface provided with sensory hairs (Figs. 7–9, 11) and a lower rounded basal end where the cell forms synaptic contacts with the terminations of the afferent and efferent nerve fibers described above. The cells are partly surrounded by supporting cells, but the "vertical" sides of the cells, especially at the outer hair cells, border onto the fluid inside the organ of Corti. This fluid has been much discussed since I (Engström 1960) presented evidence that the fluid could be distinct from peri- or endolymph. I felt that it should be regarded as a separate fluid, which I called "cortilymph," until evidence had been brought forward that it was perilymph, which was the concept of many authors (cf. PETERSON et al. 1978). In several subsequent publications evidence was presented indicating that the interior of the organ of Corti contained perilymph (VOSTEEN 1970). Then still newer evidence contradicted the results of Vosteen. Thus ANGELBORG (1974) carried out experiments similar to those of the Vosteen group but found evidence that there was a fluid barrier between the perilymph and the cortilymph. Recent experiments indicate a difference in chemical composition between cortilymph and peri- or endolymph (RYAN et al. 1980), but the true nature of the fluid is not yet clarified. Although for some time I thought the question had been settled, and that the interior of the organ of Corti contained perilymph, I have now returned to my earlier opinion that cortilymph is a very good descriptive name for the fluid inside the organ of Corti. This now seems to be the opinion of many other authors. The peri- and endolymph are less contradictory and their chemical compositions are well known, the endolymph having a much higher potassium content than the perilymph (cf. PETERSON et al. 1978).

Typical of the cochlear hair cells is that the main agglomeration of nerve endings is at the basal portion of the sensory cells, but this is especially pronounced in the case of the outer hair cells. However, even there some, mainly efferent, endings can be found along the sides of the supranuclear portion (BREDBERG 1977). This is quite commonly seen at the inner hair cells, where nerve endings can often be found along the modiolar side of the cells. According to LIBERMAN (1980a, b) these endings belong to a special group of afferent fibers. We have frequently seen efferent fibers rather high up on the modiolar side. In the vestibular sensory epithelia it is normal to find nerve endings high up, even close to the surface along type II cells; type I cells are surrounded by nerve chalices up to the reticular membrane.

1. The Sensory Hairs and Their Relation to the Tectorial Membrane

a) The Hairs

All cochlear sensory cells are provided with hairs (stereocilia) sticking up from the cuticular plate. During embryonic life there is also a kinocilium, which usually disappears or remains as a basal body in a cuticula-free zone (Figs. 7 and 9). The arrangement of the hairs on inner and outer hair cells is very different. On the inner hair cells they form two or three almost straight rows, whereas on the outer ones they form three to five or even six rows, depending on the species. They are arranged in the form of a W or M (Fig. 10), and the angle between the hair rows at the surface varies from 60° to 120° wide at the base, getting smaller higher up (ENGSTRÖM and ENGSTRÖM 1979). The hairs differ considerably in length, both between the individual rows of hairs on each cell and between different parts of the cochlea. Most pronounced are the differences in length on the inner hair cells, as can be seen in Fig. 7. It is interesting to see that the hairs on these cells also differ from the hairs in the second and third rows, which are flattened at their tips (Fig. 7). The length of the hairs also differs between the different cochlear coils. LIM (1980)

has recently made careful measurements in the chinchilla and found a regular increase from the basal coil ($\sim$2–3 μm) over the middle coil ($\sim$2–4 μm) to the apex
($\sim$3–6 μm). The hairs in the third row of cells at the top were the tallest. The hairs
on inner hair cells also vary, increasing in length from the base (2.5 μm) to the top
(4.5 μm). The hairs on the inner hair cells are considerably thicker than the hairs
on the outer ones. It has been shown that remains of hairs can be found in the
cuticular plate (Engström 1967), indicating that a greater number of hairs existed
during embryonic development. The number of hairs varies considerably in the different species (60–120).

The ultrastructure of each hair has been carefully studied by many authors
(Engström et al. 1962; Engström and Ades 1973; Kimura 1966; Engström and
Engström 1979; Flock 1965; Flock and Cheung 1977; Flock et al. 1977; Hudspeth and Jacobs 1979; Lim 1980; and others). Each hair is bordered on the outside
by a plasma membrane provided with a fine "fuzz" at the free surface. In the interior there are large numbers of microfilaments (up to 300 on outer and up to 800
on inner hair cells). According to Flock and Cheung (1977), these fibrils contain
actin. In the lower portion of the hairs a condensation of fibrils forms a tube-like
core, which continues into the hair root and is anchored in the cuticle. Whether
these rootlets can penetrate the cuticle and reach into the infracuticular region is
not yet clear. The content and distribution of actin in inner ear hair cells is today
a problem of central interest in inner ear research (Itoh 1982; Hirokawa and Tilney 1982; Engström et al. 1983).

b) The Relationship with the Tectorial Membrane

The relationship between the sensory hairs and the tectorial membrane has been
a question of extreme physiological interest, and a large number of papers deal
with this question. As it is generally believed that stereocilia mediate transduction
in vertebrate hair cells, the relation to the superimposed tectorial membrane has
been much debated. Several papers discuss this problem in detail (Kronester-Frei
1977; Engström and Engström 1979; Hudspeth and Jacobs 1979; Lim 1980;
Shotwell et al. 1981). According to most authors, the hairs on the outer hair cells
are directly in contact with the tectorial membrane (Tanaka and Smith 1975),
making imprints which can remain long after the hair cells have degenerated (Lim
1972, 1980; Hoshino 1974, 1976; Hunter-Duvar and Mount 1978). The very interesting question of how the hairs on the inner hair cells make contact with the
tectorial membrane is not definitely solved. Kronester-Frei (1977) and Lim (1980)
have tried to resolve the problem by investigating it in a milieu as closely resembling endolymph as possible. From these investigations, transmission electron microscopy carried out by my daughter and myself (Engström and Engström 1979)
and scanning electron microscopy by Hoshino (1976), there are certain indications
that inner hair cells also make contact via their hairs with the tectorial membrane,
at least in certain parts of the cochlea. Lim (1980) summarizes his results as follows:
"The inner hair cell cilia do not have the same firm attachment to the tectorial
membrane as outer hair cell cilia. This suggests that the modes of mechanical coupling between the tectorial membrane and the inner and outer hair cell cilia are dif-

ferent." This is a Solomonic conclusion on a most interesting but difficult problem. It is rewarding to follow the many controversial opinions in a field where authors using new methodology have tried to produce a correct solution. When DE VRIES and BLEEKER (1949) used deep-frozen and fractured material, they were certain they had solved the problem. BORGHESAN (1954) was even more convinced that his solution was correct, and still we are not completely certain, as can be seen from the quotation from Lim's paper.

The relation of the tectorial membrane to the whole organ of Corti is of great significance for the understanding of cochlear mechanics, and much interest has been devoted to the marginal band and marginal network, and also to the inner sulcus. The gelatinous material in the tectorial membrane has a pronounced tendency to shrink, and this considerably increases the possibility of artifacts. The marginal connection between the tectorial membrane and the organ of Corti was described by DE VRIES and BLEEKER (1949) and by NEUBERT (1952), among many others. It was stated that a fine network (*Randfasernetz*) connected the Hensen cells and the membrane. KIMURA (1966) and LIM (1972), among others, believe that the membrane is connected to the phalanges of the outermost row of the Deiters' cells.

LIM (1980) has found differences between the base and the top of the cochlea. At the base, imprints of outer hair cilia have been observed in the marginal net or band. At the top, the marginal net forms a real meshwork attached to the phalanges of the third row of Deiters' cells. In my opinion, it also forms a contact with the first row of the Hensen cells, but due to the artifact problem it is difficult to be absolutely certain. There is also evidence that there are differences between early and later life in certain animals (LINDEMAN et al. 1971; LIM 1972). In RETZIUS' (1884) paper, as in LIM's (1977) paper, the modifications of the tectorial membrane have already been well described.

LIM (1980) has devoted much interest to the stripe of Hensen. The question is whether this stripe makes contact with the organ of Corti in such a way that the inner sulcus is sealed off like a closed tube-like canal (KRONESTER-FREI 1977) and this is of great interest from the point of view that this canal could contain a separate fluid, the fourth lymph of RAUCH (1964).

2. The Sensory Cells

In Sect. B.III.1 I dealt separately with the hairs as a kind of supracellular structure; here I shall give a short description of the hair cell, from the cuticular plate down to the synaptic regions. In Fig. 7 the general form and structure of the inner hair cell can be seen. The same main principles are usually found in the structural organization of most animal species, and this is especially true for mammals. Individual variations can often be seen, however. This is, for instance, common in the distribution of glycogen in the outer hair cells, and in some animals other variations can be seen. Thus most outer hair cells are, as can be seen in Fig. 11, rich in mitochondria at the basal end. However, in the rabbit, the basal portion is practically void of mitochondria, as pointed out by several authors (OMATA and SCHÄTZLE 1980). As the mitochondria and glycogen are both important for energy turnover, this indicates that different functional modes must be present.

a) The Inner Hair Cells

The inner hair cells form one row on the modiolar side of the tunnel of Corti and the inner pillar cells. They are oblong with a rather small oval upper surface, a bent neck, and a more ovoid cell body around the nucleus. The cuticular plate is rather thick, and in many species a basal body, the remains of a kinocilium, is found in a cuticula-free region. From this basal body, or sometimes from a centriole found below the basal body, large numbers of microtubules (Fig. 8) fan out into the interior of the cells. We usually distinguish an infracuticular, a supranuclear, and an infranuclear portion. In the infracuticular region endoplasmic reticulum of the smooth type is very abundant, and many rounded mitochondria are normally seen. There are also a few multivesiculated bodies, a few lysosomes, and sometimes lipofuscin granules. In the supranuclear portion we find a well-developed Golgi complex, often forming an almost ring-shaped structure. The nucleus is rounded with a fine chromatin network.

In the infranuclear portion there are often found, at least in some species, a few or sometimes up to seven or eight cisternae of the rough endoplasmic reticulum type. In direct relation to these membranes, several rounded mitochondria with densely packed cristae are common. In light microscopy this area below the nucleus can be seen as an almost ball-shaped formation. In our studies of cochleas modified by noise exposure or ototoxic antibiotics, we have carefully studied this region, and there is reason to believe that it varies in relation to stimulation or damage. In this region and around the nucleus, the endoplasmic reticulum, which was so abundant in the infracuticular region, is less prominent. In the synaptic region it becomes well developed again. This is especially evident in specimens fixed with potassium bichromate. The synaptic region will be discussed in greater detail in relation to the innervation of the organ of Corti.

b) The Outer Hair Cells

These outer hair cells (Figs. 8–11) are very smooth cylindrical, tube-like cells with a flattened upper cuticular surface and a rounded basal end. The cuticle greatly varies in thickness, and in several mammals cuticular extensions reach far down (>15 μm) into the infracuticular region. In some animals, e.g., some species of bird, the cuticular plate has a very thick inverted cone-shaped form. In certain mammals the cuticular prolongations can be very irregular. This makes it difficult to tell whether the rootlets of the hairs sometimes penetrate the cuticle completely, or whether they are surrounded by a thin layer of cuticular matter. The cuticle has a very fine fibrillar structure and occasionally, especially in old animals, laminated structures can be seen, similar to those discussed by myself and my co-workers (Engström et al. 1977) in vestibular cells. Flock (1980) has provided evidence that the fine fibrillar structures forming the cuticle may contain actin in special arrangements. A laminated system of membranes can occasionally be seen in the cuticle.

A basal body, situated in a cuticula-free zone is common in many animals. From the basal body, cross-striated roots and thin tube-like threads reach into the interior of the cells, the tubular ones all the way down to the lower end. They seem less prominent or frequent than in the inner hair cells. They were first pointed out by von Ilberg (1969), and my co-workers and I have since described them in several publications. They are especially evident in the type I cells in the vestibular end organ. These tube-like structures reach all the way from the surface down to the vicinity of the synaptic regions. We have not seen any direct relationship to the synaptic structures but they form a very interesting part of inner ear sensory cells.

In the infracuticular region, and especially in the region below the basal body, there is an accumulation of mitochondria, lysosomes, and lipofuscin, which in old animals and especially in the old, noise-exposed guinea pigs in our studies is quite considerable. Thus we have in one cell seen an accumulation or formation 3×5 μm, almost filling the whole infracuticular portion. The nucleus of the outer hair cell is situated in the basal portion of the cell, leaving a cylindrical column for the infracuticular and supranuclear portions. At the border between these two portions, a series of discontinuous lamellae can be seen. In some animals they form several layers of irregular form, and in many of our specimens they formed round, ball-shaped bodies, called "Hensen bodies" in the early literature. We have named them "lamellar bodies," since this is a more descriptive name. Around these bodies an agglomeration of glycogen particles and mitochondria is often seen. The lamellae show a striking resemblance to the discontinuous lamellae found along the vertical sides of the outer hair cells. The arrangement of glycogen, mitochondria, and membranes indicates a center of high energy turnover, but their function is not known. From experiments with noise exposure we have found reason to believe that they become modified by noise, sometimes increasing in number or moving lower down into the cell. Thus they can occasionally be found close to the nucleus, and in a few cases we have seen lamellae of this type even below the nucleus. The discontinuous membranes inside the long sides of the cells vary in number, as stated previously. In the squirrel and rhesus monkeys, they form a single layer; in the guinea pig up to seven or eight layers can be found. These membranes have a denser outer layer and a less opaque center. Some authors have called them "cisternae." I am of the opinion that there is no hollow center but rather some kind of lighter protoplasm bordered by a denser coating, and I therefore believe "membrane" to be a more appropriate term. On the inside of the membranous sheath very long mitochondria can be seen. Agglomeration of glycogen particles (in fixed specimens) and of mitochondria at these membranes indicates some kind of special activity.

The infranuclear region is especially interesting. This is the region of synaptic contact with afferent and efferent nerve endings. It is a region rich in mitochondria. These mitochondria were observed by light microscopy by Retzius, and the agglomeration is often called the "Retzius' body." When electron microscopy was able to separate the details of the Retzius' body, it became apparent that this must be a center of high enzymatic activity. The interesting fact is that it is possible that these mitochondria belong to two different populations. In some guinea pigs, we have observed smaller mitochondria close to the synaptic region and larger mitochondria closer to the nucleus. This double population is also very evident in some other authors' publications (e.g., C. SMITH 1968; Figs. 9, 10, and 18). As far as I know, this has not been widely discussed, but it should be of great importance in those cases where we are looking for structural modifications caused by noise exposure or ototoxic antibiotics. Whereas it is true that there are two mitochondrial populations in certain animals, the squirrel and rhesus monkeys seem to have only one type, and the rabbit has almost no mitochondria at all. This speaks in favor of the fact that the activity of the structures in the infranuclear region can vary greatly between different species.

3. The Innervation of the Sensory Cells

On no other part of the organ of Corti has so much new information been produced as on cochlear innervation. Electron microscopy has generated completely new information, and has in many ways altered the direction of neurophysiological experiments.

It has long been known that the cochlea is innervated by both centrifugal and centripetal nerve fibers. The afferent system has been known for 100 years. "Descending connections of the central auditory system" as the efferent fibers were first described by RASMUSSEN (1946, 1960) were carefully investigated by him, and his descriptions form the basis for further studies. Many scientists from different countries have tried to elucidate the peripheral terminations of the nerve fibers (cf. IURATO et al. 1971). Several techniques have now contributed to a description of the innervation pattern of the organ of Corti. In 1958 I was able to use electron microscopy to distinguish two distinct systems of nerve endings at cochlear and vestibular sensory cells (ENGSTRÖM 1958). WERSÄLL (1956) had already observed nerve endings in vestibular sensory epithelia containing "densely packed granules of the same type, with diameters of 200–400 Å, embedded in a sparse intermediate substance, and occasional mitochondria or none at all." Wersäll did not describe these endings as efferent, but he understood their importance and he even says: "The presence of such efferent fibers in the epithelium does not seem to be altogether improbable." He writes in his discussion that "they may well be of fundamental importance to the conduction of impulses."

According to this concept, which is now generally accepted, inner ear sensory cells have a double innervation varying in different types of cell and in different regions. Afferent endings are found at the inner hair cells and so are efferent endings, but efferent endings also make contact with afferent fibers below the sensory cell. The junctions between nerve endings and sensory cells, or synaptic regions, are found not only at the bases of inner hair cells but also along the side surfaces of the cell and often higher up on the modiolar side. Several of these highly localized endings seem to be efferent. At the outer hair cells, the majority of synapses are found at the basal ends and the volume of neural matter forming the endings is very interesting. Thus the efferent endings at the basal end are much larger than the afferent ones. There follows a gradual reduction in the volume of efferent endings higher up in the cochlea, while the afferent endings seem to maintain a more or less standard size all the way (ENGSTRÖM et al. 1966; Figs. 75–85). A subsynaptic cistern seems to be found almost invariably when an efferent ending contacts a sensory cell, but it is almost always absent when an efferent ending contacts an afferent fiber. Why this is so is not known. For a long time it was accepted that the outer hair cells are the more sensitive and more abundantly innervated ones, and that a smaller number of nerve fibers come from inner hair cells. It therefore proved a great sensation when Spoendlin in a series of publications was able to demonstrate that this concept was wrong and that only 5%–10% of the afferent nerve fibers emanate from endings at the outer hair cells, where each fiber innervates approximately ten sensory cells. These cells are also innervated by other fibers. In a series of experiments, he was able to show that 90%–95% of afferent fibers came from the inner hair cells. His observations were first doubted but have now been accepted, and they have caused a great increase in interest in inner hair cell function. In my opinion, it is one of the most interesting observations concerning the inner ear made by morphological methods (cf. B. ENGSTRÖM, 1983).

In both morphological and physiological studies, the interaction between inner and outer hair cells is of primary importance, and many studies have been made. Contacts between afferent and efferent fibers have been observed, as well as contacts between afferent and efferent fibers in different regions, but it has been difficult to find distinct synapses, and in several of our publications my co-workers and I have been uncertain whether we have synaptic contacts or some kind of nerve–nerve junction of desmosome-like, nonsynaptic nature. We have studied our material very carefully but we have not been as successful as members of Kiang's group; LIBERMAN (1980a, b), for example, in some recent papers has followed the radial afferent and efferent fibers in serial sections. In his opinion the inner hair cells are innervated by unbranched fibers, each forming a single synapse with one inner hair cell. He has found that there are among the radial fibers one mitochondrion-rich, relatively large fiber, comprising 60% of his sample. The remaining 40% are relatively mitochondrion-poor and thinner, and terminate mainly on the modiolar side of the hair cell. He has also in serial sections followed synaptic interrelation between afferent and efferent fibers and seen large numbers of synaptic contacts which, if they are real synaptic contacts, are of great functional significance. We and others have for many years used different fixatives, as described by AKERT and PFENNINGER (1969), CHALAZONITIS (1969), and others, and know that the same fixative can produce different results. We are now reviewing our material concerning synaptic contacts. The species differences can play an important role here, as has already been pointed out. We have in our material very few cats but large numbers of guinea pigs, squirrel monkeys, and rhesus monkeys, and the species difference must always be recognized. LIBERMAN (1980a, b) reports that only 6% of the afferent fibers crossed the inner pillars into the tunnel and 94% of the afferents terminated at the inner hair cells. These figures very much resemble those found by Spoendlin and others. The publications by Liberman contain important information and enrich our knowledge of the complicated pattern of nerve fibers in the organ of Corti. Both we and Liberman have made measurements of the diameters of the different nerve fibers. Many of the fibers are "beaded" at intervals and this complicates matters. The very rich beading of the spiral tunnel bundle is still unexplained. Because of the long course of the outer spiral afferents and their irregular divisions, reconstructions over longer stretches from serial sections are very difficult to effect. However, it now seems possible by different techniques to come closer to the real innervation pattern of the cochlea.

With recent techniques using horseradish peroxidase and other tracers for axonal transport studies, it is now possible to get a much faster and better idea of neural pathways. The efferent innervation is now well described (cf. WARR 1979), and it is known that there are uncrossed and crossed fibers. According to Warr's studies in the kitten, approximately 1,800 efferent neurons project onto one

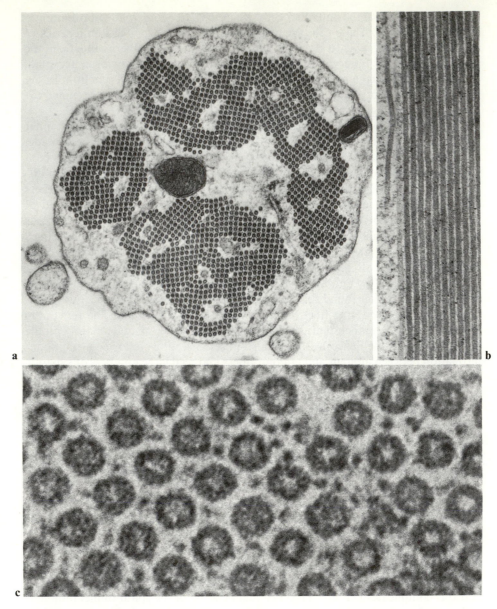

Fig. 12. a Cross-sectioned outer pillar cell. **b** Longitudinally sectioned tubular fibrils. **c** High magnification of cross-sectioned tubular and solid filaments from outer pillar

cochlea. Of these fibers, more than 50% are of ipsilateral origin. In studies using ^{35}S-methionine, Warr followed the fibers to their peripheral terminations. The recent studies by LIBERMAN (1980 a, b) add further information about the distribution of these efferent fibers from the olivocochlear bundles.

4. The Supporting Cells

The supporting cells have been the subject of several studies. IURATO (1962) provided one of the good early descriptions of the basilar membrane, the spiral limbus, and the spiral ligament. In 1975 JAHNKE described the junctional complexes in the guinea pig inner ear, and in the following year Iurato and his collaborators gave a description of the junctional complexes in the reticular membrane of the organ of Corti (IURATO et al. 1976). In this study Iurato used freeze fracture techniques and described the contacts between sensory and supporting cells and between the different supporting elements. He summarizes his findings by stating that the intercellular spaces of the organ of Corti, filled with cortilymph, are sealed from the endolymph by zonulae occludentes located at the level of the reticular membrane. At the basal portions of Deiters' cells he found only gap junctions. The high concentration of potassium ions in the endolymph is in this way sealed off by the tight junctions, while the gap junctions at the base of the organ of Corti concur with a looser form of interconnection and greater possibilities of ion transportation (GULLEY and REESE 1976). In the literature there are many good early studies on the supporting framework; HELD's (1926) excellent description has already been mentioned. Electron microscopy has made it possible to carry out more detailed analysis of the interior of the different supporting cells. Angelborg and I (ANGELBORG and ENGSTRÖM 1972) have made a thorough study of the pillar cells and the Deiters' cells, laying special emphasis on the fibrillar structures. We were able to discern two separate types of fibril, one coarser and tubular ($\sim$27 nm) and the other thinner and solid ($\sim$6 nm). The total number of tubular (1,000–3,000) and solid fibrils ($>$5,000) varies in different cochlear regions and species. They form a beautiful system of mechanical support in the organ of Corti, where the pillar cells and the Deiters' cells with their phalanges (Figs. 9 and 12) act as a kind of skeleton for the sensory cells. It has also been maintained that some of the supporting cells have a nutritive function. It is interesting to see how the pillar cells seem to be the most resistant in the cochlea to degenerative processes caused by noise. The sensory cells seem to degenerate first, then the Deiters' cells, and finally the pillar cells. B. ENGSTRÖM and BORG (to be published) have shown that pillar cell remnants can be found sticking up over the surface of the more or less damaged surface of the organ of Corti in animals, having survived the noise exposures by 10 months (Fig. 13). This has also been seen by myself and co-workers (ENGSTRÖM and ADES 1973) using transmission electron microscopy, but is much more effeciently visualized with the help of scanning electron microscopy.

IV. Concluding Remarks

It is not within the limits of this paper to cover all the details of the cochlear duct. My collaborators and I have studied and followed with interest the extensive studies by others on the membranes of the cochlear duct. Hinojosa has written several excellent papers on the organ of Corti (HINOJOSA 1972) and on the stria vascularis (HINOJOSA and RODRIGUEZ-ECHANDIA 1966), and was at an early stage my collaborator for several months. The excellent studies on the blood vessels of the inner ear by AXELSSON (1968, 1974) began in my laboratory and have contributed much

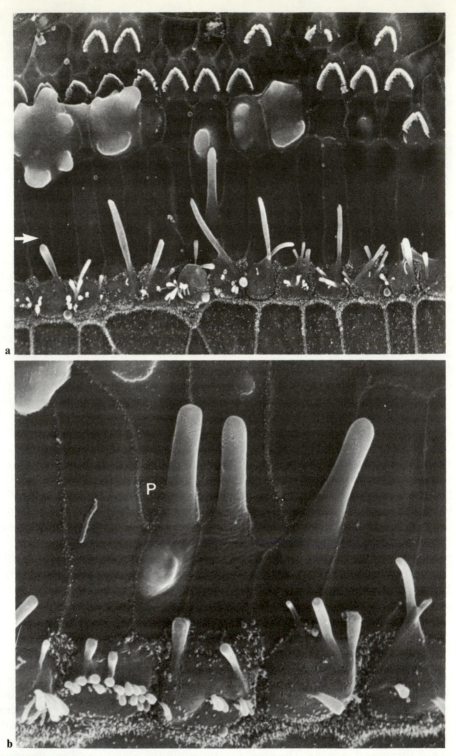

Fig. 13 a, b. These two scanning electron micrographs from the organ of Corti of a rabbit exposed to noise and with survival time 10 months show fused hairs or macrohairs (*white arrow*) and remnants of pillars (*P*). In **a** several outer hair cells have degenerated

to our knowledge of the vasculature of the inner ear. For a long time, we devoted much time to the cells of the spiral ganglion and B. KELLERHALS et al. (1967) worked for a year on an interesting project. For a long time ANGELBORG (1974) studied fluid transport in the inner ear together with me, and he wrote his thesis on this subject. He is now leading a group (Angelborg, Hultcrantz, and Larsen) doing interesting research on inner ear blood circulation. In this work they are using tracer particles, and are working in cooperation with Bill, the Head of the Physiology Department.

C. The Vestibular Sensory Regions

I. Development of Our Knowledge of the Vestibular Sensory Regions

In 1954 WERSÄLL et al. produced a preliminary description of the sensory cells in the macula utriculi of the guinea pig, and from then on Wersäll devoted considerable effort to the study of the vestibular sensory cells. This resulted in his doctoral thesis of 1956, which was a real breakthrough in our knowledge of the vestibular sensory epithelia (WERSÄLL 1956). The diagram in his Fig. 9 represents the basis for our discussions today, and although important additions have been made, his basic information has been verified by numbers of authors. It was my pleasure to be the faculty opponent at the defence of the doctoral dissertation, which was held according to Swedish tradition. Even the high regard I then had for Wersäll's book has been surpassed by its importance for our further research. The later cooperation between Wersäll and Flock, as well as with other scientists, has added much information and clarified many details.

It is interesting to note that shortly after Wersäll's publication, C. SMITH (1956) produced a corresponding description of the macular epithelium, and within a short time several publications appeared in which Wersäll's observations were verified. In 1958 I demonstrated that both the type II cells and the type I cells were provided with granulated, presumably efferent, nerve endings, as were also inner and outer hair cells in the cochlea (ENGSTRÖM 1958; Fig. 14). The series of new findings stimulated a much increased degree of activity in vestibular research, and this increase is still very evident. In the Wersäll group, FLOCK (1965–1971) started a long series of excellent publications on the lateral line organ, the macula utriculi, and the vestibular sensory cells in general. In these studies, which were paralleled by many others (LOEWENSTEIN and WERSÄLL 1959; DIJKGRAF 1960), much interest was devoted to the directional sensitivity of the sensory cells. The background to these studies is in short as follows. Even before electron microscopy came into use, it became evident that the displacement of the cupula or the tectorial membrane resulted in a decrease in the endolymphatic potential, and it was assumed that this was dependent upon a depolarization of the sensory cells. This in turn caused an increase in the action potentials of the vestibular nerve fibers. Certain unexplained facts about the frequency of these potentials had earlier been noted by neurophysiologists. It was also already known that in the maculae there was a subdivision on both sides of a line called a "striola" (WERNER 1940). Electron microscopy could now demonstrate that the sensory cells on both sides of the striola were ar-

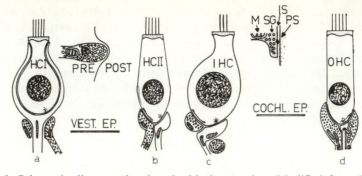

Fig. 14 a–d. Schematic diagram showing double innervation. Modified from Engström (1958)

ranged in a way which we today designate "morphological polarization." The first note on the matter of structural polarization came, as far as I can tell, in a paper by Lowenstein and Wersäll (1959), who demonstrated a structural polarization in the crista of the ray, and in a paper by Trujillo-Cenoz (1961), who demonstrated one in the crista of the fish. The first reference to a structural polarization in the maculae came from observations by myself and my co-workers (Engström et al. 1962):

In our sections we have seen that the pattern of the hairs on all the cells over a wide area is the same, with the kinocilia all facing in the same direction. Along a certain line this pattern reverses itself so that the kinocilia on opposite sides of the dividing line face each other. This arrangement apparently represents a functional polarization of the maculae, which we are investigating further.

The morphological polarization was then carefully analyzed by Flock (1965), and he related structural and functional polarization to each other in a series of ingenious experiments. Flock and Wersäll (1962) proposed a hypothesis for the function of the receptor cells in the lateral line organ, and in his thesis of 1965 Flock summarized his observations in a study with special reference to the directional sensitivity of the sensory cells (Flock 1965). His studies clearly demonstrated that an acceleration must be directed in a certain way in order to cause maximum effect. Accelerations in the opposite direction caused, on the contrary, a reduction in the action potential.

Series of studies have since then been made both from physiological and morphological points of view (Spoendlin 1965; Budelmann 1977, 1979; Bagger-Sjöbäck and Wersäll 1973, 1976; Dale 1976; Popper and Clarke 1976; and many others). In recent years, Flock (1980) and Shotwell et al. (1981) have made studies concerned with the function of the sensory hairs and the factors that are of importance in the activation of the sensory cells. In Flock's and Hudspeth's groups, morphological and functional studies are interwoven in a very interesting way.

In several groups much work has been devoted to the study of the effects of ototoxic antibiotics on vestibular sensory cells and on structural modification in genetically impaired ears. In Sect. C.II, a short survey will be presented of our present concept of the vestibular sensory cells.

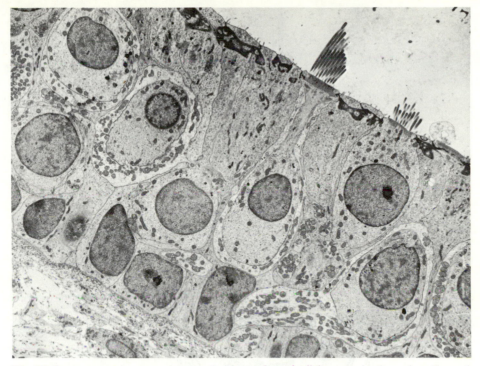

Fig. 15. Low-power electron micrograph of macula utriculi from squirrel monkey. Several type I and type II cells

II. The Vestibular Sensory Cells

The main features can be found in the basic study by Wersäll, but Figs. 15–17 represent the recently obtained small but important additions. There are, in principle, two main populations of sensory cells, type I and type II. There are also occasional intermediate cells, where one half looks like a type I and the other like a type II cell. Wersäll has pointed out that the type II cell is in reality the more primitive one and that the type I cell is a specialized type. Type II cells are most common in more primitive animals.

The type I cell is flask-shaped, as can be seen in Figs. 15 and 16. It has a rounded lower end and is surrounded by a nerve chalice. It is not uncommon that two or even three type I cells can be found in the same calyx. The cell surface is provided with sensory hairs, which are of two different types. There is one kinocilium and many stereocilia. The kinocilium is the longest and the stereocilia are of graded lengths, the longest lying closest to the kinocilium. The kinocilium and the stereocilia vary considerably in length. Scanning electron microscopy enables pleasing visualization of the hairs. In some animals the kinocilium has a bulbous tip, but usually, at least in mammals, the hairs have a rather uniform diameter from the cellular surface to its rounded outer end. At its base the kinocilium has a helical arrangement forming a short neck. Below the surface of the cell there is a basal

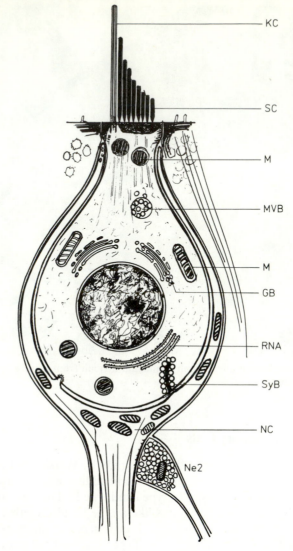

Fig. 16. Schematic diagram of type I cell with one kinocilium (*KC*) and several stereocilia (*SC*). *NC* is the surrounding nerve calyx. *M*, mitochondria; *GB*, Golgi complex; *RNA*, rough endoplasmic reticulum; *SyB*, synaptic bar; *MVB*, multivesiculated body; *Ne 2*, efferent ending on the outside of nerve calyx

body, and often, at some distance from the basal body, a centriole. The stereocilia are slightly thinner than the kinocilium. They are built like the hairs on cochlear hair cells with many microfilaments (diameter 5 nm) inside. According to the studies of Flock and Cheung (1977), these contain actin. The stereocilia are inserted in the cuticle, which has a different thickness and rests on a ring of dense material. The kinocilium has a very complicated system of cross-striated fibrillar rootlets reaching down into the interior of the cell. Such rootlets have been beautifully de-

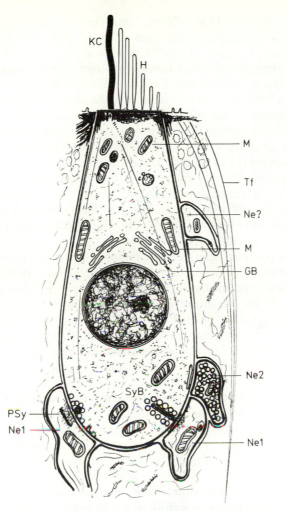

Fig. 17. Schematic diagram of type II cell. *M*, mitochondria; *GB*, Golgi complex; *SyB*, synaptic bar; *Tf*, tonofibrils in supporting cell; *Ne 1*, afferent ending; *Ne 2*, efferent ending; *PSy*, postsynaptic density

scribed by AFZELIUS and FRANZÉN (1971) in the spermatozoon of the jellyfish *Nausithoe*.

The sensory hairs have been the subject of many interesting studies during the last five to ten years. Many authors have observed a fuzz around the hairs, and HAMA (1978) has shown that this is formed by mucopolysaccharides, which stain with ruthenium red dye. According to YOSHIKA et al. (1978), all hairs are densely covered with substances having multiple electronegative charges. These authors have produced evidence that, in the lateral line organ of the tadpole, the kinocilium can adsorb cations at the hair surface. Flock and collaborators have, as has been earlier pointed out, made extensive studies of the sensory hairs, and somewhat similar experiments have been done by Hudspeth and collaborators. As pointed out, FLOCK and WERSÄLL (1962) devoted much early interest to the morphological and functional polarization of the hair cells.

In recent years, FLOCK et al. (1977), using a water immersion lens, studied the hairs in detail when the latter were moved by a microprobe. These studies disclosed that the hairs "pivot stiffly around their base with the shorter stereocilia following the longer ones." When fixatives were added, the stiffness of the cilia was reduced, and this may acount for the impression from fixed material. The kinocilium seems to be attached to the stereocilia, but there is also evidence suggesting spontaneous motility of the kinocilia. FLOCK et al. (1980), discuss the reason for the inherent attachment between the cilia, and demonstrate that the membrane charge of the individual cilia is of vital importance. This is also true of the process of fusion observed by my group (ENGSTRÖM et al. 1962, 1981) and by authors working with ototoxic antibiotics (WERSÄLL et al. 1971; B. ENGSTRÖM and BORG, to be published). Such extensive fusion is seen in Fig. 13, depicting inner hair cells from the cochlea of a noise-exposed animal.

HUDSPETH (to be published) recently reported interesting experiments where he micromanipulated away the kinocilium and yet the sensory cells retained their function. In these experiments the basal body was left, which could be an important functional factor. It is, however, extremely probable that the whole system of cilia is of importance to normal cell function. In favor of the view that the stereocilia are of great importance is the fact that they seem to be arranged in many ways, all seeming to be of functional significance. In the infracuticular region and especially in the region of the basal body, many microtubules can be seen. They run in large numbers almost parallel down toward the lower portion of the cell, and some can be seen all the way down to the infranuclear portion. Their final fate has not yet been uncovered in our studies. In the outer hair cells of the cochlea, they were regularly seen reaching down to the neighborhood of the nerve endings.

The type II cells (Figs. 17, 18 b) vary more in shape than the type I cells. They are often of the type seen in Fig. 17, but their size depends a great deal on the form of nearby cells. Thus some may be very short whereas some reach almost from the surface to the basement membrane. These cells have also been well described in the literature, and the structure is well depicted in many of the publications of my group.

There seems to be a certain amount of difference as regards the structure of the cuticle between type I and type II cells, the latter having a looser, less distinct cuticular plate. In the same way, the microtubules are not as evident in the supranuclear portion as they are in the type I cells, where the narrow neck seems to concentrate the microtubules. Another difference is the arrangement of the ribosomes. The rough membranes often seen in the infranuclear portion of type I cells are infrequent in the type II cells.

III. The Innervation of the Vestibular Sensory Cells

The main structural difference between type I and type II cells is in their relation to the terminations of the vestibular nerve. The great interest in the interrelation between the structure and function of the vestibular sensory regions has, in recent years, enriched our knowledge considerably, and FERNANDEZ and GOLDBERG

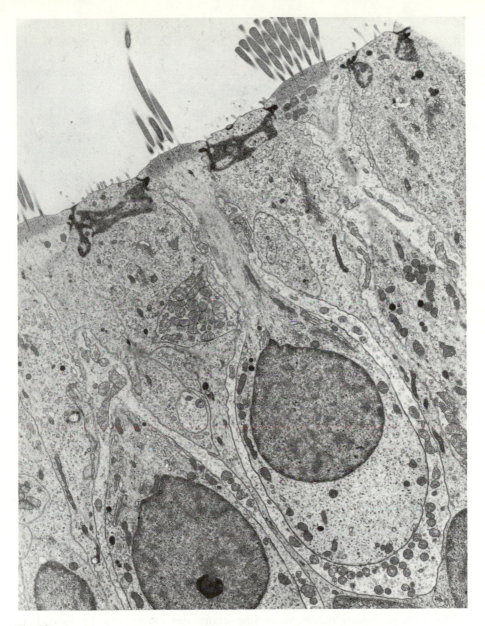

Fig. 18a

Fig. 18 a, b. Longitudinal section through type I cell from macula utriculi of squirrel monkey. The whole cell is almost surrounded by the nerve calyx, which contains many mitochondria. At the surface the reticular membrane is distinctly electron dense and rather irregular. The type I cells have often a slightly upward-pointed nucleus. **b** Longitudinal section through a type II cell from macula utriculi of the same animal as in **a.** Nerve endings and nerve fibers can be found high up along the supranuclear portion of the cells, but the major portion of the cell borders onto the supporting cell

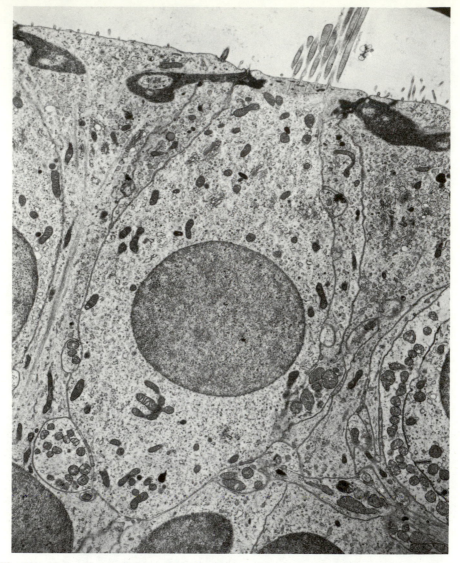

Fig. 18b. Hair cell type II from the utricular macula

(1976a–c) have, among others, made important contributions to this field. Fernandez, with whom I have had the great pleasure of collaborating on efferent endings in the cochlea, and who has received the Bárány gold medal for his work, has devoted much of his life to the study of vestibular sensory cells and nerve fibers and their function.

The sensory cells are, irrespective of type, innervated by at least two different kinds of fiber, afferent and efferent ones. This concept is to a great extent based on structural observations. As was pointed out earlier, Wersäll (1956) observed granulated endings on type II cells, and I (Engström 1958) produced evidence of

Table 1. Ratio between number of sensory cells and number of nerve fibers

	No. of cells	No. of nerve fibers	Ratio
Macula utriculi, man ROSENHALL (1974), BERGSTRÖM (1973)	33,100	5,952	5.6
Macula utriculi, guinea pig RASMUSSEN and GACEK (1961)	9,260	1,703	5.4

afferent and efferent endings on all inner ear sensory cells. The type I cells (Figs. 16 and 18) are almost completely surrounded in their intraepithelial portion by a nerve chalice, and the efferent endings reach only to the surface of the nerve chalice, not to the sensory cell itself. The type II cells (Fig. 17), on the other hand, have direct contact with both afferent and efferent endings. Endings on type II cells can typically be found very high up on the plasma membrane. It is, however, very uncommon to see typical synaptic bars, which occur regularly at the basal end, on these high endings. This is so evident that I have many times wondered if they represent something different from the lower endings with their well-developed synaptic structures. Similar high endings can also be seen along the nerve chalices of type I cells, and they are *not* granulated, which should indicate that they are not efferent endings. It was pointed out by C. SMITH (1956) that the nerve chalices in their uppermost part often contain vesicles similar to the synaptic vesicles. She therefore discussed whether this portion could be important from a synaptic point of view. We have in many nerve chalices observed an agglomeration of vesicles, very much resembling synaptic vesicles. We have tried to find evidence from our Maillet-stained specimens that they take stain like the efferent, presynaptic endings, but have not seen any clear uptake of stain.

One factor of great interest in the innervation of vestibular sensory cells is the ratio between the number of sensory cells and the number of nerve fibers. Table 1 gives the figures of ROSENHALL (1970) and BERGSTRÖM (1973) for man and the figures of GACECK and RASMUSSEN (1961) for guinea pig. This is difficult to correlate with the morphological picture, which indicates that each fiber must innervate more than one sensory cell. The ratio for the cristae is lower, as pointed out by Bergström.

In the maculae, the distance between nerve fibers which penetrate the basement is relatively large. These fibers form a rich plexus, mainly lying below the bases of the sensory cells. We have tried to follow the fibers in serial sections, but this has been very difficult because of fibers entering from the sides. There seems, however, to be evidence that many cells at least are innervated by several nerve fibers, but the type I cells by fewer than the type II cells. It is also evident that, at least in several cases, type I and type II cells can be innervated by the same fibers. It is furthermore quite clear that a nerve chalice from a type I cell can be in contact with and form synaptic structures belonging to both type I and type II cells. This has been shown repeatedly by us. We have also observed how, after the degeneration of a type I cell, the remaining chalice still forms a synaptic contact with a type II cell. In order to understand impulse formation in the vestibular nerve fibers, there can

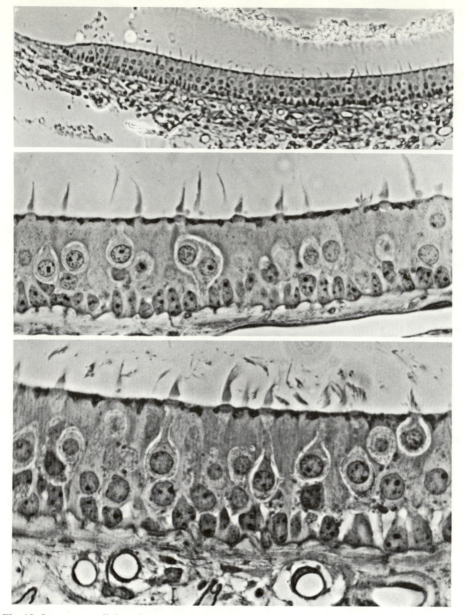

Fig. 19. Low-power light micrographs of macula utriculi of squirrel monkey. Epon embedding permits good quality light microscopy and can be followed directly by ultrathin sectioning and transmission electron microscopy

be synaptic contacts between both type I and type II cells and the same fiber. A full understanding of the frequency of this mixing of sensory cells with regard to thin and coarse nerve fibers would prove of great physiological interest. Furthermore, reference may be made to a very interesting publication by LORENTE DE NÓ

(1926). This paper has been much studied, but its full importance has perhaps not been understood. Lorente de Nó, who once worked as an assistant at the clinic from which this survey emanates, and whose excellent preparations I have studied, referred on the first page of this paper to Retzius. In translation it says: "Retzius recognized the existence of two kinds of nerve ending in the sensory epithelium of the vestibule: one in the shape of a calyx, the other in the form of ramified fibrils." As early as 100 years ago, then, there was knowledge of two kinds of neural connection between the sensory cells and the nerve terminations. Lorente's own studies verified this, and like his teacher Cajal he was able to describe regional differences in innervation. He also described extensions from nerve chalices to nearby cells, as described above, and his drawings (e.g., his Fig. 4) very much resemble electron micrographs published by my group. Lorente's paper is interesting not only as a scientific publication: his comments on other authors are very direct. About Kolmer, who carried out extensive studies of the inner ear, including a large handbook, he writes: "Kolmer has devoted many publications to this question. He has used the method of Cajal for his research, but it seems to us without great success." His comments on another publication are even more acid: this author had described some nerve branches which, according to Lorente, were nothing but "some fibrils of coagulated fibrin." My contacts with Lorente de Nó have been very pleasant and interesting. Both Retzius and Lorente de Nó brought important information concerning Wersäll's type I and type II cells, but it was not until Wersäll was able to separate and describe the two in detail that they became of real importance. In many parts of the world, scientists are producing information concerning structural polarization, innervation pattern, and ratio between type I and type II cells. Morphometric studies by LINDEMAN et al. (to be published) indicate a method of obtaining better information.

Sensory cells have accounted for most of the interest, and much less has been written about the supporting cells. These are, however, also of great interest. We are now trying to identify the chemical structure of the granules which can be observed in large numbers in the supporting cells (Figs. 15 and 18).

IV. Structural Modifications in Elderly Animals and Man

The description of the structure of the vestibular labyrinth is based upon studies of young, healthy animals. For the evaluation of long-term experiments it is, however, very important to realize that considerable structural modifications take place in elderly animals and man. Age-related modifications and hearing loss, presbyacusis, have long been well documented, and many authors have studied this problem. Excellent surveys of this problem can be found in publications by BREDBERG (1968) and by JOHNSSON and HAWKINS (1976). For a long time, very little attention was devoted to the aging of vestibular sensory epithelia. In series of clinical tests and structural studies, it has now been shown that extensive modifications also take place in the vestibular labyrinth.

These structural modifications have been studied by BERGSTRÖM (1973), ROSENHALL (1974), and myself and co-workers (ENGSTRÖM et al. 1974). The studies by Bergström and by Rosenhall showed that in elderly humans approximately 40% of the sensory cells and nerve fibers in the cristae disappeared, and about 20%

in the maculae. Our studies on an ultrastructural level demonstrated extensive modifications in the remaining cells (cf. ENGSTRÖM et al. 1977). The structural changes are of several different kinds.

V. Concluding Remarks

The increase in knowledge concerning the vestibular labyrinth, which has been promoted by electron microscopic research, has been very rewarding. In a period when some antibiotics caused problems because of vestibular and cochlear disturbances, electron microscopic research became a tool of great importance for the understanding of the nature of the damage and for the testing of new drugs. All over the world groups of scientists have devoted much time to such studies (ANNIKO 1976, 1978). The understanding of several kinds of genetic disturbance involving the inner ear has been broadened by transmission and scanning electron microscopy. Thus ERNSTSSON (1972) produced completely new findings, and FLOCK et al. (1979) demonstrated the pathological appearance of actin in certain animals. Similar studies have come from several sources. Transmission electron microscopy has also been used in animal research in relation to such special problems as space sickness (VINNIKOV et al. 1980).

D. Summary

Studies dealing with inner ear morphology have existed for more than a century, and even in publications by early scientists such as RETZIUS (1884), important information which is still of great relevance was obtained. New technological developments, depending on new inventions in the field of electronics, have revolutionized inner ear research morphologically and neurophysiologically. In the few decades that have elapsed since 1950, transmission and scanning electron microscopy have opened new pathways of understanding as regards structural components on an ultrastructural level. Other techniques and multidisciplinary approaches have brought structure and function much closer together.

In this short survey, I have attempted to present information about some of the people who have contributed in an important way. It was stipulated that the Chapter should contain details of personal experiences and relationships. This has of course biased my presentation, and many important facets have been omitted. Perhaps many things not written about may be recognized in the illustrations.

References

Names containing von are alphabetized in this list under v

Afzelius B, Franzén Å (1971) The spermatozoon of the jellyfish Nausithoe. J Ultrastruct Res 37:186
Akert K, Pfenninger K (1969) Synaptic fine structure and neural dynamics. In: Barondes SH (ed) Cellular dynamics of the neuron. Academic, New York, p 245
Angelborg C (1974) Clinical, physiological, and morphological studies on inner ear fluids and structures. Acta Univ Ups [Suppl] 200:1

Angelborg C, Engström H (1972) Supporting elements in the organ of Corti. I. Fibrillar structures in the supporting cells of the organ of Corti of mammals. Acta Otolaryngol [Suppl] (Stockh) 301:49

Anniko M (1976) The cytocochleogram in atoxyl-treated guinea-pigs. Acta Otolaryngol (Stockh) 82:70

Anniko M (1978) Atoxyl induced pathological changes of the inner ear. MD thesis, University of Stockholm

Axelsson A (1968) The vascular anatomy of the cochlea in the guinea pig and man. Acta Otolaryngol [Suppl] (Stockh) 243:1

Axelsson A (1974) The blood supply of the inner ear of mammals. In: Keidel WD, Neff WD (eds) Anatomy, physiology (ear). Springer, Berlin Heidelberg New York, p 213 (Handbook of sensory physiology, vol V-1)

Bagger-Sjöbäck D (1967) The basilar papilla of the lizard *Calotes versicolor*. Thesis, University of Stockholm

Bagger-Sjöbäck D, Wersäll J (1976) Toxic effect of gentamicin on the basilar papilla in the lizard Calotes versicolor. Acta Otolaryngol (Stockh) 87:57–65

Bagger-Sjöbäck D, Wersäll J (1973) The sensory hairs and tectorial membrane of the basilar papilla in the lizard Calotes versicolor. J Neurocytol 2:329–350

Beck C (1959) Feinere Stoffwechselreaktionen an den Sinneszellen des Cortischen Organs nach Reintonbeschallung. Arch Ohren Nasen Kehlkopfheilkd Z Hals Nasen Ohrenheilkd 175:374

Bergström B (1973) Morphological studies of the vestibular nerve. Acta Univ Ups 191:1

Borg E, Engström B (1982) Acoustic reflex after experimental lesions to inner and outer hair cells. Hearing Research 6:25–34

Borghesan E (1954) Fisiopathologia del canale cochleare. Palermo Boccone del povero

Bredberg G (1968) Cellular pattern and nerve supply of the human organ of Corti. Acta Otolaryngol [Suppl] (Stockh) 236:1

Bredberg G (1977) Scanning electron microscopy of the nerves within the organ of Corti. Arch Otorhinolaryngol 217:321

Bredberg G, Hunter-Duvar M (1975) Behavioral tests of hearing and inner ear damage. In: Iggo A (ed) Somatosensory system. Springer, Berlin Heidelberg New York, pp 261–306 (Handbook of sensory physiology, vol 2)

Bredberg G, Ades HW, Engström H (1972) Scanning electron microscopy of the normal and pathologically altered organ of Corti. Acta Otolaryngol [Suppl] (Stockh) 301:3

Breschet G (1833) Etudes anatomiques et physiologiques sur l'organe de l'ouïe et sur l'audition dans l'homme et les animaux vertébrés. Paris

Budelmann BU (1977) Structure and function of the angular acceleration receptor system in the statocysts of cephalopods. Symp Zool Soc London 38:309

Budelmann BU (1979) Hair cell polarization in the gravity receptor systems of the statocysts of the cephalopods *Sepia officinales* and *Loligo vulgaris*. Brain Res 160:261

Chalazonitis N (1969) Differentiation of membranes in axonal endings in the neuropile of *Helix*. In: Barondes SH (ed) Cellular dynamic of the neuron. Academic, New York

Corti A (1851) Recherches sur le range de l'ouïe des mammifères. Z Wiss Zool 3:109–169

Dale T (1976) The labyrinthine mechanoreceptor organs of the cod *Gadus morhua* L. Norw J Zool 24:85–128

de Vries HL, Bleeker JDJW (1949) The microphonic activity of the labyrinth of the pigeon. Acta Otolaryngol (Stockh) 37:298

Dijkgraaf S (1960) Hearing in bony fishes. Proc R Soc Lond [Biol] 152:51

Engström B (1983) Stereocilia of sensory cells in normal and hearing impaired ears. Scandinavian Audiology [Suppl.] 19:1–34

Engström H (1951) Microscopic anatomy of the inner ear. Acta Otolaryngol (Stockh) 60:1–22

Engström H (1958) On the double innervation of the sensory epithelia of the inner ear. Acta Otolaryngol (Stockh) 49:109

Engström H (1960) The cortilymph, the third lymph of the inner ear. Acta Morphol Neerl Scand 3:195

Engström H (1967) The ultrastructure of the sensory cells of the cochlea. J Laryngol Otol 81:687

Engström H, Ades HW (1973) The ultrastructure of the organ of Corti. In: Friedman I (ed) The ultrastructure of sensory organs. North Holland, Amsterdam, pp 83–151

Engström H, Engström B (1979) Ultrastruktur des inneren Ohres. In: Zöllner F (ed) Hals-Nasen-Ohren-Heilkunde in Praxis und Klinik 5. Thieme, Stuttgart, S. 3.1–3.33

Engström H, Sjöstrand FS, Wersäll J (1953) The fine structure of the tone receptors of the guinea pig cochlea as revealed by the electron microscope. In: Proceedings of the fifth international congress of Otolaryngology. Van Corcum, Assen, pp 1–5

Engström H, Ades HW, Bredberg G (1970) Normal structure of the organ of Corti and the effect of noise-induced cochlear damage. In: Ciba foundation symposium: Sensorineural hearing loss. Churchill, London, p 127

Engström H, Ades HW, Andersson A (1966) Structural pattern of the organ of Corti. Almqvist and Wiksell, Stockholm

Engström H, Ades HW, Engström B, Gilchrist D, Bourne G (1977) Structural changes in the vestibular epithelia in elderly monkeys and humans. Adv Otorhinolaryngol 22:93

Engström H, Ades HW, Hawkins JE Jr (1962) Structure and function of the sensory hairs of the inner ear. J Acoust Soc Am 34:1356

Engström H, Ades HW, Hawkins JE Jr (1965) Cellular pattern, nerve structures, and fluid spaces in the organ of Corti. In: Neff WD (ed) Sensory physiology, vol 1. American, New York, p 1

Engström H, Bergström B, Rosenhall U (1974) Vestibular sensory epithelia. Arch Otolaryngol 100:411

Engström B, Flock Å, Borg E (1983) Ultrastructural studies of damaged stereocilia in noise exposed rabbits. Hearing Research

Ernstson S (1972) The waltzing guinea pig. A study on inherited inner-ear degeneration. Thesis, University of Stockholm

Fernandez C, Goldberg J (1976a) Physiology of peripheral neurons innervating otolith organs of the squirrel monkey. I. Response to static tilt and to long-duration centrifugal force. Neurophysiology 39:970

Fernandez C, Goldberg J (1976b) Physiology of peripheral neurons innervating otolith organs of the squirrel monkey. II. Directional selectivity and force-response relations. Neurophysiology 39:985

Fernandez C, Goldberg J (1976c) Physiology of peripheral neurons innervating otolith organs of the squirrel monkey. III. Response dynamics. J Neurophysiology 39:996

Flock Å (1965) Electron microscopic and electrophysiological studies on the lateral line canal organ. Acta Otolaryngol [Suppl] (Stockh) 199:1

Flock Å (1971) Principles of receptor physiology. In: Loewenstein WR (ed) Principles of receptor physiology. Springer, Berlin Heidelberg New York, p 396 (Handbook of sensory physiology, vol I)

Flock Å (1974) Sensory transduction in hair cells. In: Loewenstein WR (ed) Principles of receptor physiology. Springer, Berlin Heidelberg New York, p 396 (Handbook of sensory physiology, vol 1)

Flock Å (1980) Contractile proteins in hair cells. Hear Res 2:411

Flock Å, Wersäll J (1962) A study of the orientation of the sensory hair of the receptor cells in the lateral organ of fish with special reference to the function of the receptors. J Cell Biol 15:19

Flock Å, Kimura R, Lundqvist PG, Wersäll J (1962) Morphological basis of directional sensitivity of the outer hair cells in the organ of Corti. J Acoust Soc Am 34:1351

Flock Å, Flock B, Murray E (1977) Studies on the sensory hairs of receptor cells in the inner ear. Acta Otolaryngol (Stockh) 83:85

Flock Å, Cheung HC (1977) Actin filaments in sensory hairs of inner ear receptor cells. J Cell Biol 75:339

Flock Å, Cheung HC, Wersäll J (1979) Pathological actin in vestibular hair cells of the waltzing guinea pig. Adv Otorhinolaryngol 25:12

Friedmann I (1968) The chick embryo otocyst in tissue culture. A model ear. J Laryngol Otol 82:185

Friedmann I (1969) The development of innervation of the inner ear. Acta Otolaryngol (Stockh) 67:224

Friedmann I, Bird ES (1967) Rudimentary kinocilia, cup-shaped nerve endings and synaptic bars. J Ultrastruct Res 20:356

Gacek RR, Rasmussen GL (1961) Fiber analysis of the statoacoustic nerve of guinea pig, cat, and monkey. Anat Rec 139:455–463

Gulley RL, Reese TS (1976) Intercellular junctions in the reticular lamina of the organ of Corti. J Neurocytol 5:479

Hama K (1969) A study of the fine structure of the saccular macula of the gold fish. Z Zellforsch 94:155

Hama K (1978) A study of the fine structure of the pit organ of the common Japanese sea eel, *Conger myriaster*. Cell tissue Res 189:375

Held H (1926) Die Cochlea der Säuger und der Vögel, ihre Entwicklung und ihr Bau. Receptionsorgane 11:467

Hinojosa R (1972) Electron microscope studies of the stria vascularis and spiral ligament after ferritin injection. Acta Otolaryngol (Stockh) 74:1

Hinojosa R, Rodriquez-Echandia EL (1966) The fine structure of the stria vascularis of the cat inner ear. Am J Anat 118:631

Hirokawa N, Tilney LG (1982) Interactions between actin filaments and between actin filaments and membranes in quick-frozen and deeply etched haircells of the chick ear. J Cell Biol 95:249–261

Hoshino T (1974) Relationship of the tectorial membrane to the organ of Corti: a scanning electron microscopic study of cats and guinea pigs. Arch Histol Jpn 37:25

Hoshino T (1976) Attachment of the inner sensory cell hairs to the tectorial membrane. A scanning electron microscopic study. ORL 38:11

Hudspeth AJ, Jacobs R (1979) Stereocilia mediate transduction in vertebrate hair cells. Proc Natl Acad Sci USA 76:1506

Itoh M (1982) Preservation and visualization of actin containing filaments in the apical zone of cochlear sensory cells. Hearing Research 6:277–289

Iurato S (1962) Submicroscopic structure of the membranous labyrinth. III. The supporting structure of Corti's organ (basilar membrane, limbus spiralis, and spiral ligament). Z Zellforsch 56:40

Iurato S (1967) In: Iurato S (ed) Submicroscopic structure of the inner ear. Pergamon, Oxford

Iurato S (1974) Efferent innervation of the cochlea. In: Loewenstein WR (ed) Principles of receptor physiology. Springer, Berlin Heidelberg New York, p 261 (Handbook of sensory physiology, vol I)

Iurato S, Luciano L, Pannese E, Reale E (1971) Histochemical localization of acetylcholinesterase (AChE) activity in the inner ear. Acta Otolaryngol [Suppl] (Stockh) 279:1

Iurato S, Franke K, Luciano L, Wermbter G, Pannese E, Reale E (1976) Fracture faces of the junctional complexes in the reticular membrane of the organ of Corti. Acta Otolaryngol (Stockh) 81:36

Jahnke K (1975) The fine structure of freeze-fractured intercellular junctions in the guinea pig inner ear. Acta Otolaryngol [Suppl] (Stockh) 336:1–40

Johnsson LE, Hawkins JE Jr (1976) Degeneration patterns in human ears exposed to noise. Ann Otol Rhinol Laryngol 85:725

Kellerhals B, Engström H, Ades HW (1967) Die Morphologie des Ganglion spirale cochlea. Acta Otolaryngol [Suppl] (Stockh) 226:1–78

Kikuchi K, Hilding D (1965) The development of the organ of Corti in the mouse. Acta Otolaryngol (Stockh) 60:207

Kimura RS (1966) Hairs of the cochlear sensory cells and their attachment to the tectorial membrane. Acta Otolaryngol (Stockh) 61:55

Kimura R (1975) The ultrastructure of the organ of Corti. Int Rev Cytol 42:173

Kolmer V (1927) In: Von Möllendorfs W (ed) Haut und Sinnesorgane. Springer, Berlin (Handbuch der Mikroskopischen Anatomie des Menschen, vol 3)

Kronester-Frei A (1977) Licht- und elektronenmikroskopische Untersuchung der Lagebeziehung der Membrana tectoria zum Cortischen Organ in Abhängigkeit von Entwicklungszustand, Fixation und Ionenmilieu. PhD dissertation, University of Munich

Liberman MD (1980a) Morphological differences among radial afferent fibers in the cat cochlea: an electron microscopic study of serial sections. Hear Res 3:45

Liberman MD (1980b) Efferent synapsis in the inner hair cells area of the cat cochlea: an electron microscopic study of serial sections. Hear Res 3:189

Lim DJ (1969) Three dimensional observation of the inner ear with the scanning electron-microscope. Acta Otolaryngol [Suppl] (Stockh) 255:1–38

Lim DJ (1972) Fine morphology of the tectorial membrane. Arch Otolaryngol 96:199

Lim DJ (1980) Cochlear anatomy related to cochlear micromechanic. A review. J Acoust Soc Am 67:5

Lindeman HH (1969) Studies on the morphology of the sensory region of the vestibular apparatus. Adv Anat Embryol Cell Biol 42:1–113

Lindeman H, Ades HW, Bredberg G, Engström H (1971) The sensory hairs and the tectorial membrane in the development of the cat's organ of Corti. Acta Otolaryngol (Stockh) 72:229

Lowenstein OE, Wersäll J (1959) A functional interpretation of the electronmicroscopic structure of the sensory hairs in the cristae of the elasmobranch raja clavata in terms of directional sensitivity. Nature 184:1807

Lorente de Nó R (1926) Etudes sur l'anatomie et la physiologie du labyrinthe de d'oreille et du VIII: e nerf. Trab Inst Cajal Invest Biol 24:53

Neubert K (1952) Zur morphologischen Erfassung der Ansprechgebiete im Innenohr. Verh Anat Ges 50:204

Omata T, Schätzle W (1980) Afferent and efferent nerve endings of the outer hair cells in the rabbit. Arch Otorhinolaryngol 229:175

Peterson SK, Frishkopf LS, Lechene C, Oman CM, Weiss TF (1978) Element composition of inner ear lymphs in cats, lizards, and skates determined by electron probe microanalysis of liquid samples. J Comp Physiol 126:1

Pfenninger K, Sandri C, Akert K, Engster CH (1969) Contribution to the problem of structural organization of the presynaptic area. Brain Res 12:10

Popper AN, Clarke NL (1976) The auditory system of the goldfish (Carassius auratus). Effects of intense acoustic stimulation. Comp Biochem Physiol 53:11

Rask-Andersen H (1979) Aqueducts and accessory canals of the inner ear. Acta universitatis uppsaliensis 338:1

Rasmussen GL (1946) The olivary preduncle and other fiber projections of the superior complex. J Comp Neurol 84:141

Rasmussen GL (1960) Efferent fibers of the cochlear membrane and cochlear nuclei. In: Rasmussen GL, Windle WF (eds) Neural mechanisms of the auditory and vestibular system. Thomas, Springfield, p 105

Rauch S (1964) In: Rauch S (Ed) Biochemie des Hörorgans. Thieme, Stuttgart

Retzius G (1884) Das Gehörorgan der Wirbelthiere. II. Das Gehörorgan der Reptilien, der Vögel und der Säugethiere. Centraltryckeriet, Stockholm

Rosenhall U (1974) The vestibular sensory regions in man. Acta Univ [Suppl] 191:1–37

Ross M (1979) Calcium ion uptake and exchange in otoconia. Adv Otorhinolaryngol 25:26

Ross M, Peacor D (1975) The nature and crystal growth of otoconia in the rat. Ann Otol Rhinol Laryngol 84:22

Ross M, Pote KG, Rarey KE, Verma LM (1981) Microdisc gel electrophoresis in sodium dodocyl sulphate of organic material from rat otoconial complexes. Ann New York Ac Sci 374:808–819

Rossi G, Cortesina G (1962) The cochleo-vestibular cholinergic efferent system. Historico-bibliographic review and personal research. Minerva Otorinolaryngol 12:173

Rossi G, Voena G, Cortesina G, Buongiovanni S (1964) Changes in the cochlear-microphonic potential due to the resection of the cochlear fibres. J Acoust Soc Am 36:1845

Ryan AF, Wickham MG, Bone RC (1980) Studies of ion distribution in the inner ear: scanning electron microscopy and X-ray microanalysis of freeze-dried cochlear specimens. Hear Res 2:1

Rüedi L, Furrer W (1947) Das akustische Trauma. Karger, Basel

Scarpa A (1789) Anatomicae disquisitiones du auditu et olfactu. Tessin

Schuhknecht HF, Churchill JA, Doran R (1959) The localization of acetylcholinesterase in the cochlea. Arch Otolaryngol 69:549

Shotwell SL, Jacobs R, Hudspeth AJ (1981) Directional sensitivity of individual vertebrate hair cells to controlled deflection of their hair bundles. Ann New York Ac Sci 374:1–10

Smith CA (1956) Microscopic structure of the utricle. Ann Otol Rhinol Laryngol 65:450

Smith C (1966) In: Zotterman Y (ed) Proceedings of the fourth international meeting of neurobiologists. Pergamon, Oxford

Smith C (1968) Ultrastructure of the organ of Corti. Adv Sci 419:419–433

Smith C, Rasmussen GL (1963 a) Ultrastructural changes in the efferent cochlear nerve endings following transection of the olivocochlear bundle in the chinchilla. Anat Rec 145:287

Smith C, Rasmussen GL (1963 b) Recent observations on the olivocochlear bundle. Ann Otol Rhinol Laryngol 72:489

Smith C, Rasmussen GL (1965) Degeneration of the efferent nerve endings in the cochlea after axonal sections. Cell Biol 26:63

Smith CA, Sjöstrand F (1961) A synaptic structure in the hair cells of guinea pig cochlea. J Ultrastruct Res 5:184

Spoendlin H (1965) Ultrastructural studies of the labyrinth in squirrel monkeys. NASA publication SP-77, 7–22

Spoendlin H (1979) Anatomisch-pathologische Aspekte der Elektrostimulation des ertaubten Innenohres. Arch Otorhinolaryngol 223:1

Spoendlin H, Brun JB (1974) The bloc-surface technique for evaluation of cochlear pathology. Arch Otolaryngol 208:137

Tanaka K, Smith C (1975) Structure of the avian tectorial membrane. Ann Otol Rhinol Laryngol 84:287

Todd RB, Bowman W (1845) In: The physiological anatomy and physiology of man, vol II. Parker, London

Trujillo-Cenoz O (1961) Electron microscope observations on chemo- and mechanoreceptor cells of fishes. Z Zellforsch Mikrosk Anat 54:654

Vinnikov JAA, Lychakov DV, Pal'mbakh LR, Govardovskii VI, Adanina VO (1980) Ipsledovanie vestibularnogo apparatr liagushki xenopus loevis i kryp v uzloviiakh dlitel'noi nevesomorti. Zh Evol Biokhim Fiziol 16:574–579

Vinnikov JA, Titova LK (1961) Kortief organ (Organ of Corti). Moskow

Vinnikov JA, Titova LK (1963) Cytophysiology and cytochemistry of the organ of Corti. Int Rev Cytol 14:157

von Ilberg C (1969) Tubuläre Strukturen in äußeren Haarzellen. Arch Klin Exp Ohren Nasen Kehlkopfheilkd 194:408

Vosteen KH (1970) Passive and active transport in the inner ear. Arch Klin Exp Ohren Nasen Kehlkopfheilkd 195:226

Warr WB (1979) Efferent innervation of the organ of Corti: two separate systems. Brain Res 173:152

Watanuki K, Dawamoto K, Katagiri S (1970) Surface structure of the cochlea. Tohoku J Exp Med 100:359

Werner CF (1940) Das Labyrinth. Thieme, Leipzig

Wersäll J (1956) Studies on the structure and innervation of the sensory epithelium of the cristae ampullares in the guinea pig. Acta Otolaryngol [Suppl] (Stockh) 126:1–85

Wersäll J, Engström H, Hjorth S (1954) Fine structure of the guinea pig macula utriculi. Acta Otolaryngol [Suppl] (Stockh) 116:298

Wersäll J, Flock Å, Lundqvist PG (1965) Structural basis for directional sensitivity in cochlear and vestibular sensory receptors. Cold Spring Harbor Symp Quant Biol 30:115

Wersäll J, Björkroth B, Flock Å, Lundqvist PG (1971) Sensory hair fusion in vestibular sensory cells after gentamycin exposure. Arch Otorhinolaryngol 200:1–14

Wilbrand H (1974) Multidirectional tomography of minor detail in the temporal bone. Experimental and clinical investigations of the facial canal, intraossicular cavities, reconstructed ossicular chain and the vestibular aqueduct. Acta Univ Ups

CHAPTER 4

Biophysics of the Mammalian Ear

JOZEF J. ZWISLOCKI

A. Introduction

I. Biographical Notes

The foundations of a science may be viewed from various aspects. To gain a better perspective, I had originally assumed in my chapter the position of a somewhat detached observer. However, the editors of the handbook have reminded me that by writing it in an almost impersonal way, as I did, I fulfilled only part of my obligation, and suggested that I make some additions concerning factors that have influenced my scientific career. In an attempt to comply with their request, I have added some autobiographical notes in this Introduction, and have personalized some descriptions of my contributions.

    Living up to the tradition of science and engineering in my family, I studied electrical engineering at the Federal Institute of Technology in Zürich, Switzerland. Although my aptitude seemed quite in tune with this discipline, I found it somewhat confining, and gradually developed a consuming interest in living organisms – much less well understood and, therefore, more mysterious than structures designed by engineers. Because of this interest, I probably would have ended by studying medicine were it not for the fact that, as a foreigner, I could not have practiced it in Switzerland.

Lady Luck smiled on me, however. In 1944, at the end of my engineering studies, the position of applied physicist was offered to me at the Medical School of the University of Basel. It happened to be in the Department for Ear, Nose, and Throat Disorders. Its Director, Erhart Lüscher, well known for his pioneering observations of stapedius muscle contractions and other contributions to otology, was looking for a research assistant. His main research interest concerned psychophysical diagnostic tests for auditory disorders, an area that now belongs to audiology. I found this fascinating, partly because it concerned the human organism and partly because it seemed to present an almost limitless array of unsolved problems. I accepted the position, choosing academic idealism and the poverty that went with it over the prosperity offered me by industry.

My first task in Basel was to acquaint myself with the multilingual literature on hearing and the auditory system. I could speak and read German and French but had to learn English in a hurry. I still see myself ploughing laboriously with heavy use of a German–English dictionary, through H. FLETCHER's (1929) *Speech and Hearing* and S. S. STEVENS and H. DAVIS's (1938) *Hearing, Its Psychology and Physiology*. However, the first research problem Lüscher assigned to me was not described adequately in any of these languages, even though its roots extended to the mid-nineteenth century. It concerned the buildup and decay times of tonal sensations and their possible dependence on inner ear pathology. By lucky coincidence I had invented a simple electronic timer and switch during my engineering studies, which came in handy in producing the required stimuli in the form of tone bursts with variable duration, interburst interval, and onset and decay times. For the main experiments I introduced a stimulus paradigm consisting of a short tone burst preceded by a longer one at a variable time interval. Its threshold of audibility was measured as a function of the interburst time interval and several other parameters. The paradigm is now used routinely for measurements of what is called "forward masking," and which we called "decay of sensation and remainder of adaptation" (LÜSCHER and ZWISLOCKI 1947).

Before leaving Zürich I had been invited by my adviser, Professor F. Tank, then Rector of the Institute, to become his assistant and work on my doctoral dissertation. Because of the Basel commitment, I could not accept the offer, but the Institute gave me a special dispensation to do my dissertation work in Basel. The psychophysical studies I was engaged in did not appear to be a subject lying suitably within the Institute's sphere of research. As a consequence, I started to look elsewhere and discovered a rich controversial literature on mechanical sound analysis in the cochlea of the inner ear. There was von Helmholtz's famous resonance theory; Ewald's standing wave model; Meyer's traveling bulge model; Rutherford's telephone theory; Fletcher's space–time pattern theory; Ranke's rectifier resonance theory; and many others, and there were von Békésy's experiments on postmortem preparations of human cochleas. In view of von Békésy's experiments and the knowledge of physics and mathematics available in the 1940s, none of those theories and physical models appeared valid, even though reviewers without an appropriate background were not certain of this and perpetuated some of the misconceptions.

The mechanics of the cochlea were in the domain of applied physics and, therefore, acceptable to the Federal Institute of Technology as a subject for a doctoral dissertation. My background appeared appropriate to deal with it, since the electrical engineering curriculum was quite different in the mid-1940s from what it is now – it included a substantial amount of theoretical mechanics, thermodynamics, and hydrodynamics. In addition, I had taken all the available electives in physics and advanced calculus.

My dissertation task, as I saw it, consisted of adapting the classic theory of hydrodynamic surface waves to the cochlear conditions. It was fundamentally accomplished in 1946, and the first article describing my mathematical theory of cochlear mechanics appeared during the same year in the Swiss scientific journal *Experientia* (ZWISLOCKI 1946). The article contained a fundamental differential equation and its approximate solution, as well as a description of validating experiments on a physical model that resembled von Békésy's models, except that an optical system allowed the obtained pattern of surface waves to be projected on a screen under high magnification.

The substance of these developments is described in the main body of this chapter. Here I should note only that the theory, published in its entirety in 1948 (ZWISLOCKI 1948), unwittingly stirred up a prolonged controversy begun by Ranke and involving even von Békésy, and also earned me an invitation to the first Speech Communication Conference held at the Massachusetts Institute of Technology in 1950. The conference initiated a new phase in my scientific career. In spite of Ranke's criticism, my paper must have been received well, since S.S. Stevens offered me the position of research fellow in his famous Psychoacoustic Laboratory at Harvard.

When I selected cochlear mechanics as my dissertation topic while working full time on auditory psychophysics, I did not suspect that the decision would set a dichotomous pattern for most of my scientific career. Even today I divide my efforts between the two fields, in addition to trying to keep abreast of auditory neurophysiology. This diversity has one unquestionable effect – it keeps me very busy. Its disadvantage is that it prevents me from becoming a consummate expert in any one field. From a basic armamentarium of scientific tools I have to select ad hoc the ones that seem the most appropriate for a given problem and try to hone them to the required perfection. Once the problem is solved, the tools may have to be abandoned, making way for another set more appropriate for the logically following problem. Experts seem to espouse an opposite attitude by choosing problems that fit the one set of well-maintained tools they own. It would be possible to debate the advantages and disadvantages of the two attitudes at length, but the first appears more satisfying to me by its potential to better preserve a logical sequence of worthwhile problems. It may have the added advantage of providing a more analytical insight into a system by illuminating its diverse aspects.

During my six years at Harvard, various powerful influences came to bear on me, and I tried to integrate them as best I could. In matters of auditory biophysics focused on the cochlea and the middle ear my most direct interaction was with von Békésy, who occupied the position of senior research fellow. Because we shared a European origin, studies in Switzerland, and a greater mastery of German than of English, I was probably closer to him than anybody else in the laboratory. Scientifically, we complemented each other in the sense that von Békésy performed experiments on animal preparations and physical models, while I attempted to account for some of his results in the mathematical terms of theoretical physics. Our research concepts diverged, however. With his empirical studies of the cochlea he started a revolution against the armchair theorizing of the nineteenth century, eventually becoming a "rugged empiricist" who rejected almost entirely any mathematical deductions. Arriving on the scene a quarter of a century later, I benefited from von Békésy's revolution but also saw its excesses. Although science since Bacon has been an empirical enterprise, mathematics, which originally evolved in close association with empirical observations, is the universal organizer of empirical data. It shows us their mutual relations and, from them, allows us to derive new data that are difficult to obtain through direct experimentation.

I attempted to counteract von Békésy's extreme empiricism by example rather than direct criticism. I used mathematics to explain his cochlear waves in terms of the general hydrodynamical theory, to pinpoint artifacts in his measurements, to resolve differences between his results and those of others, and to predict some key relationships. Only through a close coupling of experiments and mathematical theory was it possible for me to analyze the function of the intact human middle ear and to show how some of its pathologies could be diagnosed from acoustic measurements in the ear canal. While the latter effort had an immediate effect on auditory science because of its practical applications, my cochlear theory remained in obscurity until, in recent years, some of its mathematical predictions were incidentally verified and some artifacts of von Békésy's measurements became clearly apparent.

Von Békésy's empiricism was not isolated, but belonged to a Zeitgeist that still endures. It seems that every science begins by being almost entirely descriptive, and the use it makes of mathematics only gradually increases with the process of its maturation. Measured by this yardstick, auditory science must now be reaching puberty. In an attempt to speed up the maturation process, I have established at Syracuse University the Institute for Sensory Research, the objective of which is a synthesis of the life and physical sciences that use mathematics as one of their fundamental tools. It seems to me that progress in our understanding of the auditory and other sensory systems will be considerably accelerated when experimentalists and theoreticians of sensory science learn enough of a common language to begin a useful dialogue, like that of the physicists.

II. Scope of the Chapter

Biophysics is a broad interdisciplinary field overlapping with several more traditional disciplines. Clearly, it is not possible in one chapter to touch upon the wide array of its strongly divergent aspects, even within the framework of one sensory system. As a consequence, this chapter is focused on the biophysical topics most characteristic of the auditory science, irrespective of their place in the general structure of contemporary biophysics.

The main thrust of mammalian auditory biophysics has been aimed at the acoustic and mechanical processes ranging from sound diffraction at the head to the transduction of mechanical vibration into electrochemical events ending in the release of neural action potentials. Between the two boundaries, the processes include sound transmission in the outer, middle, and inner ear, and sound analysis in the latter. The various anatomical parts involved are so adapted to each other as to produce an astonishing sensitivity to sound, which has remained unmatched by man-made devices, and a resolution of sound frequencies so exquisite that it taxes the equipment used for its measurement to the limits of technical feasibility. Both phenomena have fascinated scientists for more than a century and are only partially explained by mechanisms that have become evident thus far.

In this chapter, I attempt to retrace the history of experimental discoveries and theoretical derivations pertinent to auditory sensitivity and sound analysis, which seem to constitute a chain of successive approximations leading to the current state of our knowledge. I have been fortunate enough to remain in the mainstream of the events involved for 35 years, even though my attention often wandered to other problem areas. As a consequence, most of the events included are rendered on the basis of firsthand information, in agreement with the spirit of this volume. Those that have proved themselves to be productive are emphasized; some others are mentioned because of the germinal controversies they stirred up before being discarded. The latter are used sparingly, however, so as not to obscure the main developmental process of auditory biophysics. This process is still in vigorous progress, and the chapter does not end until the most recent insights have been mentioned.

In spite of species differences, the mammalian ear shows substantial fundamental uniformity. Perhaps the greatest deviations from it are exhibited by echolocating animals, such as bats. These animals have specializations adapted for reception and extremely fine analysis of high-frequency sounds above the range of audibility for other mammals. Such specializations are beyond the scope of this chapter, which is focused on the human ear, although ears of common laboratory animals, such as domestic cats and guinea pigs, often have to be used as its models.

For the purpose of convenient reference, Section B describes the functional anatomy of the ear and introduces the main functions performed by its various parts. Section C concerns the sound transmission and analysis in the auditory part of the inner ear – the cochlea; Section D, the mechanoacoustic function of the middle ear; and Section E, the overall sound transmission in the ear. This order may appear illogical, since it goes counter to the direction of sound propagation. However, the function of the middle ear depends and is contingent upon the mechanical input properties of the inner ear, and the acoustics of the outer ear is affected in turn by the input properties of the middle ear.

If sound originated in the cochlea, its transmission to the ear canal would depend on the properties of the middle ear, which would be determined in part by the properties of the outer ear, and the order of consideration of the various parts of the ear would have to be reversed. It has been discovered recently that such an event can actually take place when the cochlea is stimulated by a short pressure pulse or sound burst – it emits an echo (KEMP 1978; KEMP and CHUM 1980).

B. Functional Anatomy

The gross anatomy of the human ear according to a classical drawing by BRÖDEL (1946) is shown in Fig. 1. To the left, the convoluted shape of the auricle, or pinna,

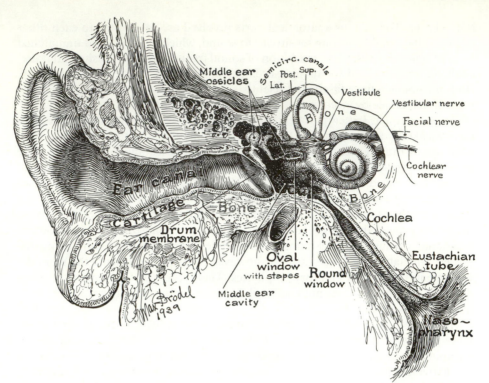

Fig. 1. Gross anatomy of the human outer, middle, and inner ear, including the proximal portion of the ear canal. Brödel (1946)

is easily recognizable. The concha, its deepest portion which can be discerned at the entrance to the ear canal, has an important acoustic function exerted through its cavity resonance. A similar effect at a somewhat lower sound frequency is produced by the ear canal, which is a somewhat irregular, rather narrow tube closed at its proximal end by the highly flexible tympanic membrane. The distal part of the ear canal, like the concha, is surrounded by cartilage and is somewhat flexible. The proximal part has bony walls and is extremely sensitive to touch. Both the pinna and the ear canal show strong interspecies variations that seem at least in part to reflect functional adaptations.

The tympanic membrane separates the outer ear from the system of middle ear cavities and is connected to the malleus, the first of three middle ear ossicles that transmit the vibration of the tympanic membrane to the inner ear. The middle ear cavities control the sound transmission through the middle ear to a degree that is often underestimated. For instance, in small mammals, the air entrapped in them provides most of the stiffness that is measured at the tympanic membrane, the stiffness of the latter by itself being almost negligible. In humans and other large mammals the air-filled space behind the tympanic membrane is enlarged by the system of interconnected pneumatic cells of the temporal bone. A small part of this system is visible in Fig. 1 above the proximal part of the ear canal. Its effect is to improve sound transmission at low sound frequencies. The middle ear cavities are con-

nected to the nasopharynx by the Eustachian tube that provides pressure equaliz-
ation, but is closed most of the time and has no direct effect on sound transmission.

The ossicles of the middle ear – the malleus, incus, and stapes, constitute a
mechanically refined lever system essential for effective sound transmission from
the air-filled ear canal to the fluid-filled inner ear. In humans and many other mammals the ossicles are connected by firm but somewhat flexible joints, the joint between the malleus and incus being much firmer than that between the incus and
stapes. In rodents the malleus and incus tend to be fused together, and the flexibil-
ity of the incudostapedial joint appears to be highly variable. A common feature
of the various ossicular chains appears to be that they oscillate around their points
of gravity during sound transmission. This motion is insured in part by the system
of ligaments attaching the ossicles to the bony walls of the middle ear cavities.

The vibration of the ossicles is regulated to some extent by two small muscles,
the tensor tympani and the stapedius, the first attached to the malleus and the second to the stapes. Both muscles are capable of providing great tension with minimal contraction, and have antagonistic orientation but are synergistic in decreasing the mobility of the ossicular chain when contracted (for review see Møller
1974).

Acoustically, the inner ear communicates with the middle ear through two
openings, the oval and round windows. The stapes is embedded in the former and
held in place by the narrow annular ligament, its foot plate occupying most of the
window space. The oval window is located at the vestibule, a cavity that serves as
a point of departure for three semicircular canals and together with them contains
sensory organs that signal accelerations and positions of our heads rather than the
presence of sound. It seems to be an accident of evolution that the spirally wound
cochlea, which does respond to sound, also opens into the vestibule. This response
is made possible by the presence and location of the round window that is covered
by a thin membrane and serves for compensation of volume displacements produced by the stapes foot plate in the oval window. Because the lymphs filling the
inner ear spaces are practically incompressible, hardly any motion of the stapes
would be possible without such compensation.

The cochlear canal, whose outer walls consist of hard bone, is divided longitudinally by the membranous cochlear duct into scalae vestibuli and tympani, as
shown in Fig. 2 (Rasmussen 1943). The division is not complete, since the two
scalae communicate through the helicotrema, a sizeable opening at the cochlear
apex. As their names suggest, scala vestibuli opens into the vestibule and scala tympani into the tympanic cavity of the middle ear, this through the round window.
The cochlear duct itself forms the scala media, separated from the scala vestibuli
by the thin Reissner's membrane, and from the scala tympani in part by the spiral
bony lamina with the spiral limbus and in part by the rather thick basilar membrane that supports the organ of Corti. The spiral lamina is wide at the cochlear
base, near the round window, and becomes gradually narrower toward the
cochlear apex. As the width of the lamina decreases, that of the basilar membrane
increases.

The transduction of mechanical signals into electrochemical ones takes place
in the organ of Corti (see Davis's chapter in this volume), which contains three
rows of sensory outer hair cells and one row of sensory inner hair cells (shaded)

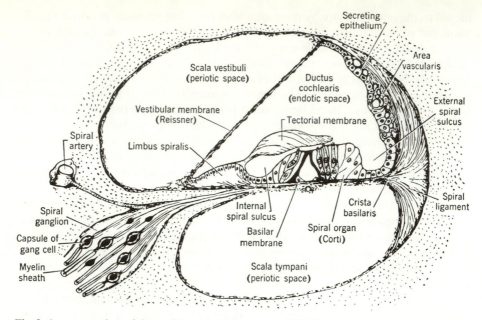

Fig. 2. A cross section of the cochlear canal. RASMUSSEN (1943)

in addition to nerve endings, supporting cells, and the stiff arches of Corti (shaded dark). Over the organ of Corti is suspended the tectorial membrane, which is anchored at the spiral limbus and attached to the organ of Corti by the stereocilia, or hairs, of the outer hair cells and by other microvilli. Its size increases considerably from the cochlear base to the apex.

The scalae vestibuli and tympani are filled with perilymph, similar to the cerebrospinal fluid. The scala media contains endolymph resembling in its ionic content the intracellular fluid. From the point of view of sound propagation in the cochlea, both lymphs may be regarded as similar to water.

C. Mechanics of the Cochlea

I. Early History

The interest in cochlear mechanics originated in pitch perception and musical scales as well as their physical correlates. As early as the sixth century B. C., Pythagoras observed relations between musical intervals and the lengths of strings. In particular, he determined that halving the length of a string produced an octave interval. He was aware of the fact that longer strings vibrated at a lower rate than shorter strings, but does not seem to have put the quantitative relation between the frequency of vibration and pitch together (cit. BORING 1942). This was discovered somewhat accidentally by Galileo one millennium later. He found that pitch did not depend directly on the length of a string but rather on the frequency of its vibration. His pupil Mersenne determined the relationships between the physical parameters of a string – such as its thickness, weight, and tension – and its vibration frequency. In their studies, Galileo and Mersenne seem to have applied the phenomenon of resonance, which was described formally about a hundred years later by John Willis (cit. BORING 1942).

The study of vibrating strings led to the discovery of overtones, or partials, by the observation that, through resonance, vibration of a short string could make a string that was twice or three or more times as long vibrate in parts. The lowest natural vibration frequency of a string was called the "fundamental," or "first harmonic," and the multiples of this frequency, its "higher harmonics." In the first quarter of the nineteenth century, Fourier (1822; cit. BORING 1942) formalized the harmonic relations and showed that vibration patterns of any form can be decomposed into their harmonics.

Just before the half-way mark of the same century, Ohm (1843; cit. BORING 1942) made the germinal observation that the ear functions as a Fourier analyzer and decomposes complex sounds into their sinusoidal components. This observation with some modifications is still valid, and is known as the auditory Ohm's law.

Simultaneously with the development of the physics of sound, progress was being made in the anatomy of the ear. It was known already in the seventeenth century that sound was conducted from the tympanic membrane through the middle ear ossicles to the bony labyrinth of the inner ear. The anatomical techniques of the time did not allow a study of its membranous contents, however. Even so, the cochlea was regarded as the organ of hearing, and Du Vérney (cit. VON BÉKÉSY and ROSENBLITH 1948) ascribed to it the capacity of sensing pitch. Knowing of the relations between the length of strings and vibration frequency and of the resonance phenomenon, he attributed resonance properties to the osseous spiral lamina. Since the lamina is relatively wide at the cochlear base and becomes gradually narrower toward the cochlear apex, Du Vérney thought that the lamina resonated with low frequencies at the base and with high ones at the apex. In the nineteenth century, on the basis of much more complete knowledge of cochlear anatomy, this order was reversed.

II. Von Helmholtz's Resonance Theory and Its Early Antagonists

When, at the beginning of the second half of the nineteenth century, von Helmholtz took up the study of hearing, the state of knowledge of the physics of sound, of some auditory effects, and of the anatomy of the ear was ready for synthesis into a comprehensive theory. VON HELMHOLTZ (1863) achieved it in his classic *Die Lehre von den Tonempfindungen als physiologische Grundlage für die Theorie der Musik* (On the Sensation of Tone as a Physiological Basis for the Theory of Music), adding many observations of his own. At the center of his theory was the resonance theory of auditory sound analysis, which incorporated Ohm's law, the physical phenomenon of resonance, the anatomy of the cochlea, and an extension of Johannes Müller's (1826; cit. BORING 1942) doctrine of specific nerve energies. On more solid ground than Du Vérney, he concluded that the only known physical system capable of implementing Ohm's law was a set of resonators tuned to different frequencies within the audible frequency range. The already known graded growth of the dimensions of the organ of Corti toward the cochlear apex, especially that of the outer rods of Corti, induced von Helmholtz to hypothesize at first that the latter acted as the resonators (cit. WEVER 1949). They appeared as more solid structures than the other parts of the organ, their length increased toward the cochlear apex, and they seemed to be innervated by the cochlear nerve fibers. However, additional anatomical knowledge revealed that the basilar membrane, whose width increased much more along the cochlea than the height of the rods of Corti, contained radial fibers resembling piano strings, and von Helmholtz became persuaded that the basilar membrane fibers rather than the rods of Corti acted as the resonators. Since the fibers were not entirely independent of each other but were embedded in the tissue of the basilar membrane, von Helmholtz envisaged that a whole region of the membrane responded to any particular sound frequency, but the maximum of vibration coincided with the fiber optimally tuned to that frequency. The amplitude distribution depended on the damping of the fibers, which von Helmholtz attempted to calculate on the basis of psychophysical evidence.

Since every sound frequency was expected to produce a vibration maximum at a different location of the cochlea, von Helmholtz's theory became classified later on as "place theory." The place principle in itself became perhaps more important than the resonance mechanism invoked to account for it, since it required an extension of Johannes Müller's doctrine of specific nerve energies. It was known that the cochlear nerve fibers were distributed over the length of the cochlea, so that it seemed plausible to conclude that every discriminable sound frequency stimulated maximally a different nerve fiber. Von Helmholtz postulated that subjective pitch was determined by which fiber was the most excited.

At this point, Hensen's (1863; cit. BORING 1942) influence on von Helmholtz's resonance theory should be acknowledged. It was he who made measurements of cochlear microstructures and showed that the width of the basilar membrane varied much more than the length of the outer rods of Corti. Hensen also studied sensory hairs in hearing sacs of crustacea and observed that they resonated with particular sound frequencies. This led him to conclude that the cilia of the cochlear hair cells might act as resonators. Because of their small size, this possibility was not taken seriously for over a century, but recent indirect evidence suggests that Hensen may have been partially right after all.

Appealing as von Helmholtz's resonance theory appeared from the point of view of auditory sound analysis, it ran into difficulties with respect to the persistence of auditory sensations. Since the analysis is astonishingly fine, it requires sharply tuned resonators. In turn, such resonators have low damping and long transient times at the onset and termination of physical sound. However, the subjective sensation of sound was observed to grow and terminate nearly as rapidly as its physical cause. The apparent paradox and other considerations led to a host of nonresonance theories in the last part of the nineteenth century, some of them attempting to preserve the place principle, others completely abandoning it. Extensive reviews of these were undertaken by BORING (1942) and WEVER (1949). Here only those that may be considered physically reasonable and have exerted considerable influence on further developments are mentioned.

The most radical departure from any resonance or even place theory was achieved by Rutherford (1886; cit. WEVER 1949), who assumed that the basilar membrane responded to every audible sound over its entire length, vibrating like a telephone diaphragm. In this way the wave form of sound was faithfully transmitted to every hair cell, and sound analysis was ascribed entirely to the nervous system. If the basilar membrane had the consistency of a sufficiently stiff plate, such a motion would be possible indeed; however, the vibration amplitude would be very small and the efficiency of the system low.

A more probable pattern of basilar membrane vibration was advocated by Ewald (1898; cit. ZWISLOCKI 1948) on the basis of model experiments. His model consisted of a thin rubber membrane stretched over a conical slit and immersed in water. When tuning fork vibration was transmitted to the model, a pattern of standing waves could be observed on the membrane. As the vibration frequency increased, the wavelengths became shorter and more waves appeared. Although physically quite plausible, the theory never gained in popularity because it had difficulties in explaining the analysis of complex sounds and the observation of hearing loss over narrow frequency ranges. It should be added that Ewald's model was not dimensionally similar to the cochlea.

TER KUILE (1900) proposed a crude traveling wave theory (cit. WEVER 1949), the details of which were physically questionable but which, in its basic concept, seems to come the closest to the modern view. He suggested that inward motion of the stapes produces a downward bulge of the basilar membrane, which he endowed with apparently nonlinear stiffness properties. The further the stapes is pressed inward, the greater becomes the extent of the bulge in the apical direction. When the motion of the stapes is reversed, the front of the bulge continues to travel toward the apex, but the extent of the bulge decreases from the side of the trailing edge. Finally, the bulge completely disappears before reaching the apical end of the cochlea. The higher the vibration frequency of the stapes, the shorter the distance over which the bulge is able to travel. Pitch is determined by this distance. Whereas the traveling front of the bulge appears physically plausible, it is difficult to see the basis for the assumption that the trailing edge catches up with it.

The most surprising aspect of all the nineteenth-century theorizing is the fact that none of the proposed hypotheses predicted the basilar membrane vibration actually observed in the next century.

III. Fundamental Experiments of von Békésy

As improvements in the compound microscope enabled the anatomists of the nineteenth century to study the fine structure of the cochlea and opened the way for von Helmholtz's theory, the development of electronic devices in the twentieth century made direct observation of sound propagation in the cochlea possible. The first man to undertake it, and the only one to do so over a time span of almost 40 years, was Georg von Békésy, a Hungarian physicist. His interest in hearing seems to have been awakened by his research on telegraph systems at the Royal Hungarian Institute for Research in Telegraphy, and was to last for the rest of his lifetime.

Von Békésy began his work on the cochlea in the late 1920s with dimensional models about four times the natural size. They represented highly simplified structures, adapted specifically for the study of the motion of the basilar membrane and

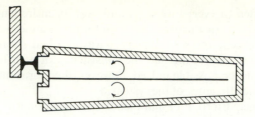

Fig. 3. A simplified hydrodynamic model of the cochlea. Von Békésy (1960)

of the fluid that surrounds it. A schematic drawing of one of them representing a straightened-out cochlea and consisting of a rather long canal divided in the middle by a simple partition is shown in Fig. 3 (von Békésy 1928). The partition was made out of a thin metal sheet containing a narrow slit of variable width and a separate round opening next to the wide end of the slit. The slit was covered by a rubber membrane mimicking the basilar membrane, and the round opening represented the helicotrema. The Reissner's membrane, the organ of Corti, and the tectorial membrane were omitted on the assumption that they did not control the basilar membrane motion.

The fundamental advantage of von Békésy's generic model over that of Ewald's was that its dimensions were roughly proportional to those of the cochlea, and an attempt was made at replicating the elastic properties of the basilar membrane. For this purpose von Békésy cleverly resorted to Wittmaack's (1917) observation on guinea pigs that a strong tone was capable of perforating the basilar membrane. The location of perforation depended on sound frequency, being near the stapes for high frequencies and near the helicotrema for the low ones. He changed the thickness of the model membrane until he could reproduce the perforations at the correct locations.

When a tone produced by an electromechanically driven tuning fork was delivered to the model through its oval window, von Békésy (1928, 1960) saw its basilar membrane vibrate in a pattern he did not expect (see Fig. 10, top). He described it in the following words: "The portion of the membrane from the stapes to the place of resonance vibrates almost completely in the same phase. At the place of resonance there appears a phase reversal, and from here on waves arise that with a uniform rubber membrane become progressively smaller in wavelength." Apparently, von Békésy thought that the vibration maximum was due to a resonance effect. "Uniform" should be interpreted as smoothly changing rather than constant.

With the help of suspended carbon powder, von Békésy was able to observe the motion of the water solution of glycerine with which his model was filled. The glycerine increased the viscosity of the fluid to make it comparable with the perilymph viscosity which he measured. The most striking feature of the fluid motion was an eddy on each side of the model membrane. Its close association with the vibration maximum made it a convenient indicator of the maximum's location, and von Békésy used it as such in later experiments. Because the vibration maxima in the models were broad and did not account for the sharp sound analysis in the ear, a possible role of the eddy as a mechanical stimulus for the auditory receptors became a subject of speculation. However, von Békésy thought that the main sharpening action of the cochlear filter was provided by the nervous system through contrast effects, like those first demonstrated by MACH (1864) in vision. Such a sequential sound analysis seemed compatible with psychophysical experiments suggesting a high damping of cochlear resonators.

Von Békésy's model experiments, although much more sophisticated than preceding ones, would hardly have had the impact on auditory science they did had they not been followed by direct microscope observations of the motion of the Reissner's and basilar membranes in preparations of human cochleae. By carefully grinding away the cochlear apex, he succeeded in making the two membranes visible over about one-third of their lengths without damaging them. Since both are almost completely transparent, he made them visible by letting some carbon or aluminum dust settle on them. After the dust had settled the cochlea was filled with saline with similar mechanical properties to those of perilymph. Observation of the membranes revealed that they moved together in phase, performing a wave motion like that seen in the models past the vibration maximum. When the sound frequency was increased sufficiently, no motion could be detected, and von Békésy concluded that the maximum of vibration must have moved further toward the stapes; in other words, that its location was frequency-dependent. The dependence was in agreement with von Helmholtz's hypothesis. Von Békésy had the impression that the damping of the cochlear waves was at least as strong as in his models, and this view prevailed for almost 40 years.

The model experiments and the preliminary observations of the basilar membrane motion were followed by over ten years of preparations for more systematic experiments on postmortem specimens of human and other mammalian cochleae. They produced an astounding number of refined preparation, stimulation, and observation techniques.

In the first experiments of the series VON BÉKÉSY (1941 a) determined the static properties of the human cochlear partition, which he identified with the cochlear duct. He found that the basilar membrane was not under tension, and had about the same stiffness in the longitudinal and radial directions. By closing the helicotrema, he could produce a static pressure differential across the partition, and succeeded in visualizing the displacements of both the Reissner's and basilar membranes. In this way he was able to determine both the compliance of the partition and the form of its deformation. In human specimens the compliance increased exponentially from the cochlear base to its apex by about two orders of magnitude, and seemed to be controlled almost entirely by the basilar membrane, although brushing aside the "gelatinous mass" overlaying the basilar membrane increased the compliance by a factor of two. Analogous measurements were made on several mammalian species ranging from mouse to elephant, and VON BÉKÉSY (1944, 1960) found a similar variation of compliance in all of them, although its absolute value decreased as the size of the animal increased (Fig. 4). By probing with fine hairs, VON BÉKÉSY (1947) confirmed his impression that the basilar membrane was the stiffest of all the structures of the cochlear partition and effectively controlled its compliance.

Having measured the static compliance of the partition, VON BÉKÉSY (1942) moved on to determine the dynamic properties of the cochlea. Because they have bearing on the understanding of mechanical processes within the cochlea, he first

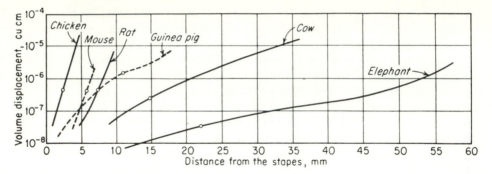

Fig. 4. Compliance of cochlear partition measured in postmortem preparations from animals of several species, and expressed in terms of volume displacement caused by pressure equivalent to that of 1 cm water. Note that the compliance increases by about three orders of magnitude between the stapes and the apex. VON BÉKÉSY (1960)

pursued its input properties. More specifically, he measured the amplitude and phase of the volume displacement of the round window membrane for a constant sound pressure at the oval window. The cochlear fluids being practically incompressible, this volume displacement is equal to that of the stapes or of the perilymph adjacent to it. As a consequence, von Békésy measured indirectly the acoustic input impedance of the cochlea, which is defined as the ratio between the sound pressure and the volume velocity. The latter is obtained when the volume displacement is multiplied by the angular frequency associated with it. Acoustic impedance is used nowadays as a standard expression of the input properties of acoustic systems. Some of the measurements were performed with the middle ear intact, and the sound pressure monitored at the tympanic membrane. Under these conditions the results reflected the properties of the whole mechanical system of the ear. In other measurements the ear was dismantled part by part – first the middle ear apparatus was taken out, then the stapes, and finally the membrane of the round window, leaving only the cochlea with its fluids. In the latter condition the impedance increased in approximately direct proportion to sound frequency and was controlled by the mass of the fluid, except at low frequencies, where friction predominated (Fig. 5). This result is inconsistent with the result von Békésy obtained with the stapes in place and was later shown to be faulty. Nevertheless, it established the order of magnitude of the input impedance of the human cochlea.

In his systematic way, VON BÉKÉSY (1942) studied the cochlear sound propagation by means of improved mechanical models and direct experimentation. In models, he found that drastic changes in the configuration of the cochlear canals had little effect on the location of the vibration maximum of the model basilar membrane. Only when one of the canals was made extremely shallow did the maximum move somewhat toward the stapes. The same was true when the viscosity of the fluid was increased. When fluid was removed completely on one side of the membrane, the maximum moved slightly toward the stapes, but the eddy accompanying it was preserved in the remaining fluid. This was true even when most of the fluid was eliminated from the model, leaving only a short column at the location of the vibration maximum. From these observations von Békésy concluded

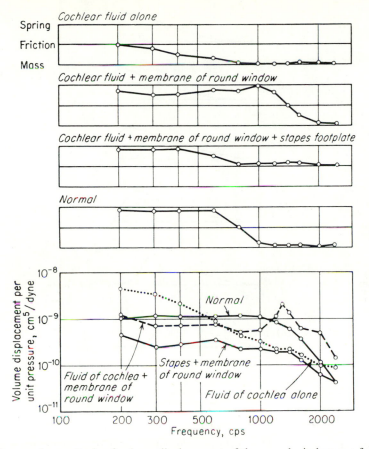

Fig. 5. Phase and magnitude of volume displacement of the round window as a function of sound frequency for a constant sound pressure at the tympanic membrane (*Normal*), stapes, or oval window, as the more distal parts of the ear were successively removed. Measurements made on a postmortem preparation of human cochlea. Note that cochlear fluid alone has the properties of a fricative resistance at low frequencies and of a mass at higher frequencies. VON BÉKÉSY (1960)

that the location of maximum vibration and of the eddy depended only on local conditions in the vicinity of the membrane. Of course, it depended critically on the elastic properties of the membrane.

One of the most startling findings was a complete lack of dependence of the location of the maximum on the place in the outer wall of the model through which vibration was introduced. In later experiments VON BÉKÉSY (1955) proved that even introducing the sound at the helicotrema end of the model did not change the mode of the membrane vibration, although the waves were forced to travel toward rather than away from the sound source. He called such waves paradoxical, and performed many experiments attempting to elucidate their nature. The stability of the vibration pattern explains the stability of our pitch perception, and especially why the pitch is the same whether sound is transmitted through the outer ear or the skull

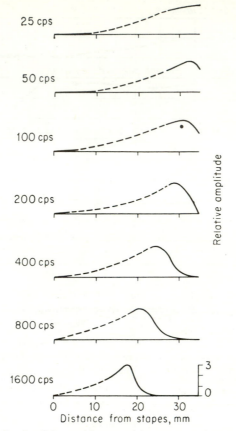

Fig. 6. Vibration amplitude of the cochlear partition measured on postmortem preparations of human cochleae for various sound frequencies as a function of the distance from the stapes. *Solid lines* indicate observation from the scala vestibuli, *dashed lines* from the scala tympani. VON BÉKÉSY (1960)

bones. VON BÉKÉSY (1932) had demonstrated this stability more directly beforehand, rendering a sound transmitted through the skull inaudible by canceling it with a sound of the same frequency delivered through the ear canal.

The model experiments had told von Békésy what to look for in the cochlea and, when he felt that he had enough preliminary information, he undertook direct microscopic studies of sound propagation in preparations of human temporal bones. The main body of observations was undertaken by gradually grinding away portions of the cochlea from the apex side and revealing successively more distant portions of the cochlear partition. From the apical end it is not possible to observe directly the basilar membrane without destroying the Reissner's membrane, and VON BÉKÉSY (1942, 1943) had to content himself at first with the observation of the latter. Another difficulty was introduced by the high sound pressures he had to use, which are known to cause distortions and damage to cochlear tissues. However, he found that the vibration amplitude of Reissner's membrane was within the linear range.

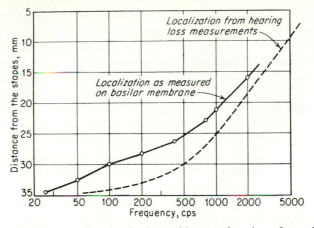

Fig. 7. Location of maximum vibration in the cochlea as a function of sound frequency, as measured directly in postmortem preparations of human cochleae (*solid line*) and as inferred from hearing loss measurements and their correlation with cochlear damage. VON BÉKÉSY (1960)

His most important findings may be summarized as follows. A pure tone produces one vibration maximum on the cochlear partition, and its location depends on sound frequency, as von Helmholtz had predicted (Fig. 6). More quantitatively, it parallels the functional relation between the frequency of maximum hearing loss and maximum damage to cochlear structures (Fig. 7). However, the maximum is rather broad and cannot by itself account for the fine frequency analysis the human ear is capable of. Therefore, further sharpening of frequency analysis in the nervous system is required, as had been suggested by VON BÉKÉSY (1928) earlier. The broad maximum is consistent with high damping determined independently by studying transient vibrations. Phase measurements show that the maximum is not produced by simple resonance, as von Helmholtz had assumed, but arises in the presence of waves that travel from the oval window toward the helicotrema with an ever-decreasing velocity and, therefore, decreasing wavelength. The waves are damped out before reaching the helicotrema at sound frequencies greater than 100 Hz. In VON BÉKÉSY's (1947) words: "These facts, taken together, clearly indicate that we are not dealing with a simple resonance but with traveling waves, whose wavelength becomes shorter as the frequency increases, and which pass by the point of measurement." The wave pattern is shown in Fig. 10, third item from the top.

What mechanism produced the maximum did not appear clear to VON BÉKÉSY (1960), since even in 1960 he wrote: "From the first observations of the vibrations of the cochlear partition it was clear that they represented a system about which physical science provided little knowledge and that many years would be required to understand it clearly ... This task is still incomplete."

IV. Understanding Cochlear Waves

When proposing his resonance theory, von Helmholtz committed a cardinal error by not including the appropriate mechanical coupling between the cochlear partition and the liquid that surrounds it. His resonators seem to vibrate as if surrounded by compressible air whose mass is negligible, although he did admit their possible loading by the liquid. If a single vibrating string is immersed in water, its natural frequency is lowered somewhat and its damping increased. These effects are not dramatic because the thin string does not displace a substantial amount of water. However, when the same is done with a membrane or a light, thin plate, the effect is much greater, due to the relatively large volume of water that has to be brought into motion. Water and its close relative perilymph have a large density, or mass taken per unit volume, and are practically incompressible in comparison to air. As a consequence, motion of membranes and light plates immersed in them depends critically on the effects of the water and perilymph. Perhaps KUCHARSKI (1930) was the first to recognize this fact and to include the hydrodynamic theory in his mathematical treatment of cochlear mechanics. Unfortunately, he assumed unrealistically high values for the stiffness and mass of the cochlear partition. As a consequence, the effects of the perilymph became minimized, and his calculations led to a vibration pattern more closely related to that postulated by von Helmholtz than to that seen by von Békésy. Kucharski's theory was followed with one year's delay by the first of RANKE's (1931) hydrodynamic theories, in which a more realistic assumption was made with respect to the compliance of the cochlear partition. However, Ranke made other unrealistic assumptions and, through flawed mathematical treatment, arrived at a standing wave pattern which not only disagreed with VON BÉKÉSY's (1928) model experiments preceding the theory but which appears physically impossible (e.g., ZWISLOCKI 1948, 1953b). An improved mathematical treatment of cochlear hydrodynamics was given by RANKE (1942) over ten years later, but even in this one he used mathematical solutions leading to physically impossible fluid motions (e.g., ZWISLOCKI 1948, 1953b). Between the two theories of Ranke appeared another one that clearly missed its target. In it (REBOUL 1938) devoted special attention to the fact that the cochlear canal becomes narrower toward the cochlear apex, and neglected the variation in the compliance of the cochlear partition. As faulty as they were, these early theories deserve mention because they attracted attention to the important role of hydrodynamics in cochlear sound propagation.

In general, transversal waves on the cochlear partition belong formally to the class of interface waves, of which waves on the surface of water are an example. The waves arise due to interaction between the inertia of a liquid and an elastic or gravitational restoring force acting on its surface. The elastic force in the cochlea arises from the stiffness of the cochlear partition; waves on the surface of an ocean are subject to gravitational force. All interface waves are governed by three physical laws. The first of them, often called "law of continuity," requires that the amount of an incompressible fluid flowing into a given space be equal to the amount of the fluid flowing out of that space. The second law is borrowed from Newton and states that the force required to accelerate a free object at a given rate is proportional to the mass of the object.

According to the third law, the force produced by the moving fluid on its surface must be balanced out by the restoring force generated there. The mathematical form of the law depends on the specific conditions prevailing at the surface. For this reason, it appears most straightforward to refer it directly to the conditions in the cochlea. The surface of interest is the cochlear partition, whose elastic properties are well approximated by those of the basilar membrane (VON BÉKÉSY 1947). The remaining surface consists of rigid walls, the helicotrema opening, and the oval and round windows. For the mathematical treatment of sound transmission in the cochlea, we can assume that the rigid walls do not move, and the wave motion does not reach the helicotrema except at very low sound frequencies, as VON BÉKÉSY (1943, 1947) was able to demonstrate. According to VON BÉKÉSY's (1942) model experiments, the conditions at the two windows do not affect the form of cochlear waves. This can also be demonstrated theoretically (ZWISLOCKI 1953 a).

Through investigation of static deformation of the basilar membrane, VON BÉKÉSY (1941 a) demonstrated that it bends like a plate rather than a stretched membrane. In an elastic plate the restoring force is directly proportional to the second power of the curvature of the plate's deformation. Since the basilar membrane is very narrow, it is reasonable to assume that the curvature in the radial direction is much greater than in the longitudinal one, so that the elastic restoring force depends only on the local deformation, irrespective of the wave pattern, as long as the half-wavelength remains larger than the width of the basilar membrane. This assumption was made in nearly all mathematical treatments of cochlear mechanics. It has been strengthened by measurements of cochlear wavelengths performed by VON BÉKÉSY (1947) and KOHLLÖFFEL (1972 a), which show that the wavelength is always considerably greater than the width of the basilar membrane. Recently, VOLDŘICH (1978) demonstrated in fresh preparations that the basilar membrane is much stiffer in the radial than in the longitudinal direction. The assumption means that longitudinal coupling within the basilar membrane can be neglected and the only coupling between its adjacent parts is provided by the fluid.

In addition to stiffness, the basilar membrane has some mass of its own and is loaded with the masses of the organ of Corti and the tectorial membrane, which produce an inertia force when the membrane is accelerated. Motion of the membrane also generates friction leading to a resistive force. The sum of all these force components must be equal to the force produced on the membrane by the surrounding lymphs.

The classical and fundamentally most accurate mathematical description of sound propagation in the cochlea consists of finding equations describing the transversal waves on the basilar membrane and the fluid motion on both sides of the membrane, which simultaneously satisfy the continuity and the Newtonian equations, as well as the boundary conditions at the membrane and the rigid walls. RANKE (1942, 1950) and some others later on took this path. Unfortunately, the problem is mathematically difficult and no exact solution has been found as yet. Because of necessary drastic simplifications, the accuracy of the approximate solutions appears questionable (e.g., GEISLER 1976; ZWEIG et al. 1976).

KUCHARSKI (1930), REBOUL (1938), myself (ZWISLOCKI 1946, 1948), and many others afterward resorted to a simplification permissible as long as the wavelength is considerably greater than the depth of the canal. As has been mentioned above, Kucharski's and Reboul's treatments were unrealistic, in part due to lack of empirical information. At the time I took up the problem in early 1946, many essential results of von Békésy's experiments had already become available, but not the cochlear wave pattern itself. Nevertheless, the wave patterns von Békésy had seen

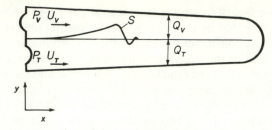

Fig. 8. A schematic representation of the straightened-out cochlea used in the derivation of the cochlear differential equation. The symbols have the following meanings: Q_V, Q_T, cross-sectional areas of scalae vestibuli and tympani; $Q_V dx$, $Q_T dx$, fluid elements of scalae vestibuli and tympani; P_V, P_T, local sound pressures in the scalae; U_V, U_T local longitudinal fluid velocities; S, displacement velocity of the cochlear partition (positive upward). ZWISLOCKI (1980a)

on his models suggested that the wavelength was sufficiently large. In addition, von Békésy's measurements of the compliance of the basilar membrane and of its damping were available. This information, together with the knowledge of gross cochlear anatomy, allowed me to derive a simplified differential equation of cochlear waves and to solve it approximately (ZWISLOCKI 1946, 1948). The equation with various modifications has been used ever since, in spite of some more or less justified criticisms it has encountered. Until recently, it provided the only means of making truly quantitative comparisons between the theoretical and empirical results, and of interpolation and extrapolation of the latter. It revealed some inconsistencies in experimental data.

The equation is obtained by applying the law of continuity to the entire cross-sectional areas of scalae vestibuli and tympani, shown in the schematic drawing of the cochlea in Fig. 8. In this configuration the difference between the inflow of the fluid into a space element dx and its outflow must be equal to the volume displacement velocity, or simply volume velocity, of the basilar membrane. When the wavelength is sufficient, the velocity of fluid flow throughout the cross section, Q, is uniform, so that the difference between the inflow and the outflow is equal to $Q_T \dfrac{\partial U_T}{\partial x} dx$ in scala tympani and to $Q_V \dfrac{\partial U_V}{\partial x} dx$ $= -Q_T \dfrac{\partial U_T}{\partial x} = S$ in scala vestibuli, where S is the volume velocity of the basilar membrane. By combining this modified law of continuity with the remaining two laws, a differential equation of the following form is obtained for sinusoidal vibration:

$$\frac{\partial^2 \Delta P(x)}{\partial x^2} = \frac{i 2\pi f \varrho}{Z_p(x)} \frac{Q_V(x) + Q_T(x)}{Q_V(x) \cdot Q_T(x)} \Delta P(x). \tag{1}$$

The symbols have the following meanings: $\Delta P(x)$, the amplitude of pressure difference across the basilar membrane; $\dfrac{\partial^2 \Delta P(x)}{\partial x^2}$, the second derivative of the pressure difference with respect to the x coordinate placed lengthwise parallel to the membrane; $Q_V(x)$ and $Q_T(x)$, the cross-sectional areas of scalae vestibuli and

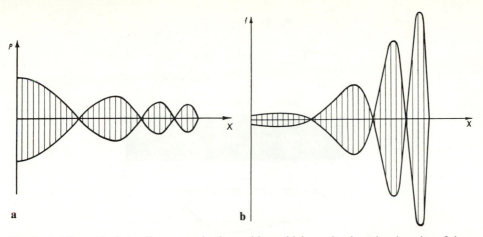

Fig. 9a, b. Theoretical standing waves in the cochlea, which result when the viscosity of the fluid and the viscosity and mass of the cochlear partition are omitted in the calculation. **a** pressure difference (p) across the partition; **b** displacement (f) of the partition. ZWISLOCKI (1948)

tympani, which depend on the distance x from the oval window; ϱ the density of cochlear lymphs; f, sound frequency; i, imaginary unit ($\sqrt{-1}$); and $Z_P(x)$, the acoustic impedance of the basilar membrane per unit of its length, defined as the ratio between the pressure difference across the membrane and the membrane's volume velocity per unit of length $\left(\dfrac{\Delta P(x)}{S(x)}\right)$. The impedance is controlled by the compliance, mass, and resistance of the membrane according to the following equation:

$$Z_P = \frac{\Delta P}{S} = i\left(2\pi f \frac{M}{b^2} - \frac{1}{2\pi f C}\right) + \frac{R}{b^2}. \tag{2}$$

The symbols ΔP and S have been defined; b, M, and R mean the effective width and mechanical mass and resistance of the basilar membrane; C is its compliance referred to its volume displacement. Remember that VON BÉKÉSY (1941 a) measured the compliance C directly; he found it to vary by a ratio of about 1 to 200 from the stapes to the helicotrema in a human cochlea. Note also that the mass M and resistance R may be expected to grow with the distance from the stapes because the dimensions of all the structures associated with the basilar membrane grow. However, the terms M/b^2 and R/b^2 should remain nearly constant because the width b of the basilar membrane also increases. The numerical values of these constants were estimated from anatomical dimensions, known densities, and VON BÉKÉSY'S (1943) damping measurements.

When the differential equation was solved for the pressure difference $\Delta P(x)$ across the basilar membrane (ZWISLOCKI 1946), a pressure wave resulted whose amplitude and wavelength decreased with the distance from the oval window (Fig. 9a). The theoretical finding that the pressure had no amplitude maximum along the cochlea was surprising at first and not predictable from von Békésy's observations. It meant that no sound analysis would take place in the cochlea if the

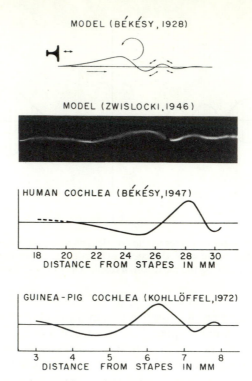

Fig. 10. Traveling waves observed in models and postmortem preparations of mammalian cochleae. *From the top:* wave drawn by von Békésy according to his early model observations; photograph of a wave seen on a model with a somewhat more compliant partition; wave reconstructed from von Békésy's magnitude and phase measurements in a postmortem preparation of human cochlea; and wave reconstructed from Kohllöffel's magnitude and phase measurements in a postmortem preparation of guinea pig cochlea. ZWISLOCKI (1974)

pressure was the adequate stimulus for the sensory cells. It follows from the definition of basilar membrane impedance that the membrane's volume displacement can be determined by dividing the pressure difference by the impedance and sound frequency multiplied by 2π. In the first solution of the differential equation the mass M and resistance R were neglected, and a standing displacement wave resulted whose wavelength decreased but whose amplitude increased with the distance from the oval window, in spite of decreasing amplitude of the pressure difference (Fig. 9b; ZWISLOCKI 1948). Maximum amplitude occurred at the helicotrema. When the resistances stemming from internal friction in the cochlear partition and from fluid viscosity were reintroduced, a traveling wave resulted exhibiting a single amplitude maximum whose location depended on sound frequency in the same way as had been seen by von Békésy in the cochlea. Since the mathematical solution did not include the mass of the basilar membrane, the theory showed that the maximum can arise without any resonance but through an interaction between the variable compliance and the resistance of the basilar membrane. The phenomenon has the following physical basis. Beginning at the basal end of the cochlea,

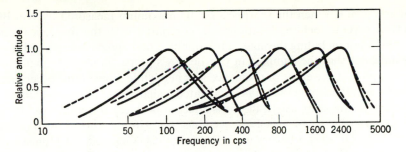

Fig. 11. Displacement amplitude as a function of sound frequency measured by VON BÉKÉSY (1943) at several locations of the cochlear partition in a postmortem preparation (*solid lines*) and analogous functions calculated by me without including the mass of the partition. VON BÉKÉSY and ROSENBLITH (1951)

the amplitude increases with distance, due to increasing compliance of the basilar membrane. As the wave progresses toward the helicotrema, the fricative resistance gradually converts its mechanical energy into heat. The greater the amplitude of motion, the faster is the conversion. Finally, the energy loss is so great that the amplitude begins to decrease in spite of continually increasing compliance. An amplitude maximum results whose location is determined by the relation between the stiffness (reciprocal of compliance) and resistance effects. Since the effect of the former decreases as sound frequency increases, the maximum moves closer to the oval window, where the stiffness is greater. In this way, always the same balance between the resistance and the stiffness effects is maintained.

The phenomenon of an amplitude maximum without resonance was confirmed by means of a simple mechanical model consisting of a canal covered with a light rubber membrane of variable width and, therefore, compliance (ZWISLOCKI 1946). The mass of the membrane was negligible. A wave pattern photographed on the model is shown in Fig. 10 (second from top). Note the difference between this pattern and the pattern described by VON BÉKÉSY (1928) on the basis of his early model experiments. Whereas in the latter the partition seems to vibrate in phase up to the amplitude maximum, this is not true in the former. Subsequently, VON BÉKÉSY (1947) found in the cochlea the theoretically predicted pattern, as is shown by the third entry in the figure. The same pattern was found much more recently by KOHLLÖFFEL (1972a), as is evident from the diagram at the bottom of the figure (for review see ZWISLOCKI 1974). Thus it was established first theoretically, then experimentally, that a traveling wave occurs in the cochlea on both sides of the maximum. Now this is taken for granted.

In a subsequent, more extensive study (ZWISLOCKI 1948), I was able to demonstrate theoretically that, even when the mass of the cochlear partition is included, the amplitude maximum cannot coincide with the location of the partition's resonance, but must occur closer to the oval window. This also is now generally accepted by all those knowledgeable in the physics of cochlear waves. The greater the damping of the partition, the further away is the amplitude maximum from the location of resonance. With a sufficient damping the maximum becomes so far removed from the resonance that the latter, and with it the mass of the partition, become irrelevant. When the sharpness of the maximum measured by VON BÉKÉSY (1943) at several cochlear locations was compared with the theoretical one obtained without including the mass, a reasonably good agreement resulted (Fig. 11). This indicates that the damping in von Békésy's preparations of human cochleae was so high that the effect of resonance was negligible. Since some other measurements of VON BÉKÉSY's (1944, 1947) indicated a sharper amplitude maximum, several theoreticians emphasized the mass effect of cochlear partition (e.g., PETERSON and BOGERT 1950; FLETCHER 1951; see GEISLER 1976 for review). As indicated by several theoretical approaches (e.g., BOGERT 1951; GEISLER and HUBBARD 1971; ZWEIG et al. 1976), the mass effect accompanied by lower damping increases the sharpness of the maximum, especially toward the higher frequencies. Nevertheless, the fundamental nature of cochlear waves remains unchanged, except that, from the resonance point on toward the apex, no wave propagation takes place, as was shown theoretically (ZWISLOCKI 1948) and confirmed experimentally (RHODE 1971). Past the resonance location, the basilar membrane moves with a constant phase and a rapidly decaying amplitude. Unfortunately, the amplitude is so small at the resonance location that the experimental demonstration of the phenomenon is difficult.

In the biological sciences we tend to give so much more credence to experimental findings than to theoretical results that we often disregard the latter entirely. For this reason it appears of some interest to mention a few key instances in which the theory was right and the experiments incorrect. Of course, a scientific theory must rely on primary experimental data, and unless they are correct, the theory cannot be. In general, my theory of 1948 agreed well with von Békésy's classical observations on the cochlea, and I regarded it as an explanation of the phenomena he had discovered. This was particularly true for the amplitude maximum in the presence of traveling waves, whether the mass of the cochlear partition was included or not. However, in two fundamental instances the experiments and the theory diverged.

As already mentioned, VON BÉKÉSY (1942) found that, after removal of the stapes and of the round window membrane, the input impedance of the cochlea was mass-controlled, presumably because of the mass of the perilymph. The theory yielded an impedance that, to the first order of approximation, had the properties of a resistance. This may seem intuitively surprising but is in agreement with the general theory of traveling waves. Perhaps the simplest explanation is that the energy imparted to the traveling waves by their source is carried away from the source and becomes lost to the source as if it were converted to heat by a fricative resistance. Later experiments showed that the input impedance of the cochlea is indeed resistive (MUNDIE 1963, MØLLER 1965; NEDZELNITSKY 1980).

The impedance is of key importance for the understanding of middle ear function and for stimulus control. A resistive impedance means that the pressure difference across the basilar membrane and with it the membrane's displacement amplitude increases in direct proportion to sound frequency when the amplitude of stapes displacement is kept constant. VON BÉKÉSY's (1943) "resonance curves" (Fig. 11) were obtained with a constant stapes amplitude. Had he kept instead the displacement amplitude of the basilar membrane in cochlear base constant, no maximum would have occurred. Such a result was obtained in fact by TASAKI et al. (1952) in their study of cochlear microphonics (ZWISLOCKI 1955, 1980). The resistive impedance also means that a rounded, triangular time pattern of stapes vibration is converted to a trapezoidal wave on the basilar membrane. This transformation was utilized in many experiments (e.g., DALLOS et al. 1972; ZWISLOCKI 1974; SOKOLICH et al. 1976). Finally, it means that basilar membrane displacement in the cochlear base must lead the displacement of the stapes by 90°. This was clearly observed by RHODE (1971). It should be noted, however, that the relations are somewhat more complicated at moderately low sound frequencies (TONNDORF et al. 1966; DALLOS 1970), where the cochlear input impedance can no longer be expected to be purely resistive.

Another point of apparent disagreement between von Békésy's experiments and my theory extended to nonlinear hydrodynamic processes (ZWISLOCKI 1948) and concerned the eddy VON BÉKÉSY (1928) had discovered on each side of the cochlear partition at the location of the vibration maximum. According to his observations, the eddy velocity increased in proportion to the vibration amplitude. According to the theory, it should increase in proportion to the square of the amplitude. Subsequently, more systematic experiments of TONNDORF (1958) confirmed the latter relationship.

The main objection to my theory was its restriction to long waves, which was not tenable in the vicinity of the vibration maximum. When I found a way of removing it in my differential equation without introducing undue simplifications (ZWISLOCKI 1953a), no fundamental effect on the theoretical wave pattern resulted. However, very recently it became clear that the vibration maximum is sharpened and wave reflection in its vicinity prevented (ZWISLOCKI 1983).

In spite of the few differences between the experimental results and the theoretical predictions, the nature of cochlear waves appeared to be reasonably well understood in the mid 1950s. In particular, the flat amplitude maximum of basilar membrane vibration seemed to be widely accepted, and efforts began to be made to explain how the sharp auditory sound analysis can be achieved in its presence. VON BÉKÉSY (1960) was suggesting neural inhibition and directional sensitivity of hair cells to vibration (VON BÉKÉSY 1951, 1953) as possible factors. He obtained direct evidence for the latter. These suggestions did not prevent much erratic speculation and experimentation until, from the research of the 1970s, a strongly modified picture of cochlear mechanics emerged.

V. The Live Cochlea

Just before the 1970s began, B. Johnstone and his co-workers introduced the Mössbauer technique to the measurement of basilar membrane vibration (JOHNSTONE and BOYLE 1967; JOHNSTONE and TAYLOR 1970). A thin, radioactive foil of small surface area is placed on the basilar membrane, and the emitted gamma rays are absorbed in a collector and counted. The collector acts as a narrow-band filter mistuned somewhat relative to the wavelength of the gamma rays. As the basilar membrane vibrates, moving toward and away from the collector, the wavelength is modulated, and with it the amount of energy absorbed in the collector. From the modulation, the amplitude and phase of the basilar membrane vibration can be derived. The Mössbauer technique makes measurements on live animals possi-

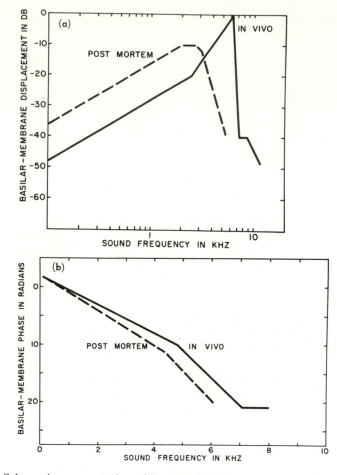

Fig. 12 a, b. Schematic representation of RHODE's (1973) measurements of **a** the amplitude and **b** the phase of basilar membrane displacement in squirrel monkey cochleae in vivo and post mortem. ZWISLOCKI (1980b)

ble, but has the drawback that only a few selected locations of the basilar membrane can be investigated. As a consequence, sound frequency rather than distance from the oval window has to be used as the independent variable.

The measurements of Johnstone and his associates performed on live guinea pigs revealed a substantially sharper filter action, or tuning, of the basilar membrane than had been found by von Békésy in postmortem preparations. The initially controversial results were soon confirmed by more extensive measurements of RHODE (1971) performed on live squirrel monkeys. KOHLLÖFFEL (1972b), using a laser method, and RHODE (1973) found the probable cause of the discrepancy between the results obtained on live and dead animals. Soon after death the vibration maximum of the basilar membrane began to become smaller and to shift toward lower sound frequencies. At the same time, the vibration amplitude at lower frequencies increased, and the wavelength decreased. These results are summarized

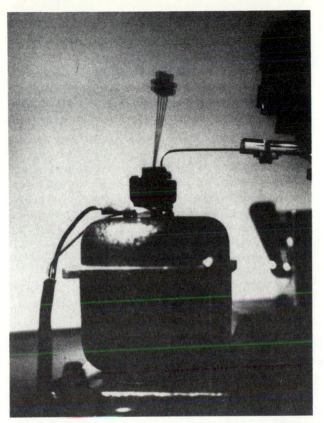

Fig. 13. A simple qualitative model of a short section of the basilar membrane with the organ of Corti and elastically attached tectorial membrane. It consists of a vibrator with a flexible reed attached at a slight angle to its armature and loaded with a small mass. The bent rod to the right of the vibrator is the fiber optic probe of the Fotonic Sensor measuring the vertical vibration. Note that the amplitude of the transversal reed vibration photographed in stroboscopic light is much larger than the vertical vibration amplitude of the vibrator armature. ZWISLOCKI (1980)

by a schematic representation in Fig. 12 (ZWISLOCKI 1980b). Interpreted in terms of the theory of cochlear mechanics, they indicate an increased damping and compliance of the basilar membrane.

RHODE's (1971) measurements revealed a nonlinearity in basilar membrane vibration. Near the vibration maximum the vibration amplitude increased less rapidly than in direct proportion to sound pressure. As a consequence, the sharpness of the maximum increased as sound pressure decreased. Because of experimental limitations, Rhode could not use sound pressures near the threshold of audibility, but KHANNA and LEONARD (1982) and SELLICK et al. (1982) achieved this feat and found the basilar membrane maximum, or tuning, to be nearly as sharp as that of the fibers of the cochlear nerve (e.g., KIANG 1965). Somewhat earlier, RUSSELL and SELLICK (1977, 1978) had shown that the receptor potentials of the inner hair cells are as sharply tuned as the fibers. This abolished the need for neural sharpening

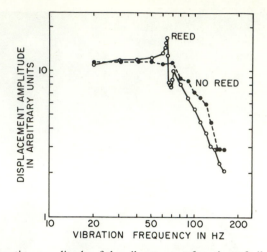

Fig. 14. Vertical vibration amplitude of the vibrator as a function of vibration frequency in the absence of the reed (*intermittent line*) and in its presence. Note the sharp peak and dip produced by the reed vibration at nearly a right angle to the vibrator motion. Zwislocki (1980b)

of cochlear frequency analysis, and the question of a sharpening mechanism interposed between the inner hair cells and the basilar membrane became controversial. Three facts speak in favor of such a mechanism, however. In the alligator lizard the cochlear hair cells and nerve fibers are reasonably sharply tuned in the absence of any tuning of the basilar membrane (Weiss et al. 1976; Peake and Ling 1980). The best neural tuning curves are substantially steeper than their best counterparts on the basilar membrane. Finally, the detailed shape of the basilar membrane characteristics appears to reflect a complicated micromechanical system in the organ of Corti, which may be expected to exert a sharpening effect (Zwislocki 1980b).

The latter deduction results from the following considerations. The measured amplitude and phase characteristics of live cochleae cannot be accounted for simultaneously by theories assuming a simple system for the basilar membrane, consisting of a compliance, mass, and resistance (e.g., Sondhi 1978; Viergever 1980). These characteristics can be explained, however, when a second mass is coupled elastically to the first (Zwislocki 1980b). It is likely that this mass consists of the tectorial membrane and the main coupling of the stiff stereocilia of the outer hair cells (Zwislocki 1980b). The system envisaged can best be explained with the help of a simple mechanical model, as shown in Fig. 13. It consists of an armature suspended elastically over a magnet and driven electrodynamically. The armature represents a short section of the basilar membrane with the organ of Corti. To it is affixed at a slight angle a flexible reed loaded at its tip with a small mass. They represent a short section of the tectorial membrane coupled elastically to the organ of Corti. When the system is driven by sinusoidal current of increasing frequency, the reed vibrates vertically together with the armature until the vicinity of its transversal resonance frequency is reached. Then it undergoes strong transversal vibration, the amplitude of which may be much greater than the vertical amplitude of

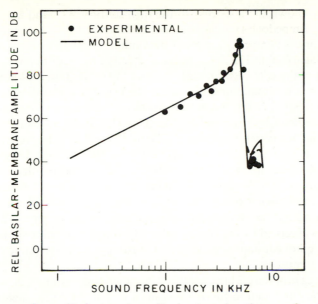

Fig. 15. Basilar membrane displacement amplitude at one location as a function of sound frequency for a constant displacement amplitude of the stapes. *Circles,* RHODE's (1971) data; *curve* calculated with the help of a mathematical model that includes a radial resonance of the tectorial membrane attached elastically to the organ of Corti. ZWISLOCKI and KLETSKY (1982)

the armature. Clearly, a strong filter effect is introduced and suggests that a similar effect could occur in the cochlea if the stereocilia tectorial membrane system were capable of transversal resonance. Just below the resonance frequency the reed strongly enhanced the vertical vibration of the armature and decreased it at the resonance frequency itself, producing a peak followed by a notch, as shown in Fig. 14. A similar pattern is evident in basilar membrane vibration, as was demonstrated by RHODE (1971, 1980), and LE PAGE and JOHNSTONE (1980). One set of Rhode's data is shown by filled circles in Fig. 15. The solid and dashed curves have resulted from theoretical calculations with slightly different parameter values. A resonating stereocilia-tectorial membrane system was assumed (ZWISLOCKI and KLETSKY 1982). A sharp peak followed by a notch is visible in both the experimental and theoretical results. Although these similarities are suggestive, the micromechanical processes in the cochlea await much further experimentation. Nevertheless, it appears evident that the mechanical processes in a live cochlea are more complex than in a dead one.

D. Mechanics of the Middle Ear

I. The Beginnings of Understanding

Because of their accessibility, some parts of the middle ear were discovered before the labyrinth of the inner ear. The tympanic membrane and the tympanic cavity were already known to the Greeks of the fifth century B.C. and were described in particular by Empedocles (cit. WEVER and LAWRENCE 1954). Not knowing the rest of the auditory system, they regarded the tympanic cavity as the seat of hearing. Although Galen (about 175 A.D.) became aware of the auditory nerve, and moved the seat of hearing centralward, real progress in the anatomical knowledge of the middle ear was not made until the sixteenth century. According to WEVER and LAWRENCE (1954), it is not clear who discovered the larger two middle ear ossicles, but they were described in detail by VESALIUS (1543). INGRESSA (1546) found the stapes and the two cochlear windows. The middle ear muscles were discovered by EUSTACHIUS (1564) and VAROLIUS (1591) (cit. WEVER and LAWRENCE 1954). Eustachius also became aware of the tube connecting the middle ear cavities with the nasopharynx, which carries his name. On the basis of the newly acquired anatomical knowledge, COITER (1566) traced the path of sound from the tympanic membrane through the ossicles to the inner ear. In the seventeenth century this pathway was accepted by DuVerney, who added to it a possible sound-amplifying effect of the outer ear and speculated on the tuning of the tympanic membrane by the middle ear muscles.

As in the case of the cochlea, we trace the beginning of our modern understanding of middle ear function to VON HELMHOLTZ [1863 (1885); 1868]. He saw the middle ear structure as a transformer increasing the transmission of acoustic energy from the light and highly compressible air to the relatively heavy and almost incompressible fluids of the middle ear. He envisaged three fundamental mechanisms: two increasing the force at the expense of the amplitude of motion, and one increasing the pressure without affecting the force or amplitude of motion. The first mechanism was assumed to result from the curvilinear shape of the tympanic membrane, and to convert the changes in this shape to a highly increased force on the manubrium of the malleus. Von Helmholtz had tried to test his hypothesis experimentally, but his experiment proved to be incorrect and it could not be confirmed (WEVER and LAWRENCE 1954). Although TONNDORF and KHANNA (1972) attempted to resuscitate von Helmholtz's hypothesis, the success of their effort appears questionable. The second mechanism was assumed to result from the difference in length between the manubrium of the malleus and the long process of the incus acting on the stapes. Although von Helmholtz did not know exactly the mode of motion of the ossicles on which the resulting lever ratio depends, the fundamental mechanism is still accepted with some modifications. According to its modern version, the malleus and incus rotate around a common axis nearly perpendicular to the plane going through the two processes, and the resulting lever ratio is smaller than one, so that the force exerted by the incus on the stapes is larger than the force produced on the tip of the manubrium by the sound acting on the tympanic membrane. Finally, von Helmholtz's third mechanism results from the ratio of the surface areas of the tympanic membrane and the stapedial foot plate. For a constant force equal to the product of pressure and surface area, the pressure acting on a surface must be inversely proportional to its area. Since the surface area of the stapedial foot plate is much smaller than the surface area of the tympanic membrane, the sound pressure acting on the latter should be enhanced many times in the cochlea. This transformer mechanism seems to be by far the most important, although von Helmholtz erroneously emphasized the first one. In any event, it is

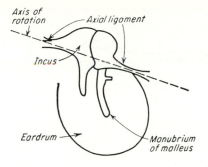

Fig. 16. Schematic drawing of the tympanic membrane and the two larger middle ear ossicles with the axis of their rotation marked by the *intermittent line*. The axis goes through the major ligamental attachments of the ossicles and through their point of gravity. VON BÉKÉSY (1960)

clear that the middle ear does act as a transformer and a substantial hearing loss ensues, when it is missing.

Many experiments on middle ear preparations and models followed von Helmholtz's publications. Two pieces of work deserve especial attention because of their relevance to contemporary research. O. FRANK (1923) came to the conclusion that the large ossicles, malleus, and incus should tend to oscillate around their point of gravity, which he determined. By letting the ossicles oscillate in this way, he was able to measure their effective mass, which was considerably smaller than the static mass.

In a different and more direct study, DAHMAN (1929, 1930) was able to determine the mode of motion of the tympanic membrane and of the ossicles with the help of little mirrors attached to them. Oscillatory rotation of a mirror produced oscillation of a reflected light beam, and the amplitude of this oscillation determined the magnitude of angular motion. For the tympanic membrane, Dahman found that the angular motion was by far the greatest near its rim, so that the amplitude of motion must have decreased rapidly there. The central portions of the membrane, including the tip of the manubrium, oscillated with nearly constant amplitude. This was not in agreement with von Helmholtz's curved membrane hypothesis but was consistent with subsequent, more accurate experiments of VON BÉKÉSY (1941 b). As for the large ossicles, Dahman found them to oscillate around an axis that goes through the short process of the incus and the anterior process of the malleus (Fig. 16). The axis passes close to the center of gravity of the ossicles and is in agreement with VON BÉKÉSY's (1941 b) observations. With reference to it, the lever ratio between the manubrium of the malleus and the long process of the incus amounts to about 1.3:1 in the human ear. In small mammals it can be substantially larger (WEVER and LAWRENCE 1954). Both the axis and the magnitude of the lever ratio are still regarded as valid.

II. Experiments on Postmortem Preparations

It is not possible to study the motions of various parts of the human middle ear directly on live people. Therefore, many postmortem experiments have been per-

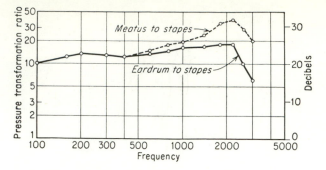

Fig. 17. Pressure transformation between the tympanic membrane, or the entrance to the ear canal, and the stapes, when the stapes is fixed. Measurement made on a human postmortem preparation. Von Békésy (1960)

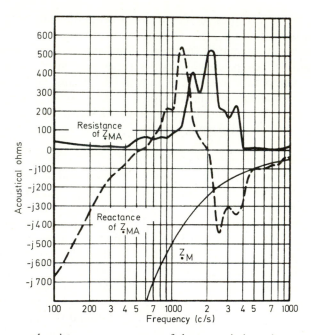

Fig. 18. Reactance and resistance components of the acoustic impedance measured at the tympanic membrane, which are contributed by the system of middle ear cavities. Onchi (1961)

formed. As in the case of the cochlea, von Békésy (1936, 1941 b, 1960) contributed some of the most fundamental information. In a crucial experiment he measured the pressure transformation between the tympanic membrane and the oval window. For this purpose, he opened and emptied the cochlea and placed a small probe microphone in front of the stapes foot plate. Sound was delivered to both the tympanic membrane and the cochlear space, the amplitude and phase of the latter being so adjusted that the stapes stood still. Were all the ossicles and the tym-

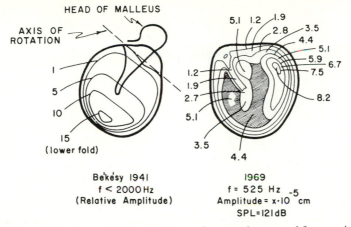

Fig. 19. Patterns of vibration of the tympanic membrane at low sound frequencies, as determined on human cadaver ears by von BÉKÉSY (1941 b) (*left*) and TONNDORF and KHANNA (1972). TONNDORF and KHANNA (1972)

panic membrane rigidly attached to each other, they would have been immobilized, the effects of their masses and elastic attachments would have been eliminated, and the measurement would have yielded the ideal, frequency-independent transformer effect. Because the attachments are not entirely rigid and the tympanic membrane is highly flexible (e.g., TONNDORF and KHANNA 1972), this is not exactly true, and the transformer effect determined by von Békésy and shown in Fig. 17 is somewhat frequency-dependent. The peak near 2,000 Hz and the following drop suggest a resonance effect in the tympanic membrane loaded by the large ossicles. The intermittent line refers to sound pressure measurement at the entrance to the ear canal and includes the effect of a quarter-wave resonance in the canal.

Von Békésy also measured in postmortem preparations with cochlear fluids present or absent the amplitude of stapes displacement as a function of sound frequency for a constant sound pressure at the tympanic membrane. His results are not mutually consistent, however, and only vaguely agree with similar measurements performed later on (ANDERSEN et al. 1962, 1963; FISCHLER et al. 1967). ON-CHI (1961) found in extensive middle ear experiments a transmission characteristic exhibiting a maximum near 1,000 Hz. He also measured the sound pressure in the ear canal at the tympanic membrane and in the tympanic cavity for various surgically induced conditions of human cadaver ears. From these measurements he derived the acoustic impedance at the tympanic membrane and the contributions of various middle ear parts to it. In particular, he found that the contribution of the tympanic membrane itself was very small, in agreement with an earlier study of von BÉKÉSY's (1936). His determination of the effect of the middle ear cavities on the impedance (Fig. 18) was unique and became useful in a subsequent analysis of the function of the human middle ear, even though the pneumatization of the temporal bone in the specimen he used was considerably smaller than average. Since the middle ear cavities cannot be expected to change much after death, these characteristics ought to hold approximately for live ears. Indeed, subsequent measurements on such ears have been found to be consistent with them.

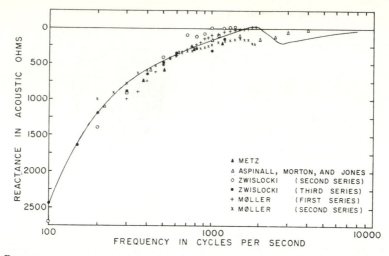

Fig. 20. Reactance component of the acoustic impedance measured at the human tympanic membrane in several studies, and as obtained by means of an electrical network analog of the middle ear (*solid curve*). ZWISLOCKI (1962)

VON BÉKÉSY (1941 b) attempted to determine the mode of vibration of the tympanic membrane and found it to move as a nearly rigid plate suspended flexibly at its oval rim and including the manubrium of the malleus. The motion was consistent with the oscillation of the ossicles around their point of gravity, so that the anteroinferior part of the membrane vibrated with the greatest amplitude, as shown on the left side of Fig. 19. It is not clear how detailed von Békésy's measurements of the vibration pattern were, but the more refined experiments of TONN-DORF and KHANNA (1972) performed with laser interferometry revealed a somewhat different pattern, as is evident on the right side of the figure. The dark and light fringes show constant vibration amplitudes and demonstrate that the manubrium of the malleus moves less than the tympanic membrane around it.

As useful as the experiments on postmortem preparations have been in giving us an insight into the mode of operation of the middle ear, the accumulated evidence shows that their quantitative results do not hold for the live middle ear. The most apparent effect of death is a highly increased acoustic impedance measured at the tympanic membrane (ZWISLOCKI and FELDMAN 1964; GUINAN and PEAKE 1967). As a consequence, experiments on live ears become of paramount importance.

III. Human Middle Ear In Vivo

The human middle ear cannot be disassembled in vivo and studied part by part. Its only reasonably accessible part is the tympanic membrane, even though it is located at the end of the long and somewhat tortuous ear canal. Therefore, practically all experiments on live human middle ears have concerned acoustic impedance measurements at the tympanic membrane; that is, measurements of the ratio between the sound pressure at and the volume velocity of the tympanic membrane.

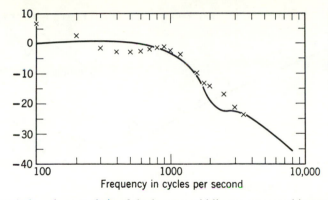

Fig. 21. Transmission characteristic of the human middle ear expressed in terms of the volume displacement of the stapes for a constant sound pressure at the tympanic membrane. The *curve* has been obtained by means of the network analog; the *crosses* are derived from ONCHI's (1961) measurements on cadaver ears. ZWISLOCKI (1965)

The early measurements of the 1930s were motivated in part by the needs of the telephone industry, but in the 1940s METZ (1946) pioneered their application to diagnosis of middle ear disorders.

It occurred to me that the mechanoacoustic function of the normal middle ear could be determined from acoustic impedance measurements at the tympanic membrane with the help of known middle ear pathologies that simplify the middle ear system. For instance, when strong adhesions practically immobilize the ossicles, the measured impedance depends entirely on the compliance of the tympanic membrane and the acoustics of the middle ear cavities. Separation between the incus and the stapes eliminates the effects of the stapes and the cochlea, etc. The analysis was performed using the theories of electroacoustic analogies and of electrical networks (ZWISLOCKI 1957b, 1962). It allowed the determination of the interactions among the various parts of the middle ear in sound transmission and of the transmission characteristic of the human middle ear shown in Fig. 21 (ZWISLOCKI 1965, 1975). The indirect determinations were validated by comparing theoretical predictions to empirical data. The comparisons are illustrated in Fig. 20 for the reactive impedance component at the tympanic membrane and in Fig. 21 for the transmission characteristic. It should be noted that the experimental data of Fig. 21 were obtained after death, and the agreement applies only to the general shape of the functions. The same type of analysis was performed for the guinea pig ear where many more comparisons were possible (ZWISLOCKI 1963). As an example, Fig. 22 shows the theoretical and experimental transmission characteristics, both for live animals.

The instrumentation used for acoustic impedance measurements in the ear prior to the 1950s was too awkward and imprecise for systematic investigations. Therefore, I was forced to develop my own. Two instruments working on entirely different principles proved useful. The first utilized the principle of a high impedance source and was implemented by means of an earplug containing two narrow tubes, one leading to an earphone and one to a microphone (ZWISLOCKI 1957a). This type of instrument is now used routinely in clinical tests (see for review FELD-

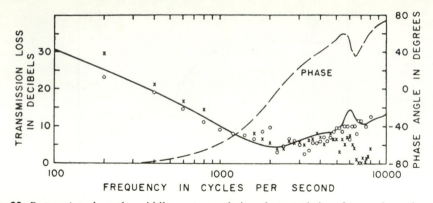

Fig. 22. *Data points* show the middle ear transmission characteristics of two guinea pigs obtained with the help of cochlear microphonics measured in the basal turn of the cochlea. The microphonics may be regarded as approximately proportional to the sound pressure across the basilar membrane. The *solid curve* shows corresponding magnitude values obtained on the electrical analog. The *intermittent curve* indicates the accompanying phase values. The measured values shown by *crosses* depart from the theoretical values at high frequencies and, according to more recent measurements, are not typical. ZWISLOCKI (1963)

MAN and WILBUR 1976). The second consisted of a radically modified Schuster bridge (for review see ZWISLOCKI and FELDMAN 1970).

Because of the involvement of ear pathology in the fundamental work on the middle ear, this work was rapidly adapted to clinical tests (ZWISLOCKI and FELDMAN 1970). Eventually, new procedures based on effects of static pressure changes in the ear canal were added (TERKILDSEN and NIELSEN 1960; for review see FELDMAN and WILBUR 1976).

IV. Animal Experiments

Many aspects of middle ear function that cannot be determined directly on humans may be investigated on anesthetized animals. So, for instance, WEVER et al. (1948 a) investigated the sound transmission through the middle ear by measuring cochlear microphonics. They also confirmed von Békésy's observation that a pressure differential across the tympanic membrane decreases the sound transmission (WEVER et al. 1948 b). This work was reviewed together with the work of others by WEVER and LAWRENCE (1954). They added some improved measurements of the transfer characteristic and of the ossicular lever ratio in the cat, finding it to be of the order of 2.5:1.

A different approach to the study of the mammalian middle ear was taken by MUNDIE (1963), who measured the acoustic impedance at the tympanic membrane of the guinea pig ear. By changing the ear surgically he was able to determine the component effects of the middle ear cavities, of the tympanic membrane, of the ossicles, and of the cochlea. Mundie found that the cochlea provided most of the resistive component of the system, thus confirming the earlier theoretical conclusion that its input impedance was essentially resistive (ZWISLOCKI 1948). He also confirmed the earlier observations that the static pressure difference across the tympanic membrane critically affected the mechanical properties of the middle ear. Mundie's experiments provided sufficient information to devise an electrical network analog with a structure corresponding to the anatomy of the guinea pig middle ear (ZWISLOCKI 1963). This theoretical work served to validate the analogous work on the human ear and became a prototype for subsequent analysis of other mammalian middle ears.

More extensive data on input impedance and transfer function were obtained on the cat's ear by MØLLER (1963, 1965) and by GUINAN and PEAKE (1967). Although Møller used a capacitive probe and Guinan and Peake microscopic observation, their results basically agree with each other and are consistent with those of Mundie. Møller found in particular that the input impedance of the cochlea was resistive and that the ossicles moved almost like a rigid body up to 5,000 Hz. He concluded, therefore, that the middle ear system could be approximated by a second-order system, more specifically, a system consisting of a resistance, mass, and compliance connected in series. However, Guinan and Peake found deviations from such a system at high sound frequencies and represented the cat middle ear function by a network analog (PEAKE and GUINAN 1967) consistent with my own for the guinea pig. Both analogs are of higher than second order and allow us to reproduce the details of the middle ear characteristics. The necessity of a higher-order system is made particularly clear by the effects of the coupled cavities of the bulla and of the complex vibration pattern of the tympanic membrane (KHANNA and TONNDORF 1972).

To generalize, the typical mammalian middle ear does function as an acoustic transformer, amplifying the sound pressure in the cochlea relative to the sound pressure at the tympanic membrane (ZWISLOCKI 1975; NEDZELNITSKY 1980) and reducing the effects of the high cochlear input impedance on the acoustic impedance measured at the tympanic membrane. In this way it increases the transfer of energy from the sound waves in the ear canal to the cochlea. The effect is particularly pronounced in the mid-frequency range, where the contribution of the middle ear's own mechanism to the impedance at the tympanic membrane is reduced to a minimum by the system's resonances. When the sound transmission to the cochlea is expressed by the ratio of sound pressures at the cochlear base and the tympanic membrane, the middle ear acts as a rather flat band-pass filter. Its stiffness reduces the transmission of low frequencies and its mass that of the high ones (e.g., ZWISLOCKI 1975). Although many details of the middle ear function still remain to be clarified, its main features seem to be known.

E. General Transmission Characteristic

The main purpose of this short concluding section is to show the amazing mutual adaptation of the various parts of the human ear to produce a nearly flat transmission characteristic for sounds in the most important frequency range for speech intelligibility. In Fig. 23 the partial transmission characteristics from the sound field to the entrance of the ear canal are shown for a listener facing the sound source (upper solid line), from the entrance of the ear canal to the tympanic membrane (intermittent line), and from the tympanic membrane to the cochlear base, the lat-

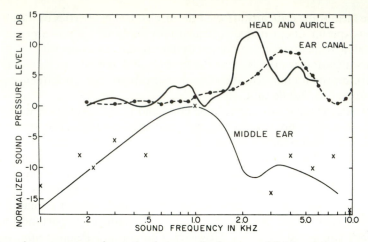

Fig. 23. Sound pressure transformation between the free sound field and the entrance to the ear canal (*upper solid curve*), between the entrance to the ear canal and the tympanic membrane (*intermittent curve*), and between the tympanic membrane and the stapes (*lower solid curve*). The *upper two curves* have been measured directly, the *lowest curve* has been obtained with the help of the network analog. For comparison, the *crosses* show values derived from measurements on human cadaver ears. ZWISLOCKI (1975)

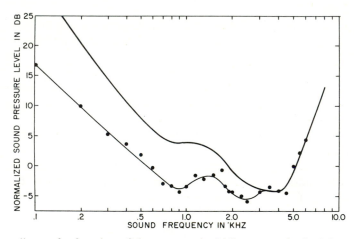

Fig. 24. Overall transfer function of the outer and middle ear synthesized from the curves of Fig. 23 in comparison with the threshold of audibility measured in a free sound field (*upper curve*). The *points* represent calculated values; the *lower smooth curve* is fitted to them by eye. The difference between the two curves must be attributed to neural processes. ZWISLOCKI (1975)

ter derived indirectly (ZWISLOCKI 1975). For comparison, the crosses show postmortem measurements of the middle ear transmission characteristics. Note that the first component characteristic, which is controlled by sound diffraction at the head and a resonance in the concha of the outer ear, has its main peak between 2,000 and 3,000 Hz, just above the high-frequency cutoff of the middle ear. The peak of the transmission characteristic of the ear canal occurs between 3,000 and 5,000 Hz and extends the effect of the former peak toward higher frequencies.

When the decibel values of all three component characteristics are added together, an overall transmission characteristic results that varies by not more than ±3 dB from 500 to 5,000 Hz. It is shown in Fig. 24, with the closed circles indicating the actually calculated values, and the curve interpolating among them and smoothing out some of their variability.

The human ear appears to be a relatively simple and beautiful example of the workings of evolution.

Acknowledgments. I thank Mrs. BETTY ZAHORA for typing and correcting the manuscript, and my wife SUNNY for her help in editing it. The work was supported by NIH grant NS-03950.

References

Names containing *von* are alphabetized in this list under *v*

Andersen HC, Hansen CC, Neergaard EG (1962) Experimental studies on sound transmission in the human ear. Acta Otolaryngol 54:511–520

Andersen HC, Hansen CC, Neergaard EG (1963) Experimental studies on sound transmission in the human ear. Acta Otolaryngol 56:307–317

Bogert BP (1951) Determination of the effects of dissipation in the cochlear partition by means of a network representing the basilar membrane. J Acoust Soc Am 23:151–154

Boring EG (1942) Sensation and perception in the history of experimental psychology. Appleton-Century-Crofts, New York

Brödel M (1946) Three unpublished drawings of the anatomy of the human ear. Saunders, Philadelphia

Dahman H (1929, 1930) Zur Physiologie des Hörens; experimentelle Untersuchungen über die Mechanik der Gehörknöchelchenkette, sowie über deren Verhalten auf Ton und Luftdruck. Z Hals-Nasen-Ohrenheilkd 24:462–497; 27:329–368

Dallos P (1970) Low-frequency auditory characteristics: species dependence. J Acoust Soc Am 48:489–499

Dallos P, Billone MC, Durrant JD, Wang C-Y, Raynor S (1972) Cochlear inner and outer hair cells: functional differences. Science 177:356–358

Feldman AS, Wilber LA (eds) (1976) Acoustic impedance and admittance – the measurement of middle ear function. Williams and Wilkins, Baltimore

Fischler H, Frei EH, Spira D, Rubinstein M (1967) Dynamic response of middle ear structures. J Acoust Soc Am 41:1220–1231

Fletcher H (1929) Speech and hearing. Van Nostrand, New York

Fletcher H (1951) On the dynamics of the cochlea. J Acoust Soc Am 23:637–645

Frank O (1923) Die Leitung des Schalles im Ohr. Sitzungsber Akad Wiss München, vol 53, S. 11–77

Geisler CD (1976) Mathematical models of the mechanics of the inner ear. In: Keidel WD, Neff WD (eds) Handbook of sensory physiology, vol V/3. Springer, Berlin, pp 391–415

Geisler CD, Hubbard AE (1971) A hybrid-computer model of the cochlea. In: Sachs MB (ed) Physiology of the auditory system. National Educational Consultants, Baltimore, Maryland, pp 39–44

Guinan J, Peake WT (1967) Middle ear characteristics of anesthetized cats. J Acoust Soc Am 41:1237–1261

Johnstone BM, Boyle AJF (1967) Basilar membrane vibrations examined with the Mössbauer technique. Science 158:390–391

Johnstone BM, Taylor K (1970) Mechanical aspects of cochlear function. In: Plomp R, Smoorenburg GF (eds) Frequency analysis and periodicity detection in hearing. Sijthoff, Leiden, pp 81–93

Kemp DT (1978) Stimulated acoustic emissions from the human auditory system. J Acoust Soc Am 64:1386–1391

Kemp DT, Chum R (1980) Properties of the generator of stimulated acoustic emissions. Hear Res 2:213–232

Khanna SM, Leonard DGB (1982) Basilar membrane tuning in the cat cochlea. Science 215:305–306

Khanna SM, Tonndorf J (1972) Tympanic membrane vibrations in cats studied by time-averaged holography. J Acoust Soc Am 51:1904–1920

Kiang NY-S (1965) Discharge patterns of single fibers in the cat's auditory nerve, Research monograph 35. MIT Press, Cambridge

Kohllöffel LUE (1972a) A study of basilar membrane vibrations. II. The vibratory amplitude and phase pattern along the basilar membrane (postmortem). Acustica 27:66–81

Kohllöffel LUE (1972b) A study of basilar membrane vibrations. III. The basilar membrane frequency response curve in the living guinea pig. Acustica 27:82–89

Kucharski W (1930) Schwingungen von Membranen in einer pulsierenden Flüssigkeit (Ein Beitrag zur Resonanztheorie des Hörens). Phys Z 31:264–280

LePage EL, Johnstone BM (1980) Basilar membrane mechanics in the guinea pig cochlea. J Acoust Soc Am 67:S45(A)

Lüscher E, Zwislocki J (1947) The decay of sensation and the remainder of adaptation after short pure-tone impulses on the ear. Acta Otolaryngol 35:428–445

Mach E (1864) Über die physiologische Wirkung räumlich verteilter Lichtreize. Sitzungsber. Akad Wiss Wien math-nat. kl. Abt. 2, 57, 11

Metz O (1946) In acoustic impedance measured on normal and pathological ears. Acta Otolaryngol [Suppl] 63

Møller AR (1963) Transfer function of the middle ear. J Acoust Soc Am 35:1526–1534

Møller AR (1965) An experimental study of the acoustic impedance of the middle ear and its transmission properties. Acta Otolaryngol 59:1–19

Møller AR (1974) The acoustic middle ear muscle reflex. In: Keidel WD, Neff WD (eds) Handbook of sensory physiology, vol V/1. Springer, Berlin, pp 519–548

Mundie JR (1963) The impedance of the ear – a variable quantity. In: Fletcher JL (ed) Middle ear function seminar, U.S. Army medical research lab, Fort Knox, Kentucky

Nedzelnitsky V (1980) Sound pressures in the basal turn of the cat cochlea. J Acoust Soc Am 68:1676–1689

Onchi Y (1961) Mechanism of the middle ear. J Acoust Soc Am 33:794–805

Peake WT, Guinan JJ Jr (1967) Circuit model for the cat's middle ear. Quart Prog Rpt 84:320–326. MIT Res. Lab. Electronics, Cambridge

Peake WT, Ling A Jr (1980) Basilar-membrane motion in the alligator lizard: its relation to tonotopic organization and frequency selectivity. J Acoust Soc Am 67:1736–1745

Peterson LC, Bogert BP (1950) A dynamical theory of the cochlea. J Acoust Soc Am 22:369–381

Ranke OF (1931) Die Gleichrichter-Resonanztheorie. Llehmann, Munich

Ranke OF (1942) Das Massenverhältnis zwischen Membrane und Flüssigkeit im Innenohr. Akust Z 7:1–11

Ranke OF (1950) Theory of operation of the cochlea: a contribution to the hydrodynamics of the cochlea. J Acoust Soc Am 22:772–777

Rasmussen AT (1943) Outlines of neuro-anatomy. Brown, Dubuque

Reboul JA (1938) Théorie des phénomènes mécaniques se passant dans l'oreille interne. J Phys Radium 9:185–194

Rhode WS (1971) Observations of the vibration of the basilar membrane in squirrel monkeys using the Mössbauer technique. J Acoust Soc Am 49:1218–1231

Rhode WS (1973) An investigation of postmortem cochlear mechanics using the Mössbauer effect. In: Møller AR (ed) Basic mechanisms in hearing. Academic, New York

Rhode WS (1980) Cochlear partition vibration – recent views. J Acoust Soc Am 67:1696–1703

Russell IJ, Sellick PM (1977) The tuning properties of cochlear hair cells. In: Evans EF, Wilson JP (eds) Psychophysics and physiology of hearing. Academic, London, pp 71–78

Russell IJ, Sellick PM (1978) Intracellular studies of hair cells in the mammalian cochlea. J Physiol 283:261–290

Sellick PM, Patuzzi R, Johnstone BM (1982) Measurement of basilar membrane motion in the guinea pig using the Mössbauer technique. J Acoust Soc Am 72:131–141

Sokolich WG, Hamernik RP, Zwislocki JJ, Schmiedt RA (1976) Inferred response polarities of cochlear hair cells. J Acoust Soc Am 59:963–974

Sondhi MM (1978) Method for computing motion in a two-dimensional cochlear model. J Acoust Soc Am 63:1468–1477

Stevens SS, Davis H (1938) Hearing. Wiley, New York

Tasaki I, Davis H, Legouix JP (1952) The space-time pattern of cochlear microphonics (guinea pig) as recorded by differential electrodes. J Acoust Soc Am 24:502–519

Terkildsen K, Nielsen S (1960) An electroacoustic impedance measuring bridge for clinical use. Arch Otolaryngol 72:339–346

Ter Kuile E (1900) Die Übertragung der Energie von der Grundmembran auf die Haarzellen. Pflügers Arch Ges Physiol 79:146–157

Tonndorf J (1958) Harmonic distortion in cochlear models. J Acoust Soc Am 30:929–937

Tonndorf J, Khanna SM (1972) Tympanic-membrane vibrations in human cadaver ears studied by time-averaged holography. J Acoust Soc Am 52:1221–1233

Tonndorf J, Khanna SM, Fingerhood BJ (1966) The input impedance of the inner ear in cats. Ann Otol Rhinol Laryngol 75:752–763

Viergever MA (1980) Mechanics of the inner ear. Delft University Press, Delft

Voldřich L (1948) Mechanical properties of basilar membrane. Acta Otolarngol 86:331–335

von Békésy G (1928) Zur Theorie des Hoerens: die Schwingungsform der Basilarmembran. Phys Z 29:793–810

von Békésy G (1932) Zur Theorie des Hörens bei der Schallaufnahme durch Knochenleitung. Ann Phys 13:111–136

von Békésy G (1936) Zur Physik des Mittelohres und über das Hören bei fehlerhaftem Trommelfell. Akust Z 1:13–23

von Békésy G (1941a) Über die Elastizität der Schneckentrennwand des Ohres. Akust Z 6:265–278

von Békésy G (1941b) Über die Messung der Schwingungsamplitude der Gehörknöchelchen mittels einer kapazitiven Sonde. Akust Z 6:1–16

von Békésy G (1942) Über die Schwingungen der Schneckentrennwand beim Präparat und Ohrenmodell. Akust Z 7:173–186

von Békésy G (1943) Über die Resonanzkurve und die Abklingzeit der verschiedenen Stellen der Schneckentrennwand. Akust Z 8:66–76

von Békésy G (1944) Über die mechanische Frequenzanalyse in der Schnecke verschiedener Tiere. Akust Z 9:3–11

von Békésy G (1947) The variation of phase along the basilar membrane with sinusoidal vibrations. J Acoust Soc Am 19:452–460

von Békésy G (1951) Microphonics produced by touching the cochlear partition with a vibrating electrode. J Acoust Soc Am 23:29–35

von Békésy G (1953) Shearing microphonics produced by vibrations near the inner and outer hair cells. J Acoust Soc Am 25:786–790

von Békésy G (1955) Paradoxical direction of wave travel along the cochlear partition. J Acoust Soc Am 27:137–145

von Békésy G (1960) Experiments in hearing. McGraw-Hill, New York

von Békésy G, Rosenblith WA (1948) The early history of hearing: observations and theories. J Acoust Soc Am 20:727–748

von Békésy G, Rosenblith WA (1951) The mechanical properties of the ear. In: Stevens SS (ed) Handbook of experimental psychology. Wiley, New York, pp 1075–1115

von Helmholtz HLF (1863) Die Lehre von den Tonempfindungen als physiologische Grundlage für die Theorie der Musik, 1st edn Vieweg, Brunswick 1863: English translation: On the sensations of tone. Dover, New York, 1885, 1954

von Helmholtz HLF (1868) Die Mechanik der Gehörknöchelchen und des Trommelfells. Pflügers Arch Ges Physiol 1:1–60

Weiss TF, Mulroy MJ, Turner RG, Pike CL (1976) Tuning of single fibers in the cochlear nerve of the alligator lizard: relation to receptor morphology. Brain Res 115:71–90

Wever EG (1949) Theory of hearing. Wiley, New York

Wever EG, Lawrence M (1954) Physiological acoustics. Princeton University Press, Princeton

Wever EG, Lawrence M, Smith KR (1948 a) The middle ear in sound conduction. Arch Otolaryngol 48:19–35

Wever EG, Lawrence M, Smith KR (1948 b) The effects of negative air pressure in the middle ear. Ann Otol Rhinol Laryngol 57:418–428

Wittmaack K (1917) Über experimentelle Schallschädigung mit besonderer Berücksichtigung der Körperleitungsschädigung. Beitr Anat Ohr 9:1–37

Zweig G, Lipes R, Pierce JR (1976) The cochlear compromise. J Acoust Soc Am 59:975–982

Zwislocki J (Zwislocki-Moscicki J) (1946) Über die mechanische Klanganalyse des Ohres. Experientia 2:415–417

Zwislocki J (Zwislocki-Moscicki J) (1948) Theorie der Schneckenmechanik. Acta Otolaryngol [Suppl] 72

Zwislocki J (1953 a) Wave motion in the cochlea caused by bone conduction. J Acoust Soc Am 25:986–989

Zwislocki J (1953 b) Review of recent mathematical theories of cochlear dynamics. J Acoust Soc Am 25:743–751

Zwislocki J (1955) The nature of auditory stimuli and their attenuation. Symposium on physiological psychology, ONR report ACR-1. Office of Naval Research, Washington, DC

Zwislocki J (1957 a) Some measurements of the impedance at the eardrum. J Acoust Soc Am 29:349–356

Zwislocki J (1957 b) Some impedance measurements on normal and pathological ears. J Acoust Soc Am 29:1312–1317

Zwislocki J (1962) Analysis of middle-ear function. Part I: Input impedance. J Acoust Soc Am 34:1514–1523

Zwislocki J (1963) Analysis of the middle-ear function. Part II: Guinea-pig ear. J Acoust Soc Am 35:1034–1040

Zwislocki JJ (1965) Analysis of some auditory characteristics. In: Luce RD, Bush RR, Galanter E (eds) Handbook of mathematical psychology, vol 3. Wiley, New York, pp 1–97

Zwislocki JJ (1974) Cochlear waves: interaction between theory and experiments. J Acoust Soc Am 55:578–583

Zwislocki JJ (1975) The role of the external and middle ear in sound transmission. In: Eagles EL (ed) The nervous system, vol 3. Raven, New York, pp 45–55

Zwislocki JJ (1980 a) Theory of cochlear mechanics. Hear Res 2:171–182

Zwislocki JJ (1980 b) Five decades of research on cochlear mechanics. J Acoust Soc Am 67:1679–1685

Zwislocki JJ (1983) Sharp vibration maximum in the cochlea without wave reflection. Hear Res 9:103–111

Zwislocki JJ, Feldman AS (1963) Post-mortem acoustic impedance of human ears. J Acoust Soc Am 35:104–107

Zwislocki JJ, Feldman AS (1970) Acoustic impedance of pathological ears, ASHA monograph 15. American Speech and Hearing Association, Washington, DC

Zwislocki JJ, Kletsky EJ (1982) What basilar-membrane tuning says about cochlear micromechanics. Am J Otolaryngol 3:48–52

CHAPTER 5

Neurophysiology of the Retina

Tsuneo Tomita

A. Introduction

When I was asked to contribute a chapter to this volume, I went through several months of hesitation before I finally made up my mind to accept the assignment. My irresolution stemmed primarily from the suspicion that my career was really not worth writing about.

To begin with, in the Department of Physiology at Keio University, which I entered soon after graduating from Keio Medical School in 1932, I did not produce any significant achievements, nor did I publish anything abroad. In 1940, I was conscripted into the army to serve as an army doctor. When I received my discharge at the end of the war in 1945 and returned to the University, I was already 37 years old. Then three more years went by before I finally began to do vision research in 1948. Thus, because of my lackluster personal history, people often ask me what on earth I did before I reached the age of 40.

However, reflecting on my life and personal experiences before and during the war, I can find several things which make me realize that not everything I did was completely meaningless (with respect to my subsequent work on vision research). Therefore, in the introduction to this chapter I would like to relate some of the circumstances surrounding my life during those years.

Enchanted by the lectures given by Genichi Kato (1890–1979), I decided to study neurophysiology in the Department of Physiology at Keio University. However, my interest at that time was in the techniques of physiology as tools for research rather than in physiology per se. Letting my intellectual curiosity follow its own course, I privately studied electronics, as well as the principles of electric network and transmission lines. In my spare time I tinkered with vacuum tubes and built an amplifier for the Einthoven string galvanometer. Also at that time, I acquired my first gas-filled, low anode voltage (300 V) oscillograph tube, which was manufactured by Western Electric Co., and was similar to the one first used by GASSER and ERLANGER (1922) about ten years earlier. Combining my homemade amplifier with that oscillograph tube, I spent many pleasant days making actual observations of voice waves and the action potential of the toad sciatic nerve.

Gradually, however, my interest turned from the Fourier analysis of voice waves to the idea of synthesizing them. My attempts to synthesize vowels at that time were carried out with a thyratron discharge used to produce damped oscillations in several (usually three) LCR resonance circuits. The natural frequency of each circuit was different, and after being properly damped, the frequencies were combined in an effort to achieve vowel synthesis. Considering the state of the art at the time, the results obtained were a relatively good imitation of natural human vowels. Consequently, several acousticians participated in an actual synthesis demonstration and a symposium broadcast by radio, which expanded my interest to include the auditory mechanism closely related to acoustics.

During this period the international situation became increasingly strained, and in 1940 I was called up for service as an army doctor of the lowest rank. For the first few months I was assigned to an army hospital on the mainland, but as I had not had any clinical experience, it was impossible for me to give the right diagnosis and treatment. Before very long I was transferred to the medical section of an ordnance depot, where my inadequate clinical ability was again called into question. At that point there was a complete change in my situation and I was ordered to work at the Army Institute of Technology in Tokyo.

At the Army Institute I was ordered to carry out research into the masking effect of sound (in connection with developing the technology to differentiate the propeller noise of enemy submarines from the noise of our ships). Before long, however, the tide of the war turned increasingly against Japan, and enemy bombers attacking from the south started to drop acoustic mines which inflicted serious damage on our vessels in the Inland Sea. I was one of the men ordered to participate in the emergency operation to sweep the Inland Sea clear of such mines.

The triggering device was removed from one of the mines that had been dropped on land by mistake; it was sent to the laboratory, where I fashioned a circuit diagram and worked out its operating mechanism. This was not a particularly difficult task for me and I finished the job in no time.

I was ordered to proceed to the local area where the mines were being gathered and to collect materials for establishing some kind of protective countermeasure. I arrived in Hiroshima in late July 1945, and upon arrival of the main squad on

3 August, I moved to a wooden schoolhouse in Hatsukaichi, a small village about 10 km from Hiroshima. Three days later, on 6 August, at 8:15 a.m., the atomic bomb was dropped on Hiroshima. By a space of only three days I escaped death, and had an opportunity of observing the disastrous moment.

On the morning of 6 August, while we were sitting at the table eating breakfast, a blinding flash suddenly illuminated the room. I ran to the window wondering what had happened; when I looked in the direction of Hiroshima I saw a mushroom-shaped cloud billowing up into the sky. Moreover, the mountains that ran along the northern side of the city were straining and undulating. Then I saw that undulation surge toward the mountains that were on our side. The moment it seemed that the undulation had engulfed me, I felt the intense blast from the explosion. In a panic I made a belated effort to hide behind something. The undulation of the mountain range was due to the lens effect produced by the compressed waves of air. The time from the blinding flash to the impact of the blast was about 30 s. During that interval, I observed the growth of that ominous mushroom-shaped cloud and the undulation of the mountains.

Nine days later, the war officially ended. I returned to Tokyo and was discharged from the army. The defeat led me first to despair, then to rouse myself to action. While studying masking effects during the war, I had fully realized the importance of basic research. Thus after the war, I decided that my first research objective would be to study the response pattern of single auditory nerve fibers to sound.

The lack of research facilities and equipment, however, presented a number of problems. There was no hope of finding a soundproof room in Tokyo, as the city had been reduced to ashes and rubble. My three associates (A. Funaishi, H. Mizuno, and Y. Torihama) and I, however, regarded these problems as challenges rather than as insurmountable difficulties.

We fashioned a manipulator for microelectrodes from an old microstage of a microscope; we made amplifiers from junk that we acquired on the black market; we modified the only electromagnetic oscilloscope that we had left so that it could be used for recording purposes; moreover, we obtained an old beat oscillator and an attenuator somehow or other and made them usable for sound stimulation.

Fortunately, at that time there were many stray cats wandering about, which meant that there was never any lack of experimental animals. We applied a stethoscope to a cat and applied sound stimulation through the stethoscope in an effort to reduce the influence of external sound, even if only by a small amount. We also limited our experiments to nights, when there was less external sound.

The experimental setup that I used in those days was extremely incomplete; even so, by inserting a micropipette electrode with a metal needle into the auditory nerve (by means of a handmade micromanipulator fixed to the occipital bone) of the cat, a fairly clean recording of the response of single auditory nerve fibers to sound stimulation was eventually obtained. In particular, the deep emotion that I felt when I clearly observed on the oscillograph the unit discharge from a single nerve fiber synchronized with the very faint tick-tock sound of the wall clock in the next room has left an indelible impression on my mind to this day.

Little did we know, however, that more advanced research based on nearly the same approach had already been carried out in the United States during the war by GALAMBOS and DAVIS (1943). Needless to say, during the war we had not been able to get scientific journals from Europe and the United States. This dearth of information continued for some time after the war. When we learned about the experiment in the United States, we were greatly disappointed, and finally decided to give up any thought of continuing our auditory research.

Subsequently, I intended to pursue olfactory research, using microelectrodes applied to the olfactory bulb. However, it proved difficult to control the stimulation, so I turned to studying the retina and have continued this research to the present day.

Having come this far in my chronicle, I feel for the first time that I am now qualified to talk about vision. However, before I go into the development of the electrophysiology of the retina, I would like to review the history of modern medicine and sensory physiology in Japan, from its late introduction into this isolated country down to the late 1940s, when I started vision research.

B. Physiology in Japan in the Past

I. The Dawn of Modern Medicine and Physiology in Japan

It is no exaggeration to say that modern medicine in Japan began with the Meiji Restoration (1868). Prior to that time the mainstream of Japanese medicine during the Tokugawa Period (1603–1867) had been Eastern (Chinese) medicine. This does not mean, however, that Western medicine was not practiced during the Tokugawa Period, as there existed several medical training academies which had been established under the influence of contact with the West, primarily Holland.

When the Meiji Restoration government was established in 1868, the government decided to adopt the German system for medical education in Japan. As a result of that decision, outstanding graduates of the medical academies were sent abroad, principally to Germany, to study for a period of two years or more. The government also invited German doctors to educate Japanese medical students in the ways of modern medicine. One of the German doctors invited by the government was Ernst Tiegel, who arrived in Japan in 1876. He was put in charge of the lectures on physiology and supervised the experimental research at Tokyo University School of Medicine (which was established by a government ordinance in 1877 as the first national university in Japan).

The first Japanese professor of physiology at Tokyo University was Kenji Osawa (1852–1927), who is regarded as the father of Japanese physiology. In 1866, at the age of 14, he entered the medical training academy in Tokyo, and in 1869 he was one of the 13 students sent by the new government to Europe to study medicine. He entered Berlin University in 1873, where he attended the lectures of Hermann von Helmholtz, Du Bois Reymond, and others, and returned to Japan in 1875. Three years later he again visited Europe, and studied at Strasbourg University. In 1882, at the age of 30, he received his MD and returned home. In the same year he was appointed Professor of Physiology at Tokyo University, replacing Tiegel.

As the textbook for the course he taught on general physiology, Osawa used *Allgemeine Physiologie* by Max Verworn (1863–1921) (VERWORN 1894), who was regarded as the authority on neurophysiology at that time. Osawa was thus instrumental in introducing Verworn's work to Japan, and as a result, many subsequent Japanese physiology students came to study at Verworn's laboratory. This is the primary reason why the mainstream of Japanese physiology has been oriented toward neurophysiology.

Among the many physiologists trained by Osawa were Toshihiko Fujita (1877–1965) and Kunihiko Hashida (1882–1945). Fujita and Hashida were actually brothers; Kunihiko, the younger brother, had his surname changed when he was adopted by the Hashida family at the age of 17. Following his graduation from Tokyo University School of Medicine in 1905, Fujita became one of Osawa's students, as did Hashida when he graduated from the same school in 1908. Since the subsequent paths these two men took are important in tracing the development of sensory physiology in Japan, I would like to describe their careers in some detail below.

1. Toshihiko Fujita (1877–1965)

Sent to Germany by the Japanese government in 1907, during his first year Fujita studied at Berlin University under W. A. Nagel. He then transferred to Freiburg University, where he continued his study of visual physiology under J. von Kries, and returned to Japan in 1910. In 1917 he was appointed Professor of Physiology in the School of Medicine at Tohoku University, which had been founded just a few years earlier. Until the later years of his life Fujita devoted himself to research and education at this institution, and worked arduously to train younger generations of physiology students. Among the many talented physiologists nurtured in Fujita's classroom was Yuji Hosoya (see Sect. B.II.2).

Fujita was a farsighted scholar who emphasized the internationality of research. Soon after he assumed his teaching duties at Tohoku University, he and Toyojiro Kato, a professor of internal medicine, were active in the foundation of the *Tohoku Journal of Experimental Medicine* (1920); both men served as chief editors. As a forerunner among the medical journals published in Western languages in Japan, this periodical went unpublished for only one year (1946) during the chaotic aftermath of World War II.

2. Kunihiko Hashida (1882–1945)

Hashida was sent to Europe in 1913 and entered M. Gildemeister's research laboratory in Strasbourg. However, World War I broke out soon after his arrival, and as a result he was temporarily imprisoned. After several months he was able to flee to safety in Switzerland, and returned to Japan when the war ended in 1918. He was appointed Professor of Physiology at Tokyo University in 1922 as Osawa's successor.

Until that time physiology courses in Japan consisted mainly of the reading of Western textbooks and work in simple student laboratories. However, Hashida was a leader in introducing more sophisticated laboratory devices for research, such as the Siemens electromagnetic oscillograph and the cold-cathode-type oscillograph, which greatly excited physiological circles. His endeavors made a significant contribution to the promotion of experimental physiology in Japan.

Many capable researchers were assembled under Hashida's tutelage. Included in the ranks of the sensory physiologists who were trained either directly or indirectly under Hashida's influence are Koiti Motokawa (1903–1971) and Naoki Toida (1911–) in visual physiology; Yasuji Katsuki (1905–) in auditory physiology; Masayasu Sato (1919–) in gustatory physiology; and Sadayuki F. Takagi (1919–) in olfactory physiology.

Hashida stressed the internationality of research as strongly as his elder brother Fujita, and in 1923 he started the *Journal of Biophysics,* published in Western languages. Unfortunately, at that time Japanese physiology circles were too undeveloped to support a Western language publication. Having run to only two volumes by 1927, the journal merged with the *Japanese Journal of Medical Science,* becoming Sect. III (Biophysics) of this government-sponsored Western language publication. In 1944, in the midst of World War II, the publication of Sect. III was discontinued, Vol. 10 being the last issue. The current *Japanese Journal of Physiology* was founded in 1950 by Yas Kuno (1882–1977) as the Western language publication of the Physiological Society of Japan.

In addition to his research on physiology, Hashida also had a deep interest in the question of "life," and he often wrote about life and science. Seeking to grasp the meaning of life in religion, he pursued a study of the Buddhist philosophy expounded by Dogen (1200–1253), a leading priest of the Zen sect in Japan. Hashida was asked to join the Konoe cabinet as the Minister of Education just before Japan became engulfed in World War II, and he served in that position for four years until, in the early years of the Tojo cabinet, Japan rushed headlong into the world conflagration. After the war, he was summoned by the Occupation Forces to appear for questioning because of his government service. Rather than comply with the summons, Hashida elected to take his own life. Even today his death is lamented as a great loss in the history of physiology in Japan.

3. Genichi Kato (1890–1979)

Genichi Kato should be mentioned because, in the 1920s when Japanese physiology was still in its infancy, he was one of the few physiologists who ardently desired to have his research recognized internationally. Kato's special field of study was neurophysiology, and thus he was not directly connected with sensory physiology. However, one of his students was Ichiji Tasaki (1910–), who has made great strides in advancing neurophysiology. Tasaki has also made significant contributions to the development of auditory physiology by plotting the response area of single auditory nerve fibers of cats (TASAKI 1954). As Kato was also my teacher, I would like to devote the following section to a discussion of his career.

Kato received his MD in 1916 and his DMS in 1920 from Kyoto University School of Medicine. For two years after receiving his MD, he stayed in the Department of Physiology at his alma mater, where he specialized in neurophysiology under the direction of his teacher, H. Ishikawa (1878–1947), who had studied in Germany under Max Verworn. In 1918, Kato was invited to Keio University as Professor of Physiology and Chairman of the Physiology Department in the Medical School, which had been founded a year earlier. After serving as Chairman for 42 years, Kato became Professor Emeritus in 1960, but held his office in the same department and continued to teach medical students until a year before his death in 1979.

Kato became internationally known for his theory of nondecremental nerve conduction. In the early part of his century, M. Verworn and his school's theory of decremental conduction prevailed in physiology circles. According to this theory, the nerve impulse, which was conducted without decrement and followed the all-or-none principle in the normal nerve, was altered in a narcotized (subnormal) region such that progressive decrement occurred in both the impulse size and conduction velocity, contrary to the all-or-none principle. Verworn's theory was based mainly on the observation that the time necessary to suspend nerve conduction depended on the length of the narcotized region. Kato and his colleagues repeated the experiment using the long nerve of the Japanese toad, *Bufo vulgaris,* and demonstrated that the suspension time was the same in longer and shorter narcotized nerves, and that conduction along the narcotized region was therefore also nondecremental and obeyed the all-or-none principle. Kato and his colleagues were successful in pointing out the sources of errors which had led to the establishment of the decrement theory.

In 1923, at the Second Annual Meeting of the Physiological Society of Japan, Kato proudly reported the above observation and his new theory, but the response of the audience was not as he expected. On the contrary, he was petrified for a while by the roar of his former teacher, Ishikawa; the former mentor opposed Kato's new concepts, basing his criticism on Verworn's theory of decremental conduction, which was like a Bible for Ishikawa. This made Kato determined to publish the results in monographs in English (KATO 1924, 1926), and also to demonstrate the experiments at the Twelfth International Congress of Physiology in Stockholm (KATO 1926). Kato and his three colleagues carried more than 150 Japanese toads all the way to the Congress via the Siberian Railway. Their painstaking task was rewarded with great success. Kato's significant contribution became well known among physiologists and was widely popularized in general physiology textbooks.

The situation within Japan regarding this controversy was not so simple as that which prevailed abroad. Beginning in 1923 and continuing for more than ten years, the Annual Meetings of the Physiological Society of Japan were mostly preoccupied by this controversial discussion, the majority of physiologists eventually being divided into two opposing camps. The controversy attained such prominence that the issue was debated in many journals and newspapers, and it not only exerted a profound influence on the development of physiology in Japan, but also directed interest toward neurophysiology.

Kato's next interest was to study the problem of nerve conduction using single fibers excised from the toad sciatic nerve. ADRIAN and BRONK (1928) had already been successful in recording single-fiber discharges in the rabbit phrenic nerve by dissecting it into a few fibers. Their aim was to obtain impulse discharges from *functionally* isolated single fibers. Kato and his colleagues improved the microdissection technique to obtain *morphologically* isolated single fibers long enough to contain three or more Ranvier nodes. Their earlier results by this technique were published as a monograph, *Microphysiology of Nerve* (KATO 1934). The microdissection technique, which was further improved by Kato's group, led Tasaki to his success in demonstrating that electrical stimuli affect nerve fibers only at the Ranvier node where the myelin sheath is interrupted. The study was essential to the discovery of saltatory conduction (Tasaki 1959).

Kato was full of enthusiasm, which was manifested in several ways: utmost devotion to research, enthusiasm in giving lectures, patriotism during the war, and love of his university. He was an excellent teacher: he often likened himself to a sculptor who bows to the statues of Buddha that he has sculpted. In his lectures he often talked with great passion, not only of his experiences in research itself but also of episodes connected with his research activities. His renowned zeal for research and scholarship attracted many students (more than 300) to his department during his academic career. Many of them later turned to clinical studies, but over 80 who remained physiologists attained posts as professors in medical colleges and university schools throughout Japan.

II. The Development of the Physiology of Vision in Japan

1. The Early Phase

As I mentioned in Sect. B.I., many Japanese physiologists received their training in Germany during the period when physiology was still in its infancy in Japan. The results of the research that they did during their training were quite often published in local medical journals.

After their return to Japan, however, they did not always continue the work they had performed during their training abroad. If they did, most of their results were published in Japanese, and thus lost the chance of receiving international attention.

In addition to the formidable language barrier, the geographical situation, requiring several months for an exchange of letters, meant that it was not easy at that time for Japanese researchers to contribute to European or American journals. Consequently, researchers who were confident of the results they had published in Japanese would summarize their findings over a certain period in a Western language monograph and then publish this monograph for distribution. This, however, represents the exception rather than the rule. Prior to World War II, competition among Japanese physiologists to come up with new findings was limited for the most part to rivalry within Japan.

Although the preceding section stressed the scientific isolation of Japan until the 1940s, the intent of that discussion was not to offer an excuse for Japan's backwardness in science. No matter how isolated an island is, if it becomes known that there is a treasure house of knowledge on the island, explorers will come from all over the world to contend for its utilization. One example of this might be the color blindness test charts developed by Shinobu Ishihara (1879–1963). After graduating from Tokyo University in 1905, he became an army doctor. Recognizing his extraordinary abilities, the army ordered him to enroll in the Graduate School of Tokyo University in 1908. Moreover, he spent two years studying in Germany from 1912 to the outbreak of World War I in 1914. He was appointed Professor of Ophthalmology at Tokyo University in 1922, while he was still in active service as an army doctor. Ishihara did not write any original papers in Western languages. Nevertheless, his charts received the highest commendation from eye specialists around the world, and today they are used as the International Standard Charts.

2. Yuji Hosoya (1897–1967)

Following his graduation from Tohoku University School of Medicine in 1923, Hosoya began to specialize in physiology under the tutelage of Fujita (Sect. B.I.1). Initially he collaborated with Fujita on psychophysical studies of dark adaptation, but soon he began to focus his research work on the biochemistry of retinal substances, and made the elucidation of their functions his life's work.

As his first research project in that direction, he investigated the fluorescent properties of tapetum lucidum (HOSOYA 1929 a). In that same year, HOSOYA (1929 b) used an ophthalmoscope to observe rhodopsin of living organisms with tapetum, particularly sharks. Hosoya's method can be regarded as the prototype of a method used about 25 years later by RUSHTON (1956) to measure human visual substances in situ.

In subsequent studies, Hosoya did comparative research on various methods of extracting rhodopsin. Sent by the government to Germany in 1932, he spent two years studying in Berlin, where he worked in collaboration with Bayerl (HOSOYA and BAYERL 1933) on the absorption spectra of rhodopsin extract and the effect of bleaching by light.

Hosoya went on to discover in 1933 that once rhodopsin had been illuminated it continued to decompose even when stored in complete darkness (HOSOYA 1933). His discovery, which he called "afterbleaching", would later afford the first clue for elucidating the existence of two phases; a photochemical reaction followed by a thermal reaction in the decomposition process of rhodopsin.

In 1936 Hosoya went to Taiwan to accept an appointment as Professor of Physiology at the new university that had just been established in Taipei. Blessed with a relative abundance of research funds and animals for research purposes, he immediately embarked on a study of the cone-dominant retina of the Taiwanese tortoise. Two years later he and his collaborators reported that they had detected red (700–670 nm), yellow (570 nm), and blue (460 nm) substances which they believed were cone visual substances (HOSOYA et al. 1938).

In his research that followed, Hosoya isolated the dark-adapted retinas from many toads (*Bufo vulgaris*) and extracted rhodopsin. His aim was to clarify the constituent elements of the retina, especially the phospholipid and protein components; however, due to the war it became impossible for him to continue his research.

Even though Taiwan was restored to China after the war, Hosoya remained at Taipei University and continued his research and teaching activities for several years. In 1949 he returned to Japan to accept an invitation to teach at Osaka City University, which had been founded that same year. At that time Tomiyuki Hara (1924–), Toru Yoshizawa (1927–), and other young researchers in the Department of Biology at Osaka University had just started doing research on visual substances, and in 1950 a retinal study group was inaugurated, under the leadership of Hosoya and of Ichijiro Honjo (1909–1974), Chairman of the Department. This created the opportunity for many researchers in Kyoto-Osaka to be influenced by Hosoya.

In 1957 a group of Hosoya's students (*Hosoya Domonkai*) gathered together all the papers that had been written by Hosoya and his colleagues in European languages, and published a total of 31 under the title of *Collected Papers in Physiology of Vision* (HOSOYA 1957) to commemorate Hosoya's 60th birthday. Included among these papers were works by Z. SAITO (1938) and E. KIMURA (1952) regarding methods of isolating rod outer segments.

With Hosoya's guidance, Saito originated the sugar floatation method, in which he shook dark-adapted frog and toad retinas in sucrose solutions of different concentrations (specific gravities). After the rod outer segments were suspended, the solutions were subjected to centrifugation. He found that when he used a 40% –45% sucrose solution, the rod outer segments would separate and collect at the top of the solution.

Around 1950, Hosoya instructed Kimura to improve Saito's 1938 sucrose floatation technique for the isolation of rod outer segments. Kimura successfully developed a multilayer sucrose centrifugation method by which he was able to collect the rod outer segments very simply and efficiently. He used three different sucrose layers of varying concentrations and found at a specific interface very clean purplish rod outer segments. In subsequent years this method has come to be widely used.

Hosoya devoted his life to the development of creative techniques. Although he initiated the development of such techniques, he was anxious for his students to get the full credit; for example, the techniques developed under his supervision by Saito and Kimura were published only under his students' names. Hosoya was chosen to become the Dean of the School of Medicine in 1955, and two years later the President of Osaka City University. He performed the duties of this office until his mandatory retirement in 1963. Not quite four years after he retired, Hosoya suffered a fatal stroke. In a message of condolence to Hosoya's wife, G. Wald wrote, "I came to know his work first as a young student and learned much from it thereafter over the years."

3. Koiti Motokawa (1903–1971)

Born into a farming family, Motokawa was the only boy among five children. Because of his outstanding elementary school record, his teacher urged his father to continue the boy's education by sending him to high school. Motokawa's father refused to give his consent, however, as he feared losing his only heir to the family farm. As a result, after Motokawa finished eight years of compulsory education, he was forced to stay at home and help his father with the farm work.

Motokawa could not give up his desire to get an education so easily, and finally at the age of 18 he ran away from home. He sought help from his cousin in Kyoto, who agreed to put up the young man in his own lodging. Shocked by his son's action, Motokawa's father used every means possible to encourage Motokawa to return home. Motokawa finally got his father's permission to study for one year by solemnly promising that if he failed to pass the special examination at the end of it, he would return home and devote himself to farming. Having secured his father's approval, Motokawa began studying intensely day and night. As promised, he took the examination at the end of the year and passed without any difficulty. Motokawa also sat for the entrance examination to Kanazawa Senior High School (under the prewar system) along with the other applicants who had studied at regular schools. This represented a true challenge to his ability, but Motokawa passed with flying colors. When his father learned the news, he finally resolved to let Motokawa leave farming for good.

As one can easily surmise from the above account of Motokawa's experiences as a youth, he was the type of person who applied himself intently to his studies, and in addition tended to have great tenacity. These traits never changed during his entire life.

After graduating from Tokyo University School of Medicine in 1929, Motokawa entered its Department of Physiology, where, under the tutelage of Hashida (Sect. B.I.2), he devoted 11 years to investigating the skin potential of frogs; during that time he published more than ten papers in German.

Motokawa was appointed to succeed Fujita (Sect. B.I.1) upon the latter's retirement from Tohoku University in 1940. When Motokawa assumed his duties, he found that the Physiology Department had very little experimental equipment. Moreover, as a war was being waged on the continent, his research funds were severely limited and he had only one assistant, Toshisada Mita (1912–), who is now President of Iwate Medical University. With Mita's help, however, Motokawa modified an old amplifier and immediately began his research on brain waves. During the next several years he published nearly 30 papers in European languages.

While he and Mita were studying brain waves, they noticed that when the waves were inhibited by a photic stimulus, another slow potential change was recorded. As a result of moving the position of the electrodes, they found that when the electrodes were attached to the frontal region, a high-amplitude slow potential change was recorded, which they identified as the electroretinogram (ERG). Moreover, they found that the ERG b-wave was preceded by a fast positive wave, which they called the "x-wave" in their report (MOTOKAWA and MITA 1942).

In subsequent research done by ADRIAN (1945), this x-wave was observed independently in the human eye, and further research (ADRIAN 1946) revealed that this was a b-wave specific to cones in the light-adapted eye.

Motokawa later collaborated with Iwama in a series of studies dealing with brain waves. While measuring the impedance of the scalp, Motokawa experienced an electric phosphene, which led him to wonder how the threshold of the phosphene changed under the influence of preceding light. He decided that he would try to follow the time course in an effort to answer this question.

The method Motokawa employed was quite simple. Using a circuit composed of a battery, several resistors, and switches, he measured the phosphene threshold that was produced when an electric current pulse was passed between a pair of electrodes, one attached to the eyelid and the other to the temple.

Let E_o represent the reciprocal of the phosphene threshold (electrical excitability) produced only by the current pulse, and E represent the reciprocal of the phosphene threshold produced by the test current pulse when the conditioning light is applied in advance. Then the percentage increase ζ in electrical excitability produced by prior application of the conditioning light can be expressed by the following equation:

$$\zeta = \frac{E - E_0}{E_0} \times 100. \tag{1}$$

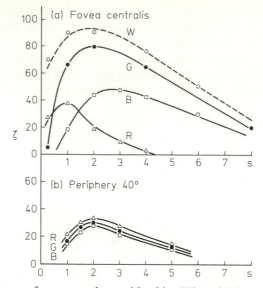

Fig. 1 a, b. ζ time curves for a normal eye with white (W), red (R), green (G), and blue (B) lights at the fovea **a** and periphery **b** of the retina. MOTOKAWA (1948)

Using this ζ value as an index, Motokawa and his collaborators proceeded vigorously with their research efforts. In less than two years after the start of his research project, Motokawa appeared to have succeeded in answering many problems that covered nearly all areas of psychophysics in vision. He presented the results of his research in a special lecture entitled "Physiological Basis of Sensation," which he delivered at the Twelfth General Meeting of the Japanese Psychological Association held in August 1948. Moreover, the outline of his lecture was published in the Japanese language journal *Kagaku* (MOTOKAWA 1948).

The first section of this paper dealt with "the discovery of a physiological process specific to light wavelengths." Since this section is a good example of Motokawa's approach, I would like to summarize it in Motokawa's own words.

Figure [1 a] shows the ζ values that were measured when the interval between the colored light pre-illumination toward the central visual field and the electrical stimulation following it were varied. As shown in this figure, when red light is used for pre-illumination the maximum value of the curve appears at about one second, for green light at about two seconds, and for blue light at about three seconds (indicated in the figure by R, G, B). If we call these maximum points peak times, the peak time is specific to each color (wavelength), and it can be proved that the light intensity does not have any effect at all. What is related to the light intensity is not the peak time but rather the height of the respective curve. It is obvious that these phenomena are related to color sensation, because the electrical sensitivity curves, as measured in the periphery of the retina [Fig. 1 b] do not show any variation due to color. The peripheral part of the retina lacks color sensation.

In subsequent sections, Motokawa proceeded to expand his method to include a critical evaluation of color sensation theories, color contrast, simultaneous contrast, visual illusions and other areas of research. Finally, he concluded his paper by saying that he was confident that the kind of research he had done succeeded in bridging the gap between physiology and psychology.

Eventually, Motokawa's work was published in Western language journals, and there is a detailed review by GEBHARD (1953) of some 40 of his papers.

Although it had appeared that recognition of Motokawa's phosphene experiment was in the ascendant, it was not long before his approach became the object of sharp criticism. RIGGS et al. (1957) reexamined Motokawa's experiment and found that there was a slight enhancement of the ζ value due to the conditioning light, but that no difference attributable to the wavelength could be detected. They pointed out that Motokawa's method of measuring the phosphene threshold was not based on the standard psychophysical procedures, and that the results obtained might thus have been influenced by the preconceptions of the experimenter.

The following year, HOWARTH and TREISMAN (1958) also criticized Motokawa's method from a psychological point of view, and presented conclusions similar to those advanced by RIGGS et al. (1957).

What was the reaction in Japan to Motokawa's work during this same period? No particular counterarguments were heard from the psychologists; however, physiologists often raised serious questions about Motokawa's work. Despite the criticism from other researchers both at home and abroad, Motokawa's faith in his approach was not shaken. In his later years, his duties as University President kept him busy, but he continued working on a monograph which dealt primarily with his phosphene studies. When his monograph (MOTOKAWA 1970) was finally published, Motokawa was already sick in bed with a painful and rapidly progressing illness, and a few months later he died.

In his obituary of Motokawa, Kyoji Tasaki wrote, "he was fond of paintings, and his childhood desire was to become an artist." Perhaps during his entire life Motokawa painted the beautiful images he cherished on the canvas of physiology, and the "paintings" he produced were a source of unlimited personal satisfaction. He died in the firm belief that some day his approach would gain public recognition. RIGGS (1973) concludes his book review of Motokawa's monograph by saying, "Perhaps some day, there may be a revival of the phosphene–light interactions when these questions can be cleared up."

C. Electrophysiology of the Retina

The historical review in the preceding sections may help the reader to appreciate the atmosphere of the developing area of Japanese neurophysiology and therefore the context in which my research, which is described below, proceeded.

I. Electroretinogram Analysis by Means of Intraretinal Electrodes

Near the end of the Introduction to this chapter, I described how my research shifted from the ear to the nose and finally, in turn, to the eye. During this transition, there was some degree of overlapping in my research, and the process of trial and error was repeated again and again. However, after having decided that I would concentrate on vision research, I devoted myself to acquiring a good grasp of the electrophysiological studies that had been done on the retina. Since this was an entirely new field for me, I resolved not to repeat the mistakes that I had made in auditory research.

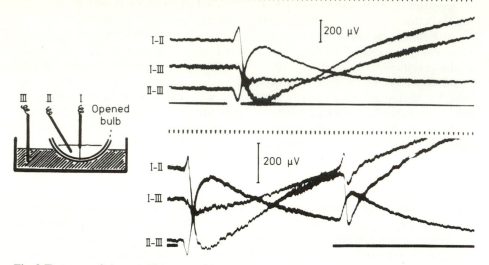

Fig. 2. Two sets of electroretinograms of the bullfrog, recorded by shorter (*upper record*) and longer (*lower record*) durations of illumination. Recordings for each set were made by three combinations of three electrodes arranged as shown in the diagram on the *left*. The duration of illumination is marked by *interruption of the bottom line*. Time marking: 0.1 s. Tomita (1950)

Initially, I read an article by Kohlrausch (1931) entitled „Elektrische Erscheinungen am Auge". About the time I finished reading it, Granit's (1947) monograph *Sensory Mechanisms of the Retina* was published.

The first half of the monograph dealt mainly with the analysis of the ERG, and the second half described in detail the results of microelectrode studies conducted on various vertebrates to investigate the activity of single optic nerve fibers, especially their spectral sensitivity. After reading it repeatedly, I arrived at the idea that in recording the optic nerve fiber response Granit had applied microelectrodes only to the surface of the retina. However, if the ERG could be recorded by a microelectrode inserted to different depths in the retina, then this would offer a more direct method of ERG analysis. Following this line of thought, I decided to assemble a microelectrode, amplifier, and recording system.

First, I made glass micropipettes by hand-pulling. Using a pair of scissors, I cut the micropipette to make a tip diameter of several micrometers. I then filled the inside with Ringer's solution. [It was the following year that Ling and Gerard (1949) reported the fabrication of a superfine microelectrode.] Next, through the goodwill of the Toshiba Electric Co., I obtained on permanent loan an electrometer tube UX-54, which I used as the preamplifier tube.

As the main amplifier I needed a dc amplifier. When I discussed this with my friend Y. Ogino (currently the President of the Nihon Kohden Co.), he took me to a small office in Tokyo, and after a short conversation with one of the people in the office, I was given what appeared to be an army surplus amplifier, which had been stacked in one corner of the room; I was told to use it for as long as I liked. It turned out to be a 650/s chopper-type amplifier, which I took home, disas-

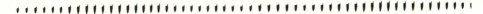

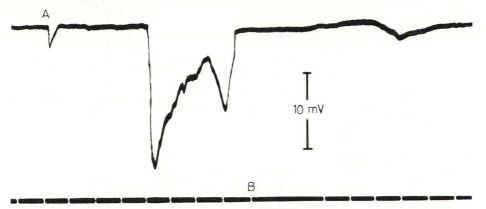

Fig. 3. Potential changes recorded by a microelectrode traveling across the bullfrog retina from its vitreal side. A small negative deflection at point A signals the moment when the electrode tip struck the inner limiting membrane, while the second, large negative deflection the moment the electrode has pierced into the retina. A sign that the electrode has penetrated through the retina to the other side is given by a rapid rise of potential to a new flat level. At point B, which is shortly after this sign, the electrode was stopped advancing and was drawn back at the same rate as it had advanced. The marking (*top*): 1 s. Marking of distance traveled (*bottom*): 35 μm. TOMITA (1950)

sembled, and then put back together. Several years later, when I looked again at the name card which I had received along with the amplifier, I discovered that the man who had given me the amplifier was Masaru Ibuka (1908–), who subsequently became the first President of Sony and is now its Honorary President, and that the small, two-room office I had visited was the precursor of the present-day Sony Company.

Having secured an amplifer, I hooked it up to the electromagnetic oscillograph I had used in my auditory research. At last I was more or less ready to record. I proceeded to prepare an eyecup from the excised eye of a bullfrog and experimented with inserting the microelectrode.

Figure 2 shows the response to both short (upper record) and long (lower record) durations of illumination, which were recorded by three different combinations of two gross electrodes (II and III) placed on the opposite sides of the retina and one microelectrode (I) placed intraretinally. The three curves for each record were not recorded simultaneously, but rather consecutively, as there was only one amplifier.

Even though the recording apparatus was extremely primitive, the condition of the retina remained stable during one series of recordings, as attested by the fact that, among the three curves, the relationship (I–III) – (I–II) = (II–III) holds up rather well.

I next proceeded to determine the relationship between the depth of the electrode and the ERG waveform. Figure 3 shows one example of the method that I employed for this purpose. The recording shown in this figure was made when the electrode was advanced slowly from the vitreous humor toward the retina without the use of any light.

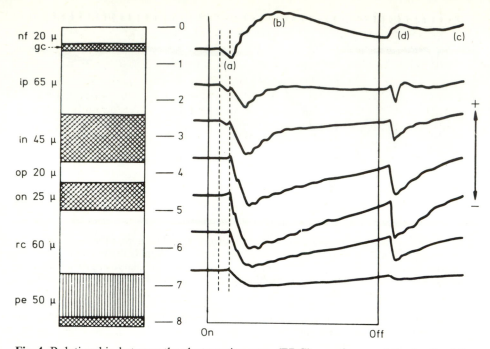

Fig. 4. Relationship between the electroretinogram (ERG) waveform and the depth of the recording microelectrode in the retina of the bullfrog. The pattern of the retinal layers is shown on the *left*, and the ERG waveforms at various depths in the retina on the *right*. The markings 0 through 8 indicate 35-µm intervals. *nf*, layer of optic nerve fibers; *gc*, layer of ganglion cells; *ip*, inner plexiform layer; *in*, inner nuclear layer; *op*, outer plexiform layer; *on*, outer nuclear layer; *rc*, layer of rods and cones; *pe*, pigment epithelium with apical processes. (*a*), a-wave; etc. TOMITA (1950)

For as long as the electrode passed through the vitreous humor, the baseline was stable. However, at a certain depth a small negative variation (A in Fig. 3) appeared. When the electrode was advanced further, slight variations continued irregularly, and at 100–150 µm from point A a large negative potential change (10–20 mV) suddenly appeared. The irregular variations were recorded again beyond this point, and then the deflection returned to near the initial baseline, at which point (B) I stopped inserting the electrode and began to pull it up. As the electrode was withdrawn, the large negative potential that had appeared when the electrode was advanced was not recorded. Even if a negative potential was recorded, it represented nothing more than residual traces.

If I tried to insert the electrode beyond point B, the electrode broke off. Comparing the distance from point A to point B with the thickness of the frog's retina, we found that there was good agreement between the two values. This led us to draw the following conclusion: Point A indicated the moment when the microelectrode struck the resistive membrane (the internal limiting membrane) covering the surface of the retina. The interval from this point to the appearance of the large negative deflection represented the distance during which the electrode was pressing on the internal limiting membrane. After that the electrode pierced the membrane and entered the retina, and at that moment a large injury potential appeared. When the electrode reached the opposite side of the retina, the deflection returned to the initial baseline (or more precisely, to the potential that was lower than the initial baseline by a value corresponding to the standing potential of the retina).

The waveforms at each depth estimated from over 100 experiments are shown on the right in Fig. 4. The left side of the figure shows the typical pattern of retinal layers obtained from the tissue specimen of the bullfrog, and the numbers from 0 to 8 in the middle mark the 35-μm intervals.

Figure 4 shows that, as the electrode penetrated deeper, polarity reversal occurred for the fast ERG components (the a- and b-waves), but the slow component (the c-wave) did not show any reversal all the way to the end. This indicated that the c-wave originated in the deepest layer. When the retina was detached from the pigment epithelium, no c-wave was recorded from either the retina side or the pigment epithelium side. From this I reasoned that the c-wave was probably caused by metabolic interaction between the pigment epithelial cells and the visual cells.

My observations were initially reported in the founding issue of the *Japanese Journal of Physiology* (TOMITA 1950), and subsequently I coauthored with my colleagues three papers that presented complementary observations. In 1952 I was awarded a fellowship by the China Medical Board of New York, and that September I left for Johns Hopkins University, where I intended to study for a year in the Department of Biophysics under the supervision of H. K. Hartline.

The years prior to my departure for the United States can probably be called the first period of my retina research. The interval immediately following World War II was a time of recovery from impoverishment. At that time I was working at both Keio University and Tokyo Women's Medical College. Keio University School of Medicine had burned down during the war, so the university rented what remained of a former airplane factory in the suburbs of Tokyo and used this building for classrooms and research. I commuted there almost every day, and left at 4 or 5 p.m. to go to Tokyo Women's Medical College in the city, where I worked until midnight on the experiments already described. As I recall, this way of life continued for about two years.

To get home I had to walk for about half an hour through the dark, fire-gutted ruins. There were many times when I was stopped and questioned by policemen who were making their nightly rounds. It was probably not unreasonable for them to have been suspicious of a man wearing a military uniform and an army field cap, of course not armed, who was walking alone through the war-ravaged rubble after midnight. In those first years after the war, that was how I looked when I went to work. Those were truly hard times, but now I have extremely fond memories of that period and regard it as the most meaningful and purposeful period of my life.

II. Study on the Lateral Eye of the Horseshoe Crab (*Limulus*) – A Year in H. K. Hartline's Laboratory

On 5 September 1952 I left Yokohama on an American freighter, and after 11 days at sea we docked in Los Angeles. From there I flew to Washington, where I transferred to a bus and went to Baltimore. I met Hartline on 18 September. After introducing me to D. W. Bronk, the President of Johns Hopkins University at that time, Hartline handed me the keys to the outside door of the Department of Biophysics and to the laboratory. Then he completely astounded me by saying, "Come when you want to, and when you don't feel like coming, you don't have to."

In the days that followed he showed me once or twice the method for excising the lateral eye of *Limulus* and isolating single optic nerve fibers. He also demonstrated how to record the response to light from the nerve fiber, but otherwise I do not remember having received any direct instruction from him. Nevertheless, the atmosphere of Hartline's laboratory was truly warm and pleasant. Even today I have a close relationship with Hartline [1] as well as with several individuals who were his students at the time, including E. F. MacNichol Jr., W. H. Miller, H. G. Wagner, and M. L. Wolbarsht. The monthly living allowance the fellowship provided was just barely enough to support a single student, but the invaluable experience I gained in that one year can never be exchanged for money. During that period I learned for the first time the utility of the binocular stereomicroscope. From MacNichol I learned the procedure for using a superfine microelectrode to make intracellular recordings from the ommatidium of the horseshoe crab.

The time of my study at Johns Hopkins was a few years after the discovery by HARTLINE (1949) that the activity of visual receptors was inhibited by illumination of nearby retinal areas in the *Limulus* eye, and people were interested in knowing the mechanisms of such lateral inhibition. One day in January 1953, I demonstrated that inhibition took place in the response to light from a single optic nerve fiber when the proximal ends of the remaining optic nerve bundle were electrically stimulated to send antidromic impulses. The patterns of inhibition resembled those produced by illumination of nearby ommatidia. Hartline was extremely pleased and said to me, "Until you go home you don't have to do anything else." The paper reporting the results of this experiment was published some years later (TOMITA 1958).

In addition to Hartline's students, I also became acquainted with many other people during the year. Among the people whose friendship I have enjoyed in subsequent years, I want to mention two individuals in particular. One is S. W. Kuffler, who was at the Wilmer Eye Institute in Hopkins Hospital, located some distance from the campus. In the early 1950s he was mapping the receptive field of single ganglion cells of the cat. Around that time, KUFFLER (1952) discovered what is known today as the concentric antagonistic center-surround organization of the receptive field. H. B. Barlow was also in Kuffler's laboratory in those days and both of them participated in the seminars that were given in Hartline's laboratory. Those seminars were a very stimulating and profitable experience for me. The other individual is L. A. Riggs, who spent half of his one-year sabbatical in Hartline's laboratory. That was the beginning of a friendship which we still maintain today.

The year that I spent studying in Hartline's laboratory was indeed pleasant and extremely beneficial. During that period, however, one event occurred which gave me quite a shock. At the Cold Spring Harbor Symposium, where the main theme was the neuron, OTTOSON and SVAETICHIN (1952) reported the results of an experiment similar to ours in which they had used retinas excised from frogs to measure

---

1 I deeply regret that, after I had finished writing this chapter, I was informed of Hartline's death (17 March 1983)

intraretinal ERG. According to their findings there was no change at all in ERG until the penetrating microelectrode reached the visual cell layer, and while the electrode passed through this layer, ERG disappeared. Consequently, they concluded that ERG originated entirely in the visual cell layer. Furthermore, they could not find any polarity reversal of the intraretinal ERG like the reversal I had reported (cf. Fig. 4). They commented that the polarity reversal which I had demonstrated was probably produced by the thick electrode damaging the retina.

It was undeniable that in their experiment Ottoson and Svaetichin had used the most advanced, superfine microelectrode, whereas we had used a thick electrode several micrometers in diameter. Nevertheless, it was impossible to believe that the polarity reversal had been caused by damage to the retina. At that time I could hardly suppress my desire to cut short my study at Johns Hopkins, return home, and redo the experiment with a superfine microelectrode. Eventually this anguish lessened as I became engrossed in the horseshoe crab experiment, and afterward I really began to enjoy my year of study.

In August 1953 I attended the Nineteenth International Congress of Physiological Sciences in Montreal, and then returned to Japan in September.

III. Discovery of the S-Potential (Svaetichin)

There were countless things that I wanted to do on returning to Japan, but there were two particular tasks that were my main concerns. First of all, I wanted to utilize the intracellular microelectrode techniques I had learned during my study at Johns Hopkins to advance my research on the horseshoe crab, *Tachypleus tridentatus*. Moreover, I wanted to find out why the conclusions advanced by OTTOSON and SVAETICHIN (1952) just mentioned had been completely different from ours. My colleagues and I worked on these two projects in a parallel fashion, but here I will confine my remarks to the latter task.

First, we repeated the intraretinal recordings applying a superfine electrode to the bullfrog's eyecup preparation. As in our earlier experiments the ERG reversal was observed, and thus we confirmed that the ERG reversal observed in those experiments had not been caused by the thick electrode.

Meanwhile, SVAETICHIN (1953) published another extremely important paper in which he reported that he had inserted a superfine electrode into single fish cones and succeeded in recording the response to white light as well as the spectral response. He explained that when the superfine electrode was inserted to the depth corresponding to the cone inner segment, a sudden negative potential change of about -40 mV was recorded. He stopped advancing the electrode at that point and proceeded to illuminate the retina. While he was illuminating the retina an additional negative potential change of -20 to -30 mV appeared, and when the light was turned off, there was an immediate return to the original resting potential level of about -40 mV. He illuminated the retina repeatedly for about an hour and was able to record the same response each time. Completely confident that these responses came from single cones, Svaetichin called the response he recorded the "cone action potential". In the same paper, Svaetichin reported that he had also tested the response to spectral light of different wavelengths, and that for the most part his findings affirmed the trichromatic theory of Young and von Helmholtz.

However, in subsequent research on the spectral response, SVAETICHIN (1956) further improved his testing apparatus and obtained results that negated his earlier hypothesis. In these later experiments, he obtained what are now called the luminosity-type (L-type) and chromaticity-type (C-type) S-potentials, which substantiated Hering's opponent color theory, and Svaetichin dedicated his paper to the deceased Hering.

I would like to digress briefly to mention an experiment that we performed in which we recorded what might be called "our first observation" of Svaetichin's potential. At the Twenty-Ninth Annual Meeting of the Physiological Society of Japan, which was held in Hokkaido in July 1952, we (TOMITA et al. 1952) read a paper entitled "A Comparative Study of the Intraretinal Action Potential (EIRG) in Several Vertebrates." In the section on freshwater fish, we presented the following:

Although the ERG for the cyprinid fish is weak, once the microelectrode is inserted into the retina a negative-dominant EIRG appears, which may be even one hundred times stronger than the surface ERG. However, in most cases it falls to less than one-tenth of the original amplitude within one minute. When the position of the electrode is changed a strong EIRG can be obtained again.

Two months after we gave that presentation I left for the United States to study under Hartline. What we had described, however, was the very potential that Svaetichin reported the following year.

About the same time that SVAETICHIN (1953) published his paper on the cone action potential, I developed a coaxial microelectrode, like the one shown in Fig. 5, and began to use it as a means of making simultaneous intra- and extracellular recordings from the eye of the horseshoe crab (TOMITA 1956), and also as a means of more accurately determining the correct position of the microelectrode in the vertebrate retina. With a special holder for the coaxial microelectrode, the internal, superfine pipette could be freely extended or retracted to any desired distance from the tip of the external pipette.

This coaxial electrode had one structural defect, in that, since the inner and outer electrodes were separated by the wall of the inner electrode, the wall served to create a capacitive coupling between them. Consequently, a rapid potential change, such as an impulse discharge, which was picked up by one electrode would affect the other electrode. To eliminate this capacitive coupling, I developed a compensating circuit (TOMITA 1956). Initially the circuit used vacuum tubes, but later it was transistorized (TOMITA 1962).

Using this coaxial microelectrode, we conducted various experiments to investigate the origin of Svaetichin's cone action potential.

Figure 6 shows the results obtained in one experiment. The internal microelectrode was extended 50 μm from the tip of the external microelectrode, and the records shown in this figure were taken when both electrodes were inserted into the retina. In order to distinguish the record made by the internal electrode from the one made by the external electrode, we arranged our equipment so that artifacts signaling the moments the light was turned on and off would be recorded only by the internal electrode.

The somewhat thick top trace in Fig. 6a is the record registered when both electrodes were near the receptor surface. The trace looks a little thick because it represents the overlapping of two similarly shaped responses. Letting this depth be

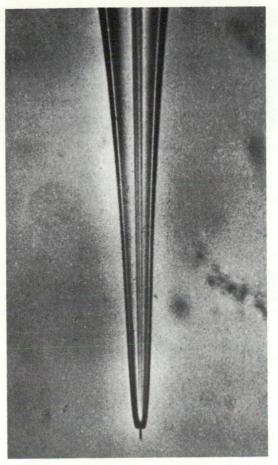

Fig. 5. Photomicroscopic picture of a coaxial microelectrode. The internal, superfine electrode, filled with 3 M KCl, is seen protruding about 12 µm out of the external electrode, which is filled with Ringer's solution and has a tip diameter of about 10 µm. The tip diameter of the external electrode could be made as small as 1 µm, depending on the experimental purpose. TOMITA (1956)

zero, the lower two tracings in Fig. 6 a show the respective responses for the internal and external electrodes when the internal electrode was inserted into the retina to a depth of 140 µm and the external electrode to 90 µm. The presence of the pips indicates that the tracing, with its large amplitude of response, was made by the internal electrode. The records made when the internal electrode was inserted to depths of 175, 210, and 245 µm are shown in Fig. 6 b–d. As can be seen in Fig. 6, both the internal and external electrodes simultaneously recorded Svaetichin's potential as the microelectrode was inserted deeper into the retina. However, with respect to the amplitude, their records interchanged as the depth increased.

Since the recorded range of Svaetichin's potential was very wide, I was convinced that the potential did not originate in single cones. Immediately after completing the experiment, I summarized the findings in a short paper which stressed

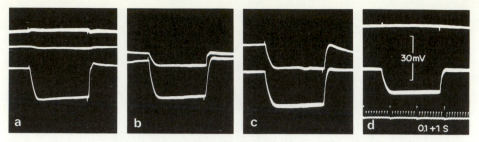

Fig. 6 a–d. Intraretinal recording from the carp retina, using a coaxial microelectrode with its internal electrode extending 50 μm out of the external electrode. Micrometer reading for the external electrode from the receptor surface: **a** 140 μm; **b** 175 μm; **c** 210 μm; **d** 245 μm. The internal electrode was 50 μm deeper at each step. To differentiate the tracings obtained by the two electrodes, an upward and a downward pip were entered at the onset and the cessation of light, respectively, only to the records made by the internal electrode. Tomita (1957)

that Svaetichin's so-called cone action potential definitely did not come from the cones, but from some structures proximal to the receptors. Furthermore, because of the wide range of Svaetichin's potential, I concluded that the recording was either extracellular or intracellular but from cells far larger than the receptors. The manuscript was submitted to the *Japanese Journal of Physiology* for publication, and at the same time I sent a copy to Hartline asking him for his comments. Shortly afterward I received an answer from him which began with the warning "Be careful!" His letter continued with the kind caution that determining the exact depth of the microelectrodes was not an easy matter. In a brief reply to his letter, I wrote that I was convinced from my own experience in using microelectrodes that it was not such an easy task to insert an external electrode 5 μm in diameter into the cone inner segment, the diameter of which had been estimated from the histological preparation to be about 8 μm. After the appearance of my paper (Tomita 1957), many researchers, including Svaetichin (MacNichol and Svaetichin 1958; Mitarai 1958; Oikawa et al. 1959; Tomita et al. 1959), began using different dyes to stain the electrode tip in an effort to pinpoint the origin of Svaetichin's potential. As a result of these experiments it was conclusively corroborated that the potential did not originate in the cones.

Consequently, at a meeting (Conference of the Microelectrode Research Project) held at Keio University School of Medicine on 6 July 1958, it was decided that the name "cone action potential" was not appropriate for the response. After discussing at some length what name would be a suitable substitute, Motokawa's proposal that the potential be called "Svaetichin's potential," or the "S-potential," using the first letter of Svaetichin, was adopted. The first paper written in a Western language to use this name was one that my colleagues and I (Tomita et al. 1959) coauthored, entitled "Further Study on the Origin of the So-Called Cone Action Potential (S-Potential): Its Histological Determination." Since then the name "S-potential" has become widely used internationally.

In the same year (1959) I attended the Twenty-First International Congress of Physiological Sciences, which was held in Buenos Aires with the late B. A. Houssay as President. This afforded an excellent opportunity for me to accept an invitation from Svaetichin to visit his laboratory. Consequently, I spent three months prior to the Congress at the Venezuelan National Research Institute (IVIC) in Caracas, where Svaetichin's laboratory was located.

The first time we met I told him, "It is now known that what you have called the cone action potential does not originate in the cones, so we have to think of another name. In Japan it has been decided to use the first letter of Svaetichin and call it the S-potential in your honor." He replied, "That's a lie. The S is probably not the S of Svaetichin, but rather the S of so-called." His response made both of us burst into peals of laughter. It is a fact that from the time it became known the source of the S-potential was not the cones, we did refer to it as the "so-called cone action potential." The title of our paper (TOMITA et al. 1959) attests to this. Svaetichin was fond of using this kind of joke to make people laugh.

IV. Simple and Complex Patterns
of the Intraretinal Electroretinogram

When the dispute concerning the origin of the S-potential was nearly over, Brindley at Cambridge published three papers (BRINDLEY 1956a–c) which were extremely important to me as far as my own work was concerned. In the introduction to his papers, Brindley stated that although the microelectrode technique seemed to be the definitive method for determining the origin of ERG, both Svaetichin and I had advanced quite different conclusions. His own research had been done from a position that was critical of the other two researchers, and the conclusions he had reached did not completely agree with either researcher's ideas.

To begin with, Brindley noted that when a fresh frog eyecup preparation was used in making intraretinal recordings, the polarity reversal that I had described could be observed. However, if a slightly stale preparation was used such a reversal could not be found. This meant that the record from a fresh preparation showed "Tomita's complex pattern," the term used later by BRINDLEY (1960) to refer to the intraretinal ERG showing reversal in polarity. Svaetichin's simple pattern was obtained from a stale preparation. He concluded from the results that the potential displaying polarity reversal had an origin different from that of ERG. As this potential was sensitive to aging, it disappeared in a stale preparation and the original ERG was manifested. The ERG thus manifested did not show a potential reversal, and it originated in the receptor layer as Svaetichin had pointed out. As evidence to substantiate his conclusion, Brindley explained that the largest ERG was recorded across the external limiting membrane (according to Brindley's explanation at that time, this was a high-resistance membrane, which he designated the "R-membrane," found approximately in the middle of the receptor layer).

This briefly summarizes the conclusions presented by Brindley. In other words, Brindley concurred with my observation regarding the existence of an intraretinal potential reversal, but he also agreed with Svaetichin in locating the origin of ERG in the receptor layer.

In response to Brindley's challenge, I carefully repeated his experiment in collaboration with Murakami and Hashimoto. Our observations turned out to be almost identical to Brindley's findings. The only reservation that remained was whether the R-membrane was in fact the external limiting membrane. As an experi-

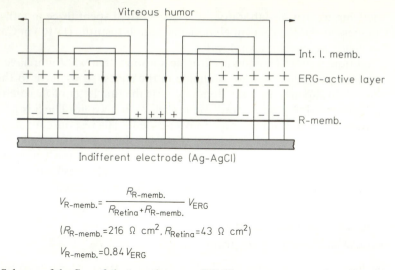

$$V_{R\text{-memb.}} = \frac{R_{R\text{-memb.}}}{R_{Retina} + R_{R\text{-memb.}}} V_{ERG}$$

$(R_{R\text{-memb.}} = 216 \ \Omega \ cm^2, R_{Retina} = 43 \ \Omega \ cm^2)$

$V_{R\text{-memb.}} = 0.84 \ V_{ERG}$

Fig. 7. Schema of the flux of electroretinogram (ERG) current across an inactive region (*central part of the diagram*) and active regions of the retina. *Int.1.memb.*, internal limiting membrane; *R-memb.*, the R-membrane, so termed primarily by Brindley for an electrically high-resistance membrane, and identified later as the pigment epithelium; $V_{R\text{-memb.}}$, amplitude of ERG recorded across the R-membrane; V_{ERG}, amplitude of ERG recorded across the retina or of the surface ERG; $R_{R\text{-memb.}}$, resistance across the R-membrane; R_{Retina}, resistance across the retina less R-membrane. Tomita et al. (1960)

ment, we tried to detect the R-membrane in an isolated retina, but failed. Brindley reported that he had made a similar attempt, and that while he was isolating the retina, the external limiting membrane ruptured, with consequent loss of its property of high resistance.

We tried various methods to find the R-membrane, and one day we finally managed to measure the resistance of an eyecup from which the retina had been removed. This eyecup consisted of the pigment epithelium, choroid, and sclera. A high resistance, corresponding to what Brindley had reported for the R-membrane, was detected in the upper surface layer or the pigment epithelial layer. This measurement indicated that the R-membrane was not the external limiting membrane inside the retina, but rather a membrane behind the retina. Later we learned that Brown and Wiesel (1958) had actually arrived at this conclusion before we did. In their investigations on cat retina they had already concluded that the R-membrane was Bruch's membrane, which was located just behind the pigment epithelium. (It has since been discovered that the R-membrane is not Bruch's membrane, but rather the pigment epithelium itself).

If it was true that the R-membrane was a membrane behind rather than in the retina, then it was necessary for us to reinterpret our data. The model that we came up with after several days of reflecting on our findings is shown in Fig. 7. In this figure the R-membrane is located behind the retina, and in addition the concept that I called "functional nonuniformity" has been introduced. The deterioration of the retina did not proceed uniformly, but rather the retina was made up of a mixture of ERG-active regions and ERG-inactive regions. Both the left and right sides of Fig. 7 show regions in which an ERG-active layer was present, and the central part of the figure shows a region in which the ERG-active layer was no longer active.

Let us consider what kind of waveform could be expected when the ERG of a retina in this condition was recorded: (a) between an electrode in the vitreous humor and an indifferent electrode placed behind the R-membrane, and (b) between an indifferent electrode behind the R-membrane and a microelectrode that pierced the retina and was advanced until it nearly reached the R-membrane.

In the case of (a), normal ERG would be recorded regardless of whether functional nonuniformity existed or not, since the electrode in the vitreous humor would record the sum of all local ERGs from active retinal region. However, in the case of (b), a significant difference would be produced in the recorded ERG, depending on whether the microelectrode was inserted in an ERG-active region of the retina or in a region that had become ERG-inactive. From an ERG-active region the microelectrode placed just in front of the R-membrane would record an ERG of reversed polarity, corresponding to what Brindley called Tomita's complex pattern. However, an inactive region (central part of Fig. 7) would merely serve as an external circuit through which the ERG current from the surrounding active regions flowed. Consequently, the microelectrode placed just in front of the R-membrane of inactive regions would record a normal ERG, corresponding to what Brindley referred to as Svaetichin's simple pattern.

Measuring the resistance of the retina and that of the R-membrane, we obtained a retina resistance of $43\ \Omega\ cm^2$ and an R-membrane resistance of $216\ \Omega\ cm^2$. Using these values and the mathematical formula given under Fig. 7, we determined theoretically what percentage of the surface ERG (V_{ERG}) was attributable to the ERG that was recorded across the R-membrane of inactive regions. This calculation produced a value of 84%. This was actually a reasonable value for the record from the inactive retinal region which displayed Svaetichin's simple pattern (see Fig. 8c).

When we found that all the results could be explained by the model shown in Fig. 7, I felt a rewarding exhilaration, as if the fog obscuring my vision had suddenly lifted. However, at that point I also thought that if the experiment could be advanced another step by artificially inactivating a special retina region and thereby proving that the complex pattern changed to a simple pattern, then our work would be complete. The two experiments that I will describe next were conducted in an effort to attain this change in pattern.

First, a thin hypodermic needle was used to inject a tiny quantity of 5% cocaine solution near the tip of the coaxial microelectrode. As time elapsed we clearly observed that the complex pattern changed to the simple pattern. The microelectrode was then moved away from the site of the cocaine injection to an untreated region of the retina which showed a typical complex pattern.

The second experiment did not involve the use of anesthetics to inactivate the region near the microelectrode. Rather, we thought that if this region was kept in the dark, it would not receive any stimulation, and thus a simple pattern could be obtained. We carried out this experiment using two lights, one of which was a light spot on the recording site (focal light), and the other a diffuse light but with a stop to keep only the recording site in darkness (nonfocal light). Using this nonfocal

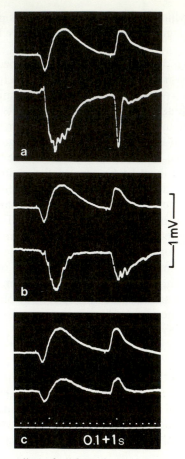

Fig. 8 a–c. Simultaneous recording of surface electroretinogram (ERG) (*upper tracing*) and intraretinal ERG at a depth just vitreal to the R-membrane (*lower tracing*), obtained with different combinations of two lights, one of which is a light spot 2 mm in diameter centered onto the recording site (focal light), the other a diffuse light but with a stop 4 mm in diameter centered on the recording site (nonfocal light). Recording by a coaxial electrode. **a** response typical of the complex pattern elicited when both lights are applied at the same time; **b** response to nonfocal light alone, which still exhibits a complex pattern because the retinal area in the shade has also been activated by scattered light; **c** response typical of the simple pattern elicited by nonfocal light in the presence of focal light as a background. TOMITA et al. (1960)

light, however, we were unable to obtain a clear simple pattern, as the recording in Fig. 8 b indicates. It seemed that even though we tried to keep one retinal region in total darkness, it was impossible to eliminate all scattered light.

Consequently, we abandoned the attempt to keep the region near the electrode in the dark, and instead we decided to steadily expose this region to focal light so as to make the region insensitive to scattered light from the nonfocal light stimulus. The result we obtained by this means is shown in Fig. 8 c, which illustrates a typical simple pattern. When the steady focal light was removed and both focal and nonfocal lights were applied simultaneously, the recording immediately returned to the complex pattern shown in Fig. 8 a. We thus learned that by applying and removing the focal background light we could repeatedly record the simple pattern (c) and the complex pattern (a), respectively, as we wished.

These results afforded complete proof that the model shown in Fig. 7 was valid. I lost no time in writing up our results (TOMITA et al. 1960), and sent a copy of the manuscript to Brindley along with a letter. In his immediate reply he wrote that since this was an extremely serious question, he was exerting every effort to repeat the experiment. In less than ten days I received a second letter in which he completely affirmed the correctness of our model.

It was not very long before the third counterargument appeared. BROWN and WIESEL (1961), in discussing the results of their research on the cat eye, contended that the PIII component of ERG, although not the other ERG components, originated in the receptor layer. In the summer of 1961, I spent three months at Brown's laboratory in San Francisco at his invitation. During that time, I became convinced that their conclusion was indeed quite sound. I puzzled over the question of why there should be such a difference between frog and cat retinas. However, subsequent research conducted by MURAKAMI and KANEKO (1966), using the coaxial microelectrode, yielded results which showed that, at least in the frog retina, the PIII component was a complex potential composed of distal PIII (receptor potential) and proximal PIII (originating in the inner layer).

V. Vertebrate Photoreceptor Potential

Recording the activity of each retinal cell type by intracellular electrodes was what I had been wanting to do since I first began applying microelectrodes to the retina. Intracellular recording was absolutely necessary in order to isolate the individual response of each cell, particularly when the retinal cells were packed densely together and most cells showed only graded responses. However, in spite of my long experience in applying microelectrodes intraretinally, I was able to obtain only two records that seemed to be intracellular: the S-potential discussed previously and potentials accompanying impulse spikes from the ganglion cells. There was no response that made me think it was an intracellular recording from the receptor layer.

To obtain the response of single photoreceptors, I concentrated my efforts on a two-pronged approach. On the one hand I looked for vertebrates with the largest possible photoreceptor cells, and on the other hand I tried to make the tip of the microelectrode as small as possible. Fortunately, since the cyprinid fish has a relatively thick cone inner segment of about 8 μm, it did not seem entirely hopeless that intracellular recordings might be obtained from such cells. Furthermore, in 1959 K.-I. Naka was sent from Kyushu University to my laboratory to study for nine months, and from him I learned how to make superfine microelectrodes with a tip diameter of less than 0.1 μm.

After fashioning such a microelectrode, I attempted to insert it into carp cones. However, each attempt ended in failure, and I spent nearly two years fruitlessly repeating one unsuccessful attempt after another. During this same period MARKS (1963) used a microspectrophotometer to measure the difference spectra of single goldfish cones. I was totally discouraged and thought that there was nothing else

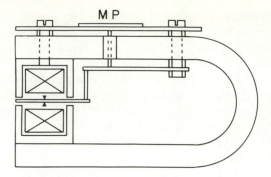

Fig. 9. Device for jolting the retina mounted on the indifferent electrode, a piece of Ag-AgCl, attached to a metal plate (MP) producing vibration. Tomita (1964b)

to do but give up my attempts at intracellular recording. Meanwhile, construction workers started driving piles into the ground directly in front of my laboratory for the new building that was to house the Departments of Biochemistry and Pharmacology. Because of the vibrations caused by the pile driver, I was forced to discontinue my microelectrode experiments. I spent day after day sunk in my chair pondering how I should proceed with my research.

One day, as I sat staring vacantly at the pile driver, an idea flashed through my mind. It occurred to me that it might be possible to tap the microelectrode vertically, and thus drive it into receptor cells in the same way as the piles were driven into the ground. A calculation of the acceleration produced a large value of 32 g (g = the acceleration due to gravity), assuming that the movement of the electrode tip caused by the shock was like a damped oscillation and letting the amplitude of the first wave be 2 μm and the frequency 2,000/s. Moreover, if it were possible to fix the amplitude at 2 μm and increase the frequency (f) further, the acceleration would become directly proportional to f^2 and would increase rapidly concomitant with f.

I was eager to begin the experiment because I felt sure it would work. However, I discovered that with a superfine electrode having a tip diameter of less than 0.1 μm, it was technically impossible to apply a purely vertical vibration to the tip without any horizontal vibration. Once again I was confronted with an impasse. It then occurred to me that instead of tapping the microelectrode to drive it into the retina, the retina could be driven against a vertically positioned microelectrode to achieve the same effect.

To carry out this experiment I fashioned the apparatus shown in Fig. 9 by removing the cone from an old electromagnetic speaker and replacing it with a metal plate (MP). Both ends of the plate were fixed fast and the plate served to produce vibration. A piece of Ag-AgCl attached to the metal plate served as the indifferent electrode. On this I placed the isolated retina with the receptor side up. The strong surge of current produced by a thyratron discharge was set to flow through the coil in synchronization with the flyback pulse of the oscilloscope.

I attempted the experiment with this apparatus and recorded for the first time in the autumn of 1963 a hyperpolarizing intracellular response from a depth cor-

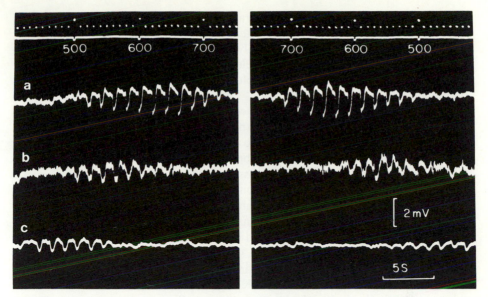

Fig. 10a–c. Three spectral response curves in the carp retina, which were likely to be from single cones with different peaking wavelengths, obtained by a return sweep run of the spectrum in steps of 20-nm wavelengths. TOMITA (1964b)

responding to the receptor layer. Encouraged by the results, I devoted all my energies to improving the experimental apparatus.

In carrying out the intracellular recording experiments I received the collaboration of J. Toyoda, H. Ito, and A. Kaneko. We decided to investigate how many spectral responses with different peaking wavelengths could actually be found in carp cones. To record the spectral response of the S-potential in earlier experiments we had fashioned a spectrum sweep apparatus with which the wavelength could be changed successively. Although the apparatus was not perfect, we were fortunately able to use it to illuminate the retina. The three records shown in Fig. 10 were selected from the records that we made in the autumn and winter of 1963. These three records were chosen because we thought they indicated maximum responses at different wavelengths.

One problem we encountered in this experiment was that most responses did not remain stable for one spectrum sweep, but deteriorated rapidly. Once deterioration appeared during one spectrum sweep, there was the possibility that the response peak would shift. To prevent peak recognition errors, once a spectral response had been obtained by sweeping the spectrum from blue to red, the direction of the spectrum sweep was reversed, and we only selected the responses showing symmetrical patterns. The three examples shown in Fig. 10 represent records that were made by a return sweep run.

The results were reported at two meetings in 1964, one in Tokyo (TOMITA 1964 a) and the other in Paris-Orsay (TOMITA 1964b), and the same report was presented the following year at the Cold Spring Harbor Symposium on sensory receptors (TOMITA 1965). In the meantime, in the United States, BORTOFF (1964) also reported intracellular recordings from mudpuppy photoreceptor cells.

In the following few years, our laboratory became better equipped, and the records (Tomita et al. 1967) obtained after these improvements were much better, as can be seen in Fig. 11. Statistical analysis of 142 such recordings revealed three classes of carp cone. Their peaking wavelengths were in close agreement with those obtained by Marks (1963) in single goldfish cones by means of a microspectrophotometer.

Our subsequent research was directed toward investigating the ionic mechanism involved in the light-induced hyperpolarization that occurs in both cones and rods, the polarity of which is the opposite of that of the ordinary receptor potentials, including those of most invertebrate photoreceptors. Since the specific details of that research have been discussed previously in several review articles (Tomita 1970a, 1972, 1973), only the conclusions, which are shown in Fig. 12, will be presented here. The model on the right side of this figure (D-type) illustrates a simplified ionic mechanism of the ordinary photoreceptor membrane of invertebrates. The resting potential is provided by a K^+ battery and the illumination reduces the resistance of the Na^+ channel, which explains the occurrence of depolarization. For the photoreceptor membrane of vertebrates (H-type in Fig. 12), the resting potential is also provided by a K^+ battery, but the resistance of the Na^+ channel is low in the dark and it is increased by the illumination to produce hyperpolarization. The response to light is thus virtually the opposite of that for invertebrates. In other words, it can be concluded that in the dark, when there is no stimulus, the photoreceptor cells of vertebrates are in an "excitatory state," and that in light they shift to a "resting state."

Initially, I had a very difficult time getting anyone to understand this idea. When I expressed this idea at symposiums and seminars, I was invariably confronted with the counterargument, "How could it be so uneconomical?" To deflect the questioner's challenge, I would ask in return, "When we reflect on our everyday life, which time is longer, that spent in the dark or the time spent in the light?"

Eventually, Hagins et al. (1970) and Korenbrot and Cone (1972) published the results of their investigations, which corroborated my hypothesis from a different perspective. At present I think it is safe to say that the conclusions shown in Fig. 12 have been completely accepted. For the sake of simplification, Fig. 12 shows only the light-induced change in the resistance of the Na^+ channel because this represents the principal change. This, of course, does not negate the existence of other ion-related secondary permeability changes.

I was greatly surprised and at the same time very happy when I learned that the photoreceptor membranes of vertebrates and invertebrates exhibited virtually diametrically opposite responses to light stimulation. In view of the fact that PIII had the shortest latency of all the ERG elements, and also considering that PIII was the most resistant to many chemicals, researchers had suspected for a long time that PIII could be the receptor potential. The largest obstacle that stood in the way of concluding that PIII was the receptor potential was that PIII had a polarity opposite to that of ordinary receptor cells. However, this obstacle was completely removed by the study mentioned above.

The preceding discussion presents a general outline of the research that my colleagues and I conducted during the 1960s in an effort to characterize the single photoreceptor potential. At this stage, with the elucidation of the ionic mechanism

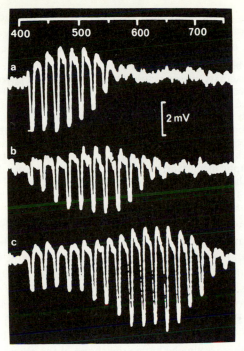

Fig. 11a–c. Three spectral response curves from single carp cones obrained by a sweep run of the spectrum of equal quantum flux. TOMITA et al. (1967)

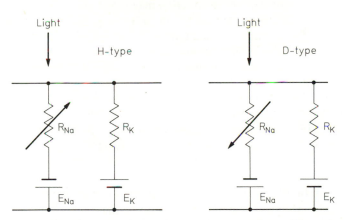

Fig. 12. Electric models of the vertebrate photoreceptor membrane (H-type) and ordinary invertebrate photoreceptor membrane (D-type). In the vertebrate the resistance of Na^+ channel is maintained low in the dark and is increased by light. R_{Na}, resistance of Na^+ channel; R_K, resistance of K^+ channel; E_{Na}, Nernst potential for Na^+ appearing across the cell membrane with the expression

$$E_{Na} = \frac{RT}{F} \ln \frac{[Na^+]_o}{[Na^+]_i} \qquad (2)$$

where $[Na^+]_o$ and $[Na^+]_i$ are extra- and intracellular Na^+ concentrations, respectively; E_K, Nernst potential for K^+. TOMITA (1972)

shown in Fig. 12, my research on the photoreceptor was concluded. In the concluding remarks of my review article (Tomita 1970a), I related my recollections of the
many difficulties we encountered and somehow managed to overcome as follows:

> What then would be the role of the intracellular micropipette technique in future studies
> of the photoreceptor activity? It seems to me that further application of this technique to
> the receptors themselves will no longer bring about very fruitful results, but that the impor-
> tance of this technique will be to record from the bipolar and horizontal cells which make
> synaptic contacts with the receptor terminals (Dowling and Werblin 1969). The analysis
> of responses in these postsynaptic neurons should serve to elucidate the synaptic events as-
> sociated with the hyperpolarizing receptor response. For instance, since the receptors are
> depolarized in the dark and polarized in the light, it is possible that a transmitter, which de-
> polarizes the postsynaptic membrane, continues to be liberated from the synaptic terminals
> of photoreceptors in the dark, and ceases to be liberated in the light (Trifonow 1968). Such
> a possibility could be tested by observing the sign of response in the postsynaptic neurons
> and the direction of changes in the membrane resistance.

I am not sure whether my colleagues were influenced by my thinking, or
whether it merely happened by chance, but at any rate, thereafter they shifted their
interest entirely from the receptor cells to more proximal cells. On the other hand,
photoreceptor research has been pursued very vigorously in Europe and especially
in the United States, contrary to my initial expectation. A few examples of the research areas that have been pursued include: (a) interreceptoral electrical connections, (b) feedback from horizontal cells to receptors, and (c) time- and voltage-
dependent permeability of the inner segment membrane. It is becoming clear that
all of the above are factors which change the shape of the receptor potential predictable from the model shown in Fig. 12.

In parallel with the photoreceptor research, steady progress has been made in
investigating the photoreceptor transduction mechanisms which occur in the interval between the light quantum absorption and the generation of the receptor
potential. At the present time, the calcium theory advanced by Hagins (1972) and
the cyclic nucleotides theory initially proposed by Bitensky et al. (1971) are rival
explanations of the transduction mechanisms. Both theories are concerned with ex-
plicating the mechanism that appears as a hyperpolarizing response when the Na^+
channel which has been opened in the dark is closed by exposure to light. Since biochemistry is far from being my area of expertise, a detailed critical evaluation of
these theories is beyond my ability. However, I enjoy learning about the present
status of the field from studies such as that by Miller (1981).

VI. Receptor-Horizontal and Receptor-Bipolar Transmission – An Unconventional Type of Subsynaptic Membrane

The horizontal cells and bipolar cells are two cell types that make direct synaptic
contact with photoreceptors. As mentioned previously, when photoreceptor cells
are stimulated, their response is exactly opposite in polarity to that of ordinary receptor cells. What then is the synaptic transmission like? Today it is common
knowledge that the transmitter substance is released when the presynaptic cells depolarize. If this theory is applied to the vertebrate photoreceptors, it can only be
concluded that in the dark there is a continued release of the transmitter substance,
but when hyperpolarization takes place with exposure to light, the release either

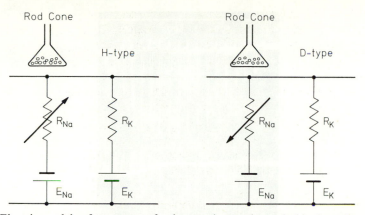

Fig. 13. Electric models of two types of subsynaptic membrane in bipolar cells: unconventional type (H-type) for the on-center response, and conventional EPS type (D-type) for the off-center response. TOMITA (1973)

stops or decreases. The following experiments, in which the response of the horizontal cells was used as the indicator, were instrumental in establishing the unquestionable validity of this idea.

In the first experiment, when the receptor synaptic ending was depolarized by transretinal current pulses, the horizontal cells depolarized (TRIFONOW 1968). In a second experiment, by application of putative transmitters (aspartate and glutamate) to the retina, depolarization of the horizontal cells occurred (MURAKAMI et al. 1972). Furthermore, in a third experiment, when the transmitter release was suppressed using high Mg^{2+} or low Ca^{2+} media or by Co^{2+}, the horizontal cells hyperpolarized (DOWLING and RIPPS 1973; CERVETTO and PICCOLINO 1974; KANEKO and SHIMAZAKI 1975 a, b). The results of these experiments show that the receptor-horizontal transmission is the conventional excitatory postsynaptic potential (EPSP) type.

Then what is the nature of the ionic mechanisms of the receptor-bioplar transmission? It has been shown by WERBLIN and DOWLING (1969) and by KANEKO (1970) that there are two types of bipolar cell: the on-center type, which responds to a spot of light on the recording site with depolarization, and the off-center type, which responds to the same stimulus with hyperpolarization. Most of these bipolar cells respond to an annulus of light with the reversed polarity, so that they make an on-center/off-surround type and an off-center/on-surround type respectively. Bridge records by TOYODA (1973) of the on-center and off-center responses in the absence of the surround effect showed that the depolarizing and hyperpolarizing responses, elicited by a spot of light, are simply accompanied by a decrease and increase in the input resistance respectively; both responses are enhanced by hyperpolarizing extrinsic current and suppressed by depolarizing extrinsic current. This suggested that both hyper- and depolarizing responses are the result of regulation of Na^+ channels, but in opposite directions. The concept is summarized in Fig. 13 by a pair of models analogous to the two types of photoreceptor membrane shown in Fig. 12. A synaptic rod or cone terminal containing vesicles is in contact with the subsynaptic membrane of a bipolar cell, where the Na^+ channel either remains

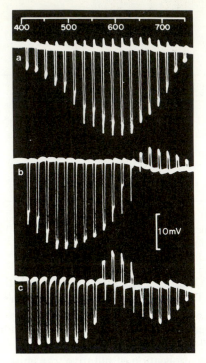

Fig. 14a–c. Three types of spectral response of carp horizontal cells: **a** monophasic, **b** biphasic, and **c** triphasic. Tomita (1965)

open when there is no transmitter release and is closed by release of the transmitter (left, H-type), or remains closed when there is no transmitter release and is opened by release of the transmitter (right, D-type). On the basis of the evidence that there is a continuous release of transmitter in the dark which is suppressed by light, the H-type should represent the membrane of the on-center response and the D-type the off-center response.

I was curious to know whether an H-type synapse such as the one shown in Fig. 13 does exist in some other parts of the nervous system, and made inquiries about it in an essay to Japanese neurophysiologists (Tomita 1970b), but with few responses. Recently, however, further pieces of evidence have been provided in the retina for the two types of bipolar cell characterized by the two types of subsynaptic membrane shown in Fig. 13. First, Murakami et al. (1975) observed that glutamate and aspartate, which mimic the transmitter action, depolarize the off-center bipolar cell, while they hyperpolarize the on-center bipolar cell. Secondly, Kaneko and Shimazaki (1975) showed that short transretinal current pulses applied in the direction to depolarize the synaptic terminals of receptors, and hence to cause transmitter release, depolarize the off-center bipolar cell but hyperpolarize the on-center bipolar cell. According to more recent studies by Saito et al. (1979), the H-type and D-type in Fig. 13 do apply to the rod bipolar transmission but not always to the cone bipolar transmission. Despite this complexity, all the above studies demonstrate the existence in the retina of an unconventional type of subsynaptic mem-

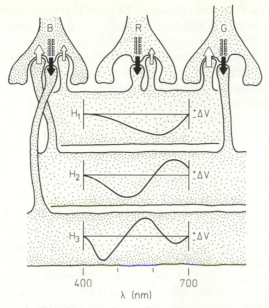

Fig. 15. Cone-horizontal cell pathways inferred from electron microscopy of goldfish retina. *B, R, G,* blue-, red-, and green-sensitive cones; H_1, H_2, H_3, monophasic, biphasic, triphasic cone-horizontal cells. Sign-inverting synapses are shown by *white arrows,* and sign-conserving synapses by *dark arrows.* STELL et al. (1975)

brane, or H-type in Fig. 13, in which Na^+ channels remain open in the absence of the transmitter and are closed by the transmitter.

Coming back to the receptor–horizontal transmission, it is well known that in animals possessing color vision a Young–Helmholtz trichromatic type process at the receptor level (see Fig. 11) is converted to a Hering opponent color type process at the horizontal cell level (Fig. 14). I had once thought that the ionic mechanisms shown by the two models in Fig. 13 might also account for this conversion. Later, however, GOURAS (1972), FUORTES and SIMON (1974), and eventually STELL et al. (1975) proposed that the conversion is the result of an interaction between cones and horizontal cells in such a manner as illustrated by the model in Fig. 15. The following experiment performed recently by TOYODA et al. (1982) supports the model in this figure. They applied two microelectrodes, one in an H_1 horizontal cell and the other in an H_2 horizontal cell, and observed that when the H_1 cell was de- or hyperpolarized by extrinsic current, the potential of the H_2 cell shifted in the opposite direction. Similarly, with a pair of electrodes, one of which was in an H_2 cell and the other in an H_3 cell, a change in the membrane potential of the H_2 cell by extrinsic current caused the potential of the H_3 cell to shift in the opposite direction.

D. Concluding Remarks

Many other important retinal functions, such as adaptation, retinal circuitry, retinal synaptology, and the detail of the color coding, have not been discussed in this chapter. All of these functions, however, lie outside the immediate area of my research, and a review of the literature on them was not the object of this chapter. Therefore, I will defer all discussion regarding them until another time.

In 1969 I was obligated to serve for a short time as the Dean of Keio Medical School, and soon after that I reached mandatory retirement age. Fortunately, through the cordial invitation of W. H. Miller, whose friendship I had enjoyed since my stay in Hartline's laboratory in 1952–1953, and M. L. Sears, the Chairman of the Department of Ophthalmology and Visual Science at Yale Medical School, of which Miller was a member, I became a member of the Yale University faculty. Thus for the past ten years I have been going back and forth between Yale Medical School and St. Marianna Medical School, located in the suburbs of Tokyo, and I have concentrated my research on reexamining the origins of the ERG waves in collaboration with my colleagues at both institutions. At one time the ERG was investigated as an important method for elucidating retinal mechanisms. In recent years, however, intracellular recording from single retinal cells and dye staining of these cells have made physiological study of individual cell function and morphological cell identification possible. Consequently, the wheel has turned a full circle, and now the origins of the ERG waves can be sought in individual retinal cell functions. This interpretation was the starting point for my reinvestigation of ERG, and already some of the relationships between retinal cell functions and ERG waves have been clarified (TOMITA 1978; TOMITA and YANAGIDA 1981).

Upon returning to ERG research, I became more fully cognizant of the invaluable contributions made by several researchers in this field, and in this regard I would particularly like to mention the following two individuals.

The first is W. K. Noell, who in 1954 had already located the origin of the ERG c-wave in the pigment epithelium (NOELL 1954), and in a later study (NOELL 1963) suggested, as I had earlier (TOMITA 1950), that the c-wave was generated as a consequence of some ionic interaction between pigment epithelial cells and photoreceptor cells. In June 1969, at the Fifth Annual Symposium on Mechanisms of Vertebrate Vision, which was held in Rochester (United States), I had an opportunity to have a personal discussion with Noell. At that time he was quite certain that the origin of both the ERG c- and b-waves was nonneuronal. He stated that the former originated in the pigment epithelial cells and the latter in the Müller cells. Since I had been familiar with his previous work, I was not at all surprised when he said that the origin of the c-wave was in the pigment epithelial cells. However, I must confess I had to suppress a feeling of discomfort with regard to his assertion that the b-wave originated in the Müller cells. When I reflect back on our discussion now, I realize that Noell had merely related to me what he regarded as valid based on the research being done in his laboratory at that time by FABER (1969). One reason Noell's group ascribed the origin of the b-wave to the Müller cells was that the transretinal distribution of the b-wave showed excellent agreement with the total extension of the Müller cells. Several questions (see TOMITA and YANAGIDA 1981) have been raised about the validity of the Müller cell theory of the b-wave, as it was proposed in its original form by FABER (1969) and shortly thereafter by MILLER and DOWLING (1970), but it is my feeling that the problems which have been pointed out do not negate the Müller cell theory; rather, they suggest the necessity of making some modifications in it.

The second individual whom I should like to mention is S. W. Kuffler, who in collaboration with his colleagues (see KUFFLER 1967) demonstrated that the glial cell membrane behaves exactly like a K$^+$ electrode. Thus Kuffler made a significant contribution to the fundamental evidence supporting the conclusions drawn by Noell's group. Today it has been established that the pigment epithelial cells function as K$^+$ electrodes and that the c-wave is generated as a result of the [K$^+$]$_o$ change which accompanies the response of the photoreceptor cells to light (see OAKLEY 1981). Kuffler's basic biological studies, which ranged over a number of different areas, have very broad applicability in helping to explain various phenomena. The explanation of the action of the glial cell membrane as a K$^+$ electrode is just one example of the many significant contributions he made, which include his discovery of the concentric antagonistic organization of the receptive field of ganglion cells. This apparently stimulated Hubel and Wiesel to initiate their research on the receptive field of neurons in the visual cortex. It is a matter of profound regret to me that, while I was writing this chapter, I was informed of his death (11 October 1980). As a token of my esteem for Kuffler's outstanding achievements, I would like to close by emphasizing my admiration for his many contributions, not merely to vision research, but also to sensory science in general.

Acknowledgements. I would like to express my gratitude to Drs. TSUTOMU WAKABAYASHI (Professor Emeritus of Tokyo University), NAOKI TOIDA (Professor Emeritus of Kyushu University), EIICHI KIMURA (Professor and President of Osaka City University), and KYOJI TASAKI (Professor of Tohoku University) for providing the data and materials for Sect. B of this chapter; to Professor RYOJI KIKUCHI and Mrs. MASAKO SHIMODA of the Department of Physiology at Tokyo Women's Medical College for their painstaking help as intermediators between the translator and me; to Mr. LARRY D. CHRISTENSEN for his excellent translation from Japanese; and finally to Mrs. DORIS JAMISON of the Department of Ophthalmology and Visual Science at Yale University for her invaluable assistance in making the manuscript final.

References

Adrian ED (1945) The electric response of the human eye. J Physiol (Lond) 104:84–104

Adrian ED (1946) Rod and cone components in the electric response of the eye. J Physiol (Lond) 105:24–37

Adrian ED, Bronk DW (1928) The discharge of impulses in motor nerve fibres. Part I. Impulses in single fibres of the phrenic nerve. J Physiol (Lond) 66:81–101

Bitensky MW, Gorman RE, Miller WH (1971) Adenyl cyclase as a link between photon capture and changes in membrane permeability of frog photoreceptors. Proc Natl Acad Sci USA 68:561–562

Bortoff A (1964) Localization of slow potential responses in the *Necturus* retina. Vision Res 4:627–635

Brindley GS (1956a) The passive electrical properties of the frog's retina, choroid and sclera for radial fields and currents. J Physiol (Lond) 134:339–352

Brindley GS (1956b) The effect on the frog's electroretinogram of varying the amount of retina illuminated. J Physiol (Lond) 134:353–359

Brindley GS (1956c) Responses to illumination recorded by microelectrodes from the frog's retina. J Physiol (Lond) 134:360–384

Brindley GS (1960) Physiology of the retina and the visual pathway. Arnold, London

Brown KT, Wiesel TN (1958) Intraretinal recording in the unopened cat eye. Am J Ophthalmol 46:91–96

Brown KT, Wiesel TN (1961) Localization of origins of electroretinogram components by intraretinal recording in the intact cat eye. J Physiol (Lond) 158:257–280

Cervetto L, Piccolino M (1974) Synaptic transmission between photoreceptors and horizontal cells in the turtle retina. Science 183:417–419

Dowling JE, Ripps H (1973) Effects of magnesium on horizontal cell activity in the skate retina. Nature 242:101–103

Dowling JE, Werblin FS (1969) Organization of retina of the mudpuppy, *Necturus maculosus*. I. Synaptic structure. J Neurophysiol 32:315–338

Faber DS (1969) Analysis of the slow transretinal potentials in response to light. PhD thesis, University of New York at Buffalo

Fuortes MGF, Simon EJ (1974) Interactions leading to horizontal cell responses in the turtle retina. J Physiol (Lond) 240:177–198

Galambos R, Davis H (1943) The response of single auditory nerve fibres to acoustic stimulation. J Neurophysiol 6:39–58

Gasser HS, Erlanger J (1922) A study of the action currents of nerve with the cathode ray oscillograph. Am J Physiol 62:496–524

Gebhard JW (1953) Motokawa's studies on electric excitation of the human eye. Psychol Bull 50:37–75

Gouras P (1972) S-potentials. In: Fourtes MGF (ed) Physiology of photoreceptor organs. Springer, Berlin Heidelberg New York, pp 513–529 (Handbook of sensory physiology, vol 7 pt 2)

Granit R (1947) Sensory mechanisms of the retina. Oxford University Press, London

Hagins WA (1972) The visual process: excitatory mechanisms in the primary receptor cells. Annu Rev Biophys Bioeng 1:131–158

Hagins WA, Penn RD, Yoshikami S (1970) Dark current and photocurrent in retinal rods. Biophys J 10:380–412

Hartline HK (1949) Inhibition of activity of visual receptors by illuminating nearby retinal areas in the *Limulus* eye (abstract). Fed Proc 8:69

Hosoya Y (1929a) Studien über das Tapetum lucidum chorioideale. Tohoku J Exp Med 12:119–145

Hosoya Y (1929b) Über den Sehpurpur im tapezierten Auge. Tohoku J Exp Med 12:146–152

Hosoya Y (1933) Absorptionsspektrum des Sehpurpurs und des Sehgelbs; Nachbleichung des Sehgelbs im Dunkeln. Pflügers Arch Ges Physiol 233:57–66

Hosoya Y (1957) Collected papers in physiology of vision. Hosoya Domonkai in Department of Physiology, Osaka City University Medical School, Osaka

Hosoya Y, Bayerl V (1933) Spektrale Absorption des Sehpurpurs vor und nach der Bleichung. Pflügers Arch Ges Physiol 231:563–570

Hosoya Y, Okita T, Akune T (1938) Über die lichtempfindliche Substanz in der Zapfennetzhaut. Tohoku J Exp Med 34:532–541

Howarth CI, Treisman M (1958) Validity of Motokawa's technique for investigating retinal function. Nature 191:843–844

Kaneko A (1970) Physiological and morphological identification of horizontal, bipolar, and amacrine cells in goldfish retina. J Physiol (Lond) 207:623–633

Kaneko A, Shimazaki H (1975a) Synaptic transmission from photoreceptors to bipolar and horizontal cells in the carp retina. Cold Spring Harbor Symp Quant Biol 40:537–546

Kaneko A, Shimazaki H (1975b) Effects of external ions on the synaptic transmission from photoreceptors to horizontal cells in the carp retina. J Physiol (Lond) 252:509–522

Kato G (1924) The theory of decrementless conduction in narcotised region of nerve. Nankodo, Tokyo

Kato G (1926) The further studies on decrementless conduction. Nankodo, Tokyo

Kato G (1934) The microphysiology of nerve. Maruzen, Tokyo

Kimura E (1952) A new method of separating the outer segments of rods from retinal tissues. Jpn J Physiol 3:25–28

Kohlrausch A (1931) Elektrische Erscheinungen am Auge. In: Handbuch der normalen und pathologischen Physiologie 12/2. Springer, Berlin, S. 1394–1496

Korenbrot JI, Cone RA (1972) Dark ionic flux and the effects of light in isolated rod outer segments. J Gen Physiol 60:20–45

Kuffler SW (1952) Neurons in the retina: organization, inhibition, and excitation problems. Cold Spring Harbor Symp Quant Biol 17:281–292

Kuffler SW (1967) Neurologial cells: physiological properties and a potassium-mediated effect of neuronal activity on the glial membrane potential. Ferrier Lecture. Proc R Soc Lond [Biol] 168:1–21

Ling G, Gerard RW (1949) The normal membrane potential of frog sartorius fibres. J Cell Comp Physiol 34:383–396

MacNichol EF Jr, Svaetichin G (1958) Electric responses from isolated retinas of fishes. Am J Ophthalmol 45:26–40

Marks WB (1963) Difference spectra of the visual pigments in single goldfish cones. PhD dissertation, The Johns Hopkins University, Baltimore

Miller RF, Dowling JE (1970) Intracellular responses of the Müller (glial) cells of the mudpuppy retina: their relation to b-wave of the electroretinogram. J Neurophysiol 33:323–341

Miller WH (ed) (1981) Molecular mechanisms of photoreceptor transduction. Academic, New York

Mitarai G (1958) The origin of the so-called cone action potential. Proc Jpn Acad 34:299–304

Motokawa K (1948) Physiological basis of sensation (in Japanese). Kagaku 18:526–537

Motokawa K (1970) Physiology of color and pattern vision. Igaku Shoin, Tokyo

Motokawa K, Mita T (1942) Über eine einfachere Untersuchungsmethode und Eigenschaften der Aktionsströme der Netzhaut des Menschen. Tohoku J Exp Med 42:114–133

Murakami M, Kaneko A (1966) Differentiation of PIII subcomponents in cold-blooded vertebrate retinas. Vision Res 6:627–636

Murakami M, Ohtsu K, Ohtsuka T (1972) Effects of chemicals on receptors and horizontal cells in the retina. J Physiol (Lond) 227:899–913

Murakami M, Ohtsuka T, Shimazaki H (1975) Effects of aspartate and glutamate on the bipolar cells in the carp retina. Vision Res 15:456–458

Noell WK (1954) The origin of the electroretinogram. Am J Ophthalmol 38:78–90

Noell WK (1963) Cellular physiology of the retina. J Opt Soc Am 53:36–48

Oakley B (1981) Light-evoked changes in retinal extracellular potassium. In: Zeuthen T (ed) The application of ion-selective microelectrodes. Elsevier, Amsterdam, pp 109–128

Oikawa T, Ogawa T, Motokawa K (1959) Origin of so-called cone action potential. J Neurophysiol 22:102–111

Ottoson D, Svaetichin G (1952) Electrophysiological investigations of the frog retina. Cold Spring Harbor Symp Quant Biol 17:165–173

Riggs LA (1973) Motokawa's monograph. Interam J Psychol 7:255–258

Riggs LA, Cornsweet JC, Lewis WG (1957) Effects of light on electrical excitation of the human eye. Psychol Mon 71:1–45

Rushton WAH (1956) The difference spectrum and the photosensitivity of rhodopsin in the living human eye. J Physiol (Lond) 134:11–29

Saito T, Kondo H, Toyoda J (1979) Ionic mechanisms of two types of on-center bipolar cells in the carp retina. I. The responses to central illumination. J Gen Physiol 73:73–90

Saito Z (1938) Isolierung der Stäbchenaußenglieder und spektrale Untersuchung des daraus hergestellten Sehpurpurextraktes. Tohoku J Exp Med 32:432–446

Stell WK, Lightfoot DO, Wheeler TG, Leeper HF (1975) Goldfish retina: functional polarization of cone horizontal cell dendrites and synapses. Science 190:989–990

Svaetichin G (1953) The cone action potential. Acta Physiol Scand 29 [Suppl 106]:565–600

Svaetichin G (1956) The spectral response curves from single cones. Acta Physiol Scand 39 [Suppl 134]:17–46

Tasaki I (1954) Nerve impulses in individual auditory nerve fibers of guinea pig. J Neurophysiol 17:97–122

Tasaki I (1959) Conduction of the nerve impulse: In: Field J, Magoun HW, Hall VE (eds) Handbook of physiology, Section 1, Neurophysiology 1. American Physiological Society, Washington, D.C, pp 75–121

Tomita T (1950) Studies on the intraretinal action potential. Part I. Relation between the localization of micropipette in the retina and the shape of the intraretinal action potential. Jpn J Physiol 1:110–117

Tomita T (1956) The nature of action potentials in the lateral eye of the horseshoe crab as revealed by simultaneous intra- and extracellular recording. Jpn J Physiol 6:327–340

Tomita T (1957) A study on the origin of intraretinal action potential of the cyprinid fish by means of pencil-type microelectrode. Jpn J Physiol 7:80–85

Tomita T (1958) Mechanism of lateral inhibition in eye of *Limulus*. J Neurophysiol 21:419–429

Tomita T (1962) A compensation circuit for coaxial and double-barreled microelectrodes. IRE Trans Biomed Electron 9:138–141

Tomita T (1964a) Attempt at intracellular recording from single photoreceptors in the vertebrate. Symposium on neurophysiology, Japan-US science cooperation program, Tokyo, p 58

Tomita T (1964b) Mechanisms subserving color coding in the vertebrate retina. IOPAB international biophysics meeting, Paris-Orsay, Abstract II, CIII, 1

Tomita T (1965) Electrophysiological study of the mechanisms subserving color coding in the fish retina. Cold Spring Harbor Symp Quant Biol 30:559–566

Tomita T (1970a) Electrical activity of vertebrate photoreceptors. Quart Rev Biophys 3:179–222

Tomita T (1970b) An inquiry to neurophysiologists (in Japanese). J Keio Med Soc 47:692–693

Tomita T (1972) Light-induced potential and resistance changes in vertebrate photoreceptors. In: Fuortes MGF (ed) Physiology of photoreceptor organs. Springer, Berlin Heidelberg New York, pp 483–511 (Handbook of sensory physiology, vol 7 pt 2)

Tomita T (1973) Electrophysiology of the receptors and postsynaptic neurons in the vertebrate retina. Nova Acta Leopold 37/2:13–30

Tomita T (1978) ERG waves and retinal cell function. Sens Processes 2:276–284

Tomita T, Yanagida T (1981) Origins of the ERG waves. Vision Res 21:1703–1707

Tomita T, Kanda M, Ida H, Hara A (1952) Comparative study of the intraretinal action potential (EIRG) in several vertebrates (in Japanese). J Physiol Soc Jpn 14:256–257

Tomita T, Murakami M, Sato Y, Hashimoto Y (1959) Further study on the origin of the so-called cone action potential (S-potential). Its histological determination. Jpn J Physiol 9:63–68

Tomita T, Murakami M, Hashimoto Y (1960) On the R membrane in the frog's eye. Its localization, and relation to the retinal action potential. J Gen Physiol 43:81–94

Tomita T, Kaneko A, Murakami M, Pautler EL (1964) Spectral response curves of single cones in the carp. Vision Res 7:519–531

Toyoda J (1973) Membrane resistance changes underlying the bipolar cell response in the carp retina. Vision Res 13:283–294

Toyoda J, Kujiraoka T, Fujimoto M (1982) The role of L-type horizontal cells in the opponent color process. Color Res Appl 7:Pt 2, 152–154

Trifonow JuA (1968) Study of synaptic transmission between photoreceptors and horizontal cells by means of electric stimulation of the retina (in Russian). Biophysica 13:809–817

Verworn M (1894) Allgemeine Physiologie. Ein Grundriß der Lehre vom Leben. Fischer, Jena

Werblin FS, Dowling JE (1969) Organization of the retina of the mudpuppy, *Necturus maculosus*. II. Intracellular recording. J Neurophysiol 32:339–355

CHAPTER 6

Recollections of Early Laboratory Experiments on Vision

Lorrin A. Riggs

A. Introduction

My task is to describe, for readers mostly younger than myself, a half century of experience in the field of vision research. But there are two formidable barriers to this communication. First, I can scarcely remember the impetuous and inexperienced person that I was so long ago; and secondly, the world itself has changed so radically since then. As André Maurois once said, "The minds of different generations are as impenetrable one by the other as are the monads of Leibniz." I never could understand Leibniz.

Perhaps the best way out – if there is one – is to emphasize whatever continuity I can discern from one stage to the next in this long journey. At each stage, after all, there are the antecedent persons, ideas, and results that lead up to the next stage: a *connectedness,* if you will. This connectedness seems real enough over the short span of one academic generation. Perhaps, with a judicious application of hindsight, it can be seen that there are even some themes and predilections that run through the whole period. With more or less difficulty I may be able to show that at least two factors have operated to shape the research from the earliest days to the most recent. One is a penchant for objective methods rather than subjective ones for measuring visual sensitivity, and the other is a preoccupation with the design and use of new devices for the recording of visual responses.

Anyway, I shall try. I shall first try to size up my indebtedness to a number of academic forbears, then thread the way through my own generation, and finally lead up to some talented younger people whom I have been privileged to know. Because so much of my academic career has been at Brown University, I shall emphasize the work in vision done at that institution.

B. Early Research at Brown University

I. The Delabarre Laboratory (1892–1927)

Edmund Burke Delabarre (Fig. 1) founded one of the earliest laboratories of psychology in America at Brown. Like most American scholars of his day, he had gone to Europe for graduate studies, earning the PhD degree under Hugo Muensterberg at the University of Freiburg in 1892. At Brown he assembled some of the standard psychological equipment of those days, (e.g., chronoscopes, tachistoscopes, and ergographs) and set it up in a laboratory room that was made available to him, primarily for the instruction of undergraduates, in the physics building. His was a one-man department, without graduate students or other colleagues. But he did have a strong interest in visual perception. He was fascinated by the possibility of using muscular activity as an indicator of sensory processes.

A notable accomplishment of Delabarre's was his development of one of the earliest attachments to the human eye for the purpose of recording eye movements. It consisted of a shell of plaster of Paris that was carefully molded to fit over the cornea. To it was attached a light piece of thread running to a recording lever, so that the movement of the eye could be recorded on the smoked drum of a kymograph (DELABARRE 1898). The idea was a good one, but far ahead of its time. Half a century later, the same idea was to be carried out much more easily by Ratliff and myself (RATLIFF and RIGGS 1950). By that time we had the benefit of plastic contact lenses to achieve a firmer and more comfortable attachment to the eye.

Delabarre, as was typical of a *Gelehrter* (scholar) of this time, had interests that ranged widely. A major fascination of his, dating from about 1914, was with Dighton Rock. This rock appears to bear historical markings carved on it by early ex-

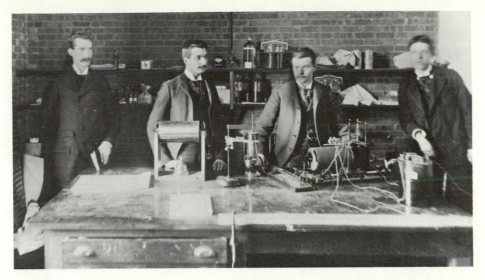

Fig. 1. Delabarre (*second from right*) with three Brown undergraduates in the laboratory of psychology in 1892/1893. The kymograph was later used in recording eye movements

plorers of the New England shores. From his summer cottage nearby, Delabarre spent many years of research unraveling these markings. He came to the conclusion that the principal inscription was by Miguel Cortereal, a Portuguese explorer, dating from 1511. As a psychologist, Delabarre was fascinated by the myriad interpretations and misinterpretations by other investigators of what they perceived to be a diversity of meaningful inscriptions. He bolstered his own theory with photographic evidence, and eventually published a book about it (DELABARRE 1928).

When I first came to Brown in 1938, Delabarre had already retired. I remember him as a gentle, soft-spoken man in his seventies. He still maintained a lively interest in human perception, and came regularly to his office in the psychology building until shortly before his death in 1945.

II. The Carmichael Years (1927–1936)

Leonard Carmichael (1898–1975) was appointed in 1927 to succeed Delabarre as Chairman and to institute a graduate program in psychology at Brown. During his tenure the Department acquired laboratory space in an old frame house at 89 Waterman Street, initially used by Carmichael as his own residence. Carmichael was a tall and imposing man; he commanded immediate attention as a lecturer of undergraduates and as a father figure for junior faculty and graduate students. My first meeting with him was in 1934, not at Brown but at Clark University, where I was a graduate student at the time. Carmichael had driven from Providence to Worcester in his large, open touring car, a huge dog riding in the seat beside him. He addressed the Clark colloquium on the experiments that he and his protégés were doing at Brown on fetal behavior of the guinea pig, reflex responses in the cat, and the maturation of swimming movements in the tadpole.

Carmichael left no doubt that the course of the Brown Department was firmly set in the direction of physiological and behavioral research. Further in that direction, he teamed up with a neurophysiologist, Herbert H. Jasper, for experiments at a neighboring institution, the Emma Pendleton Bradley Home for emotionally disturbed children. In the relatively well-equipped laboratory there they made some of the earliest American records of the newly discovered electroencephalogram. In a prophetic paper, Jasper and Carmichael (1935) concluded:

> ... it has been possible for us to confirm many of Berger's observational findings. With the improvement of recording technique and with an increased understanding of the functional relationship between the results secured and other processes of the living organism, it may well be that electroencephalograms of the sort described in this note may prove significant in psychology and clinical neurology.

Their reported findings included the suppression of alpha waves by visual stimulation, and the appearance of characteristic slow waves in a patient suffering an epileptic seizure.

Thus it was that Brown University, together with Harvard and a few other centers, became a pioneer in the pursuit of electrical records from the human brain. Carmichael did indeed get a significant research program going at Brown before leaving, in 1936, to further a career that was to include the presidency of Tufts University and later the secretaryship of the Smithsonian Institution.

III. The Hunter Regime (1936–1954)

In appointing Walter Hunter to the Chair of Psychology, Brown University secured a person who would surely continue on the course set by his predecessor. Indeed, he had strong behavioral leanings, and sought explanations in the underlying physiological and anatomical features of man and other animals. He also resembled Carmichael in presenting to the world a somewhat austere and autocratic appearance (Fig. 2). Hunter, moreover, had a directness and intolerance of sham that inspired confidence and respect on the part of his colleagues. He ran the Department like a benevolent dictator, making all the decisions alone, but only after seeking out the opinions of those who were closely concerned. He also took a fierce pride in his personal accomplishments and those of his own Department. He was at the same time a father figure and a role model for his "academic children" – faculty and graduate students alike. Perhaps by today's standards he would have been branded a chauvinist, racist, and sexist. But he knew "a good man" when he saw one, and did all he could to provide his protégés with whatever opportunities they seemed to merit for professional advancement.

With all his insistence on academic excellence, Hunter strove to minimize competitiveness and jealousies among his students and staff. At the beginning of each year he have a quiet "pep talk," telling all of us that we were to work very hard to distinguish ourselves by our academic accomplishments. But the aim was not to beat out any of our colleagues. Hunter's bitter experiences with Murchison at Clark (see Sec. CII) were perhaps still fresh in his memory when he urged us to work together as a team, to build up the recognition of the Brown Department by becoming leaders in our respective fields of teaching and research. This theme, in fact, has guided the efforts of each of Hunter's successors as chairman: Schlosberg,

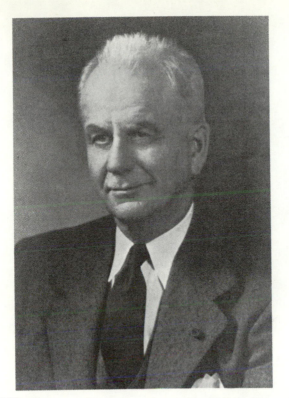

Fig. 2. Walter S. Hunter

Kling, Blough, Eimas, and Church. And it has worked well; the Department still cherishes a tradition of friendliness as well as one of sound accomplishment.

Hunter did only a few experiments of his own in the area of vision (HUNTER 1914, 1915, 1942). But he maintained a strong interest in that field, and he was the one who attracted first Clarence Graham and eventually me to join him in the Department. Hunter once told me that Harvey Carr, his PhD sponsor at the University of Chicago, had asked him to choose between two alternative projects for his dissertation. The one he chose was the "delayed reaction" in animals; but the second choice was the electroretinogram in response to flashes of light. I often wonder what might have happened, had he chosen the second instead of the first. As it was, his dissertation on the delayed reaction led to a fruitful line of comparative studies of animals, human infants, and adults. Out of it grew also two of the basic techniques for testing intelligence, namely the multiple choice and the delayed response.

C. The Background of the 1930s

I. Graham's Early Training

Clarence H. Graham (1906–1971) (Fig. 3) grew up in Worcester, Massachusetts. He remained there, going to Clark University for his undergraduate and graduate

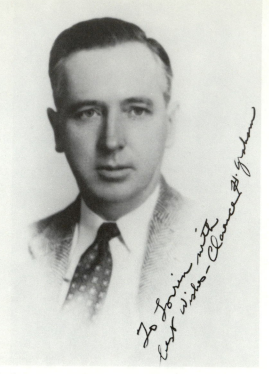

Fig. 3. Clarence H. Graham

work in psychology and receiving the PhD degree in 1930 under John Paul Nafe. After an initial year of teaching at Temple University, Graham went as a postdoctoral fellow to work in the Johnson Foundation for Medical Physics at the University of Pennsylvania. The head of that Foundation was Detlev Bronk, who had done pioneer work in the recording of nerve impulses with Adrian in England. But Graham chose to work with H. Keffer Hartline, a promising young neurophysiologist who had received the MD degree at John Hopkins and had just returned from two years of postdoctoral work in Germany.

Hartline and Graham were both perfectionists in their work habits. They also shared a penchant for applying mathematical treatment to their data. Each, too, had had to work very hard to earn the necessary money for an education. And each had a puckish sense of humor, together with a profound distrust of "the establishment" in medicine or science. But there the similarities ended. Graham craved companionship, and seldom worked alone. Hartline, on the other hand, built up his own unique equipment and planned his own experiments. Graham had episodes of self-doubt and uncertainty, Hartline never: often he was heard to mutter, "If you want something done right, do it yourself."

Hartline's early research was done principally on the excised compound eye and optic nerve of the horseshoe crab, *Limulus polyphemus*. His was an exquisite knack of carefully dissecting out a single active fiber of the optic nerve and recording from it the train of impulses initiated by flashes of light. Clarence Graham, who did not share the patience or delicacy of touch for such work, could only stand by in admiration. But he did once tell me that he believed it was his words of encouragement that first led Hartline to dissect out a single optic nerve fiber of *Limulus* (HARTLINE and GRAHAM 1932). Hartline's successful exploitation of this technique, followed by even more difficult work on single fibers in the frog retina (HARTLINE 1938), finally prepared the way for Granit, Kuffler, Tomita, and many subsequent workers to explore single-unit activity in a wide range of experimental animals.

In the early stages of the *Limulus* work, it appeared that each separate facet of the compound eye was responding in isolation to the light falling on it. The presumption was that the optic nerve was a bundle of fibers, one from each facet, that carried impulses directly to the central ganglion. There, presumably, the activity of the many hundreds of facets, each pointing in a particular direction, could be analyzed into a neural representation of the visual scene. GRAHAM (1933), much to his later embarrassment, actually published a paper at that time entitled, "The Relation of Nerve Response and Retinal Potential to Number of Sense Cells Illuminated in an Eye Lacking Lateral Connections." It was only much later, alas, that HARTLINE and RATLIFF (1957) revealed the mutual inhibition among the sense cells that must result from neural interconnections just behind them. Still later, BARLOW et al. (1977) demonstrated that the intact eye of *Limulus,* as distinct from Hartline's excised eye preparation, is subject to much greater modification of sensitivity due to dark adaptation and circadian rhythms.

But to return to the early 1930s, it was in the Hartline laboratory that Graham first encountered Ragnar Granit (see his chapter in this volume) and R. Margaria, with each of whom he did psychophysical experiments on human vision (GRAHAM and GRANIT 1931; GRAHAM and MARGARIA 1935).

After his postdoctoral year with Hartline, Graham was offered a position as Instructor at Clark University, his old alma mater. He went there in 1932, and only one year later I showed up for work in his laboratory as a new graduate student.

II. My Graduate Student Years

I went to Clark from Dartmouth College, where I had majored in psychology and had developed a strong interest in vision by working in the laboratory with Theodore Karwoski. But Karwoski was mainly a perception man, who was fascinated by subjective phenomena such as illusions and afterimages, interpreted along the lines of Gestalt theory. My own interests, though, were more in the direction of optics, electronics, and apparatus design. Not many Dartmouth graduates went on to graduate school, but Karwoski sensed that I might find satisfaction in an academic career, and advised me to go either to Clark or to Duke for further training in vision. Both universities seemed to offer the appropriate environment, but Clark was nearer by, and I had little money for travel. A final consideration was that Clark offered me a $100 research assistantship for the first year.

As I look back on it now, that first year at Clark was a difficult experience. The Chairman of the Department was Carl Murchison, no great scholar but a shrewd and successful publisher. Through the Clark University Press he brought out several journals and handbooks, together with a series of autobiographies by well-known psychologists. Walter Hunter was clearly the intellectual leader of the Department, and indeed an outstanding figure in American psychology at the time. He was also the editor of *Psychological Abstracts,* an indispensable and prestigious journal of international repute. Hunter and Murchison developed the kind of rivalry and bitterness between them that is almost inevitable when two ambitious chiefs try to govern the same tribe. There were only two others in the department, both much younger. Vernon Jones represented educational psychology, and had little influence on the graduate program; and Clarence Graham was just beginning the series of studies that would soon put him at the forefront of vision research.

Clark had always been one of the most active laboratories in American psychology. G. Stanley Hall was its founder, and many eminent scholars had participated in Clark's development. Several had done their early work under Titchener, the Englishman who had come to Cornell from the Wundt laboratories in Germany. The Wundt–Titchener influence was still apparent at the time I went to Clark. The corridors were lined with exhibits of early German brass instruments used for introspective studies of sensation and feeling. And the weekly colloquium was quite a formal occasion, with speakers from outstanding laboratories throughout the world. A particular feature of the colloquium was the afternoon tea – never coffee – that always preceded it. This was served in a little alcove off the seminar room, where people could sit on hard benches facing a narrow table. I think the tea and Wednesday colloquium tradition had come to Clark from the Titchener laboratory at Cornell. There were only about eight or ten of us graduate students, and mostly we kept silent as the speaker conversed with faculty members about what was going on in psychology at other institutions. I began to have the depressing feeling that the Clark University that I had once considered a great power in experimental psychology had dwindled to a small, tradition-bound vestige of its former eminence.

Even the graduate seminars, which were intended to broaden a student's background in experimental psychology, failed to rouse any enthusiasm on my part, and I neglected to read the reference material. The topics included animal learning, social psychology, mental testing, and the biology of plants and animals. It seemed to me that, by Dartmouth standards, they were poorly taught and devoid of interesting demonstrations or laboratory work. A seminar by Walter Hunter presented a particular difficulty. It was based on reports by the graduate students on a set of readings from his own work and that of other well-known behaviorists, championing the objective approach to psychology and casting aspersions on such subjective approaches as Titchener's structuralism and Köhler's Gestalt theory.

With my recent enthusiastic exposure to Gestalt at Dartmouth, I found Hunter's arguments hard to take. I actually filled out an application for an international exchange fellowship for the following year, a fellowship that would have permitted me to go to Berlin to study with Köhler himself. But fortunately, as the first few months passed, I began to appreciate the value of objectivity and of physiologically based theories of psychology. Talking things over with the faculty and fellow students, I decided to stay on for a doctorate at Clark, and I withdrew my application for international study. While I never adopted Hunter's strong antinativist views, I eventually became an enthusiastic advocate of objectivity and the alliance with biological sciences that Hunter had long espoused.

The saving feature of my first year at Clark was my work in the laboratory with Clarence Graham. Indeed, the feeling seemed to be mutual. When I arrived at Clark as a new graduate student, Graham was delighted to find that I had studied physics and electronics along with my psychology major in college, and he put me to work building some equipment for electrical recording. Those were the days of the great depression, when few laboratories had money for research, and our only chance of success was to build things with our own hands. At Clark we were able to borrow a string galvanometer from the Biology Department (through the kindness of Hudson Hoagland), and we could get a few experimental animals (principally white rats) from Walter Hunter's colony. So we decided to work on electric responses of this mammalian eye to light. We could not match the expertise and instrumentation of Ragnar Granit, who by this time (1933–1934) had begun his insightful studies of the electroretinogram (ERG) in frog and cat (see his chapter in this volume). We soon realized that our string galvanometer was not sufficiently sensitive to record the rat ERG. So Graham went back to Hartline's laboratory for a quick visit and to get whatever advice he could about how to solve our problem. I well remember that he returned from that trip with a paper napkin on which Hartline's electronics expert, John Hervey, over a glass of beer, had scribbled a wiring diagram for a one-tube radio amplifier. We then bought the necessary parts and batteries to wire it up, and eagerly put it in place between the animal and the string galvanometer. It worked! Not every day, not even every week, but sometimes it worked.

I shudder now to think of how we got the white rat to cooperate in these experiments. The main difficulty was in keeping it from struggling as we made contact with the eye through the tip of a saline-soaked wick electrode. Any eye or head movement would cause uncontrollable swings of the amplifier, blotting out the responses of the eye and threatening to break the delicate string of the galvanometer. So we devised a sort of straitjacket for the rat, and Graham would lace it up tight while I tried to get records from the galvanometer. What a conflict these maneuvers created, between Graham's desire for good records and his natural kindness toward animals! Every time he tightened the jacket he would mutter, "Poor damned animal; poor *damned* animal." And after a few hours of this the animal did become very quiet. Much to our surprise it always recovered, and we were able to use the same eye again and again to complete, over a few weeks' time, a series of experiments that was described in my master's thesis (GRAHAM and RIGGS 1934).

Later, the same basic equipment was used by GRAHAM et al. (1935) in experiments on the pigeon. We chose that animal because it had much better eyes than the rat, and because we could catch pigeons on the roof of our building. When finally the time came for me to undertake a doctoral thesis, I switched to working with frogs. The great advantage of that animal was that a considerable amount of its respiration occurred through the skin. Thus lung breathing became unnecessary, and a quiet baseline could easily be obtained for ERG records by simply paralyzing the muscles with curare. In fact, the frog remained in good shape for an all-day experiment, and eventually made a full recovery after the effects of the drug had worn off.

My doctoral research (RIGGS 1937) was a quantitative study of the course of dark adaptation in the frog eye. The topic had been suggested to me by Clarence

Graham, who saw in it a means of testing the photochemical theory of Selig Hecht. Hecht was a dominant figure in the vision research community of those days. His model of visual function was based almost entirely on a hypothetical breakdown by light of the visual pigment within the receptor cells, and the reverse reaction that he assumed to be the basis for restoring the pigment to its original concentration. This reverse reaction, then, was assumed to be the basis for dark adaptation. The exact time course of dark adaptation was predicted by Hecht's model, since the restorative process was assumed to involve a single, bimolecular process in the receptor outer segments. A direct test of the model could thus be provided by the frog experiments, since I could control the preexposure to light, the state of the preparation, and the times and intensities of test flash that could be used to elicit the ERG.

As it turned out, the results of my frog experiments were inconsistent with any single-process model of dark adaptation. Instead, I found the process to be unexpectedly rapid following short intervals of light adaptation, and much slower following longer intervals. Similar difficulties with Hecht's single-process theory were also found by WALD and CLARK (1937–1938) and by Granit (see his chapter in this volume). In fact, the monumental structure of Hecht's theory, which at first seemed to supply a quantitative basis for every important aspect of vision (HECHT 1934), eventually started to crumble. This was a sobering experience for all of us. Wald, who had been Hecht's student, and Graham, an ardent disciple, were no doubt shaken most. But as a young witness to all this, I quickly learned to reject "black box" theorizing based primarily upon hypothetical processes.

My own thinking has become increasingly empirical since the 1930s. But this was also the trend throughout the sciences. During World War II, especially, the vision research community broadened to include not only psychologists and physiologists, but also physicists, chemists, and mathematicians. After that it would have been shortsighted, so to speak, to rely exclusively on any one method, such as psychophysics, single-unit recording, or photochemistry. Instead it has become necessary to use all of these techniques and many more to analyze the complex retinal and central processing of pattern and color and the other visual functions.

As with vision research, the whole body of experimental psychology was maturing. The old global and polemical schools of psychology were losing their messiahs and disciples. Few psychologists were left who would claim, after Titchener, that introspection was the highroad to a systematic psychology; or that, as Watson implied, a person's behavior was best accounted for in terms of early conditioning; or that, after the Gestalters, perception and thinking were uniquely shaped by inborn patterns of activity. All these ideas had left their stamp on the American literature of the prewar years. But already a process of amalgamation was taking place, such that the new generation of psychologists adopted all the most valuable of the early concepts but rejected the extreme views of nativism, conditioning, and the like.

III. My Postdoctoral Years

The year 1936 was the end of an era for psychology at Clark University. Hunter and Graham left Clark to accept their appointments at Brown, and Murchison moved his publications office from Clark to his own home in Provincetown, Massachusetts. Mine was the last PhD awarded by the old faculty, and in the same year Graham and Hunter recommended me to Hartline for postdoctoral training. Despite the vicissitudes of my three years at Clark, there is no question that they had shaped me toward a career in the objective study of vision, and I was grateful for the recommendation.

That year, I was particularly fortunate to be awarded one of the two postdoctoral fellowships in the biological sciences by the National Research Council. Fortunately, too, the Johnson Foundation could accommodate me, and in Hartline's laboratory I learned the art of dissecting out single fibers of the optic nerve of *Limulus*. I did a series of experiments on the single unit's response to flicker. These I wrote up for publication with Hartline, but found to my dismay that he was not satisfied with them. I believe now that I know why: his ideal was to publish a paper only when it contributed a new understanding to the field. The mere reporting of experiments, no matter how comprehensive or technically sound they were, did not suffice. He certainly applied this criterion to his own research, as well as to that of other colleagues. His laboratory notebooks have in them many months and years of data that remain unreported. Nor did he have any taste for writing a monograph or book on the subject of his work. His chief joy was in applying his genius for new experimental techniques to the solution of fundamental problems. For this he was awarded a share (with Granit and Wald) in the Nobel Prize for Physiology or Medicine in 1967.

A quaint stipulation in the tenure of a postdoctoral fellowship from the National Research Council was to the effect that marriage was not permitted. This presumably lessened the danger that a fellow might spend his evenings at home rather than in the laboratory; or perhaps it was to guard against the possibility that some woman might marry him for the purpose of acquiring for her own uses a portion of his munificent stipend ($1,620 for the 12 months). Be that as it may, I dutifully waited until after the postdoctoral year to marry Doris Robinson, whom I had met at graduate school at Clark, and to accept one of only two academic positions that I heard about in psychology for the year 1937–1938. This was at the University of Vermont. I was offered a salary of $1,500, but when I stated that I was about to be married the offer was raised to $1,800. In consideration for that, I was assigned three sections (in a row) of the elementary course in psychology plus a laboratory course in experimental psychology, and in addition a course in social psychology that found me groping for subject matter before each lecture. There were no teaching assistants or laboratory facilities. But it was a job; and Burlington, Vermont was a beautiful place in which to begin married life. Academically, however, it was clearly a dead end in those days.

IV. New Opportunities at Brown

Meanwhile, at Brown University, Walter Hunter was busy strengthening the Department. The nucleus of Schlosberg, Graham, and himself was expanded to include J. McV. Hunt and Donald Lindsley. The Lindsley appointment was a part-time one, since his principal employment was a few miles away at the Bradley Home. He had gone there to succeed Herbert Jasper, who was called to the McGill University Medical School by Wilder Penfield, the renowned brain surgeon. Just as Jasper had set up some experiments at the Bradley Home with Carmichael, Lindsley now did some collaborative work with Hunter. One rather important study of theirs was one in which measurements were made of the dc polarity potential of the human eye (LINDSLEY and HUNTER 1939). From this they were able to conclude that the electrooculogram method of measuring eye movements is dependent on the eye's own polarity, arising chiefly within the retina, rather than on potentials generated within the eye muscles.

During the Hunter regime at Brown, vision research began to play the significant role that has continued ever since. Clarence Graham set up a number of optical systems in the basement of the psychology building. A former furnace room and several adjoining coal bins were partitioned off for well-controlled, if somewhat primitive, studies of human visual discrimination. Doctoral and postdoctoral students worked together on these, and this congenial team provided for Graham what he himself has called, "some of the happiest years of my life."

At this favorable sign of vigorous activity, Graham and Hunter were successful in obtaining a research grant of several thousand dollars from a private foundation to defray the costs of setting up still more projects in vision. Graham was particularly anxious to initiate experiments on the recording of optic nerve impulses, and he offered me a one-year appointment at Brown to help him accomplish this.

Although a research leave was a rare thing in those days, I was successful in obtaining one from the University of Vermont. This was after just one year of teaching (1937–1938), and I had to promise that I would return after the year at Brown. So I eagerly accepted the invitation from Graham. An attractive feature of the appointment was that he and I could share a relatively large interior basement room in which to set up our equipment. There were also funds with which to acquire a light-tight animal chamber, a moving film recording camera, a Duddell magnetic galvanometer, and a dissecting microscope.

Our plan was to do single-unit experiments of the kind that Hartline and Graham had first described a few years before. I had learned the necessary dissection technique during my postdoctoral year with Hartline, working on his favorite animal, the horseshoe crab. I now proceeded to build the amplifier, optical system, and auxiliary devices that we needed to carry out the work (Fig. 4). Fresh animals we obtained from the supply of the Marine Biological Laboratory at nearby Woods Hole, Massachusetts.

We were proud of our research setup, even though it had a somewhat primitive appearance because it included parts from radio shops and hardware stores. The windowless basement room turned out to be ideal: it was always cool and dark. The *Limulus* eye could be maintained for many hours at a constant temperature of 18 °C in a light-tight chamber surrounded by a jacket of circulating water. The temperature was adjusted by hand, simply by regulating a small valve in a tube that allowed water to flow down through the jacket by gravity from a tank containing a mixture of water and ice. The amplifier made use of a recently developed pentode tube for high amplification, plus the necessary power tube to drive the galvanometer, all run on dc from batteries that needed frequent recharging or replacement. The shutter regulating the stimulus flash was built around the synchronous motor of a 78 rpm phonograph. This motor rotated a large disk at constant speed, and a gap in the edge of the disk allowed the light to pass for a flash of known du-

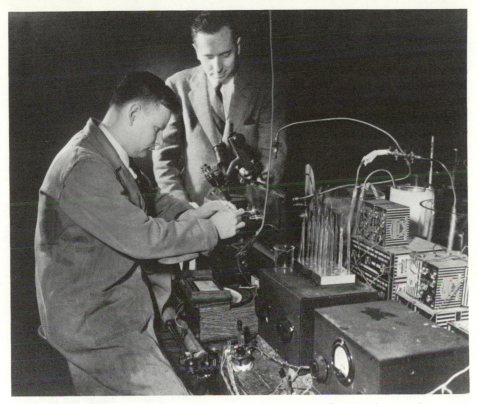

Fig. 4. Myself (*left*) and Graham with recording equipment for *Limulus* experiments at Brown in 1938. The photograph shows dissecting microscope and glass needles, cooling chamber, amplifier, and voltmeter and rheostat for regulating lamp voltage

ration. The experiments we were able to finish during the research year were of limited scope, but gave new information about the course of light adaptation in the *Limulus* eye and about a momentary refractoriness in the eye's sensitivity to light each time it discharged a nerve impulse (RIGGS 1940; RIGGS and GRAHAM 1940).

When the year ended, I returned to Vermont as I had promised. I found that the teaching load was a bit lighter, and I had a little time to think about research. Specifically, I thought how one might achieve the same objectivity with experiments on human subjects as with the work I had done on experimental animals. At about this time, plastic contact lenses first became available. They were of the scleral type, large enough to cover the entire front part of the eyeball. So it occurred to me that a silver electrode could be embedded on the inner surface of the contact lens, thereby making a relatively stable electrical connection with the fluid that it held in contact with the eyeball. Earlier work of my own, and of many still earlier experimenters, had shown that potentials developed within the retina of an experimental animal are conducted rather efficiently to the cornea, so that it is perfectly feasible to record an ERG between a corneal electrode and a reference electrode nearby on the skin. But Vermont had no laboratory and no recording equip-

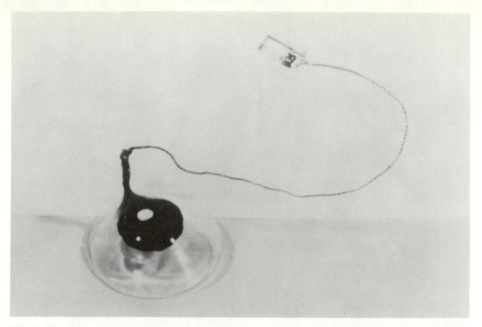

Fig. 5. The first contact lens electrode (1941). An artificial pupil is provided by a hole in the black enamel coating of the lens. A silver electrode mounted on the lens makes contact with the fluid bathing the eye. Flexible wire leads to an amplifier

ment. How could I proceed? I wrote to Graham and Hunter about my predicament, and they applied on my behalf for a research grant from the American Philosophical Society to enable me to try out my idea.

Receiving a grant of $300, I set to work building the necessary amplifier, optical system, and recording camera. A magnetic galvanometer was borrowed from the Brown laboratory. As for the contact lens, I knew that a friend (Robert Beitel) was working on preproduction models of them at the American Optical Company. He kindly allowed me to try a few on my own eye, and gave me the one that I judged to be least uncomfortable. The lens for my recording camera was also a gift, from Lloyd A. Jones at Eastman Kodak. The rest of it I built myself, the tools and parts coming mostly from the Burlington store of Sears, Roebuck, and Company.

D. The Impact of World War II

Just as I was completing my setup for the human ERG I had a call from Clarence Graham, asking me if I could come again to Brown, this time to work on military research under a large grant that had just been awarded to Graham through the National Defense Research Committee. The clouds of World War II had already spread over Europe, and it was clear that America might soon have to go to the aid of her allies.

I accepted the appointment at Brown, but first I worked intensively at Vermont to get a few representative records of the ERG from my own eye with the new contact lens electrode (Fig. 5). It became apparent that the device was a success, and the records were reliable indicators of the retinal effects of dark adaptation and variations of light intensity. I sent a report of it to *Science,* but the paper was rejected as too specialized. I have often told my graduate students and colleagues this story, when papers of theirs have been rejected. I have the satisfaction of knowing that although I had to send my report of the ERG electrode to a relatively obscure journal (RIGGS 1941), this device, with minor modifications, was subsequently adopted in many laboratories for basic research and in many hospitals for clinical diagnosis on the functions of the retina. Some 300 articles and monographs on the human ERG are listed in a recent book on the topic (ARMINGTON 1974), a dozen other books have been written on the human ERG as a clinical procedure, and there is a flourishing International Society for Clinical Electroretinography.

I. Wartime Research at Brown

From late 1941 until the summer of 1945, Clarence Graham devoted himself full time to the direction of war-related research. He put me in charge of laboratory projects at Brown, most of them having to do with stereoscopic range finders. We were asked by the National Defense Research Committee to carry out a number of experiments. Among these were the optimal design for the reticles used in these military instruments, the selection and training of personnel with the necessary accuracy of stereoscopic vision, sources of error within the instruments themselves, and methods for reducing human error in their use. Both at Brown and at military bases in which range finders were used, the research was carried out by knowledgeable persons, including several doctoral and postdoctoral students who had learned vision research techniques from Graham. The whole group included N. R. Bartlett, R. N. Berry, W. J. Brogden, R. Gagne, J. McV. Hunt, W. S. Kappauf, F. A. Mote, C. C. Mueller, R. S. Solomon, R. Stellar, W. S. Verplanck, and myself.

In the history of vision research, as in all scientific fields, World War II brought about a permanent change. The federal government became a major source of funding for personnel and equipment needed in research projects. Furthermore, scientists were brought together as never before in the common effort to solve experimental problems. Society in general, and Congress in particular, developed a new appreciation for the key role that science must play if the nation is to be kept at the forefront of industrial and military progress. The most spectacular example of this was, of course, the implementation of the atomic bomb. But there were impressive parallel advances in the production of aircraft, radar, and computers. Little new basic research was done, but the war effort required enormous expenditures of time and money for applying old scientific principles to the development of ever more complex new devices. And so it was with vision research. The Army, Navy, and Air Force each expanded the work of numerous laboratories in bases throughout the country.

Stereoscopic rangefinding was, of course, but one small aspect of this effort. Yet it was true that until radar was fully developed, the stereoscopic range finder was the most accurate means available for tracking a rapidly approaching target such as a tank or a plane. First mechanical and then electronic computers were used to convert this visual three-dimensional information into an estimate of the target's position at the probable moment of impact by a shell or rocket fired against it.

The most basic facts about stereoscopic vision were already known: under ideal conditions, angles as small as 2″ of arc could be discriminated on the basis of disparity in the right and left eye views of the target, yet only a small percentage of people were capable of this degree of precision. The precision actually attained under field conditions was much poorer than in the laboratory: the "unit of error" adopted throughout the services was 12″ of arc rather than 2″. The immediate military problems in this area included improvements in the optical display of range finders, in the dials and knobs used by the operator, and in the selection and training of personnel. Most of the work done in the Brown laboratory was reported in classified military documents. But some could later be published in regular journals. We worked on the design of reticle scales for range finders (RIGGS et al. 1948), dials for panoramic telescopes, the effects of atmospheric shimmer (RIGGS et al. 1947), and distraction of the operator by stress or fatigue.

As World War II came to a close it became clear that the era of stereoscopic rangefinding was nearly over. The detection and pursuit of moving targets was rapidly being taken over by radar. New visual problems arose, of course, in connection with the radar displays and later with their analysis by computers. Still, the fascination of research on the extraordinary precision of human stereoscopic vision persists to this day (WESTHEIMER and MCKEE 1979).

II. Federal Support of Wartime Research

During the war it was realized that the separate armed services shared many of the same problems in the efficient use of human vision. At the outset of the war many separate laboratories, including the one at Brown, were pursuing individual projects without adequate sharing of information with other laboratories. The result was a wasteful duplication of effort. Furthermore, there was often inadequate communication between the military personnel who could identify the needs of combat units and the scientists who might have the expertise to solve them.

To remedy this situation, Army and Navy officials asked the Director of the Office of Scientific Research and Development (OSRD) to set up a central agency for the coordination of vision projects. The first meeting of the resulting group, the Army-Navy-OSRD Vision Committee, was held on 7 April 1944 at the Navy Department in Washington, and 12 more meetings were held from month to month prior to the war's end. Several were held at the National Academy of Sciences, and others at individual research installations. From its beginning, the Committee had a full-time executive secretary, and a scientist who was given an office and staff in the National Academy building. Army and Navy members were chosen to represent the various agencies confronted by practical military problems, and civilian members were chosen for their scientific and engineering skills.

E. Peacetime Prosperity

I. Federal Sponsorship

After the war's end, in 1945, the Office of Naval Research (ONR) took responsibility for continuing the activities of the Vision Committee. The ONR rationale for doing so was that the Vision Committee had become a highly successful coordinating body for interaction among scientists, among military experts, and between these two groups for the promotion of vision research. Furthermore, it was realized that little basic research had been pursued during the war, and that peacetime projects could now be undertaken that would form the basis for future peacetime applications as well as those arising in times of national emergency. On this basis the Committee was expanded, separate working groups were formed, and some truly outstanding national meetings were held on particular topics. Furthermore, the ONR contracted with many universities for the sponsorship of vision research on a scale never before possible. This permitted the universities to hire additional staff members on "soft money" that could also be used for equipping their laboratories, traveling to meetings, and furnishing the University with funds for "indirect costs," such as secretarial salaries and shares in the funding of libraries and administration.

Thus the ONR was the chief architect in the creation of peacetime scientific facilities. Many civilian scientists, myself among them, accepted this support and happily adjusted to the new era of scientific prosperity. But we all shared the uneasy feeling that some day there might be an attempt by the ONR to dictate the direction in which future research should be undertaken. We were getting a large amount of "something for nothing" and we feared that our dependence on it might become an addiction. What then, if the soft money were to dry up or if its continuance were to be tied to doing research on problems of immediate military relevance?

Speaking for myself, I can state that none of these feared eventualities ever materialized. Other federal agencies, notably the United States Public Health Service and the National Science Foundation, were later created to take over sponsorship of basic and clinically applicable vision research, as a part of their huge commitment to the scientific progress of the country. The whole system of research grants, based upon councils for planning and peer review for evaluation, grew to the stature that we see today.

The current annual budget of the National Eye Institute is over 100 million dollars, a major portion of which goes to support investigator-initiated grants for vision research in universities and institutes throughout the country. While this is by far the largest source, there is also substantial support by the National Science Foundation, by other federal agencies, and by private funding agencies. The research grant of $300 that enabled me to begin work on the human ERG in 1939 seems in strange contrast to what is available to a young faculty member today. Now the smallest of grants is likely to provide $10,000 or more, and an exceptionally promising researcher can apply for a wide range of individual opportunities for research, such as a postdoctoral fellowship or, at a later stage, a Research Career Development Award. Despite a present downward trend in academic vacancies, and despite the shrinkage of the dollar, the overall prosperity of scientists in the early 1980s is incomparably better than was the case 50 years ago.

But perhaps the best feature of all to accrue from sponsored research is the degree to which scientists have become aware of each others' goals and achievements. Travel to meetings, visits to other laboratories, the sharing of costly equipment and library holdings – all these have removed much of the inbreeding and provincialism that I witnessed in my student days.

II. The Postwar Years

Graham's record of good research and good management had brought him wide recognition during the war. When peace came, in 1945, he left Brown to accept a position at Columbia University, as successor to Robert S. Woodworth. This provided him with increased facilities and personnel for research, and also the possibility of collaborative work with Selig Hecht, Yun Hsia, and others at Columbia. He went on to become one of America's most distinguished vision experts.

More than 70 PhD dissertations were done under Graham's direction at Clark, Brown, and Columbia. At the age of 40 he was elected to the National Academy of Sciences. In 1947 Hecht died, and Graham took over some of his research equipment and personnel. In 1952–1953 Graham was a scientific liaison officer in London, through the ONR. On several research visits to Japanese laboratories he introduced such topics as visual contrast discrimination and figural aftereffects. But his most lasting achievement was to bring out the book entitled *Vision and Visual Perception* (GRAHAM 1965). Graham wrote much of the book, some chapters of which were contributed by J. L. Brown, N. R. Bartlett, Y. Hsia, C. G. Mueller, and myself. He planned and edited the entire volume, which well summarized the field at the time it was written and is still among the most useful of books on the subject. Graham remained at Columbia until his death, in 1974.

1. Expansion of the Research at Brown

Although I had first gone to Brown in 1938 to set up the *Limulus* experiments, and returned in 1941 to participate in the war-related vision projects, it was not until 1945 that I became a regular member of the faculty. I did my best to fill the position left by Graham when he went to Columbia. In those postwar years several graduate students returned from war service to complete their work for the PhD degree, and most of the new graduate students had also undergone military duty. Walter Hunter could again devote a major part of his time to strengthening the Department. Starting in 1945, and continuing for the next three years, he appointed Carl Pfaffmann and several others to the staff (Fig. 6) in addition to Harold Schlosberg, J. McV. Hunt, and Donald Lindsley, the members continuing from before the war. Hunt left the Department in 1946 for the directorship of a foundation in New York; Lindsley left in 1947 to accept a professorship at Northwestern University.

The postwar years were a time of expanded opportunity for basic research. The Department had acquired two more old frame houses, at 81 and 85 Waterman Street, during the war. Thus Carl Pfaffmann and I could move our research projects out of 89 Waterman, the old headquarters building, and expand into the seemingly limitless rooms in 85 and 81. New opportunities for vision research were provided by using some of the optical and electronic equipment acquired during the war. Of major importance was a contract between Brown University and the ONR that enabled me to set up new experiments along the lines of my own interests.

Two of the graduate students who returned to Brown after the war were Parker Johnson and Richard Berry. I was delighted that they both decided to do research in human vision, and I eagerly set to work with each on experiments I had long planned to undertake. Berry's doctoral research (BERRY 1948) resulted in a precise determination of the acuity of human vision as measured by a vernier offset task

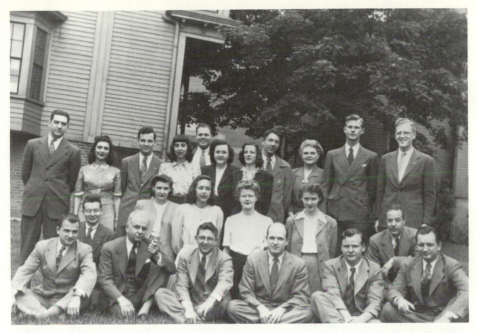

Fig. 6. Psychology Department at Brown in 1946. *Seated (left to right)* are Berry, Hunter, Kimble, Pfaffmann, myself, and Lindsley. *Standing fourth from the right* is Parker Johnson

in comparison with stereoscopic discrimination of depth. The experiments required the determination of visual thresholds, seemingly a completely subjective task for the human observations. But Berry was one of the first experimenters to use a bias-free psychophysical method, the two-alternative forced-choice procedure. His results have stood the test of time, in that the values he arrived at have been repeatedly confirmed with the most advanced modern equipment.

2. The Human Electroretinogram

With Parker Johnson I returned to the human ERG recording that I had begun five years earlier, at Vermont. This time there were great improvements. Plastic contact lenses were now being fitted to patients by optometrists and ophthalmologists. They were still the same basic type as the prewar ones: large molded shells with a central portion of spherical shape to fit loosely over the cornea, and a large outer portion to fit more snugly in contact with the scleral portion of the eyeball. Pioneering in the clinical dispensing of such lenses were the Obrig Laboratories in New York. Their practice was to provide each practitioner with a graded set of such lenses that could be tried on their patients in the attempt to provide a comfortable fit. The set covered a suitable range of corneal and scleral radii so that nearly every eye could be fitted. Since the lenses were large, it was necessary for the patients' eyelids to be opened wide in order to apply the lens to the eyeball. Furthermore, a fluid solution of "artificial tears" had to be used to fill the space between the plastic lens and the cornea. This meant that inserting the lens was a difficult maneuver. First the lens was filled like a cup from a bottle of the fluid. Then the patient leaned forward so that the eye was looking straight down at the floor. Finally, the lids were spread apart by the fingers, and the lens was applied to the eyeball in such a way that the cornea was fully covered, without air bubbles, and the outer portion of the lens fitted snugly between the lids and the scleral portion of the eyeball. All this was difficult at first, and required a skillful practitioner and a cooperative – not to say stoic – patient. Fully half those who tried to wear contact lenses gave them up as too much of a nuisance, or too uncomfortable for ordinary wear. A few patients, however, were strongly enough motivated to continue wearing them. Among these were film stars and others who did not wish to be seen with ordinary spectacles. Also swimmers, football players, and others for whom spectacles were out of the question. Also Parker Johnson and I, together with a few other hardy subjects, such as graduate students and their wives. We were all helped immeasurably by the skill and patience of Edward Troendle, an optometrist with an office nearby.

Parker Johnson's doctoral research clearly showed that the time course of human dark adaptation could be measured reasonably well by the size of the ERG b wave in response to test flashes of light. When converted into sensitivity units (i.e., reciprocal of light energy needed to elicit a minimal ERG response), the data showed a time course rather similar to (but not identical with) that of the scotopic portion of the dark adaptation curve on the same subject as obtained by conventional psychophysical threshold techniques. But the flashes needed to elicit a b wave of minimal size had to be more than a thousand times more intense than those that the subject could barely detect in the threshold experiments. Partly for that reason, the ERG was dismissed by some critics as a mere "epiphenomenon," a sort of accidental accompaniment occurring somewhere in the vicinity of the receptors, while the main business of seeing was taking place through the well-known chain of receptors, bipolars, and ganglion cells in the retina.

Looking back now at those early experiments, we can see that their main conclusion is still valid: the major part of the huge increase in visual sensitivity with dark adaptation does occur in scotopic (rod-initiated) retinal changes. Moreover, we already knew from Granit's early analysis of the cat ERG that these retinal events occurred at an early stage, without the participation of the ganglion cells or optic nerve fibers. But in those early days we did not suspect the fact that nearly all the b wave response to each test flash was originating in the "unstimulated" part of the retina. The 7° test field we were using at that time was totally inappropriate as a stimulus for the rod receptors. More than 99% of the rods lie outside that area, and it was only because of the huge blanket of much weaker light reaching them through scatter within the eyeball that they could work together to produce the ERG waves that we were recording.

The stray light problem had been uncovered in rabbits by FRY and BARTLEY (1935). The seriousness of the problem for human ERG work was finally demonstrated by ASHER (1951), Boynton and myself (BOYNTON and RIGGS 1951), and BOYNTON (1953). In these studies, light that was focused within the receptorless portion of the blind spot turned out to be as effective a stimulus for the ERG as the same light directed to a nearby region of the normal retina. This was conclusive evidence that the ERG came from light outside the focal area.

The solution to the problem of eliminating stray light turned out to be a simple one for ERG work with the scotopic system. This was the use of full-field techniques for illumination and testing. Research of this kind has narrowed or eliminated the gap between the light intensity needed for eliciting the human ERG and the intensity barely detected by the same subject in psychophysical experiments. Thus it is now possible to use the ERG for both clinical and experimental investigations of dark adaptation and other aspects of human night vision.

But the isolation of photopic (cone-initiated) activity in ERG research was far more difficult. MOTOKAWA and MITA (1942) first identified an "x wave" in response to flashes of red light. This was shown by ADRIAN (1946) to be an early (photopic) component of the b wave. It was manifested most clearly in response to flashes at the red end of the spectrum, but showed up also with other wavelengths down to about 500 nm. Its photopic nature was further attested by SCHUBERT and BORNSCHEIN (1952) and ARMINGTON (1952), who found that it was absent in the ERG of protanopes when the stimulus was a deep red light. But even with normal subjects, this early photopic component of the b wave was invariably contaminated by larger, scotopic ones. Thus it could not serve as a selective indicator of cone-mediated vision.

GRANIT (1935) had shown with experimental animals that photopic ERGs could be enhanced (and scotopic ones depressed) by using high-luminance backgrounds against which to display the test stimuli. But this turned out not to be a clean separation when applied to the human eye. Our ERG studies (RIGGS et al. 1949) showed some systematic effects of high background luminance, but failed to achieve a truly photopic spectral sensitivity curve. Later work by AIBA et al. (1967) achieved a more complete suppression of scotopic activity by the use of a strong blue background. But this expedient did not permit any systematic studies of the color-responding capabilities of the cones, since the blue receptors were always depressed.

Still other attempts to isolate cone-initiated signals in the human ERG were made by a number of investigators (e.g., ADRIAN 1945; ARMINGTON and BIERSDORF 1956) by stimulating the eye with intermittent light. Flicker rates of about 20 flashes per second failed to arouse much scotopic activity, and photopic spectral sensitivity functions were achieved. But chromatic response was lost also; rates as high as this do produce a luminance response in the cones, but they are above the fusion point for color, as is evident from the practice of flicker photometry. That technique is based on the fact that alternation of wavelengths is not perceived at rates above 20 Hz, at which complete fusion of the two colors is observed.

Again, as so often is the case, the solution to our problem was found by the use of entirely new technical developments. The first of these was computer averaging, a revolutionary procedure developed in laboratories of electronic engineering (ROSENBLITH 1962). This now familiar technique made possible the recording of signals in the microvolt range, despite a background noise level much larger than the signal itself. It requires multiple presentations (often 100 or more) of the stimulus in order to cumulate the response potential waves that are time-locked to the stimulus. The cumulation process results in an ever-increasing response wave that emerges out of the total output of the recording system. Randomly occurring positive and negative potentials tend to cancel one another. These are the unwanted potentials due to activity not correlated with the visual stimulus (heartbeat, lid twitches, electronic noise, etc.). In the human experiments, since no direct contact with the human retinal or brain cells is possible, the electrodes must necessarily be located on the surface, at such distances that "noise" is large and true visual response waves are severely attenuated. Hence the great importance of signal averaging.

The other necessary technique, first introduced in our laboratory (RIGGS et al. 1964) was that of counterphase alternation. For this, the stimulus field consisted of a grating composed of alternate stripes of two different wavelengths of light, λ_1 and λ_2. As the eye fixated steadily a point at the center of the grating, the λ_1 stripes replaced the λ_2 stripes and vice versa periodically, so that each point on the retina received a long series of stimulations of the form $\lambda_1, \lambda_2, \lambda_1, \lambda_2 \dots$ When λ_1 and λ_2 were sufficiently different, even though the two beams were carefully matched as to brightness, it turned out that each alternation produced an ERG wave. Furthermore, we were able to show (JOHNSON et al. 1966) that these waves were photopic in origin, thus representing the true chromatic response function of the human eye. We had got round the stray light problems by keeping constant at all times the total amount of light at wavelengths λ_1 and λ_2, and we had avoided the direct stimulation of the rod receptor system by using stripes sufficiently narrow and bright not to work in the scotopic domain.

Throughout the course of this work on the ERG at Brown, the summer months were nearly always the most productive. Not only were academic duties at a minimum, but also visiting scholars could often join the research team. Among the most faithful of these was Parker Johnson, who returned to Brown each summer for many years in a row: a wise and congenial experimenter, subject, and companion in ERG research.

The technique of counterphase alternation allowed us to continue a series of studies of chromatic contrast, leading to objectively determined chromaticity diagrams at the levels of the retina and the occipital cortex (RIGGS 1974). In our laboratory we also applied the technique to psychophysical studies of chromatic contrast (BUTLER and RIGGS 1978).

Many other laboratories have now adopted the phase alternation principle for a wide variety of other studies, both electrophysiological and psychophysical (see CAMPBELL and ROBSON 1968; REGAN 1972). We are proud to have initiated the phase alternation technique, but we can hardly take credit for its later application to what the engineers call the "steady state" stimulation of the visual system. This now involves sinusoidally modulated gratings of variable spatial frequency and contrast, thus permitting the application of Fourier analysis to the study of visual spatial discrimination.

As in every field, the most recent advances in the study of chromatic responding have been greatly facilitated by computer analysis. Of particular significance is the development of techniques of multidimensional scaling (KRUSKAL 1964). These have made possible a comparison of chromatic contrast sensitivity functions obtained with psychophysical procedures (BOYNTON 1979; BUTLER and RIGGS 1978) and with the human visually evoked cortical potentials (PETRY et al. 1982). The results of these experiments can now be used to construct chromaticity diagrams in which the various wavelengths are placed appropriately to indicate the distances between them as they affect the visual system.

It is now abundantly clear that computer techniques will shape the future of both basic research and clinical measurement of responses within the human visual system. Computers can be programmed to adjust and present the visual stimuli, to record and display the responses from the eye or brain, and to perform the appropriate analyses of the data. It is no exaggeration to say that a single experimental session can now yield more comprehensive and reliable results than could have been obtained, 50 years ago, by many months of painstaking research.

3. Involuntary Eye Movements

We have seen that the advent of plastic contact lenses opened up the possibility of convenient and reliable records of the human ERG. But there was another use for contact lenses that soon occurred to us and later to several other investigators. This was to use the contact lens as a basis for precise measurements of the movements of the eye. For the first time it was possible to achieve a relatively firm and comfortable attachment of a plane mirror to the eyeball. The mirror could then be used to provide an optical lever for the precise determination of eye movements. All previous methods (corneal reflection, cine photography, electrooculogram) had been much less sensitive.

It is true that earlier investigators had devised schemes for putting a mirror on the eye. But without a contact lens the attachment was insecure and uncomfortable. In addition to the work of DELABARRE (1898), ORSCHANSKY (1898), and MARX and TRENDELENBURG (1911) each used a carefully fabricated attachment to the eye, in this case a thin metal shell with a hole in the middle, over the cornea. A mirror attached to the shell reflected light to a moving film camera. Despite the pain and danger to the eye, enough records were taken to show that the eye was never motionless, but was able to maintain fixation for brief intervals to an accuracy of a few minutes of arc. ADLER and FLIEGELMAN (1934) placed a small mirror directly on the eye of one hardy subject, who used his forefinger to prevent the upper lid from closing over it. Even with this limitation, they were able to identify three of the principal types of eye movement that normally occur during attempted steady fixation (rapid flicks, slower wavy excursions, and fine tremor).

The first attempts to mount a mirror on a contact lens revealed the advantages of this procedure, so Floyd Ratliff pursued the eye movement recording. Using well-fitted contact lenses and high-quality mirrors he and I were able to confirm the qualitative findings of Adler and Fliegelman. But we showed that their reported amplitudes of motion were unaccountably high. We also added a fourth category to their description of the eye movements, that of a relatively slow "drift" occurring between the rapid flicks. But our main conclusion was that the eye was remarkably good at holding steady under favorable conditions (RATLIFF and RIGGS 1950). Consequently, we were forced to take extraordinary care to prevent our records from being contaminated by vibration of the building or of the motor used to drive the camera film. Even the subjects' own breathing and heartbeat were a problem, and they had to learn not to blink. Our final recording setup was mounted on a heavy steel H-beam, supported by concrete columns rising from the cement foundation of the basement. The subject's head was held in place by the use of a dental impression plate and forehead rest bolted to the steel beam. And the contact lenses were especially selected for a tight fit. Only in this way could we measure with some confidence the true capacity of the eye for holding still.

A few years later, Ditchburn, a distinguished physicist in England, likewise saw the possibilities for using a contact lens for eye movement recording (DITCHBURN and GINSBORG 1952). From that time on, he and his colleagues contributed many innovative experiments and improved optical devices for the study of the involuntary eye movements. This has culminated in a fine monograph on the subject (DITCHBURN 1973), written after the author's retirement from the Chair of Physics at the University of Reading.

It is hard to realize now that so little was known, in the early 1950s, about the stability of the eye during fixation. HARTRIDGE and THOMSON (1948) had concluded that the eye was essentially motionless. LORD and WRIGHT (1948) had found that some small movement was present, but they had looked in vain for the fast tremor that ADLER and FLIEGELMAN (1934) had described as having average amplitudes of more than 2' of arc. Our (RATLIFF and RIGGS 1950) experiments, confirmed by DITCHBURN and GINSBORG (1953) showed why: the true tremor amplitudes are seldom higher than 20″ of arc, and require very sensitive methods of recording for their measurement. Moreover, the tremor of the right eye is uncorrelated with that of the left (RIGGS and RATLIFF 1951). This finding definitely supported an old idea that the visual system must perform a good deal of averaging over space and time (ANDERSON and WEYMOUTH 1923). The most precise experiments have achieved stereoscopic resolution thresholds as low as 2″ of arc (ANDERSON and WEYMOUTH 1923; WALLS 1942; BERRY 1948). The brain thus has the formidable task of putting together, with that degree of precision, the retinal information from two eyes that are wandering separately through distances at least ten times as great.

4. The Stabilized Image

But even monocular vision leads to a fundamental question which could not be answered up to that time: Are the involuntary eye movements good or bad for vision? A direct answer to that question could be found, it would seem, if the eye movements could somehow be stopped while tests of acuity and other visual functioning could be carried out. Floyd Ratliff and I had thoughts about paralyzing the eye muscles, but realized that this would be uncomfortable, and possibly hazardous, for the subject. A different solution finally occurred to us, and independently to Ditchburn and his colleagues in England: instead of stopping the eye movements, we could devise an optical system that would counteract them by stabilizing an optical image on the retina. RATLIFF (1950) planted the germ of this idea in his doctoral dissertation.

But how to achieve a motionless retinal image? Could we reflect a beam of light from the contact lens mirror to a screen in front of the eye, so that the image on the screen would move exactly with the eye at all times? No, it would not work because the beam would be reflected through twice the angular excursion of the eye itself. But finally we thought of how to do it: look at the screen through a set of

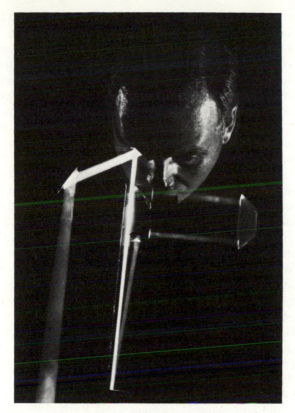

Fig. 7. Light beams used for stabilizing the retinal image (1952)

mirrors that would double the length of the viewing path. To our delight, this trick was successful, and we could go ahead with our research on vision without motion of the retinal image (Fig. 7).

Almost immediately the principal result was apparent: rapid fading and then disappearance of any object that is imaged without motion on the retina. We had the thrill of exploring a new perceptual domain. Never before, we realized, had people gone temporarily blind while staring intently at a test pattern that was initially sharp and clear. We made our first report of these effects at a meeting of the Optical Society of America (RIGGS and RATLIFF 1952). This caused quite a stir, and a crew from *Life* magazine came to Brown to take pictures of subjects wearing contact lens mirrors and looking into our novel optical apparatus. By that time Floyd Ratliff had gone to an academic appointment at Harvard, and Tom Cornsweet had come to Brown as a graduate student. He and his wife conducted many of the early experiments on rate of disappearance of acuity test objects.

By the time we had published a full account of our work (RIGGS et al. 1953), we had heard about the DITCHBURN and GINSBORG (1952) observations of stabilized images. It was apparently one of those common occurrences in scientific work, the simultaneous and independent discovery of a new phenomenon because the time was right and the tools had just become available.

I have mentioned that Ditchburn and his colleagues continued for many years to work on involuntary eye movements and the stabilized image. The same was true of our own laboratory. RATLIFF (1952) contributed evidence against the currently popular "dynamic" theory of visual acuity. That theory supposed that the eye must make use of its small, involuntary movements to scan a visual pattern in order to sharpen up its contours. The analogy is with the tactile sense, in which a feel for the texture of cloth can best be obtained by rubbing it between finger and thumb. In the same way, a blind person identifies the raised dots of the Braille alphabet by movement of the fingers across them. But Ratliff's experiments showed that a line is best seen by the eye during moments of time when the involuntary eye movements are at a minimum as shown by records from the contact lens mirror. A line presented during a moment of greater movement is less successfully resolved. Thus the analogy with the sense of touch seems not to be a valid one, and instead the visual effect was more like that of a camera, where motion during the exposure results in blur on the film.

Later experiments by RIGGS et al. (1954) provided evidence that the contact lens mirror method of recording was a valid one, not showing any appreciable slippage on the eye during the measurement of small, involuntary eye movements. It also provided information on the total amount that a fixating eye may typically be expected to move during any particular interval of viewing (covering a range from 5 ms to 1 s). Tom CORNSWEET (1956) made a pioneering study of the role of microsaccades in the correction of the direction of fixation.

Within a few years, a new "generation" of researchers was attracted to the field of stabilized image experiments. These included YARBUS (1967) in Russia, FENDER (1955) in the Ditchburn laboratory, and Tulunay-Keesey (RIGGS and TULUNAY 1959) and Krauskopf (KRAUSKOPF and RIGGS 1959) at Brown. Many more have entered the field since then, and progress is still being made with respect to the refinement of methods and the application of image stabilization to specific visual problems. In our own laboratory, stabilized viewing was used to test hypotheses about the role that involuntary eye movements were alleged to play in such diverse visual functions as the aftereffects of motion (SEKULER and GANZ 1963), the Mach band phenomenon (RIGGS et al. 1961), and even visual acuity (KEESEY 1960). In all these cases it came out that stabilized viewing was as good as unstabilized. The involuntary eye movements may eventually prevent disappearance, but they do not affect the initial appearance of a test field.

F. A New Era: Experiments in the Walter S. Hunter Laboratory

By the time of these later experiments, both new and old equipment for vision research had been properly installed in the basement floor of a new laboratory. Walter Hunter had died in 1954, and Harold Schlosberg had succeeded him as Chairman of the Psychology Department. It was largely through Schlosberg's careful and insightful planning that the new building came to fruition, in 1958, and gave us real laboratory facilities instead of the makeshift ones of the old frame houses (SCHLOSBERG 1958). The vision research group had the new luxuries of built-in shielded cubicles, darkrooms, storage shelves, and its own repair shop.

Old series of experiments were continued and new ones begun in the new Hunter Laboratory. Of the latter, I shall detail only two: saccadic suppression, and the McCollough effect. There were many others, but these two eventually became rather major projects. They also bring out the fact that many vision researchers were becoming interested in phenomena that related to the rapidly expanding knowledge of brain physiology.

I. Saccadic Suppression

Frances Volkmann brought this topic to my attention in the late 1950s. She was a graduate student at the time, searching around for an appropriate topic for her doctoral dissertation. She pointed out that, as early as 1900, Dodge had noted a marked impairment of vision that accompanies a saccadic eye movement, and that ever since that time the topic had been a controversial one.

1. The Hypothesis of a Neural Inhibition

On the one hand, it was obvious that some loss of visual acuity must accompany eye movements that are as rapid and extensive as a typical saccade, simply because the retinal image must be swept across thousands of receptors and must therefore produce a temporal blur for all its contours. Just so a photograph is blurred if the camera is moved during the exposure. But is there more to it than that? HOLT (1903) had thought so, and introduced some evidence of a visual "anesthesia" during a saccade that seemed to have a physiological basis in addition to the optical one. Volkmann thought there was a good chance that there was indeed a significant neural inhibition, and proposed that she explore it for her doctoral research.

My own attitude was one of skepticism. I felt that optical blur could account for a large part of the visual failure that had been found in the saccade research. Furthermore, I knew that vision during a saccade can clearly be demonstrated. All one needs to do is to make a saccade across a flickering source of light, such as an ac. operated neon bulb, and the multiple stroboscopic images are clearly seen throughout the course of the eye movement. I suspected that if there were any more than optical blur to account for visual loss during an eye movement it would probably turn out to be the result of some artifact such as a faulty experimental procedure or some bias or inattention on the part of the subject. So I told Volkmann that I was afraid it was a risky topic to choose for a doctoral thesis. She might waste a lot of time controlling for all possible errors and then wind up with inconclusive or negative results instead of a definite answer. Perhaps it is characteristic of Volkmann that this kind of advice made her all the more determined to try it. And I like to think that it is characteristic of me that I let her go ahead with what she wanted most to do. In fact, once the matter was decided I did all I could to provide her with the best equipment available to carry out the kind of thorough investigation that would remove all doubts about the matter.

2. Problems of Equipment

We decided that several improvements needed to be made on anything previously available for this kind of experiment. The background must be a large, uniformly bright field with fixation guides outside the fovea so as to guide the subject in making saccades from one to the other, but not to interfere with detection by the finest cone receptors. The test pattern must be so extensive that some part of it could be seen with foveal vision wherever the eye was looking in the course of a 6° saccade. And most important, the test pattern must be exposed for such a short time that, as in stroboscopic photography, the motion of the retinal image could be "stopped" and thus prevented from causing any blur due to the rapid eye movement.

These were formidable requirements, but again we were fortunate. The necessary items of equipment had recently been developed, although never put to this particular use. We used ultraviolet light to reflect an invisible beam from the cornea of the subject's eye. A multiplier phototube, with 900 V supplied by a battery of hundreds of tiny dry cells, was actuated by the ultraviolet beam as it was swept across the tube by the eye movement. Finally, the multiplier tube output was amplified and fed into a Schmitt trigger circuit to discharge a strobe lamp that gave an instantaneous presentation of the test pattern against the steady background.

I do not wish to give the impression that the above equipment was taken off the shelves of any apparatus companies and simply installed for use in the experiments. The Schmitt trigger circuit and amplifier we made ourselves from parts obtained in Dandreta's radio store, and the optical system was put together with military surplus mirrors and lenses from the Edmund Salvage Company. The lens and mirror mounts were made in our little machine shop by Volkmann, who is very good at metal work. The 900-V battery, in the days before stabilized dc power supplies, was indeed a commercial unit designed for the multiplier tube. But it was not long before one after another of the cells of the battery began to fail. And since the cells were in series connection, failure of one meant failure of the entire battery. We grew very skilled at locating, and eventually correcting, all the numerous trouble spots in the whole complex of none-too-reliable equipment.

3. Interpretation of the Results

And it worked! VOLKMANN'S (1962) doctoral research provided convincing evidence that visual detection is very significantly impaired during a saccade. She had controlled for optical blur and the other factors that had plagued earlier experimenters. By elimination, then, she was left with clear evidence that some sort of neural inhibition – ZUBER and STARK (1966) were later to call it "saccadic suppression" – accounted for a two- to fivefold elevation of the detection threshold. The experiments involved many long hours of careful psychophysical testing on three subjects, and the development of hundreds of feet of camera film to verify the timing and amplitude of the saccade in relation to the test flash. But it was a really admirable dissertation that taught me not to prejudge the significance of any new line of research. My early doubts had been completely wiped out, and I now accepted the idea of a central inhibition.

As in so many cases of new ideas, the saccadic suppression experiment was thought up independently by another researcher, this time in the Netherlands (LATOUR 1962). His work was apparently carried out with dark surrounds and was simpler in design, but led to a similar conclusion. Indeed, a number of experimenters have confirmed the basic phenomenon in the succeeding two decades, whenever care has been taken to eliminate optical blur, the masking of test stimuli by fixation points or other features of the background, and other contaminating factors.

The saccadic suppression research is of particular interest because it illustrates scientific attitudes and bias. My own initial reluctance to accept the existence of a neural inhibitory component has apparently been a bias widely shared by others, even in the face of the best contrary evidence. Somehow the issue has degenerated into one of feeling compelled to decide between peripheral and central explanations of the impairment of vision during saccadic eye movements. This is reminiscent of other questions which have aroused heated controversy in the past. Does light consist of particles or waves? Are there three primary colors or four? Is depth perception learned or innate? Questions such as these, seemingly important at the time that they are first raised, have a way of fading away as more facts become known and the full complexity of the issue begins to be appreciated. Just so it is with the impairment of vision during a saccade. CARPENTER (1977) has given a succinct review of the current turmoil: evidence that retinal blur, masking of test by background, and changing retinal illumination can each contribute to visual impairment under various experimental conditions. But he also summarizes the evidence that Volkmann, Latour, and many succeeding investigators have amassed for suppression that cannot be explained in this way. He concludes with the observation that, "If all the observations described here are correct, it is difficult to avoid the conclusion that all the methods by which saccadic suppression might conceivably occur do in fact contribute to it, insofar as they have been tested at all."

Fortunately, we have been able to go on with many aspects of the saccadic suppression experiments at Brown. Volkmann herself has spent vacation time and sabbatical leaves with us. The research has included a series of studies of the time course of the suppression (VOLKMANN et al. 1968) and its dependence on luminance, pattern, wavelength, contrast, and other aspects of the test situation.

4. Suppression During Blinks

Most recently we have discovered that blinks, as well as saccades, are accompanied by a momentary rise in the visual threshold (VOLKMANN et al. 1980). To find this out we had to devise a scheme for getting the test stimuli into the eye without interference by the lids. We succeeded in doing this by delivering light through a fiber optic cable to the roof of the mouth (Fig. 8). This light reaches the lower nasal portion of the retina by traversing the intervening tissues, and is seen by a dark-adapted subject as a diffuse cloud of light localized in the upper temporal part of the field. Just as with saccades, the effect of this light is considerably reduced at the time of a voluntary blink. We think that this helps to explain the fact that people scarcely notice the visual effect of a blink, even though the usual blink shuts out the visual scene for several tenths of a second.

5. Psychophysical Methods

In doing the saccade and blink experiments, the basic question was: "How much more light does a subject need to see the test stimulus during a saccade or a blink

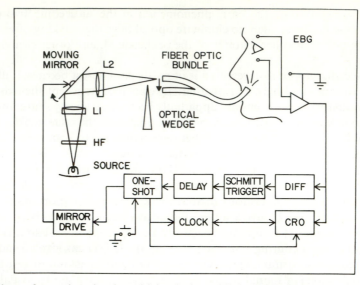

Fig. 8. Scheme for testing visual sensitivity during a blink (1980). Electrodes above and below the eye are used to record the lid closing and actuate a trigger circuit. This causes a momentary deflection of the moving mirror during the blink. The effect of this is to produce a brief decrement in light entering the fiber optic bundle and reaching the eye through the mouth. Amplitude of the decrement, varied by an optical wedge, must be high enough during a blink to overcome the neural suppression that accompanies it. *EBG*, electrodes for recording the electroblepharogram (lid closure); *Diff*, differentiating circuit to actuate the trigger as lid closure begins; *CRO*, cathode ray oscilloscope; *HF*, heat filter; L_1 and L_2, achromatic lenses to focus rays from the source onto a branch of the fiber optic bundle

than when the eye is at rest?" This would seem to require a subjective judgment. But fortunately the answer can be obtained by an almost completely bias-free psychophysical method, the same one used by BERRY (1948) so many years before. It is the two-alternative forced-choice procedure. The subjectivity of the method is greatly reduced by the fact that the subject is not required to say whether he sees anything or not, but simply to guess which of two temporal intervals contains the stimulus. The experimenter randomly delivers the stimulus during the first or second interval of each pair, and a sufficient number of pairs is used to ascertain the percentage of correct choices. This percentage rises from chance (50%) to near certainty (100%) as stronger and stronger stimuli are presented. Threshold is found by a statistical treatment that yields an estimate of the stimulus required for 75% correct choices. This threshold stimulus is always found to be significantly higher when evaluated for the time during a saccade or blink than in the condition of rest. This is the index of the amount of suppression. The forced choice procedure has two distinct advantages. First, it is "bias-free" in the sense that the subject has no prior knowledge of when the stimulus will be present, and has no need to set for himself a criterion of certainty of judgment. Secondly, it fulfills BRINDLEY's (1960) condition for "class A" psychophysical judgments, namely that no qualitatively different stimuli are to be discriminated.

One curious aspect of forced-choice procedures is that the subject can be performing far above the chance level of correct choices, and yet state that he is not aware of seeing the stimulus. As a subject, one develops the feeling that the whole procedure is going on automatically: pairs of intervals are judged, the percentages of correct choices reach levels far above chance, and still the subject is not "aware" of the stimuli. Could it be that some lower center of the brain is used for making such judgments, so that conscious awareness is somehow bypassed? In any case, the whole procedure ultimately is a satisfying one, because highly orderly and reliable relationships emerge between stimulus intensity and correctness of choice. So little possibility is there that observer bias will influence these results that we do not hesitate to use ourselves, along with more naive observers, in the course of these experiments. It is probably not too strong a statement to make at this time that all present-day determinations of visual thresholds should make use of forced-choice or other bias-free procedures wherever possible.

Perhaps I should digress and say a few words about the improvement I have witnessed in psychophysical research over the past 40 years. It is now abundantly clear that the psychophysical "threshold" is not any fixed value of a stimulus, but a statistical estimate based upon concepts that are now best understood through the emergence of information theory in the 1940s and the decision aspects of detection in the 1950s (see GREEN and SWETS 1966). These developments showed that a threshold is governed not only by the intensity of the stimulus but also by observer bias, such as any instructed or self-imposed criterion of certainty of judgment. Signal detection theory has now given us an estimate, d', of the intrinsic detectability of a stimulus after correction for bias. This consideration shows that classic methods of psychophysics, based on "yes–no" judgments, are open to some criticism. This is not to say that all the classic experiments in vision are wrong. Far from it, especially when very large effects are observed and a sufficient degree of subject agreement is found. We have no present need to discard most of the generally accepted data on such functions as spectral sensitivity, dark adaptation, acuity, wavelength discrimination, and many others.

A particularly noteworthy experiment may serve as an example, namely that of HECHT et al. (1942). The purpose was to determine the minimum number of quanta of light required for seeing a light under optimal conditions. Brief flashes of light were used, and the subject made a judgment of "yes" or "no" for the seeing of each flash. Frequencies of seeing varied from zero to 100% over the intensity range that was used. Independent calculations were made, from measurements of the energy of the light, that from 54 to 148 quanta must have been incident on the cornea for the subject to say "yes" 60% of the time. Correcting for intraocular losses, this was estimated to represent an upper limit of 5–14 quanta absorbed by the rod receptors in a region of the retina containing about 500 rods.

In analyzing their results, the authors concluded that when so few quanta were actually effective, the number of quanta per flash must have varied considerably, in accordance with the Poisson distribution of small numbers of randomly occurring events. They therefore fitted Poisson curves to the frequency of seeing data for their three observers and came out with the conclusion that the slopes of these curves indicated that from 5 to 8 quanta represented the minimum needed for vision at threshold. They then drew two further conclusions: first, that "biological variation" must be small in comparison with the physical variation of quanta per flash; and secondly, that only a single quantum is needed to stimulate each of 5–8 rod receptors at threshold.

Looked at from the perspective of the 1980s, it seems to me that several aspects of this classic experiment are clear. First, the modern way would have been to use a forced-choice procedure, or to have included a goodly number of "no-light" trials so that an estimate could have been made of each observer's rate of "hits," "misses," "false alarms," and "correct rejections." Secondly, the fact that zero false alarms were obtained indicates that the observers were setting a rather high criterion for their "yes" judgments. Thirdly, the disregard of biological variation was not realistic. We know now that random and systematic errors of judgment are always found and that "... a smaller number of quanta will appear to be required, the greater the variability in the biological mechanism" (BARTLETT 1965). Nevertheless, if all these things had been taken into account, the major conclusions would have been the same: physical variation in the number of quanta per flash would still have proven to be an important determinant of the results; and although the high observer criterion may have led to too high a threshold [DE VRIES (1943) and BOUMAN (1950) have argued that 2–8, rather than 5–8 is the minimum number of quanta that must be absorbed for a subject to report seeing a flash], the conclusion is still the same: the number of quanta required to trigger a rod response is just one.

Perhaps it is because vision research is so well advanced, with respect to the control of the stimulus and knowledge of the underlying physiology, that the principal findings have held up well over the years. In the course of my own career I have admired the carefully conducted and monumental experiments of Hecht, Graham, Stiles, Crawford, deLange, Bouman, and many others whose principal research effort has been psychophysical, much of it involving the determination of thresholds. For the most part they have used the classic methods of limits, constant stimuli, or adjustment. Their findings have been confirmed in many cases by parallel physiological or behavioral work on animals or human subjects. My purpose is not to question their achievements, but simply to urge that future investigators take advantage of the superior reliability of the bias-free procedures. They may take longer than the more primitive procedures such as yes-no determinations of threshold or magnitude estimation at higher levels, but they can almost always be used by a researcher who is careful to set up the appropriate conditions.

If any reader has stayed on to this point in my discourse, he or she deserves an assurance that it is soon to end. Together we have journeyed from the past into the present, and it is probably presumptuous on my part to predict or even advocate anything for the future. Nor is there room for me to expound on the many fine vision research projects of my successors at Brown: Mitchell Glickstein, Billy Wooten, and Steven Lehmkuhle. But I cannot refrain from describing one more project that has intrigued me since 1972, when I first encountered it. I refer to our series of experiments on the pattern-contingent aftereffects of color.

II. The McCollough Effect

Celeste MCCOLLOUGH (1965) at Columbia published a provocative report of visual phenomena showing that an unmistakable link between line orientation and color can be established in a few minutes' time in normal human adults. Her procedure was simple: expose the subject to a few seconds of viewing a pattern of orange vertical lines, then shift for a few seconds to blue horizontal lines, and continue the alternate presentation for 2–4 min. The result is unmistakable: achromatic test lines now appear bluish green if they are vertical, and orange if horizontal. Most intriguing of all is the fact that these aftereffects outlast any typical afterimages consisting of colors or patterns alone.

1. Interpretations of the Effect

What is the meaning of these novel aftereffects? McCollough herself recognized that they might involve edge-detecting mechanisms such as those revealed by microelectrode studies in the brains of cats or monkeys. These are exquisitely tuned for line or edge orientation (HUBEL and WIESEL 1962, 1968). She also called attention to relatively long-lasting color aftereffects that had been reported as a result of prolonged wearing of strong prismatic spectacles (KOHLER 1964). She apparently had the insight to put these earlier findings together, and thus to generate her novel demonstration. A significant feature of this work is that the aftereffect colors are self-originated, occurring long after all similar colors have been removed from the visual field. Furthermore, these subjective colors are seen whether the test field is achromatic or monochromatic. They are therefore a new manifestation of what von Helmholtz called "sensations in the brain." Von Helmholtz argued that motion aftereffects, electric phosphenes, and other subjective phenomena represent the purely spontaneous operations of the brain's machinery, in the absence of input from sense organs. He thus recommended them to psychologists as being true indicators of the manner in which the brain functions to analyze incoming sensory messages. In this age of the rapid accumulation of facts about single unit activity, we would do well to heed von Helmholtz' advice – and McCollough's exemplification of it – to relate subjective effects to neurophysiological events.

2. Psychophysical Procedures

The major contribution of our Brown laboratory to a rapidly growing body of research on the McCollough effect was our quantification of it. This took a little doing, because instead of getting the subject's qualitative judgment about the aftereffect colors we put together a testing device in which the subject could cancel these subjective colors by the use of variable amounts of real colors of complementary hue. The result was a reasonably reliable specification, in standard colorimetric units, of the amount and direction of the effect (RIGGS et al. 1974).

3. Major Conclusions

As I look back on the McCollough effect experiments, I have to admit that they did not reveal any new explanation of how the effect takes place, but they established the following points.

1. Although completely subjective, the effect was scaled with considerable precision by a nonverbal, unambiguous matching technique.
2. This matching procedure, while perhaps not literally an objective test, nevertheless clearly met BRINDLEY's (1960) criterion for a class A experiment. It was bias-free, in that no estimates were required of the subject. He simply had to adjust a knob to a point at which two panels containing the oppositely oriented lines appeared identical in hue.

3. A relatively simple mathematical equation described the decay of the aftereffect with time. When measured as above, the aftereffect decayed at a rate proportional to its strength measured immediately after inspection.

4. The equation held true regardless of absolute amounts of the effect due to a wide range of experimental conditions and individual subjects, leading to the presumption of an underlying physiological process.

5. The aftereffect strength decayed linearly over a logarithmic scale of time after inspection, in nearly all cases approaching zero strength at from 4 to 6 days.

6. An occasional subject was found with a "built-in" effect. That is, achromatic lines of a particular orientation had a slightly different chromaticity from oppositely oriented lines at all times. This leads to the presumption that orientation-tuned visual mechanisms may have become permanently different in their sensitivities to color in these few subjects, perhaps through genetic, neurochemical, or environmental influences.

4. Research Teams

The most extensive of our McCollough effect experiments went better because the work of apparatus building, experimenting, and observing was shared among several people (RIGGS et al. 1974; WHITE et al. 1978). This brings me to say that I have derived great satisfaction, over the years, in laboratory team work. No one, I suppose, can predict just what group of individuals may find themselves to be working together most felicitously. I have particularly happy memories of working together with Ratliff, Cornsweet and Cornsweet, Armington and Johnson, Johnson and Schick, Blough and Schafer, Merton and Morton, White and Eimas, and Volkmann and Moore. More complete evidence of my good fortune in regard to research companions is provided by the festschrift volume on the occasion of my academic retirement (ARMINGTON et al. 1978).

G. Conclusion

I have tried to convey in this chapter some personal experiences that illustrate the great progress that has taken place over the last five decades in the study of vision. Some of this is due, no doubt, to instrumentation. It is hard to realize that in my student days there were, for example, no oscilloscopes, tape recorders, microelectrodes, solid state amplifiers, xerox copiers, or computers. But perhaps even more impressive is the progress toward scientific rigor and objectivity that I have witnessed. Hunter, Graham, and Hartline pushed me strongly in that direction, and since then I have continued to urge the same course on my students.

I like Floyd RATLIFF's (1962) version of this theme:

Of course, objectivity and quantitative measurement are not absolutely necessary at all times and in all aspects of science. Indeed, as we have attempted to show, it is a historical fact that many major concepts stem from originally nonobjective and nonquantitative observations. But it is clear that all such concepts have been abandoned as soon as they could be replaced by more rigorously formulated ones.

I like to think that the behavioral sciences, which were successfully overthrowing structuralism and Gestalt theory as I first came on the scene, will continue to reject all forms of mentalism. But perhaps, in some quarters, we are now witnessing a return swing of the pendulum. It seems again acceptable, indeed even fashionable, to attempt to observe specifically verbal and logical mental processes, without reference to underlying neural events, in order to account for complex aspects of human cognition. Thus it would appear that history is repeating itself, and in a field that is evidently enjoying a rapid expansion among philosophers, mathematicians, linguists, and psychologists. Does this trend toward subjectivity now extend into our field of sensory science? I think not; and I confidently expect that the story told by other chapters in this *Foundations* volume will lend support to that conclusion.

References

Adler FH, Fliegelman F (1934) Influence of fixation on the visual acuity. Arch Ophthalmol 12:475–483

Adrian ED (1945) The electric response of the human eye. J Physiol 104:84–104

Adrian ED (1946) Rod and cone components in the electric response of the eye. J Physiol 105:24–37

Aiba TS, Alpern M, Maaseidvaag F (1967) The electroretinogram evoked by the excitation of human foveal cones. J Physiol 189:43–62

Anderson EE, Weymouth FW (1923) Visual perception and the retinal mosaic. I. Retinal mean local sign. Am J Physiol 64:561

Armington JC (1952) A component of the human electroretinogram associated with red color vision. J Opt Soc Am 42:393–401

Armington JC (1974) The electroretinogram. Academic, New York

Armington JC, Biersdorf WR (1956) Flicker and color adaptation in the human electroretinogram. J Opt Soc Am 46:393–400

Armington JC, Krauskopf J, Wooten BR (eds) (1978) Visual psychophysics and physiology: a volume dedicated to Lorrin Riggs. Academic, New York

Asher H (1951) The electroretinogram of the blind spot. J Physiol 112:40P

Barlow RB, Bolanowsky SJ, Brachman ML (1977) Efferent optic nerve fibers mediate circadian rhythms in the *Limulus* eye. Science 197:86–89

Bartlett NR (1965) Thresholds as dependent on some energy relations and characteristics of the subject. In: Graham CH (ed) Vision and visual perception. Wiley, New York, pp 154–184

Berry RN (1948) Quantitative relations among vernier, real depth, and stereoscopic depth acuities. J Exp Psychol 38:708–721

Bouman MA (1950) Peripheral contrast thresholds of the human eye. J Opt Soc Am 40:825–832

Boynton RM (1953) Stray light and the human electroretinogram. J Opt Soc Am 43:442–449

Boynton RM (1979) Human color vision. Holt, Rinehart,and Winston, New York

Boynton RM, Riggs LA (1951) The effect of stimulus area and intensity upon the human retinal response. J Exp Psychol 42:217–226

Brindley GS (1960) Physiology of the retina and visual pathway. Arnold, London

Butler TW, Riggs LA (1978) Color differences scaled by chromatic modulation sensitivity functions. Vision Res 18:1407–1416

Campbell FW, Robson JG (1968) Application of fourier analysis to the visibility of gratings. J Physiol 197:557–566

Carpenter RHS (1977) Movements of the eye. Pion, London

Cornsweet TN (1956) Determination of the stimuli for involuntary drifts and saccadic eye movements. J Opt Soc Am 46:987–993

Delabarre EB (1898) A method of recording eye-movements. Am J Psychol 9:572–574

Delabarre EB (1928) Dighton Rock. Neale, New York

DeVries H (1943) The quantum character of light and its bearing upon the threshold of vision, the differential sensitivity and visual acuity of the eye. Physica 10:553–564

Ditchburn RW (1973) Eye movements and visual perception. Oxford University Press, London

Ditchburn RW, Ginsborg BL (1952) Vision with a stabilized retinal image. Nature 170:36

Ditchburn RW, Ginsborg BL (1953) Involuntary eye movements during fixation. J Physiol 119:1–17

Fender DH (1955) Torsional motions of the eyeball. Br J Ophthal 39:65–72

Fry GA, Bartley SH (1935) The relation of stray light in the eye to the retinal action potential. Am J Physiol 111:335–340

Graham CH (1933) The relation of nerve response and retinal potential to number of sense cells illuminated in an eye lacking lateral connections. J Cell Comp Physiol 2:295–304

Graham CH (ed) (1965) Vision and visual perception. Wiley, New York

Graham CH, Granit R (1931) Comparative studies on the peripheral and central retina: VI. Am J Physiol 98:664–673

Graham CH, Margaria R (1935) Area and the intensity relation in the peripheral retina. Am J Physiol 113:299–305

Graham CG, Riggs LA (1934) The visibility curve of the white rat as determined by the electrical retinal response to lights of different wavelengths. J Gen Psychol 12:279–295

Graham CH, Kemp EH, Riggs LA (1935) Analysis of the electrical retinal responses of color-discriminating eye to lights of different wave-lengths. J Gen Psychol 13:275–296

Granit R (1935) Two types of retinas and their electrical responses to intermittent stimuli in light and dark adaptation. J Physiol 85:421–438

Green DM, Swets JA (1966) Signal detection theory and psychophysics. Wiley, New York

Hartline HK (1938) The response of single optic nerve fibers of the vertebrate eye to illumination of the retina. Am J Physiol 127:400–415

Hartline HK, Graham CH (1932) Nerve impulses from single receptors in the eye. J Cell Comp Physiol 1:277–295

Hartline HK, Ratliff F (1957) Inhibitory interaction of receptor units in the eye of *Limulus*. J Gen Physiol 40:357–376

Hartridge H, Thomson LC (1948) Methods of investigating eye movements. Br J Ophthalmol 32:581–591

Hecht S (1934) Vision. II. The nature of the photoreceptor process. In: Murchison C (ed) Handbook of general experimental psychology. Clark University Press, Worcester, MA

Hecht S, Shlaer S, Pirenne MH (1942) Energy, quanta, and vision. J Gen Physiol 25:819–840

Holt EB (1903) Eye-movement and central anaesthesia. I. The problem of anaesthesia during eye-movement. Psychol Monogr No. 17

Hubel DH, Wiesel TN (1962) Receptive fields, binocular interaction, and functional architecture in the cat's striate cortex. J Physiol 160:106–154

Hubel DH, Wiesel TN (1968) Receptive fields and functional architecture of monkey striate cortex. J Physiol 195:215–243

Hunter WS (1914) The after-effect of visual motion. Psychol Rev 21:245–277

Hunter WS (1915) Retinal factors in visual after-movement. Psychol Rev 22:479–489

Hunter WS (1942) Visually controlled learning as a function of time and intensity of stimulation. J Exp Psychol 31:423–429

Jasper HH, Carmichael L (1935) Electric potentials from the intact human brain. Science 81:51–53

Johnson EP, Riggs LA, Schick AML (1966) Photopic retinal potentials evoked by phase alternation of a barred pattern. Clinical electroretinography. Vis Res [Suppl]:75–91

Keesey UT (1960) Effects of involuntary eye movements on visual acuity. J Opt Soc Am 50:769–774

Kohler I (1964) The formation and transformation of the perceptual world. International Universities Press, New York

Krauskopf J, Riggs LA (1959) Interocular transfer in the disappearance of stabilized images. Am J Psychol 72:248–252

Kruskal JB (1964) Multidimensional scaling. Psychometrika 29:1–27, 115–129

Latour PL (1962) Visual threshold during eye movements. Vision Res 2:261–262

Lindsley DB, Hunter WS (1939) A note on polarity potentials from the human eye. Proc Nat Acad Sci USA 25:180–183

Lord MP, Wright WD (1948) Eye movements during monocular fixation. Nature 162:25–26

Marx E, Trendelenburg W (1911) Über die Genauigkeit der Einstellung des Auges beim Fixieren. Z Sinnesphysiol 45:87–102

Maurois A (1935) Ariel, a Shelley romance. Penguin, London

McCollough C (1965) Color adaptation of edge-detectors in the human visual system. Science 149:1115–1116

Motokawa K, Mita T (1942) Über eine einfachere Untersuchungsmethode und Eigenschaften der Aktionsströme der Netzhaut des Menschen. Tohoku J Exp Med 42:114–133

Orschansky J (1898) Eine Methode, die Augenbewegungen direkt zu untersuchen (Ophthalmographie). Zentralbl Physiol 12:785

Petry HM, Donovan WJ, Moore RK, Dixon WB, Riggs LA (1982) Changes in the human visually evoked cortical potential in response to chromatic modulation of a sinusoidal grating. Vision Res 22:745–755

Ratliff F (1950) The role of physiological nystagmus in visual acuity. PhD dissertation, Brown University

Ratliff F (1952) The role of physiological nystagmus in monocular acuity. J Exp Psychol 43:163–172

Ratliff F (1962) Some interrelations among physics, physiology, and psychology in the study of vision. In: Koch S (ed) Psychology: a study of a science, vol 4. McGraw-Hill, New York

Ratliff F, Riggs LA (1950) Involuntary motions of the eye during monocular fixation. J Exp Psychol 40:687–701

Regan D (1972) Evoked potentials in psychology, sensory physiology, and clinical medicine. Wiley, New York

Riggs LA (1937) Dark adaptation in the frog eye as determined by the electrical response of the retina. J Cell Comp Physiol 9:491–510

Riggs LA (1940) Recovery from the discharge of an impulse in a single visual receptor unit. J Cell Comp Physiol 15:273–283

Riggs LA (1941) Continous and reproducible records of the electrical activity of the human retina. Proc Soc Exp Biol Med 48:204–207

Riggs LA (1974) Responses of the visual system to fluctuating patterns. Am J Optom Physiol Opt 51:725–735

Riggs LA, Graham CH (1940) Some aspects of light adaptation in a single photoreceptor unit. J Cell Comp Physiol 16:15–23

Riggs LA, Ratliff F (1951) Visual acuity and the normal tremor of the eyes. Science 114:17–18

Riggs LA, Ratliff F (1952) The effects of counteracting the normal movements of the eye. J Opt Soc Am 42:872–873

Riggs LA, Tulunay SU (1959) Visual effects of varying the extent of compensation for eye movements. J Opt Soc Am 49:741–745

Riggs LA, Mueller CG, Graham CH, Mote FA (1947) Photographic measurements of atmospheric boil. J Opt Soc Am 37:415–420

Riggs LA, Mote FA, Mueller CG, Graham CH (1948) Two devices for evaluating stereoscopic reticle-patterns. Am J Psychol 41:542–552

Riggs LA, Berry RN, Wayner MJ (1949) A comparison of electrical and psychophysical determinations of the spectral sensitivity of the human eye. J Opt Soc Am 39:427–436

Riggs LA, Ratliff F, Cornsweet JC, Cornsweet TN (1953) The disappearance of steadily fixated visual test objects. J Opt Soc Am 43:495–501

Riggs LA, Armington JC, Ratliff F (1954) Motions of the retinal image during fixation. J Opt Soc Am 44:315–321

Riggs LA, Ratliff F, Keesey ÜT (1961) Appearance of Mach bands with a motionless retinal image. J Opt Soc Am 51:702–703

Riggs LA, Johnson EP, Schick AML (1964) Electrical responses of the human eye to moving stimulus patterns. Science 144:567

Riggs LA, White KD, Eimas PD (1974) Establishment and decay of orientation-contingent aftereffects of color. Percept Psychophys 16:535–542

Rosenblith WA (ed) (1962) Processing neuroelectric data. MIT Press, Cambridge

Schlosberg H (1958) The psychological laboratory of Brown University. Am J Psychol 71:768–776

Schubert G, Bornschein H (1952) Beitrag zur Analyse des menschlichen Elektroretinogramms. Ophthalmologica 123:396–413

Sekuler RW, Ganz L (1963) Aftereffect of seen motion with a stabilized retinal image. Science 139:419–420

Volkmann FC (1962) Vision during voluntary saccadic eye movements. J Opt Soc Am 52:571–578

Volkmann FC, Schick AML, Riggs LA (1968) Time course of visual inhibition during voluntary saccades. J Opt Soc Am 58:562–569

Volkmann FC, Riggs LA, Moore RK (1980) Eyeblinks and visual suppression. Science 207:900–902

Wald G, Clark A (1937/1938) Visual adaptation and chemistry of the rods. J Gen Physiol 21:93–105

Walls GL (1942) The vertebrate eye and its adaptative radiation. Cranbrook Press, Michigan

Westheimer G, McKee SP (1979) What prior uniocular processing is necessary for stereopsis? Invest Ophthalmol Vis Sci 18:614–621

White KD, Petry HM, Riggs LA, Miller J (1978) Binocular interactions during establishment of McCollough effects. Vision Res 18:1201–1215

Yarbus AL (1967) Eye movements and vision. Plenum, New York

Zuber BL, Stark L (1966) Saccadic suppression: elevation of visual threshold associated with saccadic eye movements. Exp Neurol 16:65–79

CHAPTER 7

The Perception of Light and Colour

W. David Wright

This chapter is very much a personal assessment of some of the developments in visual research, especially those dealing with the sensitivity of the eye to light and colour, in the period of the 1920s to 1940s. My instructions from the editors may be summarised by the following quotation from a letter from one of them, in which I was asked to recount "how W.D. Wright interacted with other scientists, with the forces of the period and with the tools available in 1926 to produce what is currently available." This is my only justification for the frequent references to my own involvement in many of the activities which I describe.

When I started as a research student in 1926, I set out to make a redetermination of the colour mixture curves for an average normal observer, and my first task was to dismantle the colour-patch apparatus which Sir William Abney had built at Imperial College (ABNEY 1905). I then had to design and construct my own colour-mixing instrument. For several years I was concerned primarily with colour-matching and colour-measuring experiments, and it was some years before I carried out experiments on the spectral sensitivity of the foveal and extrafoveal areas of the retina. From a logical point of view I should, perhaps, have started with these measurements, and that is the order in which I shall deal with the subject in this chapter: first with the various aspects of the perception of light, and then with the perception and measurement of colour, with a final section on defective colour vision.

A. The Response of the Eye to Light

In the 1930s the incentive for much of the visual research came from a desire to relate psychophysical measurements of the response of the eye to light with the growing body of information provided by visual photochemists and electro-physiologists (WRIGHT and GRANIT 1938). LYTHGOE (1937), for example, was the leading physiologist in England to study the absorption curve of visual purple, paving the way for DARTNALL's (1972) very extensive programme of retinal photochemistry. Meanwhile, GRANIT (1933) in Sweden was recording and analysing retinal action potentials and HARTLINE (1934) was making his remarkable recordings from single optic nerve fibres of the *Limulus* crab.

Illuminating engineering problems, especially the problem of the glare from the headlights of an oncoming car, provided a more applied stimulus to visual research, and STILES (1929) at the National Physical Laboratory was a leading figure in this field. Headlight glare has many different visual ingredients, including the veiling effect of the light scatter in the atmosphere and in the observer's eye; the local light adaptation of that part of the retina on which the image of the headlight falls, the rate of recovery of the light sensitivity of the retina once the headlight has passed out of the field of view; the brightness contrast between the luminance of the headlight and the luminance of other objects in the field of view; the inhibitory effect induced laterally across the retina by the headlight glare; and the role played by subjective brightness relations in determining the visibility problems facing a driver. Equally complex problems existed in night flying in those pre-radar days, and the interaction between the engineer and the visual scientist was a very important stimulus to visual research in the 1930s.

I. The Sensitivity of the Eye to Light

The most obvious way to determine the sensitivity of the eye to light in any given viewing situation is to measure the smallest amount of radiant energy that the observer can just detect. This has the merit of being unambiguous in concept but can involve many different experimental variables, depending on how the threshold stimulus is presented to the observer and the criterion adopted to define when the observer can actually perceive the test light.

The experiment also involves some quite sophisticated radiometry, not an easy branch of technology even now, but very much more difficult 40 or 50 years ago. I can bear this out from my own experience when faced with the task of measuring the spectral energy distribution emerging from the exit pupil of my colorimeter. The light had to be focused with a microscope objective onto the small area of the junction of a Kipp and Zonen vacuum thermocouple and the output from the thermocouple was measured with a Paschen galvanometer. This type of galvanometer was a most frustrating instrument to use, especially when the extremely delicate suspension got broken, as it often did, and a new one had to be mounted by passing it down a long narrow glass tube. What a contrast to modern microprocessors!

The classic determination of the absolute sensitivity of the retina was carried out by HECHT et al. (1942). In their experiments they used a test patch having an angular subtense of 10′ of arc, and this was focused on an area of the retina located

20° from the fovea. The test light was a monochromatic radiation of wavelength 510 nm, and it was flashed on for an exposure time of 0.001 s. They also, incidentally, used a thermopile and Paschen galvanometer for their energy measurements. From a statistical analysis of the frequency of seeing of the flash for a fully dark-adapted eye, they deduced that only about six quanta were needed to react with the visual purple in the rod receptors for the response to be detected as a visual sensation.

Subsequent experiments by other workers led to claims that only one or two quanta could lead to a detectable visual response. Some fairly heated arguments were generated at the time about the precise number of quanta involved, but most of us were satisfied to know that the number was quite small!

II. The Spectral Sensitivity of the Rod Receptors

From the biological point of view, the interest in determining the spectral sensitivity of the rod receptors lies in its relation to the absorption curve of visual purple or rhodopsin, the photopigment in the rods. Threshold measurements are the most likely to give results directly related to the photochemical absorption process, and experiments carried out by WALD (1945) typify the kind of results that can be obtained. In his experiments he measured the energy required to detect a circular patch of monochromatic light subtending 1° on the retina, with an exposure time of 40 ms, when the patch was viewed on an area of the retina located 8° above the fovea. (He also carried out similar experiments with the patch viewed at the fovea, but we are not for the moment concerned with those results.) His results provided convincing evidence that the spectral sensitivity of the retina under truly scotopic conditions is governed by the spectral absorption of rhodopsin.

For rod vision at least, the same function can also be measured by direct brightness matching, provided the matching is carried out at near-threshold brightness levels. This is a valid type of observation because scotopic vision is achromatic; colour does not, therefore, intrude to confuse the nature of the brightness match which the observer is asked to make. The curve adopted by the Commission Internationale de l'Éclairage (CIE) in 1951 to define the spectral sensitivity of the eye at low brightness levels for use in scotopic photometry (the V' curve) was, in fact, based on results obtained by CRAWFORD (1949) using direct brightness matching. He used a large photometric field subtending 20°, and the observers were asked to fixate on its upper edge, so that the bulk of the field was imaged on the extrafoveal area of the retina. The luminance level at which the observations were made, 3.2×10^{-9} stilb, was approximately 15 times the absolute threshold. Crawford's mean results for 50 observers agreed closely with Wald's threshold measurements for 22 observers except at the red end of the spectrum, where Wald's values were lower. This is the type of discrepancy to be expected, since the cones would almost certainly be making a small contribution to the visual response at the long-wave end of the spectrum under the conditions used by Crawford.

These major studies by Wald and by Crawford, supplemented by other less ambitious investigations, have provided a firm foundation for our understanding of the perception of light in scotopic vision. The situation in photopic vision is much less clear, involving as it does the perception of both brightness and colour. This not only affects the precision with which brightness matches can be made, but also raises serious questions as to how far brightness (or lightness) can be identified as a separate entity when viewing a coloured source or surface. This is a subject which is being even more hotly debated now than it was 50 years ago.

III. The Spectral Sensitivity of the Cone Receptors

The curve which is most widely regarded as specifying the spectral sensitivity of the eye at photopic levels is the V_λ curve defined in 1924 by the CIE for use in heterochromatic photometry at high brightness levels. We will review the work leading up to this curve shortly, but it is more appropriate to refer first to later studies in which the foveal sensitivity was determined by the threshold technique, since, as has already been noted, this gives the most unambiguous and visually most meaningful measurement.

The results obtained by WALD (1945) for the fovea using the same 22 subjects and the same size of test patch as for his extrafoveal measurements quoted above showed the characteristic shift in sensitivity maximum from a wavelength of about 500 nm for scotopic vision to about 560 nm for photopic vision. At the long-wave end of the spectrum he found little difference in absolute sensitivity between the two processes, but at a wavelength of 492 nm the rods were found to be almost a thousand times more sensitive than the cones. This, however, was for the particular viewing conditions used in Wald's experiments.

The number of wavelengths at which Wald's subjects made their observations was insufficient to bring out clearly the irregularities which have been found in the cone sensitivity curves for individual observers, for example, by HURVICH and JAMESON (1953) and by HSIA and GRAHAM (1952). Thus all five subjects tested by Hsia and Graham gave sensitivity curves with the main maximum at a wavelength of about 560 nm and subsidiary maxima at about 440 nm and 610 nm. Absorption in the ocular media could be partly responsible for these irregularities in the curves, but it seems more likely that these three maxima are evidence for the three types of cone receptor responsible for our colour perception. It is relevant here to recall some foveal threshold measurements made by STILES and CRAWFORD (1933) under rather special viewing conditions, in which a small test field was viewed foveally in a dark central aperture subtending 1.3° in a white surround field, this field having a luminance of 300 cd per sq ft (32 cd per m²). Here again, as shown in Fig. 1, the sensitivity curve they obtained had three peaks with clearly defined maxima at wavelengths of about 440 nm, 530 nm, and 600 nm.

The alternative method of determining the spectral sensitivity curve of the cone receptors is to measure the relative brightness of the colours in the equal-energy spectrum. This is the equivalent of the observations which Crawford carried out for the rod receptors, except that the observer now has the exacting task of equating the luminous content of the two colours being matched while ignoring their colour content. This whole problem of heterochromatic photometry was investigated exhaustively by H. E. Ives in the United States between 1912 and 1923, and his conclusions were well summarised by GUILD (1926). Thus Ives established the viewing conditions (angular size of field, field brightness, and field environment) under which two different methods of measuring the relative brightness of the spectrum,

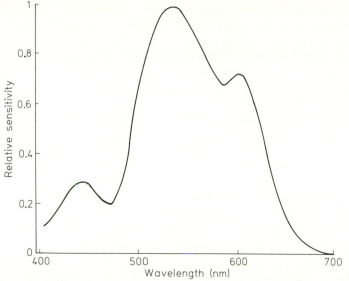

Fig. 1. A typical spectral sensitivity curve as measured by Stiles and Crawford, using the threshold method, for the particular viewing condition of a small test field viewed foveally and located in a dark central aperture (subtending 1.3°) in a white surround field, the surround having a luminance of 300 cd per sq ft (32 cd per m²). After STILES and CRAWFORD (1933)

namely by step-by-step direct brightness matching or by flicker photometry, gave comparable results and under which additivity of photometric quantities held.

In the step-by-step method the spectral sensitivity curve is built up from a series of matches through the spectrum as λ_1 is matched against λ_2, λ_2 against λ_3, and so on. By this means brightness matches between widely different colours are avoided. In flicker photometry, on the other hand, the two wavelengths to be matched are seen in rapid succession and at a frequency sufficiently high to eliminate the flicker due to their difference in colour, but not too high to eliminate the flicker due to any difference in brightness that might be present. The observer then has the task of adjusting the brightness of one field relative to the other until the flicker disappears, and this setting is considered to be the point at which the two fields are equally bright.

Because the "visibility curve of the equal-energy spectrum," as it was called then, was becoming of increasing importance in the lighting industry, a number of independent investigations to determine the curve for an average observer were carried out in the United States, either at the Bureau of Standards or in industrial lighting laboratories. Some of these studies used the step-by-step direct brightness-matching technique, while the others used flicker photometry, but in general they adhered to the viewing conditions recommended by Ives. GIBSON (1926) presented a paper to the CIE in 1924 entitled "The Relative Visibility Function," in which he recommended a mean set of values for adoption to define the V_λ curve, as we will call it, for an internationally agreed standard observer.

The approval of this recommendation by the CIE was a landmark in the history of photometry, since it now became possible to specify light intensity, luminous flux, luminance, and illumination on an internationally agreed basis. This 1924 V_λ curve, in fact, became the bridge between radiometry and photometry, making it possible to convert radiant flux expressed in radiometric units (watts) into luminous flux expressed in photometric units (lumens). In spite of the recognition some years later that the V_λ values at the violet end of the spectrum were too low, this 1924 curve has survived to the present day as the international standard observer for photometry.

As, however, we shall be noting later in connection with the definition of the 1931 standard observer for colorimetry, these standards were established as technological standards for use in the lighting and colour industries. Their use in visual research is an altogether different matter. I have the impression that visual researchers have been almost bemused by the authority of the CIE and have too readily assumed that the visual processes themselves were being standardised by the CIE. GUILD (1931) was under no illusions about this. In the paper in which he was recommending the adoption of data defining a standard observer for colorimetry based on his and my experimental results, he wrote:

> The international photometric scale, which governs the output of large industries concerned with the production of illuminants, necessitates the elevation of some particular set of visibility data to the dignity of a standard, to be used universally in all computations carried out for technical purposes. ... Hopeless confusion would arise if every lamp manufacturer, or every photometric standardising laboratory, employed units based on individual judgment as to the most accurate visibility data available at any particular time. ... But from the point of view of our knowledge of the behaviour of the human eye, there can be no question of standardising data; no question of *defining* any set of experimental results as "true," or as representing the performance of the average eye.

I am not sure that I always bore this dictum of Guild's in mind in the early years of my visual research, but if our interest in measuring the spectral sensitivity of the eye derives from a desire to relate the results to the biological processes in the retina, we are more likely to be successful if we use the sensitivity curves of individual observers rather than the standard observer curve, the curves obtained by the threshold technique almost certainly being the most meaningful.

IV. The Transition from Rod to Cone Spectral Sensitivity

My involvement with night-time visibility problems was the main stimulus to the study I made with Walters (WALTERS and WRIGHT 1943) on the spectral sensitivity of the eye at illumination levels intermediate between pure scotopic and pure photopic vision. Much of our perception on the roads at night operates at these mesopic levels, and photometry at these levels is fraught with real difficulty because of the shift in the sensitivity curve to shorter wavelengths as the illumination level falls. This shift in the curve had been known since 1825, when Purkinje first reported the relative darkening of red colours at very low levels of illumination (PURKINJE 1825), but few reliable studies appeared to have been made on the transition from the cone to the rod sensitivity curve when tested for an area of the retina containing both rods and cones.

Our measurements had to be made with the direct brightness-matching technique between the two halves of a 2° field of view, in which successive wavelengths illuminating one half of the field were matched against a red of wavelength 630-nm

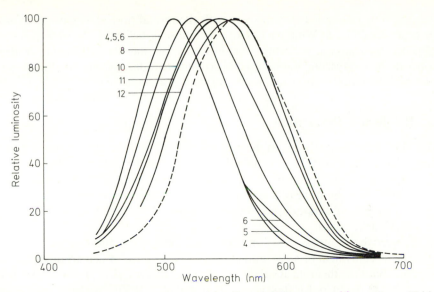

Fig. 2. Spectral sensitivity curves as measured by direct brightness matching, using a 2° bipartite field centred on a retinal area 3° from the fovea, matches being made at retinal illumination levels ranging from near threshold level (4) to near photopic level (12). Foveal photopic curve shown dotted. WALTERS and WRIGHT (1943)

in the other half of the field. The various illumination levels at which the sensitivity curves were measured were specified in terms of the energy density of the 630 nm comparison field set up for each curve. The use of a radiometric specification avoided any ambiguity that would have been associated with a photometric definition.

Figure 2 illustrates a typical set of curves obtained for a retinal area located 3° from the fovea for an illumination range from near threshold to fully photopic vision. For the first few levels the response is dominated by the rod response, with no shift in the maximum of the curve. However, at longer wavelengths above about 570 nm, the curves do begin to rise as the cone receptors come into action. At higher levels, the cone response gathers momentum, leading to a broadening of the curve and a shift of the maximum to longer wavelengths. Eventually, the response is dominated by the cones until a purely cone sensitivity curve emerges.

Results of this kind provided the lighting engineer with the information he needed in order to deal with visibility problems at light levels in the mesopic range. They also illustrate the difficulties, still not fully resolved, of establishing a system of photometry for use at these levels. They raise, too, a number of questions of importance to the visual scientist concerning the interaction between the rod and cone processes. How do the rod and cone responses combine? Does the cone response inhibit the rod response as the illumination level increases? At what level do the rods cease to function? Is their response suppressed by the cones at this level, or is the rod photopigment fully bleached, or does the rod response become saturated, as suggested by the increment threshold experiments of AGUILAR and STILES (1954). What contribution, if any, do the rods make to our perception of colour?

Are the rods associated in some way with the retinal process responsible for our perception of blue, as WILLMER (1946) would have us believe?

There was never any shortage of questions about the interaction of the rods and cones in those days, and the same is no doubt true today, except that the questions now have a more structural and neurophysiological slant.

B. Brightness Perception

One very significant element in the perception of light is the apparent or subjective brightness of any object or scene at which we may be looking. While apparent brightness is dependent on the luminance of the object (the photometric measure of the amount of light the object is reflecting), it is also very dependent on whether the eye is light- or dark-adapted and on whether the object is seen against a light or a dark background.

Subjective brightness in vision is the equivalent of loudness in hearing, just as glare is the equivalent of noise, and in the 1930s there was much argument and discussion about the theoretical validity of trying to derive a scale of subjective brightness (GUILD 1932a, b; RICHARDSON 1932; CAMPBELL 1933; CAMPBELL and MARRIS 1935). As has so often been the case in both vision and hearing, the motives behind these studies were two-fold, academic and applied, since adequate subjective brightness and the absence of glare are essential items in the successful design of lighting installations in offices, homes, factories, and on the roads. My own involvement in this field arose from my application of a binocular matching technique to the study of light and dark adaptation, a technique which was subsequently put to very good use by Schouten and by Craik.

I. The Binocular Matching Technique for Studying Light Sensitivity

GUILD's (1932 a, b) and RICHARDSON's (1932) papers on subjective brightness were presented at the Discussion on Vision organised by the Physical Society and held at Imperial College, and it was at this same meeting that I reported some initial experiments using the binocular matching technique (WRIGHT 1932; a more complete account of a wide range of experiments which I carried out with the technique is given in WRIGHT 1946). The observation consisted essentially of using the right eye to observe a test field, first with the eye dark-adapted and then after the eye had been exposed to an adapting light of some given luminance, colour, and duration. Meanwhile, the left eye was maintained in a constant state of dark adaptation and used as a reference to view a comparison field which could be matched against the test field seen in the right eye.

There is no occasion here to describe the instrumental details of the experiment, but it proved possible to carry out a wide variety of observations for various colours and intensities of both adapting light and test colour, and to record not only the loss of sensitivity produced by the adaptation but also the course of its recovery. I was certainly not the first to use this technique of interocular comparison, but its particular merit that appealed to me was that it provided a method of measuring the light and colour sensitivity of the eye when it was operating well above the threshold level. As I made clear at the beginning of this chapter, the most unambiguous and meaningful method of determining the sensitivity of the eye to light is to measure the threshold energy that the observer can just detect, but additional information can be obtained from supra-threshold measurements. As an illustration of this, we may note the experiments of J. F. SCHOUTEN (1937), who took up and extended my binocular matching technique.

He obtained his doctorate at the Rijks University of Utrecht with a thesis the object of which "was to investigate the mechanism by which the visual impression of the foveal and of the parafoveal part of the retina is affected by the presence of other light sources in the field of view." And he described his experimental method in the Summary to his thesis as follows:

The binocular method, as described by Wright, is used throughout the experiments. The application of the method has been considerably extended by an experimental arrangement in which the test objects did not coincide in the field of vision with the adapting light source (indirect blinding). For indirect blinding it thus becomes possible to take measurements both during the time of exposure and during the time of recovery.

The first I knew of these experiments was when Schouten sent me a printed copy of his thesis. This was a moment of considerable significance for me and initiated a friendship which we maintained throughout our professional careers. Schouten's interests moved over to acoustics and hearing, in which he became a leading authority, and his wide experience in sensory perception led in due course to his appointment as Director of the Institute of Perception in Eindhoven.

The main features of Schouten's thesis were published in a paper written jointly with L. S. Ornstein in the *Journal of the Optical Society of America* in 1939 (SCHOUTEN and ORNSTEIN 1939). Sadly, Ornstein became a victim of the Nazi regime during the war. Reading this paper again after more than 40 years, it still seems to me to be one of the most important psychophysical studies of adaptation to have been reported. Thus, in his experiments on indirect blinding, the time of exposure of the glare source in the right eye was varied between 0.02 and 0.2 s by means of a rotating slit-wheel, while the test object seen by the right eye and the comparison field seen by the left eye were exposed for 0.01 s at the end of each of the exposure periods of the glare source. It was thus possible to measure the drop in sensitivity for various times of exposure of the glare source. Schouten also measured the rate of recovery of sensitivity after the glare source had been removed, and it is worth quoting the conclusions reached from these experiments as given in the Summary of Schouten and Ornstein's paper:

The binocular method, generalised for the measurement of indirect adaptation, makes it possible to obtain quantitative data on the adaptive processes in the retina. When a small area of the retina is illuminated, the sensitivity of this area and also of the surroundings drops to a considerably lower level within 0.1 s. This sudden fall is followed by a gradual drop in brightness of the light source, indicating a gradual drop in sensitivity. In the surroundings, however, the sensitivity remains practically constant during exposure. Notwithstanding this fact, some processes must be going on in that part of the retina because the rate of recovery of the sensitivity after exposure is dependent upon the time of exposure. Hence the state of adaptation of the retina is determined by at least two independent parameters.

Just as my experiments had been the stimulus to Schouten to take up the binocular matching technique, so Schouten's experiments on indirect adaptation encouraged me to modify my apparatus so as to repeat some of his observations and confirm his main findings. In this kind of experiment it is difficult to disentangle the effects due to light scatter in the eye, which produces a veil of light extending some distance from the image of the glare source on the retina, from lateral inhibitory effects in the retinal tissue and possibly at higher levels along the visual pathway. Schouten and Ornstein made the very definite statement: "Indirect adaptation can neither be accounted for by assuming a lateral diffusion of photo-sensitive substances or of photolytic products over the retina, nor by assuming a strong adaptive influence of the stray light within the eye." Stiles, on the other hand, tended to place more weight on the effect of stray light, and his use of the equivalent background brightness as a means of defining the level of adaptation and the loss of sensitivity due to a glare source fitted in well with this approach (STILES 1929). Certainly, the effect of stray light cannot be ignored, but this is an area where there has been some creative tension between different viewpoints. Subsequent experimentation has been unsuccessful so far, I think, in resolving this conflict of ideas.

Schouten was not the only researcher to take up binocular matching, as another brilliant young scientist, K. J. W. Craik, was inspired by Schouten and Ornstein's paper to use the technique to study the effect of adaptation on subjective brightness (CRAIK 1940). Craik's initial experiments were concerned with the measurement of subjective brightness and the level at which the response saturates. Later, as he reported at a discussion on a paper which I gave in 1941 (WRIGHT 1941) on vision in very weak light (a topic of some practical importance at that time when wartime black-out conditions prevailed), he had been asked by the Medical Research Council to carry out some work similar to mine and he described a portable instrument for the measurement of subjective brightness, a rival to the portable "brillmeter" which I described in my paper.

All the signs indicated that Craik was destined for an outstanding career in the Psychology Department at Cambridge, as he turned his attention to brain models and in 1943 wrote a small book, *The Nature of Explanation* (CRAIK 1943). But in 1945 he was killed in a cycling accident in Cambridge at the age of 31. As a tribute to his contribution to psychology at Cambridge the Kenneth Craik Laboratory has been named after him. It was a privilege to have been associated with some of his work, and from my point of view it was gratifying to have had two scientists of the calibre of Schouten and Craik take up the binocular matching technique in their studies on adaptation.

II. Hecht's Contribution to the Study of Light Perception

Selig Hecht was such a leading figure among visual scientists in the 1930s that it is fitting to close the first half of this chapter, which deals with the perception of light, with some comments about the influence which he exerted. My own relations with Hecht varied from the extremely cordial to the decidedly strained. My first meeting with him was a very exciting one. It occurred at a meeting of the Optical Society of America (OSA) in 1929 at Cornell University, when Hecht gave one of the invited lectures on Young's theory of colour vision (HECHT 1930). In the course of the lecture, he quoted the very recent results of mine giving new trichromatic colour mixture data. Unbeknown to Hecht, I was in the audience, and as a very young research worker in a foreign country, it was an unexpected surprise to find that my results were already being quoted by one of the leading visual scientists of the time. This established a very friendly start to our relationship, but as I became disillusioned with some of his theories, the relationship cooled off. He was, though, an inspiring lecturer and many of us, including Craik, came under his spell.

One example of my disillusionment concerned Hecht's interpretation of brightness discrimination, in which he postulated that a discrimination step involved a constant additional amount of photosensitive substance to be decomposed to produce a just-noticeable difference in brightness (HECHT 1935). I was satisfied that discrimination experiments which I carried out with a bipartite field having a given luminance, with the eye successively adapted to a range of retinal illuminations between 1,000 and 40,000 trolands, effectively disproved this theory (WRIGHT 1935, 1946), although I do not think Hecht ever accepted this (HECHT 1936).

That Craik reacted similarly is illustrated in a recent Craik Memorial Lecture given in 1978 by O. L. Zangwill (ZANGWILL 1980). He recalls Craik's fellowship dissertation at St. John's College, Cambridge, and comments:

It still has a freshness and intellectual inciseness hard to fault. True, his enthusiasm at times outruns his judgement, most notably in his over-estimation of Selig Hecht's photochemical theories at that time much in vogue. Even so, he expresses on occasion distinct doubt as to how well Hecht's theoretical structure really held together in a satisfactory quantitative fashion. In this connection, it is apposite to note that in the copy of his Fellowship dissertation that he presented to our Departmental Library, there is a pencilled note in the margin of Hecht's theory: "I now disagree with this and hold other views."

Nevertheless, although many of Hecht's contributions now seem dated and many of his ideas have been discarded, I would consider him fully justified in pressing his photochemical concepts to the limit to see how far various aspects of visual perception could be explained in those terms. From 1929, when I first met him at the OSA meeting at Cornell, until 1947, when he participated in a conference on colour vision which we had organised in Cambridge (HECHT 1949), he was the most active and stimulating of the visual researchers whom I knew. As an indication of the influence which he exerted on the subject of vision, his papers appear to be the most quoted by any of the authors in the volume *Vision and Visual Perception* edited by C. H. Graham (1965). In spite of the differences which we had, I very much enjoyed showing him (and also George Wald, who inherited Hecht's gifts as a lecturer) something of the countryside around Cambridge in 1947, especially as this proved to be the last time we should see him, as he died soon after returning to the United States from the Cambridge meeting.

C. The Perception of Colour

Colour has proved such a fascinating subject of study to such a variety of people that there has never been any need to search for an incentive to carry out research in the field or to justify the expenditure of time or money on its investigation, other than the sheer incredibility of the colour vision process. Yet colour technology has proved of such commercial importance to so many industries that much of the research on colour during the past 50 or 60 years has been carried out in response to demands from industry. Further, in the last 20 or 30 years the theorists among our scientific colleagues have come to realise that the biological processes from retina to visual cortex provide a remarkable system of information processing, so that a rather different motive than the love of colour has stimulated their contributions to the subject.

I shall be dealing almost entirely with the visual rather than the technological studies, except for the establishment of the 1931 CIE system of colour measurement. This was a landmark in the history of colorimetry, just as the 1924 V_λ curve was a landmark in the history of photometry. From 1931 it was possible to specify a colour on an internationally agreed system, and this had advantages but also dangers for colour vision research. We shall need to comment on this in due course, but first we will deal with colour discrimination. This is where colour vision starts, since the most striking colour phenomenon in nature is the spectrum, with its brilliant variation of hues from red at the long-wave end to violet at the short-wave end.

I. Colour Discrimination

The spectrum is not only the most striking colour phenomenon in nature but is also the one example where the light stimuli generating the colour sensations that we see can be specified in the simplest possible physical terms, namely by their wavelength λ. As a corollary to this, if we can just detect the difference in hue between two wavelengths λ_1 and λ_2, this just-noticeable wavelength difference can be specified in equally simple physical terms, namely by $\Delta\lambda$. For this reason I shall be restricting our discussion of colour discrimination almost entirely to the discrimination of the colours in the spectrum, since not only can we specify a spectral stimulus by its wavelength, but we also know that the light will be unaffected in spectral quality by absorption in the optic media of the observer's eye. With non-spectral stimuli, the spectral composition of the light reaching the retina will depend on the density of the yellow macular pigment and the degree of yellowing of the crystalline lens.

It is fitting here, I think, to quote the description of the spectrum which NEWTON (1730) gave in his *Opticks:*

The Spectrum did appear tinged with this Series of Colours, violet, indigo, blue, green, yellow, orange, red, together with all their intermediate Degrees in a continual Succession perpetually varying. So that there appeared as many degrees of Colours, as there were sorts of Rays differing in Refrangibility.

We normally associate Newton with the statement that there are just seven hues in the spectrum, but this quotation shows that he recognised that there is a continuous variation of hue between one main hue and the next.

If we are prepared to accept that the first stage of the colour perception process consists of three types of colour receptor in the retina, we can obtain a first understanding of the mechanism underlying our colour discrimination in the spectrum if these three receptor processes have spectral sensitivity curves such as those shown in Fig. 3. We have to assume further that each of the three processes generates signals in the retina which are identifiable, after whatever coding takes place along the visual pathway, when they reach the visual cortex and give rise to the appropriate colour sensation. On these assumptions we then see from Fig. 3 that as we move along the spectrum, so there is a continuous variation in the relative sen-

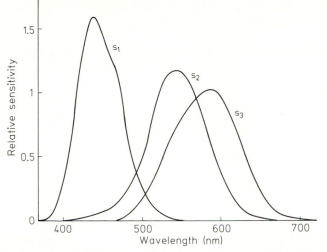

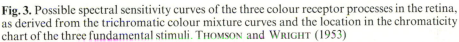

Fig. 3. Possible spectral sensitivity curves of the three colour receptor processes in the retina, as derived from the trichromatic colour mixture curves and the location in the chromaticity chart of the three fundamental stimuli. THOMSON and WRIGHT (1953)

sitivities of the three receptor processes, and therefore in their responses, leading to a pattern of signals arriving at the visual cortex which can generate a continuous variation of colour sensations through the spectrum.

To put this explanation of colour discrimination on a firm theoretical basis, we need experimental data on the variation of the just-noticeable wavelength difference $\Delta\lambda$ for a series of wavelengths λ through the spectrum. KÖNIG and DIETERICI (1884) were the first to determine a reliable wavelength discrimination curve, using von Helmholtz's colour-mixing apparatus. In their experiments the observer was not, in fact, asked to say when there was a just-noticeable difference (jnd) between the two wavelengths illuminating the two halves of the field; instead, he was asked to adjust the wavelengths so that the fields matched in colour and to repeat the match 50 times. The spread in the 50 wavelength settings was then analysed to give a measure of the discrimination sensitivity at the mean wavelength setting. This is a very sound technique, although more arduous for the observer than the jnd technique; it gives a discrimination step equal to about one-third of a jnd.

Several other determinations of the wavelength discrimination curve were carried out in the 50 years following König and Dieterici's experiments, until the measurements which I made with Pitt in 1934 (WRIGHT and PITT 1934). The mean curve which we obtained for five observers is shown in Fig. 4, and this still seems to be regarded as the definitive function. [This is the curve which BOYNTON (1979), for example illustrates in his *Human Color Vision*.] I am surprised that more studies of this curve have not been made, but the intense commercial interest in the specification of colour tolerances has meant that most of the recent researches on the detection of small colour differences have been carried out with coloured samples rather than with spectral lights.

A major theoretical paper on colour discrimination was written by STILES in 1946 on the basis of the line element concept of von Helmholtz (VON HELMHOLTZ

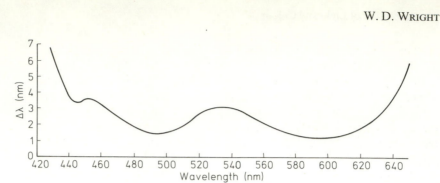

Fig. 4. The wavelength discrimination curve, showing the variation of the just-noticeable wavelength difference $\Delta\lambda$ as measured at a series of wavelengths through the spectrum. WRIGHT and PITT (1934)

1896). More recently, STILES (1972) has given a historical review of the line element in colour theory. The concept in effect applies the Weber-Fechner brightness discrimination ratio $\Delta B/B$ to each of the three sensitivity curves of Fig. 3 and sums their contributions to the colour difference by a formula originally proposed by von Helmholtz but which was modified by Stiles to give a closer fit to the experimental data.

My personal criticism of this type of analysis (a criticism which does not seem to be shared by anyone else), is that the whole responsibilty for the colour discrimination process is placed on the spectral sensitivity curves of the three colour receptor systems in the retina. They must clearly play a major role and it is not difficult to deduce a general relation between the sensitivity curves (s_1, s_2, and s_3) of Fig. 3 and the wavelength discrimination curve of Fig. 4. Thus, where s_1 and s_2 cross around 490 nm, we have a region of maximum wavelength discrimination (minimum $\Delta\lambda$ in Fig. 4); where the proportions of s_2 and s_3 are changing very rapidly in the region of 580–600 nm, we have another region of maximum wavelength discrimination; and where the proportions of s_2 and s_3 are changing relatively slowly, the discrimination in the green and in the red is poorer. Yet this cannot be the whole story.

As I understand it, the magnitude of the jnd must be determined in part by neural fluctuations in the signals, by spontaneous discharge in the receptors, and by other sources of biological noise along the visual pathway. In addition, any coding of the signals that occurs in the retinal network and in the lateral geniculate nucleus could influence the ability of the eye to detect small colour differences. What worries me most about the line element concept is that it does not seem to take any account at all of the actual colour quality of the sensations that we perceive. Our ability to distinguish red from yellow, for example, depends on the vividness of the redness that we perceive. Thus an observer who experiences a very intense redness when viewing the spectrum at a wavelength of, say, 650 nm, will record more jnd's between that wavelength and a yellow at 580 nm than an observer for whom 650 nm generated only an orange-red sensation. It seems to me that we cannot afford to ignore these possible variations in our actual colour perceptions if we wish to achieve a full understanding of the very considerable differences in colour discrimination that exist between one observer and another.

Then again, the discrimination observation itself is not just dependent on the mechanics of the receptor mechanism, but is governed also by the nature of the colour change and the rate at which the colour changes. This is illustrated by the observing technique that we had to adopt to obtain valid discrimination values, especially at the red end of the spectrum. Suppose, for example, we wished to measure the discrimination step at a wavelength of 630 nm. We would illuminate both halves of the field with monochromatic light of this wavelength, match them for brightness, and then slowly turn the wavelength control of one of the fields to a shorter wavelength until that field was just noticeably more orange than the 630 nm field. This might occur at a wavelength of, say, 628 nm, corresponding to a jnd of 2 nm. Repeat observations would, of course, give slightly different values, but the setting would be quite critical because the hue changes fairly rapidly towards the yellow. If, however, the observation had been made in the opposite direction, that is, by turning the wavelength control towards longer wavelengths, the setting would have been much more uncertain. There is a two-fold reason for this. In the first place, as we have already noted, the hue changes quite slowly at the red end of the spectrum, so a rather large wavelength change is needed before the observer can be certain that he can see a hue difference. In the second place, as you make this wavelength change, the brightness of the field falls because of the lower sensitivity of the eye to the longer wavelengths. With the darker field, a bigger wavelength difference is required before the observer can see a hue difference. So the wavelength control has to be turned still further, causing the field to become darker still and calling, perhaps, for yet a further increase in wavelength.

In this situation, we would always make the observation in the direction in which the hue is changing more rapidly with wavelength. In some regions of the spectrum, for example in the yellow, there is no problem, as the hue changes almost equally rapidly both in the long-wave and in the short-wave directions. It could be argued that the measurement of jnd's is not the best way to study wavelength discrimination, and there is something in this argument. König and Dieterici, as we have seen, used a "match spread" technique, while a third alternative is the so-called forced-choice technique, in which the observer is presented by the experimenter with a succession of pairs of wavelengths and has to decide from their hue difference which is the longer or shorter wavelength. Yet in both these techniques there is some difficulty in ensuring that equality of brightness is maintained and the influence of the rate at which the hue varies with wavelength is hidden but not eliminated.

I suspect that these theoretical and experimental uncertainties are at the root of the failure to develop an acceptable colour difference formula such as industrial colorimetrists have been searching for during the past 50 years or more. They may also help to explain some rather unexpected discrimination data that have sometimes been reported (see, for example, LE GRAND 1971).

I made the statement earlier that colour discrimination is where colour vision starts, and I would justify this by emphasizing that a reduced ability to discriminate colours is the primary characteristic of defective colour vision. We shall be considering studies that have been made on the different types of congenital colour-defective observers in the final section of this chapter, but in all cases there is some loss of colour discrimination. For a very small number of observers the loss is complete, so that all their vision is in monochrome. For those with two retinal receptor processes instead of three, wavelength discrimination will be good at some wavelengths in the spectrum but will be lost or greatly reduced at other wavelengths, depending on which process is missing. For example, if the s_3 process is missing (Fig. 3), as in protanopia, discrimination in the red-to-green range of wavelengths is almost non-existent.

One of the more unexpected investigations with which I became involved followed the rediscovery by WILLMER (1944) that the centre of the fovea was tritanopic, that is, that the s_1 process of Fig. 3 was missing. This had first been reported by KÖNIG (1894), but had been ignored and then forgotten. (How often König's name recurs! He must have been an outstanding experimenter.) Willmer, both a histologist and an artist, was looking for evidence in support of his idea that the rods might be responsible for our blue perception, and since the rods are absent from the fovea, we should be blue-deficient in the central fovea. This he found to be true when experimenting with small painted discs in yellow and blue, as when the discs were viewed from a distance, it was impossible to distinguish the yellow discs from white or the blue discs from black.

This observation obviously called for more detailed investigation, and he and I carried out colour discrimination and colour-matching experiments on my colorimeter, when the field of view was reduced to an angular subtense of about 15′ of arc and was fixated at the centre of the fovea (WILLMER and WRIGHT 1945). We found that colour matching was dichromatic, as König had, and we also found a break in the wavelength discrimination curve in the region of 440–490 nm, where no hue differences could be detected.

This phenomenon plumbed greater depths and raised many more questions than seemed likely at first (WRIGHT 1971). Was it really due to the absence of blue receptors at the centre of the fovea or was it merely a small-field effect? When I carried out further experiments with L. C. Thomson with 15′ fields located at a distance from the fovea of 20′ and 40′ of arc, we found some loss of discrimination in the blue and blue-green wavelengths, but the loss was relatively less striking than at the foveal centre (THOMSON and WRIGHT 1947).

Was the effect due essentially to steady fixation and consequent local adaptation in the foveal centre? McCree, for example, found that with observers who could maintain very steady fixation there was a marked loss of colour discrimination even with field sizes subtending 80′ of arc, and that the type of loss that occurred most readily was in the blue-green, corresponding to tritanopia (MCCREE 1960).

Was the effect associated in any way with the role of eye movements in colour perception? As a result of his experiments with stabilised retinal images, Ditchburn has suggested that colour information is generated at the boundary between one coloured area and another by the fine scanning movements of the eye. He has also shown that with partial image stabilisation, colour discrimination is reduced and leads to colour confusions which are symptomatic of tritanopia (DITCHBURN 1973).

Another possible explanation is the need for the summation of the response from a considerable number of blue receptors before the perception of blueness is generated. Since there is little neural convergence and summation among the receptors in the central fovea, this could lead to a type of tritanopic loss of wavelength discrimination even though some blue receptors were present.

This is one of those delightful problems where several alternative explanations are almost equally plausible. My own assessment of the evidence makes me believe that there is at least a small central area of the retina which is devoid of blue-sensitive cones. So I would go along with the conclusion which Wald reached in his Frederick Ives Medal Address to the Optical Society of America (OSA), "Blue-Blindness in the Normal Fovea," namely that blue-sensitive receptors are absent from a central area of the fovea subtending a visual angle of 7′ or 8′ of arc (WALD 1967). Yet we could both be wrong!

II. Three-Colour Mixture and Matching

As I mentioned in the Introduction to this chapter, my first task as a research student was to build a colour-mixing apparatus with which to make a redetermination of the colour mixture curves for an average normal observer. MAXWELL (1860) made the pioneer determination of these curves using his "colour box," followed by KÖNIG and DIETERICI (1892) using VON HELMHOLTZ'S (1896) colour-mixing apparatus and ABNEY (1905) with his "colour-patch" instrument. I had to learn as I went along what kind of instrument was needed to improve on the results of these early workers, but I was fortunate in that very up-to-date literature was available for me to consult. As it turned out, the year when I started, 1926, proved to be the ideal moment to set out on my colour vision research.

The basic facts of three-colour mixture and matching had been established very effectively by Maxwell, although the actual colour mixture curves that he obtained were of only limited value because of the rather rudimentary construction of his colour box. Nevertheless, his experiments confirmed that by making a series of colour matches through the spectrum, three spectral mixture curves could be obtained corresponding to the trichomatic response curves of the Young–Helmholtz theory. (It is now clear that Maxwell contributed as much as, if not more than, von Helmholtz did to the formulation of this theory, and a more appropriate name would be the Young–Maxwell theory or the Young–Helmholtz–Maxwell theory.) Maxwell was also responsible for the colour triangle, an equilateral triangle with the red, green, and blue primaries at the corners, within which a colour could be located according to the proportions of red, green, and blue required to match it. This was, of course, the forerunner of the modern CIE chromaticity chart.

The determination of the colour mixture curves of an individual observer was of fundamental importance to the understanding of the colour perception process and for establishing the spectral sensitivity curves of the retinal receptors. If, also, the colour mixture curves could be measured for a group of observers, then a mean set of curves for an average observer could be adopted as a standard and provide the framework for an international system of colour measurement.

At an Optical Convention held at Imperial College in 1926, Guild from the National Physical Laboratory gave a masterly review of modern developments in colorimetry (GUILD 1926), and in this review he emphasised the need for further progress in the science of colorimetry and most urgently of all, accurate information on the chromatic properties of the average human eye, in order that a "normal" eye for the purpose of colorimetry may be established by an agreed set of spectral mixture curves in the same way as a "normal" eye for photometry has been established by an agreed visibility curve.

This, then, was the background against which I set out to build my colorimeter (WRIGHT 1929, 1946) and I could hardly have asked for greater motivation to design the right kind of instrument and to produce an accurate set of colour mixture curves. The major decision which I had to make regarding the colorimeter concerned the relative merits of an instrument with red, green, and blue filters as the instrument primaries, or a spectroscopic type of instrument from which narrow wavebands could be selected from the red, green, and blue regions of the spectrum to serve as the instrument primaries. I was probably influenced by Abney's use of spectral primaries in his colour-patch apparatus, which I had to dismantle, in opting for this type of primary in preference to filter primaries, and I am sure this proved to be the right choice. For one thing it led to a much more flexible instrument, which I was able to adapt for measurements of the V_λ curve, for measuring the wavelength discrimination curve, for use as a visual spectrophotometer, and for a number of other uses, in addition to its use as a trichromatic colorimeter for measuring the spectral mixture curves. It was also an advantage when the time came to compare the results which GUILD (1925–1926) obtained with his "filter" colorimeter and my results obtained with my "spectral primaries" instrument. The very close agreement between the two sets of measurements which Guild was able to report (see WRIGHT 1929–1930, p. 213) had a greatly enhanced significance because we had used entirely different types of apparatus.

Since I want to emphasise in the next section the limited use which should be made in visual research of a colour specification based on the CIE Standard Observer, I need to describe in this section the differences which individual observers may make in their colour matches. I must, therefore, give a brief description of the optical system of my colorimeter, but this has been described in detail elsewhere (WRIGHT 1946).

A prism system was used to produce two spectra, one of which provided the red, green, and blue instrument primaries and the other the monochromatic test colour to be matched. The red-green-blue mixture illuminated one half of the 2° field of view, and the observer had three knobs to operate to vary the amounts of the primaries in the mixture. The test colour seen in the other half of the field could be set at any wavelength in the spectrum, while a small amount of one or other of the primary wavelengths could also be selected from that spectrum and added to the test colour.

The wavelengths I chose as the instrument primaries were a red at 650 nm, a green at 530 nm, and a blue at 460 nm. They were chosen for their practical convenience, as their additive mixture embraced a wide range of colours at a reasonably high luminance. The units on which the amounts of the primaries should be measured posed a more difficult question. Three possibilities existed, namely to use radiometric units (watts), photometric units (lumens) or colorimetric units in which the amounts of the red, green, and blue primaries were normalised to be equal in a match on some defined white illuminant. Radiometric units are physically the most unambiguous but experimentally the most difficult to calibrate.

(They certainly were in 1926!) Photometric units are rather unsatisfactory because the blue values in a colour match are usually very much smaller than the red and green values when they are expressed in terms of lumens. They also immediately raise uncertainties for an individual observer, since his eye is unlikely to have exactly the same spectral sensitivity as the standard V_λ curve.

I decided to use colorimetric units, but in a modified form in which I normalised the red and green primaries to give equal values in a match on a monochromatic yellow of wavelength of 582.5 nm, while the green and blue were adjusted to be equal in a match of a spectral blue-green of wavelength 494.0 nm. I adopted this unit system in the first place merely as a temporary measure while I was waiting for my standard white illuminant to be delivered from the National Physical Laboratory, but I retained it when I discovered that it was possible to analyse the observer differences in colour matching as due either to absorption in the ocular media or to differences in the spectral sensitivity of the retinal receptors.

The reason for this is that the spectral quality of a monochromatic radiation is unaffected by absorption in the optic media, as explained in Sect. C.I.; it is merely reduced in intensity. With a white illuminant, on the other hand, the energy distribution reaching the retinal receptors will vary from observer to observer depending on the density of the macular pigment and the degree of yellowing of the crystalline lens. It therefore hardly provides a very satisfactory standard on which to base the units of the red, green, and blue primaries. Yet with the system of units which I adopted, the colour co-ordinates of the white illuminant gave a direct indication of the absorption in the optic media, varying from a blueish white to a yellowish white depending on the absorption in the observer's eye. Further, any difference in the colour co-ordinates of the colours in the spectrum between one observer and another could only be due to differences in spectral sensitivity of the retinal receptors and not to absorption in the eye. (See WRIGHT 1946, for more detailed discussion of this unit system.)

Looking back over the years, I think it is very unfortunate that so few spectral colorimeters have been in existence with which an individual observer's colour mixture curves could be measured. I built the first model of my colorimeter in 1926 and a greatly improved version in 1938. We also built a similar model at about the same time for use in Sweden. Since then further models have been made in Japan, Norway, and Argentina. Subsequently, the need to determine colour mixture curves for large-field (10°) viewing conditions led to the construction by STILES (1955) of his very elaborate trichromator at the National Physical Laboratory, and other models of this equipment have been built in Japan and Canada. So far as I know, however, no other models of either Stiles' or my type of instrument are in use in the United States or elsewhere in Europe, but a new instrument is being developed at The City University in London by P. W. Trezona.

My concern at so few facilities of this kind being available arises from my conviction that the laws of colour mixture and colour measurement, and the differences between observers, can only be fully understood from laboratory experience with spectral trichromatic colorimeters. I will quote only two experiments to illustrate what I have in mind. One of the first observations I would ask a new research student to make would be to match a spectral blue-green colour, say of wavelength 490-nm. He would soon find that to get anywhere near a match, he would have to turn the knob controlling the red 650 nm primary down to zero. Yet as he adjusted the amounts of the 530-nm green primary and the 460-nm blue primary to give something like a close match so far as the hue was concerned, the mixture would still be too desaturated to match the monochromatic 490-nm test colour. The mixture would appear to be diluted with white compared to the vivid blue-green test colour. I would then advise him to add some of the red 650-nm primary to the test colour until he could obtain a satisfactory match, this time using all three, red, green, and blue, primaries. He would then take the readings for this match and also measure how much of the red primary he had added to the blue-green test colour to make it matchable with a red-green-blue mixture. By subtracting this amount from the first match, he would then have the negative amount of red, together with the positive amounts of blue and green, which would be the trichromatic specification of the 490-nm test colour itself.

A negative amount of a primary sounds nonsense, and it has caused much heart-searching to many people in the past, yet the explanation is quite simple. It occurs merely because the sensitivity curves of Fig. 3 are broad overlapping curves, so that the 530 nm primary stimulates not only the s_2 process but also the s_3 process to quite a considerable extent. On the other hand, the 490-nm test colour hardly stimulates the s_3 process at all, so that there is no possibility of obtaining a colour match without desaturating 490-nm by adding a wavelength such as 650-nm to increase the response of the s_3 process. There is, therefore, nothing mysterious about the negative red value; it is a necessary consequence of the shape of the spectral sensitivity curves of the retinal receptors.

The second instructive observation I would like to quote follows directly from the match of 490 nm when desaturated with a suitable addition of the red 650-nm primary. With the 2° size of field of my colorimeter, this match could be made by foveal vision, the fovea being an area of the retina covered by the yellow macular pigment. Having made a good match, it is possible to view the two halves of the matched field on an area of the retina outside the fovea, say 5° from the foveal centre, merely by fixating in a direction 5° to one side of the field. For most observers the two halves of the field will no longer appear to be an exact match when seen by extrafoveal vision, the half of the field containing the red-green-blue mixture looking too blue. This is because the field is now being imaged on a part of the retina beyond the macular pigment, so that more of the blue primary is reaching the retinal receptors. On the other hand, while more of the 490-nm test colour may also be reaching the receptors, it will still have the same blue-green hue, although it may look a little brighter.

This observation is instructive for several reasons. In the first place, it is a direct demonstration of the influence of the yellow macular pigment on colour matching. Then it can bring out the difference between one observer and another, because a person with a dense macular pigmentation will notice a much bigger change in the colour match than an observer with only a slight pigmentation. If the observer actually makes an extrafoveal match, this will give a measure of the density of his pigment. Further, the observation explains why, in his determination of the large-field colour-matching functions, Stiles instructed his observers to ignore the central 3° or 4° area of the field and to make the match for the annular portion of the field lying outside the pigmented area (STILES 1955).

The experiment is also a forcible reminder that the retina is not a uniform structure even in the central few degrees covering the fovea. This was already implicit in the evidence for foveal tritanopia discussed in Sect. C.I., and sections of the retina through the fovea and parafovea illustrate very clearly how the shape and dimensions of the cones vary from very long, narrow and closely packed cones in the very centre of the fovea to shorter, fatter and more cone-like structures in the parafovea. This variation in cone shape and dimensions must almost certainly imply some variation in spectral sensitivity, not only because the light will have to pass through varying depths of photopigment, depending on the number of laminations or discs in the cones, but also because the variation in shape will affect their wave-guide properties. Attempts have been made to explain the colour sensitivity of the cones entirely in terms of their wave-guide action, but although this is a very improbable explanation, there could be some variation in concentration of energy for different wavelengths along the length of the outer segments of the cones. In that event the spectral sensitivity of individual cones could be affected by their length and their shape.

Hence, while the colour mixture curves obtained from making a series of trichromatic colour matches through the spectrum must be closely related to the spectral sensitivity curves of the three colour receptor processes in the retina, we have to recognise that we are almost certainly dealing with a large number of individual receptors grouped into three types according to their photopigments, but with significant variations in spectral sensitivity among the receptors in each group. We are probably wrong, therefore, in expecting to be able to derive an exact relation between the colour mixture curves and the spectral absorption curves of the three photopigments.

III. The 1931 Commission Internationale de l'Éclairage System of Colorimetry

I referred in the previous section to the call made by Guild in 1926 for a more reliable set of colour mixture curves. Guild had already built his filter colorimeter in 1922 (GUILD 1925–1926) and had used it for the colour specification of samples in terms of his filter primaries. By the time of his 1926 survey he had recognised the need for a new set of colour mixture curves and had almost certainly set up the equipment to measure the curves at the National Physical Laboratory. He did not report his results for some years (GUILD 1931), although his experiments were completed almost before I had started. I remember going to see him, probably early in 1927, to discuss how I should set about my own experiments and generally to benefit from his help and advice, and by then he was able to show me illustrations of the spectrum locus in the chromaticity chart for some, if not all, of his observers.

His colorimeter provided a 2° square field of view in which one half of the field was illuminated by the mixture of his red-green-blue filter primaries. He also had to make provision for a small amount of one or other of the three primaries to be added to the test colour in the other half of the field. The spectral test colour was provided by two monochromators in series, the second monochromator serving to filter out any stray light that might be included in the light emerging from the exit slit of the first monochromator. The observer then made a series of colour matches of some 35 wavelengths between 400 nm and 700 nm, with supplementary measurements of the amounts of the desaturating primary that had to be added at each wavelength measured.

Guild based the units of his primaries on a match on a standard white illuminant and the colorimetric equation for each wavelength was then calculated in terms of his filter primaries expressed in these units. The filter primaries which Guild used in his colorimeter had been chosen for their practical convenience in providing saturated red, green, and blue colours with as high light transmission as possible. To that extent their actual colours were quite arbitrary, so that colour mixture curves expressed in terms of his instrument primaries would have had no merit for defining the standard observer. Instead, Guild transformed his curves so that they were expressed in terms of three spectral primaries which could be defined with precision, namely a red of wavelength 700.0 nm, a green at 546.1 nm and a blue at 435.8 nm. The green and blue wavelengths corresponded to strong lines in the mercury arc spectrum, while at 700 nm the hue changes very slowly with wavelength, so that the red primary was also defined with certainty. The colour mixture curves subsequently used by the CIE to define the standard observer were also specified in terms of these primaries.

The procedure for transforming colour mixture data from one set of primaries to another had been developed by Ives (1915, 1923) and by Guild (1924–1925 a, b). The legitimacy of the procedure depended on the assumption that colour matches obeyed the ordinary laws of arithmetic, such as additivity, so that if a colour C_1 was matched by a certain mixture of the red, green, and blue primaries, and a second colour C_2 was matched by a different red-green-blue mixture, then the additive mixture of $C_1 + C_2$ would be matched by the additive mixture of the two red-green-blue mixtures. This assumption can be shown experimentally to hold to within reasonable limits, close enough at least to be an acceptable convention for use in technical colorimetry.

The possibility of being able to transform colour-mixture curves from one set of primaries to another was very important for the development of colorimetry. For one thing, it enabled colour-mixture data obtained with different instruments and primaries to be compared on the same basis; for example, I had to transform my results and express them in terms of the 700-nm, 546.1-nm, and 435.8-nm primaries (Wright 1929–1930) before Guild could compare my results with his. Then it freed colorimetry from any link with particular colour vision theories, such as the Young–Helmholtz three-components theory. In some quarters it had been held that colorimetry would only be valid if the colour mixture curves corresponded to the actual spectral sensitivity curves of the three retinal receptor processes, for example, to the curves in Fig. 3. It cannot be denied that when the CIE established trichromatic colorimetry on an international basis in 1931, this gave a boost to supporters of the Young–Helmholtz theory, although it should have been seen as a technological development enabling colours to be specified in terms of a mixture of colorimetrically specified primaries, with no direct reference to the physiological processes going on in the eye.

When Guild rather belatedly discovered in 1930 that the mean colour mixture data of his seven observers and my ten observers were in very close agreement (Wright 1929–1930), he set to work to prepare a paper describing his experiments and deriving an average set of colour mixture curves for consideration as the definition of a standard observer for colorimetry (GUILD 1931). Since the CIE was due to meet in Cambridge in September 1931, time was running very short for international approval to be given to Guild's proposal at that meeting, especially as very different ideas prevailed between I. G. Priest of the Bureau of Standards in the United States, representing American opinion, and Guild, representing British opinion, on how an international system of colorimetry should be defined.

I have described elsewhere the drama that immediately preceded the CIE meeting, and there is no occasion to repeat that account here (WRIGHT 1981). Suffice it to say that following a week of intensive discussions at the National Physical Laboratory prior to the meeting, Priest and Guild were able to appear at Cambridge with an agreed set of resolutions for consideration by the CIE. The compromise that emerged was that the standard observer should be defined in terms of the three spectral primaries that Guild had adopted as standard at the National Physical Laboratory, while a separate co-ordinate system should be used for actual colorimetric specifications. This second system was obtained by transforming the mean Guild–Wright colour mixture data from the spectral primaries to a new set of primaries, (X), (Y), and (Z), giving all-positive mixture curves. For this selection of primaries they were indebted to an important paper by Deane B. Judd of the Bureau of Standards (JUDD 1930), in which he developed a concept first enunciated by SCHRÖDINGER (1925) of choosing two of the nonphysical primaries, (X) and (Z), to have zero luminosity. The corollary of this was that all the luminosity information was provided by the mixture curve associated with the (Y) primary and this curve was also adjusted to be in agreement with the 1924 standard V_λ curve. In this way it was ensured that the standard observer for photometry and the standard observer for colorimetry were one and the same person.

To the non-specialist, these rather unusual properties of the (XYZ) system must have been almost as difficult to understand as mixture curves with negative quantities, but they were quickly accepted by colour technologists and it is not too much to claim that the 1931 system unleashed a flood of activity in the colour industries. Perhaps its most spectacular use occurred in the development of colour television in the United States in the late 1940s and early 1950s, since the colorimetric framework on which the American National Television System Committee, or NTSC system (and subsequently all other colour television systems) was defined was the 1931 CIE system of colorimetry (FINK 1955). The one failure, or partial failure, of the system has been in the derivation of a universally acceptable colour difference formula for the specification of colour tolerances. As I suggested in Sect. C.I., a colour discrimination judgement involves additional elements in the visual process compared with colour-matching judgements, so that we may have been at fault in trying to extract a colour difference formula from a colorimetric system based on colour matching.

While the 1931 colour-matching functions, as they are now generally called, are still in very active use, they were supplemented by the CIE in 1964 by an additional set of functions for large-field, 10° viewing conditions. In some industries, such as the textile industry, colour matching is often carried out by viewing large areas of cloth, so that functions based on observations made with instruments using 2° fields of view are not necessarily relevant to such industrial applications. These new functions were based mainly on a major study by STILES and BURCH (1959) at the National Physical Laboratory using STILES' (1955) new trichromator, with additional data obtained by SPERANSKAYA (1959) in Russia. Since, as mentioned in Sect. C.II., Stiles had to instruct his observers to ignore the central macular area of the field (Speranskaya actually blocked out this area), the 1964 large-field functions were actually based on colour matches made with annular fields, which are different again from the viewing conditions used in industry. Also, there has been a rather bigger question mark concerning additivity with the large-field data, probably because of the influence of the rod receptors in the extrafoveal retina. Nevertheless, the 1964 10° functions have proved generally acceptable in those industries where their use is appropriate and they are, I believe, being widely used.

IV. Defective Colour Vision

Once I had built my colorimeter and had measured the colour mixture curves and wavelength discrimination curves for observers with normal trichromatic vision, it was natural to try to obtain comparable data for subjects with defective colour vision. I was able to collect some initial colour-matching data for six dichromats (WRIGHT 1929), but these were little more than preliminary experiments to work out a more detailed programme of measurements. PITT (1935) was the first researcher in our laboratory to undertake such a programme, in which he measured the luminosity curves, the colour mixture curves and the wavelength discrimination curves for six protanopes and six deuteranopes. He, in his turn, obtained some preliminary observations on three anomalous trichromats.

Perhaps the two most reproduced diagrams ever to come out of our laboratory are those in Figs. 5 and 6, in which Pitt showed the colours which the protanope and deuteranope would confuse by plotting their respective confusion loci in the chromaticity chart. These charts have proved of much practical value, as they provide the basic information needed to select the correct colours for use in diagnostic colour vision tests. For example, in the Farnsworth–Munsell 100 hue test (FARNSWORTH 1943), the location of the colours round the hue circle which the different types of colour-defective observer will most confuse can be deduced from these confusion loci. Then the convergence of the protanopic confusion loci onto a point in the chromaticity chart just beyond the red end of the spectrum locus is a strong pointer to the defect being due to the absence of the red-sensitive receptors in the retina (PITT 1944).

However, so far as this chapter is concerned, my special interest in these diagrams is that they really owe their origin to a question put to me by Sir Ronald Fisher, Professor of Eugenics at University College, London. He had come to see me about our results, probably sometime in 1934, and pressed me to explain where the colours confused by a dichromat would be located in the normal observer's chromaticity chart. This is a question which I should have been asking myself, but it often takes someone not too involved in the details of a subject to ask the questions which are at the same time both simple and profound. I should also have known that Maxwell and von Helmholtz had asked themselves the same question and had suggested an answer. But PITT (1944) was the first to provide the experimental confirmation of their explanation.

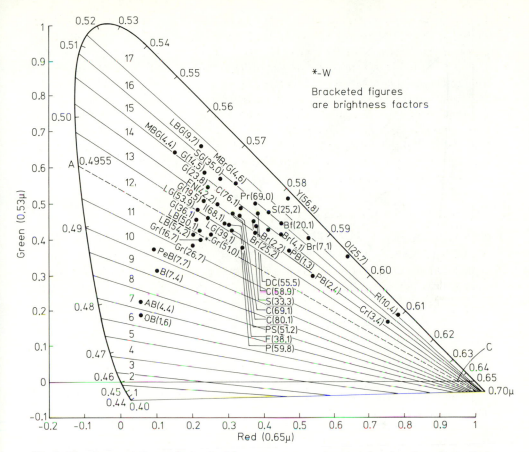

Fig. 5. The chromaticity confusion loci for an average protanope, showing the colours that the protanope would confuse when their protanopic luminances (or brightness factors) are the same. PITT (1935)

OB, Oxford blue	PS, Portland stone	DC, Deep green
AB, Azure blue	F, Fawn	SG, Sea-green
B, Blue	I, Ivory	MBrG, Mid-bronze green
PEB, Peacock blue	S, Stone	PR, Primose
GR, Grey	BR, Brown	BF, Buff
LB, Light blue	C, Cream	LBG, Light Brunswick green
G, Green	EN, Eau-de-nil (G)	CR, Crimson
LG, Light green	MBG, Mid-Brunswick green	Y, Yellow
P, Pink	PB, Purple brown	O, Orange
AC, Confusion locus through white point W (CIE source B)		R, Red

Subsequently, NELSON (1938) investigated anomalous trichromatism, more especially deuteranomalous vision, while McKeon and I reported on protanomalous vision (MCKEON and WRIGHT 1940). It was not, however, until 1952 that I was able to use a popular illustrated weekly magazine to discover a number of the quite rare type of dichromat, the tritanope, and to investigate their characteristics (WRIGHT 1952) on much the same lines as Pitt's study of protanopes and deuter-

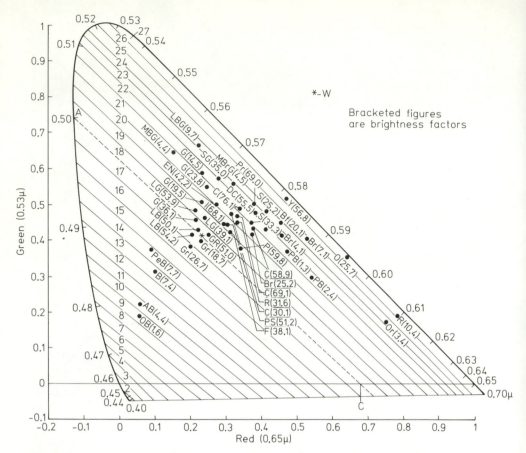

Fig. 6. The chromaticity confusion loci for an average deuteranope, showing the colours that the deuteranope would confuse when their deuteranopic luminances (or brightness factors) are the same. For key to letters see Fig. 5 legend. PITT (1935)

anopes. In the case of the tritanope, the confusion loci converged onto a point just beyond the violet corner of the spectrum locus in the chromaticity chart, in this case being a strong pointer to the defect being due to the absence of the blue-sensitive receptors in the retina.

With the so-called red and blue fundamental stimuli being located in the chromaticity chart with a good deal of precision, and using other evidence for the likely location of the green fundamental stimulus, I collaborated with L. C. Thomson to transform the colour mixture curves in terms of these fundamental stimuli to determine a possible set of sensitivity curves which could correspond to the actual sensitivity curves of the three retinal receptor processes (THOMSON and WRIGHT 1953). The curves in Fig. 3 are, in fact, these curves. I am not, however, concerned here with the correctness or otherwise of these particular curves but with the principle on which their derivation is based.

The main assumption that has to be made is that dichromatism is a reduced form of trichromatism. By this is meant that dichromatism is due to the absence of one or other of the three retinal receptor processes possessed by the trichromat; the justification for this assumption is that dichromats accept the trichromat's colour matches. On that assumption MAXWELL (1890) showed that the colours confused by the dichromat would, when plotted in his colour triangle, lie on lines radiating from the point in the triangle corresponding to the missing colour process. This principle was elaborated by VON HELMHOLTZ (1924) and is, indeed, often attributed to him (SHERMAN 1981).

PITT (1944) used his data on dichromatic vision to derive what he called the fundamental sensation curves, applying the Maxwell–Helmholtz principle to the results for his average protanope and average deuteranope, together with KÖNIG's (1897) data for tritanopia, by plotting their confusion loci in the chromaticity chart of the average trichromat. This procedure does, however, raise the major question of whether it is legitimate to use average observer data in this way.

FARNSWORTH (1961) criticised Pitt's derivation of the sensation curves on the grounds that if you plotted the confusion loci of Pitt's individual observers, they converged, if at all, onto very different points in the chromaticity chart. Now just as trichromatic observers differ among themselves in the density of their lens and macular pigment coloration, so too will dichromatic subjects. This means that dichromatism is only a reduced form of trichromatism, provided we compare dichromats and trichromats with the same degree of pigmentation. Any attempt, therefore, to represent the colour confusions of a dichromat with some given lens and macular coloration in the chromaticity chart of a trichromat with a different degree of coloration is mathematically invalid. Not only will the confusion loci not be straight or converge onto the expected point in the chart, they will not exist at all, since stimuli with different spectral compositions but the same chromaticity for the trichromat could have different chromaticities for the dichromat.

All this means that average or standard observer data should only be used in visual research with the greatest caution, since it cannot be assumed that they specify the characteristics of any given individual observer. So far as Pitt's analysis was concerned, I would consider he was correct to relate average dichromatic data with average trichromatic data, in the reasonable expectation that pigmentation differences would more or less average themselves out. In fact, I do not see what else he could have done. ALPERN (1976) made a somewhat similar criticism to Farnsworth's when he examined the individual confusion loci of the six tritanopes on whom I had reported in 1952 (WRIGHT 1952). I have replied to these criticisms elsewhere (WRIGHT 1982), but as a warning about the risk of using the standard observer defined for use in colour technology as if he were also the standard observer for visual research, it is perhaps fitting to close this chapter by quoting the closing sentence of Alpern's paper: "The present analysis suggests that the common practice of attempting to derive the fundamental response functions from the tritanope's confusion locus and the color matches of the standard observer is subject to serious objections."

References

Names containing *von* are alphabetized in this list under *v*

Abney W de W (1905) Modified apparatus for the measurement of colour and its application to the determination of the colour sensations. Philos Trans R Soc Lond Ser A 205:333–355

Aguilar M, Stiles WS (1954) Saturation of the rod mechanism at high levels of stimulation. Opt Acta 1:59–65

Alpern M (1976) Tritanopia. Am J Optom 53:340–349

Boynton RM (1979) Human color vision. Holt, Rinehart and Winston, New York

Campbell NR (1933) The measurement of visual sensations. Proc Phys Soc Lond 45:565–571

Campbell NR, Marris GC (1935) The measurement of loudness. Proc Phys Soc Lond 47:153–170

Craik KJW (1940) The effect of adaptation on subjective brightness. Proc R Soc Lond Ser B 128:232–247

Craik KJW (1943) The nature of explanation. Cambridge University Press, Cambridge

Crawford BH (1949) The scotopic visibility function. Proc Phys Soc Lond 62:321–334

Dartnall HJA (ed) (1972) Photochemistry of vision. Springer, Berlin Heidelberg New York

Ditchburn RW (1973) Eye-movements and visual perception. Clarendon, Oxford

Farnsworth D (1943) The Farnsworth-Munsell 100 hue and dichotomous tests for color vision. J Opt Soc Am 33:568–578

Farnsworth D (1961) Let's look at those isochromatic lines again. Vision Res 1:1–5

Fink DG (ed) (1955) Television engineering handbook. McGraw-Hill, New York

Gibson KS (1926) The relative visibility function. Compte rendu, commission internationale de l'éclairage, 1924. Cambridge University Press, Cambridge, pp 232–238

Graham CH (ed) (1965) Vision and visual perception. Wiley, New York

Granit R (1933) The components of the retinal action potential in mammals and their relation to the discharge in the optic nerve. J Physiol (Lond) 77:207–240

Guild J (1924–1925 a) The transformation of trichromatic mixture data: algebraic methods. Trans Opt Soc Lond 26:95–104

Guild J (1924–1925 b) The geometrical solution of colour mixture problems. Trans Opt Soc Lond 26:139–172

Guild J (1925–1926) A trichromatic colorimeter suitable for standardisation work. Trans Opt Soc Lond 27:106–128

Guild J (1926) A critical survey of modern developments in the theory and technique of colorimetry and allied sciences. Proc optical convention, London, pp 61–141

Guild J (1931) The colorimetric properties of the spectrum. Philos Trans R Soc Lond Ser A 230:149–187

Guild J (1932 a) Some problems of visual reception. In: Discussion on vision. Physical Society, London, pp 1–22

Guild J (1932 b) The interpretation of quantitative data in visual problems. In: Discussion on vision. Physical Society, London, pp 60–86

Hartline HK (1934) Intensity and duration in the excitation of single photoreceptor units. J Cell Comp Physiol 5:229–247

Hecht S (1930) The development of Thomas Young's theory of color vision. J Opt Soc Am 20:231–270

Hecht S (1935) A theory of visual intensity discrimination. J Gen Physiol 18:767–789

Hecht S (1936) Intensity discrimination and its relation to the adaptation of the eye. J Physiol (Lond) 86:15–21

Hecht S (1949) Brightness, visual acuity and colour blindness. Doc Ophthalmol III:289–306

Hecht S, Shlaer S, Pirenne MH (1942) Energy, quanta, and vision. J Gen Physiol 25:819–840

Hsia Y, Graham CH (1952) Spectral sensitivity of the cones in the dark adapted human eye. Proc Natl Acad Sci USA 38:80–85

Hurvich LM, Jameson D (1953) Spectral sensitivity of the fovea. I. Neutral adaptation. J Opt Soc Am 43:485–494

Ives HE (1915) The transformation of color-mixture equations from one system to another. J Franklin Inst 80:673–701

Ives HE (1923) The transformation of color-mixture equations from one system to another. II. Graphical aids. J Franklin Inst 195:23–44

Judd DB (1930) Reduction of data on mixture of color stimuli. J Res Natl Bur Stand 4:515–548

König A (1894) Über den menschlichen Sehpurpur und seine Bedeutung für das Sehen. In: König A (ed) Gesammelte Abhandlungen zur physiologischen Optik. Barth, Leipzig, 1903, S. 338–363

König A (1897) Über „Blaublindheit". In: Konig A (ed) Gesammelte Abhandlungen zur physiologischen Optik. Barth, Leipzig, 1903, S. 396–415

König A, Dieterici C (1884) Über die Empfindlichkeit des normalen Auges für Wellenlängenunterschiede des Lichtes. In: Konig A (ed) Gesammelte Abhandlungen zur physiologischen Optik. Barth, Leipzig, 1903, S. 23–33

König A, Dieterici C (1892) Die Grundempfindungen in normalen und anomalen Farbensystemen und ihre Intensitätsvertheilung im Spectrum. In: Konig A (ed) Gesammelte Abhandlungen zur physiologischen Optik. Barth, Leipzig, S. 214–321

Le Grand Y (1971) Unsolved problems in vision. In: Pierce JR, Levene JR (eds) Visual science. Indiana University Press, Bloomington, pp 305–319

Lythgoe RJ (1937) The absorption spectra of visual purple and of indicator yellow. J Physiol (Lond) 89:331–358

Maxwell JC (1860) On the theory of compound colours and the relations of the colours of the spectrum. Philos Trans R Soc Lond Ser A 160:57–84

Maxwell JC (1890) The scientific papers of James Clerk Maxwell. Cambridge University Press, Cambridge

McCree KJ (1960) Colour confusion produced by voluntary fixation. Opt Acta 7:281–290

McKeon WM, Wright WD (1940) The characteristics of protanomalous vision. Proc Phys Soc London 52:464–479

Nelson JH (1938) Anomalous trichromatism and its relation to normal trichromatism. Proc Phys Soc (Lond) 50:661–697

Newton I (1730) Opticks, 4th edn. Reprint, Bell, London, 1931

Pitt FHG (1935) Characteristics of dichromatic vision. Med Res Counc Spec Rep Ser No. 200. H. M. Stationery Office, London

Pitt FHG (1944) The nature of normal trichromatic and dichromatic vision. Proc R Soc Lond Ser B 132:101–117

Purkinje JE (1825) Neue Beiträge zur Kenntnis des Sehens in subjectiver Hinsicht. In: Beobachtungen und Versuche zur Physiologie der Sinne, vol. II. Berlin, pp 109–110

Richardson LF (1932) The measurability of sensations of hue, brightness or saturation. In: Discussion on vision. Physical Society, London, pp 112–114

Schouten JF (1937) Visueele Meting van Adaptatie en van de Wederzijdsche Beinvloeding van Netvlieselementen. Thesis, Utrecht University, Schotanus and Jens, Utrecht

Schouten JF, Ornstein LS (1939) Measurements on direct and indirect adaptation by means of a binocular method. J Opt Soc Am 29:168–182

Schrödinger E (1925) Über das Verhältnis der Vierfarben- zur Dreifarbentheorie. Sitzungsber Akad Wiss Wien 134 IIa:471–490

Sherman PD (1981) Colour vision in the nineteenth century: the Young-Helmholtz-Maxwell theory. Hilger, Bristol

Speranskaya NI (1959) Determination of spectrum color coordinates for twenty-seven normal observers. Opt Spectrosc 7:424–428

Stiles WS (1929) The effect of glare on the brightness difference threshold. Dept Sci Ind Res Illum Res Tech Paper No. 8. H. M. Stationery Office, London

Stiles WS (1946) A modified Helmholtz line-element in brightness-color space. Proc Phys Soc London 58:41–65

Stiles WS (1955) The basic data of colour matching. Physical Society Year Book. Physical Society, London, pp 44–65

Stiles WS (1972) The line element in colour theory: a historical review. In: Vos JJ, Friele LFC, Walraven PL (eds) Color metrics. Association Internationale de la Couleur, Soesterberg

Stiles WS, Burch JM (1959) N.P.L. colour-matching investigation: final report (1958). Opt Acta 6:1–26

Stiles WS, Crawford BH (1933) The liminal brightness increment as a function of wavelength for different conditions of the foveal and parafoveal retina. Proc R Soc Lond Ser B 113:496–530

Thomson LC, Wright WD (1947) The colour sensitivity of the retina within the central fovea of man. J Physiol (Lond) 105:316–331

Thomson LC, Wright WD (1953) The convergence of the tritanopic confusion loci and the derivation of the fundamental response functions. J Opt Soc Am 43:890–894

von Helmholtz HLF (1896) Handbuch der physiologischen Optik, 2nd edn. Voss, Hamburg

von Helmholtz HLF (1924) A treatise on physiological optics, Optical Society of America, Rochester

Wald G (1945) Human vision and the spectrum. Science 101:653–658

Wald G (1967) Blue-blindness in the normal fovea. J Opt Soc Am 57:1289–1301

Walters HV, Wright WD (1943) The spectral sensitivity of the fovea and extra-fovea in the Purkinje range. Proc R Soc Lond Ser B 131:340–361

Willmer EN (1944) Colour of small objects. Nature 153:774–775

Willmer EN (1946) Retinal structure and colour vision. Cambridge University Press, Cambridge

Willmer EN, Wright WD (1945) Colour sensitivity of the fovea centralis. Nature 56:119–120

Wright WD (1929) A re-determination of the trichromatic mixture data. Med Res Counc Spec Rep Ser No. 139. H. M. Stationery Office, London

Wright WD (1929–1930) A re-determination of the mixture curves of the spectrum. Trans Opt Soc (Lond) 31:201–218

Wright WD (1932) The significance of colour-fatigue measurements. In: Discussion on vision. Physical Society, London, pp 117–124

Wright WD (1935) Intensity discrimination and its relation to the adaptation of the eye. J Physiol (Lond) 83:466–477

Wright WD (1941) The fundamental principles of vision in very weak light. Trans Illum Eng Soc 6:23–34

Wright WD (1946) Researches on normal and defective colour vision. Kimpton, London

Wright WD (1952) The characteristics of tritanopia. J Opt Soc Am 42:509–521

Wright WD (1971) Small-field tritanopia: a re-assessment. In: Pierce JR, Levene JR (eds) Visual science. Indiana University Press, Bloomington, pp 152–163

Wright WD (1981) The historical and experimental background to the 1931 CIE system of colorimetry. In: Golden jubilee of colour in the CIE. Society of Dyers and Colourists, Bradford, pp 3–18

Wright WD (1982) Dichromatic colour confusions and the spectral sensitivity of the retinal receptors. In: Colour vision deficiencies VI. Junk, The Hague, pp 281–286

Wright WD, Granit R (1938) On the correlation of some sensory and physiological phenomena of vision. Br J Ophthalmol Monogr [Suppl] 9:5–80

Wright WD, Pitt FHG (1934) Hue-discrimination in normal colour vision. Proc Phys Soc London 46:459–468

Zangwill OL (1980) Kenneth Craik: the man and his work. Br J Psychol 71:1–16

CHAPTER 8

Binocular Vision

GLENN A. FRY

A. Introduction

I began my career in vision as a graduate student in psychology (1929–1932) under William McDougall, who introduced me to the problems of binocular fusion and rivalry. In learning to paint, I had already encountered the problems of stereopsis and space perception. In my home was a stereoscope and a set of cards. Just a few years before in 1924, Southall had completed the translation of VON HELMHOLTZ'S (1924) *A Treatise on Physiological Optics*. The volumes of the *Treatise* were high on my reading list.

At Washington University (1932–1935) I continued working on binocular fusion and rivalry, but after becoming familiar with the work at Dartmouth, I proceeded to build a haploscope to measure aniseikonia and cyclophoria. I made my first visit to Dartmouth in 1936. Ames explained to me that he had discovered aniseikonia by noting distortions which occurred when walking through wooded areas covered with underbrush. He had to wear spherocylinders to correct his ametropia. He deduced that such an array was devoid of geometrical perspective cues and that this permitted the stereo distortions to become manifest. He was wearing aniseikonic lenses at the time. He used overall and meridional size lenses to demonstrate to me stereo distortions by having me look at the grass on which we were standing.

These observations had led to the development of the leaf room for demonstrating distortion, but the induced size effect made it unsatisfactory for prescribing aniseikonic lenses. A great deal of effort was expended on the development of the direct comparison eikonometer, which involved a direct comparison of sizes. Measurements were made in the vertical and horizontal meridians, but this did not suffice. Fixation disparity and anisophoria also presented problems. The work with tilting planes led eventually to the development of the space eikonometer, which incorporated a provision for making allowance for cyclophoria. This remains today the accepted way of making measurements of aniseikonia.

Bielschowsky and Burian were part of the staff, and this provided a link with Hering and his followers. Various aspects of binocular vision were investigated. The distortions produced by prisms were studied. An attempt was made to analyze the causes of anisometropia and the anomalous distribution of photoreceptors over the two retinas. Verhoeff's (1902) model was adopted to explain the neural connections for binocular vision. Fixation disparity and cyclophoria were studied in depth. The fundamentals of stereopsis were explored, as well as the relation of stereopsis to other cues of depth. The horopter and the apparent frontoparallel plane had been investigated previously but were further investigated at Dartmouth. Luneburg came to Dartmouth in 1946 and, as a result, developed a general formulation of the relation between physical and binocularly perceived space. This received wide attention.

The major contributions of the Dartmouth Eye Institute have been summarized by Ogle (1950, 1962) and Burian (1948, 1974).

The overall size lens was regarded as a form of Galilean telescope. Telescopic spectacles had been used before but primarily for low-vision patients and for viewing sports events. These had high magnification and only small amounts up to about 5% were needed for correcting aniseikonia. The monocular aphakic presented a special type of problem which had to be treated separately.

Meridional size lenses involved a combination of two cylindrical surfaces. I am not certain who first had the idea of using these lenses for measuring and correcting aniseikonia. A single lens which would correct ametropia and aniseikonia required toric surfaces on both sides. At about the same time that bicylindrical and bitoric lenses were introduced for measuring and correcting aniseikonia, von Rohr and Boegehold (1934) and Boegehold (1935) recommended the use of bitoric lenses for dealing with the problem of torsions associated with oblique directions of regard. In 1947 the Dartmouth Eye Institute ceased to exist, but fortunately, the art of measuring and correcting aniseikonia had been perfected to the point that it could be practiced by others. The American Optical Company also abolished its facility for producing aniseikonic spectacles, but here again, the art of fabricating bitoric and bicylindrical lenses was perfected to the point that it could be entrusted to local optical laboratories.

I have divided what follows into five topics, which cover more or less the problems of binocular vision:

1) Maintaining the images of an array of stimuli on corresponding parts of the two retinas
2) Binocular fusion and rivalry
3) Perception of direction
4) Perception of distance
5) The seam.

Under each topic I have explained the contributions which I have tried to make and the basic concepts which I have used in trying to build an overall view of the problems of binocular vision. The art of measuring and correcting aniseikonia has been soundly established by the Dartmouth group and the points to which I object do not affect that at all. I have objected to the Dartmouth concept of single vision with disparate points. I have objected to the notion that the horopter must coincide with the apparent frontoparallel plane, and also to the notion that the perception of depth associated with disparity is a unique sensation. I regard it to be an experience akin to that generated by geometrical and aerial perspective cues. Perceived depth is a learned interpretation of disparity and other cues. I have not accepted the notion that a fusional movement is a psycho-optic reflex: I regard it as a simple reflex. Ogle used rectangular coordinates to develop analytic expressions for the traces of the apparent frontoparallel plane and the horopter in the plane of regard, whereas I have used polar coordinates and parallax angles. My formulas presented in this chapter can be compared to those used by Ogle. I have also used polar coordinates for relating physical and perceived space. These points will be discussed at greater length under the appropriate topics.

Ogle also used rectangular coordinates to analyze the effect of size lenses on the appearance of complex objects like the walls and ceiling and floor of a room. For this purpose he assumed that the lenses and the eyes were free from distortion and mounted on parallel axes. These simplifying assumptions are helpful for this purpose and also for analyzing stereoscopic and other binocular displays.

B. Maintaining Stimuli on Corresponding Points

I. Rotations of the Two Eyes

One of the first things I undertook, beginning in 1935, was to develop a system of planes, lines, and points fixed with respect to the head, in terms of which I could specify directions of regard and cyclorotations of the eyes around the lines of sight.

The key points in the system are the two centers of rotation. Each of these is the point of intersection of the different directions of the primary line of sight. The line connecting these two points and the binocular point of fixation determine the plane of regard (Fig. 1). The baseline and plane of regard are concepts taken directly from VON HELMHOLTZ (1924, Vol. III, p. 42). I also followed von Helmholtz in specifying the direction of regard in terms of angles of azimuth and elevation. A change in azimuth is a rotation around an axis through the center of rotation per-

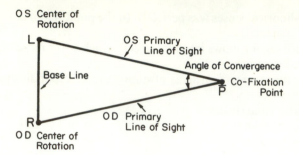

Fig. 1. The plane of regard containing the point of cofixation (P̄) and the baseline (RL). OS, oculus sinister, OD, oculus dexter. FRY (1941 b)

pendicular to the plane of regard. A change in elevation is a rotation of the plane of regard around the baseline. Cyclorotation occurs around the primary line of sight.

Zero elevation occurs when the plane of regard is perpendicular to the face plane. The head is erect when the face plane touching the chin and two ciliary ridges is vertical and the baseline horizontal. Zero cyclorotation was defined as that which occurs when the eye is fixating straight ahead and accommodation is relaxed and the opposite eye is occluded. Rotation from this zero position is positive if it is counterclockwise to a second person looking at the first person's face. Zero azimuth occurs when the line of sight is perpendicular to the baseline.

The Committee on Nomenclature and Standards of the American Academy of Optometry, of which I was Chairman, succeeded in getting these reference points and planes approved by the Academy (FRY et al. 1945). These standards are more far reaching than appears on the surface, because the same system can be used to specify the position of a pair of glasses on the face, the cylinder axis, prism axis, size lens axis, field of fixation, and axes of rotation of devices which are designed to present stimuli to the eyes at different directions of regard.

II. Binocular Displays

In ordinary vision the two eyes are exposed to the same array of objects and the primary lines of sight converge on a common fixation point. In some cases, separate displays are used for the two eyes and each eye has its own fixation point. The two displays to be fused may be presented in the two halves of a Wheatstone- or Brewster-type stereoscope or they may be projected on a screen. In this case, there are several ways to keep the right eye from seeing what the left eye is supposed to see, and vice versa.

III. Fusional Movements

Binocular vision involves getting the two primary lines of sight to converge at the common fixation point. This requires vertical and horizontal fusional movements of the two eyes. These are reflex movements. Were it not for the continuous operation of this reflex, the eyes would revert to their phoria position. If the eyes start slipping out of alignment, reflex movements bring them back.

This reflex is strongest at the center of the fovea and hence, whatever the subject looks at controls the operation of the fusional reflex. Switching the direction of fixation invokes a fixational movement which uses a separate neural mechanism.

If there are two objects in the field of view which lie at different distances, the subject can use voluntary accommodative convergence to switch convergence from one distance to another. This is a third kind of eye movement. After fixation gets switched from right to left or from far to near, reflex fusional movements have to take over and get the images precisely on corresponding parts of the two retinas.

The two eyes not only have to converge on a common fixation point, but they have to cyclorotate to get the images properly registered on the two retinas. This requires cyclofusional movements. The eyes generally fail to converge precisely on the intended fixation point, and this is known as "fixation disparity." In spite of this, it is possible for the two eyes to generate a unified impression of what lies in front of them.

My concept of the neural mechanism for fusional movements is based on Kleist's concept, set forth in 1926 (DUKE-ELDER 1934, p. 271); the signals from corresponding parts of the retinas maintain separate pathways through the lateral geniculate body and do not interact at that level, but the pathways end in layers of the cortex on opposite sides of the layer of Gennari (with pathways from corresponding points on the retinas ending at points which are opposite each other in the two layers). If the signals arrive by way of pathways from corresponding points, the stimulus to a fusional movement is zero. But if the signals come from noncorresponding points and arrive at disparate points on the two sides of the layer of Gennari, that generates the combination of lateral and vertical movements necessary to bring the two stimuli onto corresponding points. Cyclofusional movements have to be generated by opposite disparities in adjacent parts of the cortex.

C. Sensory Fusion and Rivalry

At Washington University in 1932–1935, I set out to explore the mechanisms of fusion and rivalry with all possible combinations of stimuli. I was impressed, at the outset, that borders play a dominant role and I identified four fundamental combinations (FRY 1936 a, b; FRY and BARTLEY 1933):
1) A border in one eye pitted against a uniform field in the other
2) Borders crossing each other
3) Borders parallel to and near each other
4) Congruent borders.

I believed that any binocular display, no matter how complicated, could be broken down into these elements. I used stimuli continuously presented to the two eyes. The use of momentary and intermittent stimuli introduces special effects which we shall need to consider, but for the moment let us keep temporal manipulation of the stimuli in abeyance.

Most of the important facts about fusion and rivalry had already been pointed out by PANUM (1858, 1861), VON HELMHOLTZ (1924, Vol. 3, pp. 493–530), SHERRINGTON (1906), MCDOUGALL (1910), TRENDELENBURG (1923), HECHT (1928), DAWSON (1917), EDRIDGE-GREEN (1920), and others.

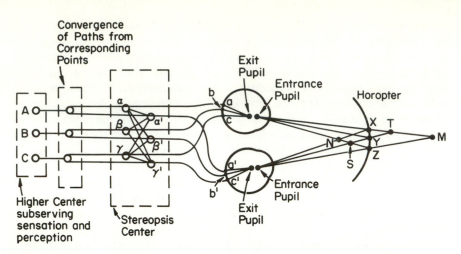

Fig. 2. A schematic representation of the neurological mechanisms subserving stereopsis and fusional movements. This diagram was used in my class notes as early as 1941 to explain stereopsis and fusion and rivalry but was not used until later to explain fusional movements. The pathways from points on the retinas to the cortex do not show the synapses in the retinas and lateral geniculate bodies. Two sets of points (α, β, and γ and α', β', and γ') are assumed to lie on opposite sides of the layer of Gennari. This is a convenient way of visualizing the two layers of elements, but is not essential for the model. Interaction between elements in the two layers generates both the stereo signals and the signals for fusional movements (FRY 1941 b). *Capital letters* represent points in the field of view of the two eyes; *lower-case letters* represent points on the retinas

A complete discussion of this topic is out of the question here, but it suffices to say that in some instances true fusion or integration occurs, but in others the impression of one eye dominates and the impression generated in the other eye is not seen at all. It is actually possible to combine the images of a bright disk on a dark background seen through a red filter with one eye and seen through a green one with the other eye and produce a yellow impression. This finding is important for color vision.

Suppose the eyes are cofixating a small black disk on a white background. In this case, one of the images is suppressed. If one of the eyes is viewing the disk through a pair of rotary prisms, and if the power is gradually increased, the fusional mechanism keeps the eyes converged on the disk but not perfectly. Single vision is maintained but this is because the impression generated by one eye is inhibited. How can the fusional mechanism operate when the image generated by one eye is suppressed?

My concept of the neural mechanisms involved is illustrated in Fig. 2. Let us assume that a small black disk on a white background lies at y. As long as the eyes stay converged on the small black disk, the stimulus to fusional movements is zero. In order to explain the rivalry between the impressions initiated at b and b′, we have to assume that binocular fusion and rivalry occur at a higher level than the layer of Gennari, at which signals for fusional movements are generated.

I have proposed that pathways coming into layers IV a and IV c from corresponding points of the retinas are connected to a higher level, at which fusion and

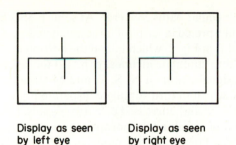

Display as seen   **Display as seen**
by left eye   **by right eye**

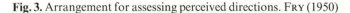

Fig. 3. Arrangement for assessing perceived directions. FRY (1950)

rivalry occurs. If rivalry occurs, this means that information about color (hue, brightness, and saturation) from one eye is being blocked, but this does not interfere with the generation of the signals for fusional movements at the lower level.

A most important combination of stimuli is illustrated in Fig. 3. It is basic not only for understanding fusion and rivalry but also for understanding stereopsis. The lower vertical line is on a sheet of paper which is held in front of a second sheet with a vertical line, so that for each eye the two lines can be compared for vertical alignment. The amount of disparity for the upper line can be varied by moving the cofixated lower line in a fore and aft direction (FRY 1950). There is no way of telling if the lower line is actually being cofixated so that the images of the lower line may not fall on corresponding points, but this is not important. The question is: Where is the upper image located relative to the lower when the disparities are small enough to permit a single image for each line?

Ames and his associates at Dartmouth, following Verhoeff, claimed that the images of the upper line are fused and shifted toward a point intermediate between where the monocular images would be expected to be seen. It has been my claim in this case that there is no fusion or shifting. Single vision depends upon the inhibition of one of the images, and hence the observer sees only one member of each pair of images.

A more important aspect of what is seen with the pair of lines in Fig. 3 is that the lower line is perceived as lying in a less remote plane than the upper. If one of the monocular components of the upper line and also of the lower line is inhibited, how is it possible to assess the difference in distance?

If the separation between the two pieces of paper in Fig. 3 is large, an actual diplopia of the upper line is seen and the depth effect still persists. This proves that it is not dependent on the fusion of disparate images.

It is my belief that the same interactions that generate fusional movements also generate disparity signals which are used in assessing distances from the eyes. We have to assume that binocular rivalry and fusion occur at a higher level.

In terms of Fig. 2, the disparity signals are generated at the stereopsis center. Rivalry and fusion occur at the level at which pathways from corresponding points converge. When rivalry occurs, information about color (hue, brightness, and saturation) from one retina is blocked. The disparity signals generated at the lower level still get through.

It must be assumed that duplicate information about disparity is being transmitted over the right eye and left eye channels from the IV a and IV c layers to the level at which the monocular paths converge. At some higher level these lateral disparity signals get reinterpreted in terms of farness and nearness.

Stimuli X, Y, and Z in Fig. 2, which fall on the horopter, stimulate corresponding points, which in turn stimulate identical points at the layer of Gennari and generate zero disparity signals. Stimuli N, S, T, and M stimulate noncorresponding points at the retinas, which in turn stimulate disparate points at the layer of Gennari and generate crossed and uncrossed disparity signals. Consequently, N, S, M, and T are seen in front of or behind the horopter, as the case may be.

It was not until after I developed the model in Fig. 2 that I discovered that VERHOEFF (1902) had developed a very similar model. He was not specific about the cortical layers at which the pathways from the separate retinas terminate. He postulated an intermediate layer of elements to explain fusion with noncorresponding points. Ames and his associates at Dartmouth adopted Verhoeff's model (AMES et al. 1932).

If we measure the amount of disparity in different directions (up, down, right, and left) which permits single vision, this maps out what is known as Panum's area (PANUM 1858).

D. Correspondence Between the Two Retinas

I. Measurement of Aniseikonia and Cyclophoria

I have used a simple haploscope to measure aniseikonia and cyclophoria (FRY 1941 a). The target presented to each eye is mounted on a flat disk which is normal to the primary line of sight. The direction of a point on one of these disks from the center of the entrance pupil can be specified in terms of meridian and eccentricity. This makes it easy to deal with problems of magnification and distortion.

The arms of the haploscope can rotate around vertical axes through the centers of rotation of the eyes to simulate any amount of symmetrical or asymmetrical convergence of the primary lines of sight.

Optical devices are provided for continuous changes in the overall magnification of each target. The targets can be rotated around the lines of sight to measure and compensate for cyclophoria and for measuring aniseikonia in various meridians.

The targets used by von Helmholtz and Volkmann (VON HELMHOLTZ 1924, Vol. III, pp. 413–415) for measuring aniseikonia are shown in Fig. 4. The subject cofixates the centers of the crosses and using peripheral vision adjusts magnification of one target to obtain vernier alignment between the two spurs. The problem with this target is that of maintaining fusion with the crosses while making the vernier adjustment. Furthermore, it is difficult to make vernier settings with peripheral vision.

The magnification required is recorded as the *aniseikonia ratio* for the lower half of the vertical meridian. The targets are rotated through 180° and a similar measurement is made for the second half of the same meridian. The average of the two measurements is the *aniseikonia ratio* (S) for that meridian. Averaging the results tends to compensate for errors due to fixation disparity. Aniseikonia may also

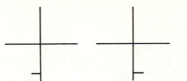

Fig. 4. Targets used by von Helmholtz and Volkmann to measure size differences between the images of the two eyes. FRY (1941 a)

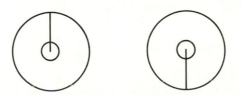

Fig. 5. Targets for measuring cyclophoria. FRY (1941 a)

be expressed as a percentage difference in size (s), as well as the ratio of the sizes of the two stimuli which appear equal in size.

$$s = 100 (S-1) \tag{1}$$

S has a value of unity when s is zero; s is negative when $S < 1$ and positive when $S > 1$.

The percentage aniseikonia for the various meridians can be analyzed to determine the size lenses required to correct the aniseikonia. If the aniseikonia is the same in all meridians, it is called "overall aniseikonia" and can be corrected with an overall size lens worn over one eye. It may, however, manifest differences in the various meridians. In such cases, the meridians of minimum and maximum aniseikonia ratios lie approximately at right angles. The aniseikonia can be corrected with an overall size lens combined with a meridional size lens.

The two targets shown in Fig. 5, which are presented to the two eyes, can be used for measuring cyclophoria. The circles control the fusion in the vertical and horizontal directions but leave the eyes free to cyclorotate to the cyclophoria position. The targets can be rotated around their centers to make the lines correspond to the various meridians. With the OS (oculus sinister) line set in a given meridian, the OD (oculus dexter) target is rotated until the two lines appear continuous.

Cyclophoria represents the angular separation between the OS meridian and the corresponding OD meridian, and is specified as the cyclophoria for the meridian corresponding to the OS line. The condition is excyclophoria when the OD pattern is displaced counterclockwise, encyclophoria when clockwise. Data for the various meridians can be obtained. If the cyclophoria is the same in all meridians, it is called myologic, because it depends upon a rotation of one eye around its line of sight relative to the other eye.

The measurements of cyclophoria may, however, involve meridional differences. The two meridians which manifest the greatest difference in cyclophoria lie approximately 90° apart. The average of the values for these two meridians gives

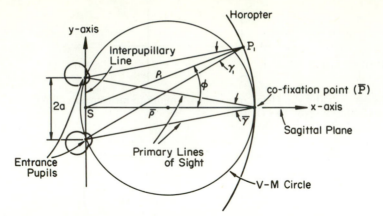

Fig. 6. The trace of the horopter in the plane of regard for symmetrical convergence. The horopter passes through the point of fixation (P̄) and is tangent to the *V-M* circle. P, is one of the points that lie on the horopter. Fry (1941 b)

a measure of the myologic cyclophoria, and the difference between the values gives a measure of the meridional difference in cyclophoria. The meridional cyclophoria can be corrected with a meridional size lens, which at the same time will correct the meridional difference in aniseikonia. The direct comparison eikonometer (Ogle 1950, pp. 243–247) measures the aniseikonia in the vertical and horizontal meridians.

II. The Horopter

The *horopter* is the locus of points at which corresponding lines of sight converge. Points on the horopter are seen in the same direction by both eyes. Some investigators have tried to visualize the horopter as a three-dimensional surface. If we define it as the locus of points which stimulate corresponding points on the two retinas, we soon realize that if such a surface existed for any given position of the two eyes, such a surface would cease to exist as soon as the eyes turned to the right or left. Points above or below the plane of regard could no longer stimulate corresponding retinal points.

It is possible to talk about the trace of the horopter in the plane of regard (Fig. 6). Even this requires that the eyes are free from cyclotropia and hypertropia and that points on the horizontal meridian of one eye have corresponding points on the horizontal meridian of the other eye. This trace was the limit of Ogles's concern with the horopter (Ogle 1950, pp. 14–17). In what follows I shall refer to this trace as the horopter.

It is helpful in the study of the horopter to compare it to the Vieth–Mueller circle, which is also illustrated in Fig. 6. It is the circle through the cofixation point and the centers of the entrance pupils. As pointed out by Vieth (1818) and Mueller (1826), any two points on this circle will subtend equal angles at the centers of the entrance pupils. It is referred to as the "geometrical horopter."

Ogle (1950, pp. 20–22) used a horopter device to locate the horopter. Vertical rods could be moved along paths that converged at the midpoint (S) of the interpupillary line. The paths represented different angles of azimuth, with the path perpendicular to the interpupillary line representing zero azimuth for symmetrical convergence. The position of each rod could be measured in terms of its distance (ϱ) from the origin and the angle of azimuth (ϕ). This is a simple polar coordinate system.

Ogle had the eyes cofixate a target (F) in the plane of regard on the line of zero azimuth and then used a binocular vernier technique (pp. 36–40) to locate various points on the trace of the horopter. He also used a technique for measuring the limits of the zone of single vision (pp. 40–44). The position of the horopter can be deduced from such data.

The data for the horopter can be fitted by the following formula:

$$\frac{\gamma_1 - \bar{\gamma}}{\phi} = \frac{s}{100} + H_1 \phi, \tag{2}$$

where γ_1 is the parallax angle for the point P_1 on the horopter at an angle ϕ from $\bar{P}$ which is the point on the horopter at $\phi = 0$ and $\bar{\gamma}$ is the parallax angle at $\bar{P}$. The term s is a constant which represents the percentage aniseikonia in the horizontal meridian, and H_1 is the Hering-Hillebrand deviation. The angles $\gamma_1, \bar{\gamma}$, and ϕ are expressed in radians. Note from Fig. 6 that

$$\gamma_1 = \frac{2a \cos \phi}{\varrho_1}, \tag{3}$$

where $2a$ is the length of the interpupillary line.

The constant s is related to the angle at which the horopter crosses the V–M circle at $\bar{P}$. If s = zero, the horopter is symmetrical and tangent to the V–M circle at $\phi = 0$. H_1 is a measure of the extent to which the curvature of the horopter deviates from that of the V–M circle. If $H_1 = 0$, the horopter coincides with the V–M circle. The lines of sight converging at various points on the horopter are corresponding lines of sight. The value of H_1 must be constant in order for the retinal correspondence to be constant for various values of $\bar{\gamma}$.

Let us describe in a qualitative way what would happen to the horopter if H_1 were constant. At the distance at which $H_1 = 2a/\bar{\varrho}$, which is called the "abathic distance," the horopter would be a straight line. At greater distances the horopter would be convex to the observer, and at shorter distances it would be concave. If H_1 does not remain constant as $\bar{\varrho}$ changes, this could be explained by assuming that converging the eyes distorts the retinas relative to the optical systems. Ogle (1950, p. 34) found that H_1 does vary with $\bar{\varrho}$.

III. Effect of Asymmetrical Convergence on the Horopter

It is possible to use the horopter apparatus to locate the horopter with asymmetrical convergence. To achieve asymmetrical convergence, the head is rotated around a vertical axis at S so that the y-axis of the apparatus forms an angle ω with the interpupillary line (see Fig. 7). The horopter is then measured in the same way as for symmetrical convergence. If there is no aniseikonia in the horizontal meridian and if there is no fixation disparity, the horopter is tangent to the V–M circle

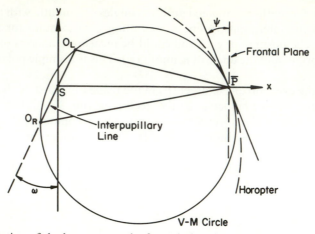

Fig. 7. The relation of the horopter to the frontal plane in asymmetrical convergence. The interpupillary line $O_L O_R$ is rotated around S from the y axis. $\bar{P}$ is the point of convergence of the primary lines of sight. Fry (1941 b)

at P and the plane tangent to these two surfaces makes an angle Ψ with the frontal plane through $\bar{P}$ which is equal to ω. The proof of these relations is given elsewhere (Fry 1941 a).

E. Perception of Distance

The use of two eyes contributes to the perception of depth or distance through convergence and stereopsis.

I. Convergence

If the eyes converge on a single point in a dark environment, can the observer be aware of the amount of convergence in play and from this assess the distance to the point? The subject can be aware of the distance at which he must concentrate his attention to avoid diplopia, but this does not provide a precise basis for assessing the distance of the point.

II. Stereopsis

Stereopsis is a form of depth perception which makes use of disparity as a cue for judging objects to lie at the same distance or at different distances. In Fig. 8 the two points $\bar{P}$ and P lie at different distances [m and $(m+\Delta m)$] from the pupillary plane. $\bar{P}$ is the point of convergence of the primary lines of sight; let us assume that the convergence is symmetrical. The lines from $\bar{P}$ to the entrance pupils of the two eyes (O_L and O_R) form an angle at $\bar{P}$ which is called the binocular parallax ($\bar{\gamma}$) of that point. There is a similar binocular parallax angle (γ) for the point P. The lines of sight from $\bar{P}$ and P to the entrance pupil of the left eye form a sinistrocular visual angle (α_L), and there is a similar dextrocular visual angle (α_R) for the right eye. Let

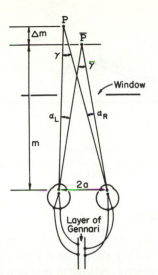

Fig. 8. Howard–Dolman peg test (HOWARD 1919) for measuring the threshold of stereopsis. $\bar{P}$ is the point of fixation upon which the primary lines of sight converge. P represents some other point in the field of view. In this case it lies more remote from the eyes than $\bar{P}$. The distance of 2a represents the separation between the entrance pupils

us assume that the point $\bar{P}$ stimulates corresponding points and hence these points are connected to two points just across from each other on the two sides of the layer of Gennari. The disparity is zero. Because the visual angle (α_R) at O_R differs from the visual angle (α_L) at O_L, the images of P fall on noncorresponding points; the signals generated go to two points obliquely across from each other at the layer of Gennari. The disparity for point P is finite, but there is no way to assess the amount of it except to say that it is proportional to ($\alpha_R-\alpha_L$) when point $\bar{P}$ falls on corresponding points.

It follows from simple geometry that

$$(\bar{\gamma}-\gamma)=(\alpha_L-\alpha_R)=\eta=\frac{\Delta m}{m^2}(2a) \tag{4}$$

where the angles are expressed in radians.

III. The Threshold of Stereopsis

It is possible to define the threshold of stereopsis as:
1) The minimum perceptible difference in binocular parallax ($\gamma-\bar{\gamma}$)
2) The minimum perceptible difference in distance (Δm) at the distance (m), or
3) The minimum perceptible disparity signal ($\alpha_R-\alpha_L$) generated by the point P at the layer of Gennari when $\bar{P}$ falls on corresponding points.

The symbol η, which is used to specify the threshold of stereopsis, is usually expressed in seconds of arc instead of radians.

For a normal observer, a typical value for the threshold of stereopsis is about 10″ of arc, which amounts to about 3 cm at 6 m (FRY 1944).

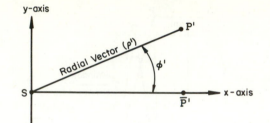

Fig. 9. Coordinates of the point P' in visual space. P̄' is the perceived image of the point of convergence of the primary lines of sight and S is the center of projection located midway between the pupils of the two eyes. FRY (1941 b)

IV. The Nature of Stereopsis

It must be made clear that the signal generated at the layer of Gennari by points P̄ and P can carry no information about the distance of P̄ or P from the subject. The signal generated can, however, be interpreted as a cue of the relative displacement of P in front of or behind P̄.

OGLE (1950, p. 133) appears to me to have made a mistake by insisting that "through vision with both eyes there emerges an entirely new sensation, namely, stereopsis." He also writes: "We can attribute the visual localization in space, on the one hand, to certain factors which are primarily empirical and, for the most part, monocular in origin; and on the other hand, to stereopsis, the unique sensation of depth which is solely binocular in origin." I believe that the experience of remoteness is an innate characteristic of all things visually perceived. The assessment of a specific distance has to be based on cues like geometrical perspective, and I put the signals of disparity generated at the layer of Gennari in the same category.

Many arguments may be advanced in support of its being learned. The experience of depth generated by geometrical perspective is qualitatively the same as that generated by stereo cues and can be just as strong. The process of learning can be demonstrated in squinters (FRY 1940). Under certain conditions the effect is reversible, just as in the case of Necker's cube (FRY 1972). Its dependence on lateral disparity is unique and vertical disparity is interpreted in a different way. Monocular and stereo cues are interrelated.

The reader must look elsewhere for a discussion of these effects as well as the relation of stereopsis to various stimulus variables (OGLE 1962).

V. The Relation of Perceived Distance and Direction to Physical Distance and Direction

For the moment, consideration will be limited to symmetrical convergence of the primary lines of sight at a cofixation point P̄ on the sagittal line which is perpendicular to the interpupillary line at its midpoint (S). The sagittal line represents the x-axis of physical space and S represents the origin; $\bar{\varrho}$ represents the distance from S to P̄ (see Fig. 6).

The point S also represents the center of projection in perceived space, and since the perceived image P̄' of P̄ is seen in the same direction as P̄, the x-axis of perceived space (see Fig. 9) corresponds to the x-axis of physical space. The point P′ in Fig. 9 represents the perceived image of any point P, which lies at a distance ϱ from S, which may put it on the horopter or in front or behind it. It lies in the direction ϕ' from the x-axis. The symbol $\bar{\varrho}'$ will be used to designate the distance of the point $\bar{P}'$ in perceived space (see Fig. 9).

FRY (1950, 1962) and BAILEY (1954) have attempted to locate the center of projection and have found justification for assuming that in observers with two normal eyes, the center of projection does in fact lie at the midpoint of the interpupillary line.

1. The Perceived Direction of Objects

The visual perception of direction has to be broken into two parts. One concerns the perceived direction of $\bar{P}'$ and the other perceived directions of other objects in the field of view relative to the cofixation point.

We have time only to consider the problem of relative directions for the case of symmetrical convergence. It is my belief that the relation between ϕ and ϕ' is learned. Although the relation is not perfect, we can accept as an approximation that $\phi' = \phi$, but for large angles it must be assumed that

$$\phi' \text{ (in radians)} = \sin \phi. \tag{5}$$

Large squares are perceived as barrel-shaped (FRY 1956b).

2. The Perceived Distance of Objects

I believe that the relation between perceived distance (ϱ') and physical distance (ϱ) is learned by looking at objects held in the hands and by watching the changes in perceived size and shape associated with the movement of three-dimensional objects in a fore and aft direction.

The subject has to learn how the perceived distances of various points on the horopter are related to the perceived distance of the point of fixation, and how crossed and uncrossed disparity can be interpreted in terms of perceived distances in front of and behind the horopter. This also varies with the perceived distance of the point of fixation.

I have derived the following equation relating ϱ' to ϕ and ϱ (FRY 1956a).

$$\frac{1}{\varrho'} = \frac{\cos \phi}{\varrho} + k, \tag{6}$$

where

$$k = \frac{1}{\bar{\varrho}'} - \frac{1}{\bar{\varrho}}. \tag{7}$$

3. The Locus of Points Perceived to Lie in a Frontal Plane

In a person free from aniseikonia, it may be shown (FRY 1956a) that the locus of points in the plane of regard which are perceived to lie in a frontal plane conforms to

$$\gamma_2 - \gamma = \frac{a}{\bar{\varrho}'} \phi^2, \tag{8}$$

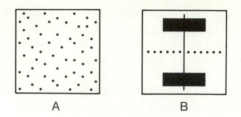

Fig. 10. Patterns for demonstrating the induced size effect. FRY (1941 b)

OGLE called this the "apparent frontoparallel plane". I shall call it the "apparent frontal plane". The term $a/\bar{\varrho}$ is the Hering-Hillebrand deviation (H_2) for the apparent frontal plane; it varies with $\bar{\varrho}$.

If a meridional size lens with the axis vertical is worn over one eye, this will rotate the apparent frontal plane around a vertical axis through the cofixation point. The horopter apparatus used for locating the horopter can also be used to locate the apparent frontal plane and a similar formula can be used to fit the data:

$$\frac{\gamma_2 - \bar{\gamma}}{\phi} = \frac{s}{100} - H_2\phi. \tag{9}$$

It does have a different value for the Hering-Hillebrand deviation.

VI. Induced Size Effect

If either one of the patterns in Fig. 10 is placed in a frontal plane and viewed with symmetrical convergence with a meridional size lens (axis 90°) mounted over one eye, the pattern will appear rotated around a vertical axis. This is the *geometric* effect. If the axis is at 180°, the effect is reversed (*induced* effect), and if an overall size lens is used, the two effects cancel. The vertical disparity is interpreted as a rotation around a vertical axis (OGLE 1950).

VII. Asymmetric Convergence

If the pattern in Fig. 10A is placed tangent to the horopter in Fig. 7 with its center at $\bar{P}$, the distance from O_L to $\bar{P}$ is shorter than the distance from O_R to $\bar{P}$ and this is equivalent to placing an overall size lens over the left eye. The geometric and induced effects cancel and the pattern is not perceived as rotated. This explains the advantage to the observer in being able to make use of the induced effect.

VIII. Space Eikonometer

The space eikonometer (OGLE 1950, pp. 247–254) is a device which uses a combination of targets A, B, and C in Fig. 11 and a meridional magnifier with the axis at 90° or 180° or one at 45° over one eye and at 135° over the other, together with the distance correction, to acquire information for designing a pair of lenses which will correct the ametropia and be free from unwanted magnification.

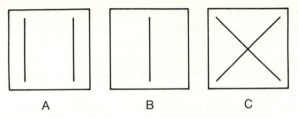

Fig. 11. Elements of the space eikonometer target. FRY (1941 b)

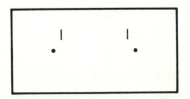

Fig. 12. Stereogram for studying the stereopsis and fusional movements induced by stimuli applied to the right and left halves of the retinas. The *lines* are on a piece of transparent plastic which can be moved sidewise relative to the *dots*. FRY (1941 b)

As long as the patient can make the necessary stereo judgments, this eikonometer is much more satisfactory than one based on direct comparisons of sizes and cycloalignments.

The meridional magnifier ×90 rotates the cross and the pair of lines around a vertical axis. A magnifier ×180 will rotate the cross around a vertical axis but not the pair of lines. The oblique magnifiers will rotate the vertical lines around the horizontal axis but will not affect the cross.

F. The Seam

One of the major problems of binocular vision (commonly referred to as the problem of the "seam") is how the binocular field of view is split between the cortices. We have to explain how the array of colors in the visual field appears to be uninterrupted in the transition from one cortex to the other. It is only when one cortex is destroyed that we can examine the border of the remaining part and wonder how it could mesh with the missing part. If there is a sharp dividing line between the two halves, we have the problem of explaining how interaction can occur between elements in the separate cortices. There is some evidence for bicerebral representation of both maculas. In this event it becomes a problem to know if a person sees simultaneously with both cortices or with one at a time.

The basic problem relative to stereopsis and fusional movements can be demonstrated with the stereogram shown in Fig. 12. The two dots are on a piece of white cardboard and constitute the cofixation points. The two lines are on a sheet of clear plastic which can be moved sidewise. The plastic sheet is moved sidewise to find a point or region in which the stereo effect produced by the lines breaks down. This would indicate that one is projected on one cortex and the other on the other. One can cover quickly the points with a piece of white cardboard and thus have the lines free to induce a fusional movement, but if the images are formed on separate cortices, they could not interact to produce a fusional movement. I have not been able to find in this way any impairment of stereopsis or fusional movements in normal subjects.

The corpus callosum is supposed to provide communication between the two cortices. There are persons in whom the corpus callosum has been severed and interference with fusional movements and stereopsis in such cases has been studied (BRIDGMAN and SMITH 1945; MITCHELL and BLAKEMORE 1970). Further studies along these lines combined with electrophysiological studies have to be depended upon for further answers.

References

Names containing *von* are alphabetized in this list under *v*

Ames A, Ogle KN, Gliddon GH (1932) Corresponding retinal points, the horopter and size and shape of ocular images. J Opt Soc Am 22:538–631
Bailey NJ (1954) Determination of the location of the center, or centers, of projection in anomalous correspondence. PhD dissertation, Ohio State University
Boegehold H (1935) Doppeltorische Linsen ohne Astigmatismus. Z Ophthalm Optik 23:41–55
Bridgman CS, Smith KU (1945) Bilateral neural integration in visual perception after section of the corpus callosum. J Comp Neurol 83:57–68
Burian HM (1948) The history of the Dartmouth Eye Institute. Arch Ophthalmol 40:163–175
Burian HM (1974) The Dartmouth Eye Institute. Survey of Ophthalmol 19:101–106
Dawson S (1917) The theory of binocular color mixture. Br J Psychol 8:510–551
Duke-Elder S (1934) Text-book of ophthalmology, vol I. Mosby, St. Louis
Edridge-Green FW (1920) The physiology of vision. Bell, London
Fry GA (1936a) The binocular integration of hue and brilliance. Arch Ophthalmol 15:443–456
Fry GA (1936b) The relation of accommodation to the suppression of vision in one eye. Am J Ophthalmol 19:135–138
Fry GA (1940) Orthoptic procedure with the royal rotoscope, Chapt 1–12. The Wottring Instrument Co, Columbus, Ohio
Fry GA (1941a) Class notes on binocular sensory mechanisms. College of Optometry, The Ohio State University
Fry GA (1941b) Class notes on visual perception. College of Optometry, The Ohio State University
Fry GA (1944) The measurement of the threshold of stereopsis. Optom Wkly 33:1029–1032
Fry GA (1950) Visual perception of space. Am J Optom 27:531–553
Fry GA (1956a) The discrepancy between physical and perceived curvature. Am J Optom Arch Am Acad Optom 33:147–154
Fry GA (1956b) The relation between perceived size and perceived distance in the periphery. Am J Optom Arch Am Acad Optom 33:477–482
Fry GA (1962) Eye-body coordination in the perception of space. In: Transactions of the International Optical Congress. Crosby Lockwood, London, pp 16–33
Fry GA (1972) Reversible stereopsis. Optom Wkly 63:300–302
Fry GA, Bartley SH (1933) The brilliance of an object seen binocularly. Am J Ophthalmol 16:687–693
Fry GA, Treleaven CL, Baxter RC (1945) Specification of the direction of regard. Special report No. 1. Committee on nomenclature and standards. Am J Optom Arch Am Acad Optom 22:351–360

Hecht S (1928) On the binocular fusion of colors and its relation to theories of color vision. Proc Natl Acad Sci USA 14:237–241

Howard HJ (1919) A test for the judgment of distance. Am J Ophthalmol 2:656–675

McDougall W (1910) On the relation between corresponding points of the two retinae. Brain 33:371–388

Mitchell DE, Blakemore C (1970) Binocular depth perception and the corpus callosum. Vision Res 10:49–53

Müller J (1826) Zur vergleichenden Physiologie des Gesichtssinnes des Menschen und der Tiere. Cnobloch, Leipzig

Ogle KN (1950) Binocular vision. Saunders, Philadelphia

Ogle KN (1962) The optical space sense. In: Davson H (ed) The eye, vol 3. Academic, New York

Panum PL (1858) Untersuchungen über das Sehen mit zwei Augen. Schwers, Kiel

Panum PL (1861) Über die einheitliche Verschmelzung verschiedenartiger Netzhauteindrücke beim Sehen mit zwei Augen. Physiol 63–111, 178–227

Sherrington CS (1906) The integrative action of the nervous system. Yale University Press, New Haven

Trendelenburg W (1923) Weitere Versuche über binokulare Mischung von Spektralstrahlen. Arch Gesamte Physiol 201:235–246

Verhoeff FH (1902) A theory of binocular perspective. Annals of Ophthalmol 11:201–229

Vieth GVA (1818) Über die Richtung der Augen. Ann Phys (Leipzig) 58:233–253

von Helmholtz H (1924) A treatise on physiological optics. Optical Society of America, Rochester

von Rohr M, Boegehold H (1934) Das Brillenglas als optisches Instrument. Springer, Berlin, S. 113–121

CHAPTER 9

Optics and Vision

Glenn A. Fry

A. Introduction

When I began teaching the optics of the eye to optometry students in 1935, most of the basic concepts of light and vision had already been discovered. In order to explain the developments which have occurred in my time, it will be helpful to review some of the early history. I have not tried to provide specific references in my review of the early history of the various topics; I have merely given dates for specific events and the years spanned by the lives of the various contributors. I want to identify as follows the historical reviews from which I have drawn material: SOUTHALL (1922, 1933, 1937), VON HELMHOLTZ (1924), TSCHERNING (1924), PRESTON (1928), BENNETT (1968), and JENKINS and WHITE (1957).

B. Basic Concepts

I. The Basic Laws of Optics

The basic laws of optics have been established for many years. The law of propagation of light along straight lines and the laws of reflection were formulated by the Greeks. Lenses were first used as burning lenses and as magnifiers, but around 1490 were also worn as spectacles. Galileo built his telescope in 1609; the pinhole camera was invented by Della Porta around 1600. He later converted it into a real camera by covering the hole with a lens. However, photographic plates for recording the image were not available until after 1800. Kepler (1571–1630) pointed out that the eye works like a camera with an inverted image on its retina. In 1625 Scheiner, using an excised eye, demonstrated that such an image is actually formed on the retina.

The law of refraction

$$n \sin \alpha = n' \sin \alpha' \tag{1}$$

was formulated by Snell in 1621. The terms α and α' are the angles of incidence and refraction and n and n' are the indices of the first and second media. Newton discovered dispersion produced by a glass prism around 1672. Huygens (1629–1695) formulated a wave theory of light which assumed a finite speed of light. In 1676 Rømer measured the absolute speed of light. The dispersion of light was attributed by Huygens to the fact that lights of different color travel at different speeds. Grimaldi (1618–1663) discovered diffraction, and Young (1773–1829) demonstrated interference between two diffracted beams, which led to the concept of periodic emission of waves; he considered the waves to be longitudinal. Fresnel (1788–1827) used the polarization phenomena discovered by Malus (1775–1812) to prove that the waves of light are transverse. Fraunhofer (1787–1826) used diffraction by a grating to measure the wavelengths of lights of different color. This gave us the fundamental relation between frequency, wavelength, and speed: frequency = speed/wavelength. The speed of light in a vacuum was found to be a constant and is recognized to be one of the fundamental constants of nature. Newton could have used his fringes produced by interference between beams reflected at two surfaces to assess wavelength, but his concepts about light included nothing that corresponds to wavelength. Michelson's (1852–1931) interferometer based on this principle has been used since 1960 to define the meter, the fundamental unit of length.

II. Geometrical Optics

By 1935 the fundamentals of geometrical optics had also been well established. Southall gives Huygens (1629–1695) credit for having established the conjugate foci formula for a single spherical refracting surface.

$$\text{Refracting power} = \frac{n'-n}{r} = \frac{n'}{u'} - \frac{n}{u}, \tag{2}$$

where u and u' are the object and image distances measured along a line normal to the surface and r is the radius of curvature and n and n' are the indices of the first and second media.

Since the index varies somewhat with the wavelength, it is necessary to specify a reference wavelength for each assessment of refracting power. Unless specified otherwise, this may be assumed to be 589.3 nm, which is the average value for the two sodium lines in the spectrum. At the moment, the International Standards Organization (ISO) has under consideration the change to a different wavelength.

Gauss (1777–1855) derived equations for computing the location of the principal and focal points of a system of refracting surfaces centered on a common axis (the *optic axis*), which could be used to locate images of objects that lie close to the axis (GAUSS 1838–1843). The aperture stop must be assumed to be small. Formulas for angular and lateral magnification and the concepts of nodal points, field stops, aperture stops, and chief rays were established at about the same time.

The formula for refracting power F is as follows:

$$F = \frac{n'}{u'} - \frac{n}{u}, \tag{3}$$

where u' is the distance from the second principal plane to the image and u the distance from the first principal plane to the object. The index of the first medium is n and that of the last n'. F is expressed in diopters. The diopter is a unit invented by Monoyer in 1872.

A ray of a given wavelength can be traced from surface to surface through such a system by the simple use of Snell's law at each surface. By tracing the rays from a given object point, one can assess the failure of the rays to pass through a single image point. This failure is described as an aberration which impairs image quality (FRY 1969).

In the case of a point on the axis, the paraxial rays do focus at a common point. If the paraxial focus does not fall at the retina of the eye or at the film of a camera, the image is said to be out of focus.

Distortion is a different kind of aberration which applies to an array of object points. The array of image points on the retina or on a film is a distorted replica of the array of object points.

In 1951 FEDER developed a new way of tracing rays through an optical system. It makes use of direction cosines to trace a ray from one surface to the next and Snell's law to assess the change in direction at each surface.

III. Physical Optics

If the rays from a given object point, after passing through an optical system, converge at a point, the image is said to be free from aberration. The waves passing

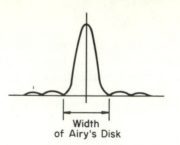

Fig. 1. Fraunhofer (in-focus) image of a monochromatic point source

through the exit pupil have a spherical wave front. The hypothetical geometrical image is a point, but the actual image is still blurred because of diffraction and interference. This blurred distribution is called the "physical image."

Fresnel (1788–1827) was the first to develop a usable concept of what happens. Instead of assuming that diffraction is produced by the edge of the aperture stop, which had been done by Young, he assumed that each element of the wave front transmitted through the exit pupil diffracts light in different directions. The diffracted waves of light from the different elements overlap and summate or interfere, and thus control the flow of light toward the image.

Fresnel computed the intensity only at the center of the image, but AIRY (1835) derived a formula for the entire distribution in the plane at which the rays converge. This is the plane conjugate to the object point. This is called the "Fraunhofer image" in order to differentiate it from Fresnel images formed in planes in front of and behind the conjugate plane. The distribution of flux found in the Fraunhofer image is illustrated in Fig. 1. It represents the irreducible blur for an optical system in focus and corrected for spherical aberration. LOMMEL (1884) extended Airy's approach to cover images out of focus. The same principles apply to aberrated wave fronts.

C. The Eye

I. The Optical System

The eye is in many respects like a camera. The optical system of the eye forms an image on the retina, whereas the camera lens forms its image on the film. The camera has to be focused by changing the distance from the lens to the film.

YOUNG (1801) was the first to demonstrate that a change in the configuration of the lens can be used to change the focus (or accommodation). He also showed that a change in the length of the eye is not involved.

VON HELMHOLTZ (1924) constructed a schematic eye with accommodation relaxed by substituting a single refracting surface for the cornea, as shown in Fig. 2. The lens was assumed to have a front and back surface with a uniform index in between. The vitreous was assumed to have the same index as the aqueous.

Von Helmholtz invented a special device to measure the index of the aqueous and vitreous, which he found to be 1.339. He used exocised eyes to determine the axial length. He invented the ophthalmometer for measuring the curvature of the front

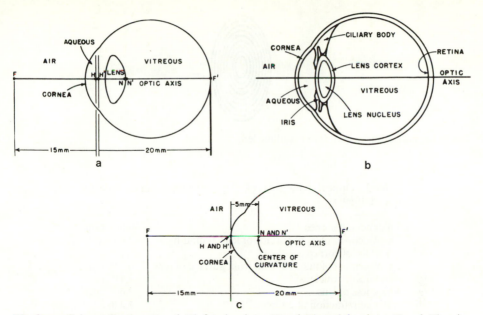

Fig. 2 a–c. Schematic eyes. F and F', focal points; N and N', nodal points; H and H', principal points. FRY (1959 a)

Table 1. Optical constants of the von Helmholtz schematic eye (FRY 1959a)

Distance from cornea to front of lens	3.6 mm
Thickness of lens	3.6 mm
Radii of curvature	
Cornea	8 mm
Front surface of lens	10 mm
Back surface of lens	6 mm
Indices of refraction (sodium light)	
Aqueous	1.333
Lens	1.45
Vitreous	1.333

surface of the cornea, and he used a device which he called the "ophthalmophakometer" for measuring the curvatures of the front and back surfaces of the lens and the distances of these surfaces from the front surface of the cornea when accommodation was relaxed. He also measured the curvature of the two surfaces of an excised lens and the thickness and the focal length. From this he assessed that the index of the lens must be about 1.455 if it is assumed to be uniform from front to back.

The von Helmholtz schematic eye illustrated in Fig. 2a is one modified by LAURANCE (1926, pp. 452–455) by changing the indices of the media slightly from the values used by von Helmholtz in order to have round numbers of −15 and +20 mm for the primary and secondary focal lengths. The constants used by LAURANCE are given in Table 1.

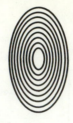

Fig. 3. Isoindicial surfaces of the crystalline lens

Table 2. Optical constants of the Gullstrand schematic eye (FRY L 1959a)

Thickness of cornea	0.5	mm
Displacement of front surface of lens behind front surface of cornea	3.6	mm
Displacement of nucleus from front surface of lens	0.546	mm
Thickness of nucleus	2.419	mm
Thickness of lens	3.6	mm
Index of refraction of cornea	1.376	
Index of aqueous and vitreous	1.336	
Index of lens cortex	1.386	
Index of lens nucleus	1.406	
Radius of front surface of cornea	7.7	mm
Radius of back surface of cornea	6.8	mm
Radius of front surface of lens	10.0	mm
Radius of front surface of nucleus	7.911	mm
Radius of back surface of nucleus	− 5.76	mm
Radius of back surface of lens	− 6.0	mm

Abbe's refractometer was used by FREYTAG (1907) to measure the index of the various layers of the lens from front to back. Gullstrand believed the lens to be constructed of layers or shells bounded by isoindicial surfaces conforming to the paths of the lens fibers, which run from a point near the axis on the front side of the lens to a point on the back. Figure 3 is an illustration of his concept of isoindicial surfaces.

It was found that the epithelium of the cornea has an index of 1.416 and that the rest of the cornea has an index of 1.377. The indices of the aqueous and vitreous are the same and are equal to 1.336.

GULLSTRAND's (1924) data for the relaxed eye are given in Table 2. He assumed that the lens can be considered to be divided into a nucleus and a core of different index as illustrated in Fig. 2b. Gullstrand used a brighter source for the ophthalmophakometer and was able to measure the thickness of the cornea and the curvature of the back surface. The Blix ophthalometer was also available at this time for making these measurements.

Figure 2b shows a reduced eye that has one medium and one refracting surface. The radius of the cornea is 5 mm and the index of the medium is 1.333. The focal lengths are the same as those of the von Helmholtz schematic eye. I have used the reduced eye in dealing with chromatic aberration. I have assumed that the exit pupil lies at the same distance (18.66 mm) from the secondary focal point as in the von Helmholtz schematic eye.

II. The Concept of Refraction

Since at the time the length of an intact eye could not be measured directly, there was no precise way to assess the focal length of an individual intact eye, and hence DONDERS (1864) invented the concept of *refraction* to describe the refractive state of an eye. This represents the reciprocal of the distance from some reference point fixed with respect to the eye to the point conjugate to the retina. Since in practice refractionists use the back surface of the spectacle lens as the reference surface for prescribing refractive corrections, it is appropriate to use as the reference point for refraction the point where the back surface of the correcting lens intercepts the primary line of sight. This is called the *spectacle point* and is assumed to lie 14 mm in front of the cornea. This point lies close to the primary focal point, which falls on the optic axis.

In what follows it is assumed that accommodation is assessed in terms of diopters of change in refraction at the spectacle point. *Static* refraction is the refractive state at the zero level of accommodation. *Dynamic* refraction refers to the maximum level.

III. Mechanism of Accommodation

The early theories about the mechanism of accommodation have been reviewed by VON HELMHOLTZ (1924), TSCHERNING (1924), and FINCHAM (1937). It is agreed now that the major factor is the change in the configuration of the lens. This also involves a change in thickness and a forward movement of the front surface. Tscherning believed that a contraction of the ciliary muscle increased tension on the zonule, whereas von Helmholtz proposed that it relaxed tension. Fincham's demonstrations appear to have settled this controversy in favor of von Helmholtz. Fincham based his theory on the elasticity of the zonule and the variation in thickness from zone to zone on the front surface. He considered the layers inside the lens to be malleable and hence to submit to the molding force of the capsule. FISHER (1971) and BROWN (1973) have demonstrated that the interior layers of the lens are also elastic and contribute to the form of the lens. GULLSTRAND (1924) emphasized the role played by the tensile strength of the fibers which arch out from the axis of the lens. Fincham used an optical section of the lens to observe the changes in the internal structure, and Brown has extended this approach.

IV. Control of Accommodation

The voluntary control of accommodation is mediated through the JAMPEL (1960) center in the brain, which simultaneously produces changes in convergence (accommodative convergence) and changes in pupil size, as well as changes in accommodation. This is called the "triad response." If the subject can be made aware of the size of his pupil with aid of a Broca pupillometer he can exercise precise control over his pupil size. At the same time, the accommodation and convergence drift with the change in pupil size. On the other hand, as explained elsewhere (FRY 1983, Fig. 12.3) one can use a stereogram which permits a subject to monitor changes in convergence by voluntary control of the triad response. The associated drifts in accommodation and pupil size go unnoticed. One can actually prevent the lens from responding to the ciliary muscle by using a presbyope as the subject or by temporarily paralyzing the ciliary muscle with a cycloplegic agent.

Furthermore, one can cover one eye, which eliminates any clue of the amount of convergence in play, and then demonstrate that one can, at will, focus on the wires of a screen or an object which lies at some distance beyond the screen. The accommodation is accompanied by changes in accommodative convergence and pupil size.

In the ordinary use of the eyes, one is aware of focusing at this or that distance but pays no attention to the pupil size or the amount of convergence in play. One is using one's Jampel center to control accommodation. The associated accommodative convergence may not be of the right amount to make one's eyes converge on what one wants to see, and reflex fusional convergence has to supplement the accommodative convergence. Without the subject's being consciously aware of it, the accommodative convergence can be utilized as an aid in maintaining single vision, but whenever it is used for this purpose, this throws the eyes out of focus.

When an eye or a pair of eyes is accommodating on a near object, there occurs what is called "microfluctuation of accommodation." It is not known for sure whether this is involved in maintaining the focus or is a form of noise. It disappears at the *zero level of accommodation.*

At the ordinary reading distances the accommodation tends to lag behind the level required for sharpest vision. On the other hand, when the eyes have nothing to focus on, as in total darkness or in looking at a cloudless sky or into a mass of fog, one might expect accommodation to relax, but in this case a small amount of it is kept in play. The zero level of accommodation has to be induced by having the eye focus on a target such as a visual acuity chart and then forcing the eye to relax as much as possible by using plus lenses. We regard this as the zero level of accommodation, and in terms of this zero it may be assessed that about 1.5 diopters of accommodation come into play when the stimulus to accommodate is removed. This is called "night" or "sky" myopia.

It is always necessary to ask what constitutes a stimulus to accommodation. Awareness of the nearness of an object and the need for concentrating attention on it can evoke a response in the JAMPEL (1960) center. In total darkness, one can evoke changes in accommodation by concentrating attention on imaginary points at this or that distance. In a lighted environment with visible objects at different distances, one can switch accommodation from one to another by noting the perceived difference in distance and shifting concentration of attention from one to the other. Any clue to distance, such as stereopsis or geometrical perspective, may be used in assessing the difference in distance.

The precise amount of accommodation used for any specific distance is determined by the level of accommodation required for clear vision. This can be shown by suddenly placing a minus one sphere in front of one open eye and noticing the blur clear up without any awareness of a change in the perceived distance of the object.

This raises the problem of whether the observer can differentiate the blurs produced by over- and underaccommodating. CAMPBELL and WESTHEIMER (1959) showed that with a 4-mm pupil an eye can use either spherical aberration or axial chromatic aberration to make the differentiation. The subject could not detect that his attention was concentrated at the wrong distance; all he could perceive was the need to increase or decrease accommodation to get in focus. AMES (1925) assumed that the blur produced by chromatic aberration could be used as a clue to distance, and recommended that artists paint blue and red fringes on objects to accentuate the illusion of difference in distance. ALLEN (1955) pointed out that uncorrected astigmatism might provide a clue to over- and underaccommodation, and used an objective recording of changes in accommodation to explore whether the subject searches by trial and error, or knows ahead of time the direction of the change required. In an objective recording, an experimenter can tell whether the subject is searching by the direction and timing of the adjustments. The findings of STARK (1968) indicate that searching dominates the response to blur.

V. Accommodation and Age

The range of accommodation decreases with age. At about the age of 40 the near end of the range recedes to the point that plus lens (presbyopic reading addition) has to be added in the form of segments in order to see near objects with comfort. The range of accommodation eventually drops to zero as age increases.

DONDERS (1864) worked out a set of data showing the relation of the amplitude of accommodation to age. He failed to make allowance for the depth of focus, which can make a person 60 years of age appear still to have a range of about 1 diopter. HAMASAKI et al. (1956) used a precise method for measuring the level of accommodation, and showed that the range drops to zero at about 54 years of age.

What determines the upper limit of accommodation? FLIERINGA and VAN DER HOEVE (1924) and others have held that the ability of the lens to respond to the tension of the zonule reaches its limit before the muscle reaches its limit, and that this leaves the lens dangling if the muscle is pushed beyond this point. VAN HOVEN (1959) has shown that this conception is not correct and that the lens can respond at the upper levels of contraction of the muscle. The ability of accommodative convergence to continue increasing after accommodation stops increasing is interpreted as a form of saturation of the output of the midbrain to the ciliary muscle.

There is also controversy about the relation of ciliary effort to the amount of accommodation generated. Some claim that it takes no more ciliary effort to produce 2 diopters at 45 years of age than at 20 years of age, although the total range of accommodation is lower at 45 years of age. It is my belief, based on the effect of age on the accommodative-convergence to accommodation ratio (FRY 1959 b), that the ratio of the response of accommodation to ciliary effort is proportional to the amplitude. The thing at stake is whether, as presbyopia approaches, a larger and larger central portion of the lens gets hard and unresponsive while the cortical portion remains unchanged, or whether the cortical portion as well as the nucleus becomes less responsive with age.

VI. Astigmatism

Astigmatism of the human eye was discovered by Young (1773–1829). A cylindrical lens with a cylinder surface on one side and a plano surface on the other was first used by Fresnel in 1819 to create a luminous line, but in 1827, Airy used a spherocylindrical lens to correct the myopic astigmatism of one of his eyes (Airy 1827). In 1864 Donders published his work on astigmatism and cylindrical lenses, and after this combination of spheres and cylinders was placed in trial frames to correct for both astigmatic and spherical errors. It was not uncommon in the early days for prescriptions to be written for a combination of two cylinders with axes at an oblique angle. Such a combination is equivalent to a combination of a sphere and cylinder, and this equivalent combination had to be computed and used in designing a spectacle lens which had to be mounted in the pair of spectacles. Formulas for making this conversion were worked out by Prentice (1900). Before toric surfaces came into use for spectacle lenses, it was necessary to have a sphere on one side and a cylinder on the other.

Toric surfaces were first generated for use on spectacle lenses around 1860. This was a step of major importance because it made possible the design of spherocylindrical lenses which could be corrected for radial astigmatism. This is true because it made it possible to change the base curve of a lens without affecting the power. This was already possible for spherical lenses.

In writing a prescription for a cylindrical or spherocylindrical lens, it is necessary to specify the location of the axis. When I began my career at Ohio State University in 1935, it was the custom to define the zero meridian as the horizontal meridian when the sagittal plane of the head is vertical. This had been recommended by the International Ophthalmological Congress in 1907. One of my first acts was to standardize on using the line connecting the centers of rotation of the eyes as the direction for the zero meridian. In my notes on the use of trial frames, refractors, and keratometers, I worked out procedures for insuring that the line connecting the centers of rotation was horizontal.

The Ophthalmological Congress had recommended that the angular displacement of the cylinder axis from the zero meridian be specified in degrees clockwise for the right eye and counterclockwise for the left (from the point of view of a person looking at the face of the spectacle wearer). In 1935 it was the custom to specify the displacement as counterclockwise for both eyes, and nothing has been done to change that.

Also it was recognized that a minus cylinder combined with a sphere is equivalent to a plus cylinder of the same power with its axis rotated 90° and combined with a new sphere, and rules were worked out for transposing prescriptions from the plus cylinder form to the minus cylinder form and vice versa.

Stokes (1849) invented a cross cylinder in which two cylinders of equal power are rotated in opposite directions. The resultant axis remains constant but the resultant sphere and cylinder both change. The Stokes cross cylinder is still not routinely used, but it does have unique properties and will undoubtedly enjoy a wider use in the future. (See Bennett 1968, p. 144).

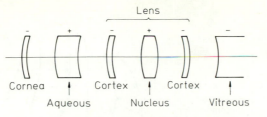

Fig. 4. Exploded diagram showing each medium of the eye as a separate lens in air. FRY (1959 a)

VII. Keratometers

VON HELMHOLTZ (1924) invented the keratometer but used it solely for making measurements of power in the horizontal direction. (The word *"keratometer"* is now synonymous with *"ophthalmometer,"* but at one time it was used as the name of an optical device for measuring the distance from the spectacle lens to the cornea.) JAVAL (1891) invented an ophthalmometer using the Wollaston prism as a doubling device which would locate the axis as well as measure the power. He demonstrated that the major source of astigmatism is the cornea. He developed a formula for predicting the cylinder to be found by measuring the refraction of the whole eye from the measurements made with the keratometer. MOTE and FRY (1939 a, b) showed that a major basis for the difference arises from the fact that the keratometer finding uses the cornea as the reference plane, whereas the skiascopic and subjective findings use the spectacle point.

Mote and Fry pointed out that part of the astigmatism can be attributed to the obliquity of incidence of the primary line of sight. In the typical eye, the line of sight is directed nasalward about 5° from the pupillary axis (normal to the cornea and passing through the center of the pupil). The obliquity of the line of sight at the cornea alone produces about 0.37 diopter of astigmatism against the rule in adult eyes.

VIII. The Basis for Spherical Ametropia

Mote and I (MOTE and FRY 1939) advocated that the keratometer finding be used to assess whether the spherical component of the ametropia is axial or refractive. I was not aware that RUSHTON (1938) had just developed the X-ray technique for measuring the length of the eye (cornea to sensitive layer of the retina) (DUKE-ELDER 1949, pp. 4253–4255). Up to this time it was not possible to measure this distance in an intact eye. Provision was also made for measuring the distance from the second nodal point to the retina. Since then an ultrasonic technique (MUNDT and HUGHES 1956) has been developed for measuring the length of the eye.

DONDERS had pointed out that the spherical component of ametropia must be attributable to axial length, curvature of the refracting surfaces, or the indices of the media. Figure 4 is an exploded diagram of the eye in which each medium is treated as a separate lens in air. One can quickly see what kind of effect a change in index of any of the media will have on the overall refraction of the eye.

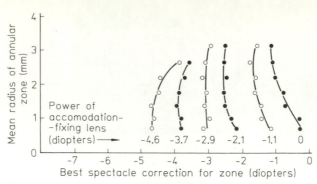

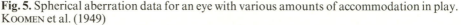

Fig. 5. Spherical aberration data for an eye with various amounts of accommodation in play. KOOMEN et al. (1949)

Availability of data on the axial lengths of the two eyes should be helpful in analyzing the size differences between the images of the two eyes. Furthermore, the distance from the cornea to the center of rotation varies with the refractive error (FRY and HILL 1962), and this affects the design of a spectacle lens in connection with unwanted sphere and cylinder in the periphery of a lens.

If a difference in the axial lengths of the two eyes is corrected with spectacle lenses mounted at the primary focal points, there is no difference in the sizes of the optical images formed on the retinas. This is known as Knapp's law (KNAPP 1869).

D. Eyewear

If a person has eyes with refractive errors, it may be necessary to wear glasses. If the lenses are properly designed and mounted before the eyes, his vision should be equivalent in most respects to that of a normal person. Instead of spectacles or in addition to spectacles, contact lenses or ocular inserts may be worn.

E. The Aberrations of the Eye

I. Spherical Aberration

A number of people have measured the spherical aberration of the eye. KOOMEN et al. (1949) have demonstrated that it switches from positive to negative as the eye accommodates (see Fig. 5). This may be attributed to the change in configuration which the lens has to undergo. From the data, one can compute the configuration of the wave front emerging at the exit pupil and then use the Lommel approach to compute the distribution of intensity on the retina. In using this approach, I have assumed that the wave front is radially symmetrical (FRY 1955).

Placido's disk, a pattern of concentric rings, was invented to study the irregularities in the curvature of the cornea. GULLSTRAND (1924) used the same principle in connection with the photokeratometer. Various modifications of this device have been invented since then, and it is now possible to make a detailed study of the contribution that the cornea makes to the spherical aberration of the eye. Other devices and procedures can be used to supplement the data.

Just as Young imbedded the front of the eye in water to neutralize the cornea to demonstrate that the lens can, by itself, generate the full range of accommodation, SIVAK and MILLODOT (1975) and MILLODOT and SIVAK (1979) have used the same approach to study the spherical and chromatic aberration produced by the lens in isolation.

A hard contact lens essentially neutralizes the cornea by sandwiching it between tear fluid in front and aqueous behind. It is possible, therefore, with an aspherical surface, to correct the spherical aberration for any level of accommodation. This can also be done with a soft contact lens when the front surface of the cornea is radially symmetrical.

II. Peripheral Vision

Since the spacing between cone photoreceptors increases rapidly as the distance from the center of the fovea increases, the visual acuity drops rapidly to a level where the eye could not benefit from a sharp optical image. There is little concern about the optical quality of the images formed on the peripheral retina so far as helping a person to see is concerned.

It is useful to know when impaired vision in the peripheral retina is due to pathology and, before assessing the effect of pathology, it is helpful to ascertain if the image is out of focus or blurred for other reasons. Various tests of peripheral vision are made with a perimeter, and when the findings are abnormal, it is helpful to assess the error of refraction for specific peripheral lines of sight. This can be done with a skiascope or a coincidence optometer. Measurements of this kind can provide information on the distoration of the eyeball in staphyloma associated with high myopia. A crude assessment of these refractive errors can be made with an ophthalmoscope.

POMERANTZEFF (1975) has been designing fundus cameras which aim at providing a clear image of the entire retina. Although the patient may not be able to appreciate a clear image formed on his peripheral retina, it is still necessary to produce a clear image of the peripheral retina on the film of the camera. Furthermore, when a beam of light (such as a laser beam) is used to photocoagulate a spot on the retina, it is necessary to keep the beam sharply focused on the retina.

LE GRAND (1967, pp. 126–130) has made a study of the astigmatic image surfaces for oblique bundles for the optical system of the eye. He used a schematic eye which differs slightly from that of von Helmholtz. The CODDINGTON (1829) equations were used to compute the astigmatic image surfaces. These surfaces are illustrated in Fig. 6. The retina (the surface of elements which respond to light) falls in between the two astigmatic image surfaces, and this is the best possible arrangement. It is assumed that the object points used in this calculation lie at an infinite distance from the eye.

III. Chromatic Aberration of the Eye

In 1955 I used the data of WALD and GRIFFIN (1947) on the axial chromatic aberration of the eye to study the effect of changing pupil size and throwing the eye

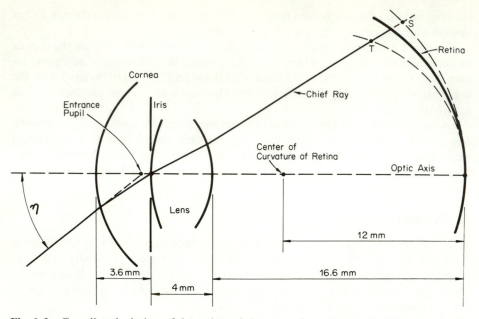

Fig. 6. Le Grand's calculation of the astigmatic image surfaces (*S* and *T*) of the eye relative to the retina. The data for the schematic eye are as follows: radius of cornea = 8 mm; radius of front surface of the lens = 10.2 mm; radius of back surface of the lens = 6 mm; index of aqueous = 1.3374; index of lens = 1.42; index of vitreous = 1.336. LE GRAND (1967)

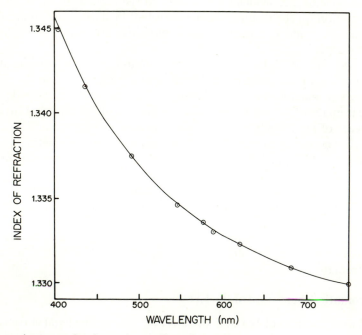

Fig. 7. Dispersion curve for the ocular medium. FRY (1976)

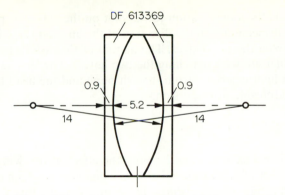

Fig. 8. The Bedford–Wyszecki lens for correcting the axial chromatic aberration of the human eye. BEDFORD and WYSZECKI (1957)

out of focus. These data were expressed in terms of the distance from the cornea to the point conjugate to the retina. I used a reduced eye, which is shown in Fig. 2, and computed the indices for the medium (Fig. 7). The radius of the cornea was 5 mm and the length of the eye 20 mm. BEDFORD and WYSZECKI (1957) generated additional data and obtained results in substantial agreement. I found that the Wald-Griffin data could be fitted with Cauchy's equation, and this analytical expression has proved useful in computing the effects of axial chromatic aberration on blur (FRY 1976, 1977).

The reduced eye helps to explain lateral chromatic aberration. In the reduced eye the nodal point falls at the center of curvature of the cornea. If the pupil were centered at this point, the eye would be free from lateral chromatic aberration. If the pupil were to move forward toward the cornea, this would produce a chromatic difference in magnification in which the blue image of a disk would be larger than a red one and the edge of a white disk would have color fringes. If the eye fixated the center point of a row of three, the images of the center point would be concentric but the images of the two flanking points would be dispersed in opposite directions. If the pupil were decentered laterally with respect to the center of curvature of the cornea, the images of a point on the primary line of sight would be dispersed and this would be pure dispersion for a single point.

In an actual eye the pupil falls in front of the center of curvature of the cornea, and since the pupil is centered on the pupillary axis, which makes an angle of about 5° with the foveal chief ray, the pupil is decentered temporalward about 0.5 mm from the foveal chief ray. The image of a point on the primary line of sight is subject to dispersion, but this is usually ignored except in dealing with chromastereopsis, which is discussed in my chapter on binocular vision in this book.

It should be noted that it is possible to construct a lens which will compensate for the axial chromatic aberration of the eye. My co-workers and I (FRY et al. 1943) constructed such a lens in 1943. WRIGHT (1947, pp. 347–348) refers to having used one in conjunction with his colorimeter. BEDFORD and WYSZECKI (1957) have described a design for such a lens in detail; it is shown in Fig. 8. The three glasses have the same index for sodium light; the lens acts as a plus lens for red light and a minus lens for blue light. I have used such a lens for viewing a bipartite stimulus in a colorimeter. It provides compensation for a point on the axis. For points on the dividing line, the dispersion is in the direction of the line and there is no blurring of the border between the two halves. The margin of the disk has color fringes but this does not interfere with matching the two halves. The lens has to be centered on the beam of light emerging from the exit pupil and the head has to be shifted sidewise to avoid chromatic dispersion.

IV. Blur

Under this topic we have to consider both the effect of throwing the eye out of focus and the effect of aberrations. Toroidal astigmatism, which occurs mostly at the cornea, and astigmatism produced by obliquity of the foveal chief ray at the refracting surfaces, can affect blur of the foveal image if these defects are not corrected with a spectacle lens. Spherical errors of refraction can also affect blur, but once these defects are all corrected with a spectacle lens, we can treat the eye as if it were equivalent to an emmetropic eye with a radially symmetrical centered optical system.

What is really meant by "throwing the eye of focus" is increasing or decreasing the level of accommodation, or adding plus or minus lenses to the distance correction, or changing the distance of the target. I have tried to deal with astigmatism at the level of blur circle theory (Fry 1955). Throwing the eye out of focus can also be dealt with in terms of blur circle theory based on concepts of ray tracing and geometrical images. The results obtained by this approach are approximate, but in most cases can be substituted for assessments based on the physical image which take into consideration diffraction and interference. In dealing with blur circles all we need to know is the radius, and I have explained elsewhere (Fry 1955) how to compute this both for the natural pupil and for an artificial pupil.

In an eye free from spherical aberration it can be assumed that the waves from a point source have spherical wave fronts as they emerge from the exit pupil, and I have used the Lommel equations to compute the distributions of intensity in images in focus and out of focus (Fry 1955). The equation for out-of-focus (Fresnel) images is complicated, but becomes much simpler when it is reduced for the in-focus (Fraunhofer) image. As a matter of fact, the equation for the Fraunhofer image is identical with that derived by Airy (1835). The distribution of intensity across the image is shown in Fig. 1. The central bright spot is called "Airy's disk."

I have found it useful to substitute the Gaussian distribution for the Fraunhofer distribution for the image of a point. I have done this for demonstrating the relation between the blur in the image of a point and that in the image of a line, border, or grating; it could be done for a pattern of any configuration for that matter. Figure 9 shows the Fraunhofer image and the distribution of intensity across the center of the Gaussian distribution, which I recommend as a substitute to simplify calculations in certain applications (Fry 1965 b).

Figure 10 illustrates the distribution of intensity in the physical image of a point out of focus. The rectangular distribution is the distribution for a blur circle computed from blur circle theory. It demonstrates that for an eye out of focus the blur circle is a reasonable approximation, and this justifies the use of blur circle theory for most out-of-focus problems.

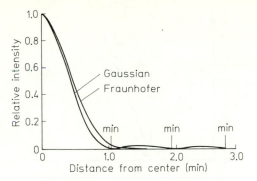

Fig. 9. Fraunhofer (in-focus) image of a point. F<small>RY</small> (1965 b)

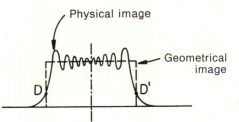

Fig. 10. Fresnel (out-of-focus) image of a point. D and D' are the points at which the borders of the physical and geometrical images cross. F<small>RY</small> (1976)

Once the distribution of intensity for a point is known, that for a line or a border or a sine wave grating can be easily computed. It involves the process known as "convolution" (F<small>RY</small> 1970).

With Cobb, I (F<small>RY</small> and C<small>OBB</small> 1935) introduced an index of blur for the purpose of being able to specify the amount of blur. It can be described best in terms of the distribution of intensity across the image of a blurred border. This is illustrated in Fig. 11. The gradient at the border levels off on both sides. The index is the ratio of the difference between the two levels and the slope at the midpoint. It can also be defined in terms of the point spread function, the line spread function, or the modulation transfer function for a sine wave grating.

We (F<small>RY</small> and C<small>OBB</small> 1935) described a procedure for assessing the index of blur by measuring contrast thresholds for bars of different width (Fig. 12a). It was based upon the notion that the contrast threshold depends on the contrast in the retinal image, which varies with the width of the bar. From the same kind of data it is possible to derive the line spread function (F<small>RY</small> 1946). It turns out that these measurements have to be made at a high level of luminance. At lower levels, neural spread as well as optical spread is involved (F<small>RY</small> 1965a). This index has been used to study the effect of such things as the size of the pupil, wavelength composition of the stimulus, and throwing the eye out of focus on the amount of blur (F<small>RY</small> 1955).

The use of the index to assess the effect of axial chromatic aberration on blur (F<small>RY</small> 1955, 1976) may be explained as follows. First of all, it is necessary to com-

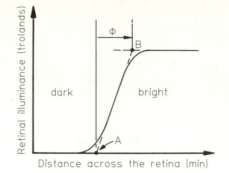

Fig. 11. Fry–Cobb index of blur ϕ as related to the gradient of retinal illuminance across the retinal image of a border between a bright and a dark area. FRY (1976)

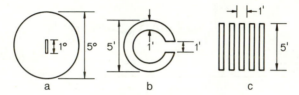

Fig. 12 a–c. Targets for measuring blur, acuity, and resolving power

pute the extent to which the eye is out of focus for the different wavelengths. The next step is to compute ϕ for the Fresnel image for each wavelength and pupil size. The third step is to summate for a given pupil size the contributions made by the separate wavelengths to the integrated value of ϕ.

I have used this procedure for comparing the blur produced by monochromatic and heterochromatic sources of light. One can determine the wavelength on which to focus to get the minimum blur and one can also assess the depth of focus. The Optical Society of America (OSA) had recommended the spectral centroid as the proper wavelength on which to focus, and the soundness of this recommendation has been confirmed. I have used the technique to check on the relative merits of high-pressure and low-pressure sodium lamps for illuminating highways (FRY 1976). I have also investigated the choice of light sources for measuring visual acuity (FRY 1977); the recommendations about light sources included in the visual acuity standard adopted by Working Group 39 of the Committee on Vision of the National Research Council (1980) are based on this study.

The Fry–Cobb index can also be used to demonstrate the effect of blur on such things as the visibility of lines, borders, and gratings, but it must be recognized that factors other than optical blur may be involved. Such factors include the length and curvature of borders and the effect of one border on another. They also include physiological spread of excitation and inhibition. Gradients that produce Mach bands involve inhibition. In connection with the quality of photographs, a different index, acutance, has been invented, which takes into account other aspects of the shape of the gradient than the slope at the midpoint (FRY 1983 b).

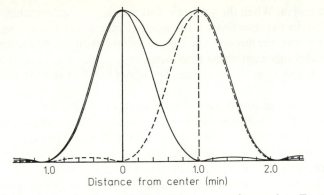

Distance from center (min)

Fig. 13. Rayleigh's criterion for the resolution of the images of two points. FRY (1970)

Since a normal eye can resolve two points separated by 1' of visual angle, and since it should be possible for two Fraunhofer images of a point to be resolved when the separation is equal to the radius of Airy's disk, RAYLEIGH (1888) argued that a telescope selected to resolve two points should have an objective large enough in relation to the focal length to produce an Airy disk 1' in diameter (see Fig. 13). In order for the von Helmholtz schematic eye looking at a remote point of monochromatic light (492 nm) to produce an Airy disk 1' in diameter measured at the second nodal point, it would have to have an entrance pupil 1 mm in radius. The resolution threshold for a pair of points is often used as an index of blur.

Mention should be made of other indices of blur, such as Strehl's ratio (GU-BISCH 1967) and BYRAM (1944).

A measurement of visual acuity is also an index of blur. Measurements made with Snellen letters or Landolt rings (Fig. 12 b) can be compared to measurements with normal subjects under standard conditions. Measurements made without a correction can be used in estimating the size of the refractive error to be corrected if there is no evidence of pathology which might impair vision. If the acuity measured with the best correction is less than normal, it is assumed that the eye is amblyopic or that vision is impaired by pathology. The level of acuity can be specified in terms of the stroke width of the smallest letter or character that can be seen. The width of the stroke is specified in minutes of arc. It is more customary to specify the performance in terms of the Snellen fraction, which is the ratio of the testing distance to the distance at which the stroke width subtends 1', e.g., 4/4 when distance is measured in meters. It is assumed that visual acuity is normal when the threshold is 1' of arc.

The visual acuity can also be measured with a square wave grating (Fig. 12 c) of high contrast having bars of equal width. This is called "resolving power" if the performance is measured in terms of cycles per degree of visual angle. The performance can also be expressed in terms of visual acuity by specifying the width of a single black or white bar at the threshold. It must be kept in mind in converting from cycles per degree to visual acuity that a cycle includes one white bar and one black bar.

At the standard level of luminance for visual acuity measurements, the results with the grating are comparable to those obtained with Snellen letters in a case of spherical ametropia. When the subject is astigmatic, the performance with a grating depends upon the direction of the bars. If measurements are made in three meridians 60° apart, the amount and axis of astigmatism can be estimated, as well as the spherical component of the ametropia. In a similar way measurements made with the Fry–Cobb target at directions 60° apart can be used for assessing astigmatism.

If a square wave grating is used at high levels of luminance it may be possible, according to von Helmholtz, to assess the coarseness of the retinal mosaic. A better method for assessing this is to use a double-slit diffraction pattern formed on the retina. Measurements of this type have been made by LE GRAND (1935), BYRAM (1944), WESTHEIMER (1960), and CAMPBELL and GREEN (1965).

A technique has been developed for assessing the line spread function for the image of a line formed on the retina by using the optical system of the eye to reimage the line in space in front of the eye and then scanning it with a slit. The most successful use of this method was made by CAMPBELL and GUBISCH (1966). The results are very reasonable in view of the fact that the results are complicated by scatter in the retina, pigment epithelium, and choroid. RÖHLER (1962) used a similar arrangement for measuring objectively the modulation transfer function for the line spread function for the eye.

A good deal of attention has been paid to the effect of blur on the modulation threshold function for a sine wave. If the modulation thresholds are determined for the neural mechanisms of the eye and brain for the different spatial frequencies by using Young interference fringes, one can subtract the contributions made by the neural mechanisms. This leaves the component due to optical blur. CAMPBELL and GREEN (1965) have used this approach to assess the blur produced by change in pupil size, focus error, and wavelength composition.

V. Perception of Direction

In this chapter I propose to limit consideration to a person with one eye. The problems with two eyes are much more complicated, and I have dealt with them in the chapter on binocular vision. The perception of direction of a one-eyed man is divided into two parts. On the one hand, we must explain how the image formed on the *anchor point* (see below) is projected from the center of projection in a given direction with respect to the head and eyes.

The object whose image is formed on the anchor point is the point of fixation, and the line connecting this point with the center of the pupil and the center of rotation of the eye is the primary line of sight. The effort to make the image of the point of fixation fall on the anchor point controls the fixational innervation, which in turn controls the direction in which the primary line of sight is pointing and provides the observer with information about the direction in which the eye is pointing. A complicating problem is that changing accommodation makes the eye turn in toward the nose (accommodative convergence), even though the effort to look in a given direction remains unchanged. This would make the observer see near-point objects in the wrong direction, were it not for the fact that the center of projection falls between the two eyes. This tends to compensate the error in perceived direction produced by accommodative convergence. The second part of the problem is learning to project an image initiated at a given part of the peripheral retina in a given direction relative to the direction of the anchor point image.

VI. Distortion of Perceived Relative Directions

It would be possible to trace rays from various objects in the field of view through the center of the entrance pupil to locate the points on the retina where the images are formed. It is pointless to do this, however, because there is no logical connection between location on the peripheral retina and perceived direction. This connection has to be learned. In order for perceived direction of a peripheral image relative to the anchor point image to be flawless, the angle subtended at the center of projection must correspond to the angle at the entrance pupil between the point of fixation and the peripheral object. Although discrepancies do exist, the one-eyed observer under ordinary conditions is not aware of them. As long as a one-eyed man does not have to wear a spectacle lens, there is no distortion of his perceived relative directions.

Since the spectacle lens is fixed with respect to his head but his eye can point in various directions, the one-eyed man cannot trust his perception of directions when he looks through the periphery. The prismatic effects in the various parts of the lens differ from those encountered when the eye looks straight ahead. He must turn his head rather than his eye and ignore the errors in perception of directions when his eye is turned.

"Metamorphopsia" is a localized distortion resulting from a displacement of the visual receptor cells of the retina. It may be due to detachment, tumor, exudative or inflammatory process, or cicatricial changes. These effects are also called "retinal micropsia" and "retinal macropsia."

F. Electromagnetic Theory

The electromagnetic theory of light formulated by Maxwell in 1867 has had an impact on visual science. It eliminated the need for the hypothetical medium ether, which was postulated to explain the propagation of waves. It helped us understand the mechanisms for generating light and such things as molecular scatter and scatter by larger particles. It has helped us to understand reflection at polished surfaces of metals and dielectrics and transmission of light along fibers which have a diameter smaller than the wavelength of light. It has helped us to understand the absorption of light and the conversion of light to heat and the various photoelectric and photochemical responses. Faraday (1791–1867) had paved the way with his experiments in electricity and magnetism. Hertz (1857–1894) did crucial experiments confirming the theory.

G. Quantum Theory

The quantum theory of light formulated by Planck in 1901 has also had a profound effect on visual science. A beam of light can be divided into a finite number of quanta. Each quantum has its own wavelength and a given amount of energy, and it is customary to assess the intensity of a stimulus in terms of so many quanta per second. The energy per quantum is given by the following formula.

$$\text{Energy per quantum} = h\nu, \tag{4}$$

where ν is the frequency per second and h is Planck's constant and energy is expressed in ergs. This is important in the photochemistry of the retina, where the change in density is proportional to the number of quanta absorbed.

I. Retinal Densitometry

One outstanding achievement in visual science was the development of devices at Cambridge University and the Institute of Ophthalmology for measuring the density of the photopigment in an intact eye (RUSHTON 1962; WEALE 1965). This made it possible to trace the bleaching and recovery and to assess the amount of bleaching required to produce a visual response. This technique has been used also to identify and study the characteristics of the visual photopigments such as rhodopsin, erythrolabe, and chlorolabe. There is known to exist a fourth one – cyanolabe – but the densities are too low to permit measurement. The densities measured by this method apply to an area of the retina larger than a photoreceptor and tells little about how the pigment is distributed in the different photoreceptors.

II. Microspectrophotometry

By the use of the microspectrophotometer (MARKS et al. 1964; BROWN and WALD 1964), it is possible to identify three kinds of cones, each of which has one of three photopigments. These experiments have confirmed the Young–Helmholtz theory about the mechanisms of color vision, which was formulated in the nineteenth century.

III. The Quantum and the Absolute Threshold

At low levels of stimulus intensity the absorption of quanta by a photoreceptor becomes infrequent and random, and if flashes are applied to the retina, the number of quanta absorbed per flash varies from flash to flash. This affects the probability of a flash being seen. Visual scientists (HECHT et al. 1942) have tried to find out how many quanta have to be absorbed for a flash to be seen. The quanta do not have to be absorbed by a single receptor, since summation over an area 10′ in diameter can occur. According to HECHT et al. 5 to 14 quanta suffice at a point 20 ° temporal from the fovea.

I have made an effort to determine the level of irradiance at which a "steady" stimulus can be treated as if it were steady (FRY 1984 b). It is my estimate that about 29 quanta per second falling randomly on a 10′ disk-shaped area 6.3° from the fovea may be considered equivalent to steady stimulation.

H. Coherence

An ordinary incandescent source involves many independent small sources of radiation. The radiation given off is composed of packets which are out of phase, and is a summation of random phases. At a given point in the path of a beam, the phase is shifting from moment to moment. To put it another way, the phase is not maintained over a large distance. The interferometer had to be invented before it was possible to assess the size of the interval along a beam at which the phases become completely random. This explained why it was necessary to use biprisms and mirrors to generate two images of the same source to produce interference between two beams.

The laser changed all this because it generates a beam that remains coherent over readily useful distances. When CAMPBELL and GREEN (1965) used the laser to generate a double source diffraction pattern on the retina, it was not necessary to keep the laser source and its mirror image at the same distance from the eye.

Another feature of the laser is its ability to concentrate a large amount of energy at a very small point, and hence it is now used by eye surgeons instead of the xenon arc to photocoagulate the retina.

The major importance of coherence lies in connection with the quality of the image falling on the retina. This is not fully appreciated and the problems are often ignored. In ordinary seeing the points in object space which we talk about can be regarded as point sources of coherent light, and the images formed on the retina are Fraunhofer or Fresnel images, which can be computed using Lommel's formulas.

In setting up an arrangement for viewing a transparency it is common to focus an image of the source of light in the plane of the pupil and an image of the transparency on the retina as shown in Fig. 2 b. In this case, Lommel's equations no longer apply. There is also a host of other arrangements to which the Lommel equations will not apply (FRY 1984 a).

J. Photometry

Space does not permit us to review the origin and development of all the concepts and units of photometry, but there are a few basic things that ought to be mentioned.

I. Light Defined as a Physical Concept

In 1953 the OSA Committee on Colorimetry defined light to be a psychophysical concept, and this began the struggle to differentiate between physical, psychophysical, and psychological concepts. I was finally persuaded that we need only to distinguish between the physical things and things perceived. I am pleased that the 1980 American National Standard Nomenclature and Definitions for Illuminating Engineering defines light as "radiant energy that is capable of exciting the retina and producing a visual sensation."

II. Light Defined as Energy

The OSA Committee on Colorimetry in 1953 debated whether energy or flux should be used for defining light. For continuous exposure the eye responds to flux, but for short flashes it responds to energy. The American National Standard (1980) RP-16 regards energy as a measure of the quantity of light.

III. Definition of Candela

From 1909 to 1948 the candle, which was the unit of luminous intensity, was based on the output of a bank of 45 carbon filamet lamps. In 1948, the ISO changed the name to candela and defined it in terms of the light emitted per unit of solid angle from a square centimeter of the surface of platinum at its freezing point (PAGE and VIGOUREX 1974).

Improvement in the ability to assess the absolute amount of flux led the ISO in 1979 to redefine the candela in terms of the output of a monochromatic source having a frequency of 540×10^{12} Hz (approximately 555 nm)[1]. This definition and the luminous efficiency curve make it possible to assess the luminance of a stimulus from its wavelength composition.

IV. Lambert Units

When I began my career, the intensity of a distal stimulus was specified in terms of footlamberts or millilamberts and these were regarded as units of luminance. In those days, luminance was called "brilliance" or "photometric brightness." Strictly speaking, the definitions given to lambert units made them units of what we now call "exitance." The reason we got by with this looseness is that in the case of a lambertian surface, exitance is proportional to luminance. At least we now know to specify luminance in candelas per square meter (cd/m² or nit), and these units apply to luminous surfaces, reflecting surfaces, and things like the sky and images produced by optical instruments.

V. Transmittance, Scatter, and Polarization

The media of the eye absorb and scatter some of the light being transmitted through the eye to the retina. Specular reflection occurs at the surfaces bounding the media. Certain layers diffusely transmit and scatter the light. Certain polarization effects also occur. These phenomena have been covered elsewhere (FRY 1984 a), and I shall not discuss them further here.

VI. Retinal Illuminance

In the early days, people who tried to relate the response of the eye to the distal stimuli placed in front of it ignored the fact that the intensity of the proximal

---

1 This figure is contained in a resolution adopted by the 16th General Conference on Weights and Measures in October 1979

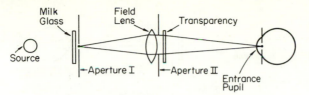

Fig. 14. Use of an aperture (*Aperture I*) to make a beam entering the eye smaller than the natural pupil

stimulus applied to the retina is affected by the size of the pupil. It should be said, however, that a human engineer may want to know how well a person can perform a task using his natural pupil, and in this case, the size of the pupils is deliberately ignored.

TROLAND (1917) showed that the illuminance on the retina is proportional to the product of the area of the pupil and the luminance of the distal stimulus, and he recommended that the product be regarded as a measure of the retinal illuminance. He specified that if the area were expressed in square millimeters and the luminance in candelas per square meter, the retinal illuminance would be expressed in photons. Since quanta were also called photons, the name was changed to "troland" in 1953 (OSA Committee on Colorimetry 1953, p. 231).

WESTHEIMER (1966) pointed out that it is possible to define the troland in terms of lumens per square minute, and this concept is very useful in dealing with blur of the retinal image.

An artificial pupil placed in front of the eye is often used to control the size of the beams entering the eye, and this in turn affects both the retinal illuminance and the quality of the image. The natural pupil becomes a field stop and this restricts the field of view. The arrangement shown in Fig. 14 is often used in visual testing. Aperture II is the field stop. If the image of aperture I formed in the plane of the entrance pupil of the eye is smaller than the entrance pupil, aperture I becomes the aperture stop. The size of the beam entering the eye is constant and unaffected by fluctuations in the natural pupil. If aperture I is large, the natural pupil becomes the aperture stop. The arrangement in which the beam entering the eye is smaller than the natural pupil is sometimes referred to as "Maxwellian viewing," but this term refers to the size of the field provided by the field stop and the field lens and the uniformity of the color across the field stop. It has nothing to do with whether aperture I is large or small.

K. The Stiles–Crawford Effect

STILES and CRAWFORD (1933) demonstrated that a narrow beam of light admitted to the eye near the margin of the pupil is less effective in stimulating the retina than a beam through the center. If allowance is made for this effect, the light admitted through a large pupil is less effective than for a beam confined to the center of the pupil. Allowance for this effect is made by multiplying the trolands of retinal illuminance by a factor to give the effective retinal illuminance for each pupil size (FRY 1983 b).

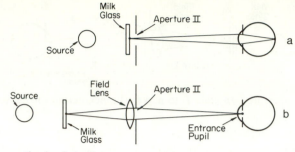

Fig. 15 a, b. Two methods of viewing

The effect depends on the angle of incidence of the light from different parts of the pupil relative to the direction of the axes of the photoreceptors and also the configuration of the receptors. The cones at the center of the fovea differ from the cones in the periphery and these in turn differ from the rods. By adapting the eye to different wavelengths, the responses of these elements can be segregated. When light enters the periphery of the pupil, hue and saturation changes are noted in addition to the change in brightness. This is known as the Stiles–Crawford effect of the second kind.

The wavelength of the light used for testing the effect can be varied, and wavelengths at the center of the spectrum are found to be more effective. If the same wavelength is used for beams at the center and the periphery, there is found to be a shift in hue which Vos and WALRAVEN (1962) interpret as evidence that the effects differ for the three types of cone, which are sensitive to different parts of the spectrum.

A discovery of major importance is that made by Enoch and his associates that the receptors are phototropic. BEDELL and ENOCH (1979) showed that in the periphery of the retina 35° from the fovea the photoreceptors are aligned on the average with the center of the exit pupil, even though this makes their axes oblique to the retina. ENOCH et al. (1979) occluded an eye for about a 2-week period and the directional effect was reduced. ENOCH (1957) showed in a study of certain amblyopes that the directional effect was reduced and that the position of the peak was shifted from the center of the pupil. Using a displaced aperture, ENOCH and BIRCH (1981) showed a shift in the peak of the directional effect towards the new apertures.

Polystyrene models have been used by O'BRIEN (1951) and Enoch and myself (ENOCH and FRY 1958) to study the receptor directionality. Microwaves of wavelengths of 3.2 and 2.42 cm have been used with cone models 70,000 times larger than a cone. O'Brien used a cluster of seven, whereas we used only a single cone, or a single cone with one neighboring cone added.

We used a point source producing a spherical wave. Orienting the cone at various angles to the wave front produces a typical Stiles–Crawford effect, with a maximum for the direction normal to the wave front. A concave mirror was used to produce a Fraunhofer image and the model was placed at different parts of the pattern. At each point the response was maximum when the cone was normal to the wave front.

From these data we would anticipate that the Stiles–Crawford effect would differ with the two methods of illuminating the pupil illustrated in Fig. 15. In both Fig. 15a and 15b the aperture is conjugate to the retina. In Fig. 15b the milk glass, which is an array of point sources, is conjugate to the pupil, and spherical waves from the different parts of the pupil approach the retina and their summated effects should conform to the Stiles–Crawford effect. In Fig. 15a points at various parts of the milk glass form overlapping Fraunhofer images with their wave fronts parallel to the retina, and the effects would be expected to summate. DRUM (1975) tested this theory by using an annular pupil compared with a small round aperture of the same area. He found a Stiles–Crawford effect for both methods of viewing. This calls for further study.

O'BRIEN (1945) formulated a theory of the Stiles–Crawford effect based on laws of transmission and reflection for different angles of incidence at the walls of the inner segment, but TORALDO DI FRANCIA (1949) pointed out that the small size of receptors requires the application of waveguide theory. This has been explored by ENOCH (1963), who observed waveguide modal patterns in a variety of vertebrate receptors, including human rods and cones.

References

Names containing *von* are alphabetized in this list under *v*

Airy GB (1827) On a peculiar defect in the eye, and a mode of correcting it. Trans Camb Philos Soc 2:267–271
Airy GB (1835) On the diffraction of an object glass with circular aperture. Trans Camb Philos Soc 5:283–291
Allen MJ (1955) The stimulus to accommodation. Am J Optom Arch Am Acad Optom 32:422–431
American National Standards Institute (1980) Nomenclature and definitions for illuminating engineering. (ANSI/IES RP-16-1980). Illum Eng Society of North America, New York
Ames A Jr (1925) Depth in pictorial art. The Art Bulletin 8:4–24
Bedell HE, Enoch JM (1979) A study of the Stiles-Crawford (S-C) function at 35° in the temporal field and the stability of the foveal S-C peak over time. J Opt Soc Am 69:435–442
Bedford RE, Wyszecki GW (1957) Axial chromatic aberration of the eye. J Opt Soc Am 47:564–565
Bennett AG (1968) Emsley and Swaine's ophthalmic lenses, vol I. Hatton, London
Brown N (1973) The change in shape and internal form of the lens of the eye on accommodation. Eye Res 15:441–459
Brown PK, Wald G (1964) Visual pigments in single rods and cones of the human retina. Science 144:145–151
Byram GM (1944) Physical and photochemical basis of visual resolving power. J Opt Soc Am 34:571–591, 718–738
Campbell FW, Green DG (1965) Optical and retinal factors affecting visual resolution. J Physiol 181:576–593
Campbell FW, Gubisch RW (1966) Optical quality of the human eye. J Physiol 186:558–578
Campbell FW, Westheimer G (1959) Factors influencing accommodation responses of the human eye. J Opt Soc Am 49:568–571
Coddington H (1829) A treatise of the reflection and refraction of light. Simpkins and Marshall, London
Committee on Vision Working Group 39 (1980) Recommended standard procedures for the clinical measurement and specification of visual acuity. Adv Ophthalmol 41:103–148
Donders FC (1864) Accommodation and refraction of the eye. New Sydenham Society, London

Drum B (1975) Additivity of the Stiles-Crawford effect for a Fraunhofer image. Vision Res 15:291–298

Duke-Elder (1949) Text-book of ophthalmology, vol IV. Mosby, St. Louis

Enoch JM (1957) Amblyopia and the Stiles-Crawford effect. Am J Optom Arch Am Acad Optom 34:298–308

Enoch JM (1963) Optical properties of the retinal receptors. J Opt Soc Am 53:71–85

Enoch JM, Fry GA (1958) Characteristics of a model retinal receptor studied at microwave frequencies. J Opt Soc Am 48:899–911

Enoch JM, Birch DG, Birch EE (1979) Monocular light exclusion for a period of days reduces directional sensitivity of human retina. Science 206:705–707

Enoch JM, Birch DG (1981) Inffered positive phototropic activity in human photoreceptors. Phil Trans Roy Soc Lond Sci B. 291:323–351

Feder D (1951) Optical calculations with automatic computing machinery. J Opt Soc Am 41:630–636

Flieringa HJ, Van der Hoeve J (1924) Accommodation. Br J Ophthalmol 8:97–106

Fincham E (1937) The mechanism of accommodation. Br J Ophthalmol Monograph Supplement VIII

Fisher RF (1971) The elastic constants of the human lens. J Physiol 212:147–180

Freytag G (1907) Vergleichende Untersuchungen über die Brechungsindizes der Linse und der flüssigen Augenmedien des Menschen und höherer Tiere in verschiedenen Lebensaltern. J. F. Bergmann, Wiesbaden

Fry GA (1946) Blurredness of the retinal image. Optom Wkly 37:1521–1523, 1537

Fry GA (1955) Blur of the retinal image. Ohio State University Press, Columbus

Fry GA (1959a) The image-forming mechanism of the eye. In: Field J (ed) Handbook of physiology, Neurophysiology I. Am Physiol Soc 1:547–670

Fry GA (1959b) The effect of age on the ACA ratio. Am J Optom Arch Am Acad Optom 36:299–303

Fry GA (1965a) Physiological irradiation across the retina. J Opt Soc Am 55:108–111

Fry GA (1965b) Distribution of focused and stray light on the retina produced by a point source. J Opt Soc Am 55:333–335

Fry GA (1969) Geometrical optics. Chilton, Philadelphia

Fry GA (1970) The optical performance of the human eye. In: Wolf E (ed) Progress in optics, vol 8. North-Holland, Amsterdam, pp 51–131

Fry GA (1976) Blur of the retinal image of an object illuminated by low pressure and high pressure sodium lamps. J Illum Eng Soc 5:158–164

Fry GA (1977) Sources suitable for use in illuminating visual acuity charts. In: Cool SJ, Smith EL III (eds) Frontiers of visual science. Springer, Berlin Heidelberg New York, pp 253–263

Fry GA (1984a) The eye as an optical system. In: Grum F, Bartleson JC (eds) Optical radiation measurements, Vol V, Ch. 2. Academic Press, New York

Fry GA (1984b) The eye as a detector. In: Grum F, Bartleson JC (eds) Optical radiation measurements, Vd V, Ch. 3. Academic Press, New York

Fry GA (1983) Basic concepts underlying graphical analysis. In: Schor CM, Ciuffreda KJ (eds) Vergence eye movements: basic and clinical aspects. Butterworth, Woburn, MA, pp. 403–437

Fry GA, Cobb PW (1935) A new method for determining the blurredness of the retinal image. Trans Am Acad Ophthalmol Otolaryngol 423–428

Fry GA, Hill WW (1962) The center of rotation of the eye. Am J Optom Arch Am Acad Optom 39:581–595

Fry GA, Bridgman CS, Ellerbrock VJ, Allen MJ (1943) Means for measuring and compensating chromastereopsis with special reference to the MI height finder. Report from The Ohio State Univ. Res. Foundation Project 117 to the Natl Def Res Com

Gauss KF (1838–1843) Dioptrische Untersuchungen. Abh Koen Ges Wiss Göttingen 1

Gullstrand A (1924) Appendices to Part I. In: von Helmholtz H (1924) Treatise on physiological optics, vol I. Optical Society of America, Rochester

Gubisch RW (1967) Optical performance of the human eye. J Opt Soc Am 57:407–415

Hamasaki D, Ong J, Marg E (1956) The amplitude of accommodation in presbyopia. Am J Optom Arch Am Acad Optom 33:3–14

Hecht S, Shlaer S, Pirenne MH (1942) Energy, quanta, and vision. J Gen Physiol 25:819–840

Jampel RS (1960) Convergence, divergence, pupillary reactions, and accommodation of the eyes from faradic stimulation of the macaque brain. J Comp Neurol 115:371–399

Javal LE (1891) Memoires d'ophthalmométrie. Paris

Jenkins FA, White HE (1957) Fundamentals of optics. McGraw-Hill, New York

Knapp H (1869) The influence of spectacles on the optical constants and visual acuteness of the eye. Arch Ophthalmol Otolaryngol 1:377–410

Koomen MJ, Tousey R, Scholnik R (1949) The spherical aberration of the eye. J Opt Soc Am 39:370–376

Laurance L (1926) Visual optics and sight testing. School of Optics, London

Le Grand Y (1935) Sur le mesure de l'acuité visuelle au moyen de franges d'interférence. C R Acad Sci 200:490–491

Le Grand Y (1967) Form and space vision. Indiana University Press, Bloomington

Lommel E (1884) Die Beugungserscheinungen einer kreisrunden Öffnung und eines kreisrunden Schirmchens. Abh K. Bayer. Akad Wiss 15:229–328

Marks WB, Dobelle WH, MacNichol EF (1964) Visual pigments of the primate retinal cones. Science 143:1181–1183

Millodot M, Sivak JG (1979) The spherical aberration of the eye. Vision Res 19:685–687

Mote HG, Fry GA (1939 a) The significance of Javal's rule. Am J Optom 16:362–365

Mote HG, Fry GA (1939 b) Relation of the keratometric findings to the total astigmatism of the eye. Am J Optom 16:402–409

Mundt H Jr, Hughes WF Jr (1956) Ultrasonics in ocular diagnosis. Am J Ophthalmol 41:488–498

O'Brien B (1945) A theory of the Stiles-Crawford effect. J Opt Soc Am 36:506–509

O'Brien B (1951) Vision and resolution in the retina. J Opt Soc Am 41:882–894

OSA Committee on Colorimetry (1953) The science of color. Crowell, New York

Page CH, Vigoureuv P (1974) The international system of units (SI). National Bureau of Standards special publication 330. National Bureau of Standards, Washington

Pomerantzeff O (1975) Equator-plus camera. Invest Ophthalmol 14:401–406

Prentice CF (1900) Ophthalmic lenses, dioptric formulae for combined cylindrical lenses. The prism-dioptry and other optical papers. Keystone, Philadelphia

Preston T (1928) The theory of light, 5 th edn. Macmillan, London

Rayleigh JWS (1888) Wave theory of light. Encyclopedia Britannica, 9 th ed. 14:421–459

Röhler R (1962) Die Abbildungseigenschaften der Augenmedien. Vision Res 2:391–429

Rushton RH (1938) The clinical measurement of the axial length of the living eye. Trans Ophthalmol Soc 58:136–142

Rushton WAH (1962) Visual pigments in man. Sci Am 207:120–132

Sivak JG, Millodot M (1975) Axial chromatic aberration of the crystalline lens. Atti Fond Giorgio Ronchi 30:173–177

Southall JPC (1922) The beginnings of optical science. J Opt Soc Am 6:293–311

Southall JPC (1933) Mirrors, prisms, and lenses, 3 rd ed. Macmillan, New York

Southall JPC (1937) Introduction to physiological optics. Oxford University Press, London

Stark L (1968) Neurological control systems. Plenum, New York

Stiles WS, Crawford BH (1933) Luminous efficiency of rays entering the pupil at different points. Proc R Soc London [B] 112:428–450

Stokes GG (1849) On a mode of measuring the astigmatism of a defective eye. Rep Br Ass Advmt Sei, Part II, p. 10

Toraldo Di Francia G (1949) Retina cones as dielectric antennas. J Opt Soc Am 39:324

Troland LT (1917) On the measurement of visual stimulation intensities. J Exp Psychol 2:1–33

Tscherning M (1924) Physiologic optics. Keystone, Philadelphia

Van Hoven RC (1959) Partial cycloplegia and the accommodation-convergence relationship. Am J Optom Arch Am Acad Optom 36:21–39

Von Helmholtz H (1924) A treatise on physiological optics, vol I. Optical Society of America, Rochester

Vos JJ, Walraven PL (1962) The Stiles-Crawford effect. A survey. Atti Fond Giorgio Ronchi 17:302–318

Wald G, Griffin DR (1947) The change in the refractive power of the human eye in dim and bright light. J Opt Soc Am 37:321–336

Weale RA (1965) Vision and fundus reflectometry. Doc Ophthalmol 19:252–286

Westheimer G (1960) Modulation thresholds for sinusoidal light distributions on the retina. J Physiol 152:67–74

Westheimer G (1966) The Maxwellian view. Vision Res 6:669–682

Wright WD (1947) Researches on normal and defective colour vision. Mosby, St. Louis

Young T (1801) On the mechanism of the eye. Philos Trans R Soc Lond 91:23–88

CHAPTER 10

A Personal Vision

RAGNAR GRANIT

A. Introduction

Invited to describe the field of vision as I experienced it 60 years ago, when I began to take an interest in it, I feel as I did while writing my book on Sherrington (GRANIT 1966) – that it is virtually impossible to make a reader of today understand what was exciting to a worker so far back in time. My findings are *vieux jeux* and to the intelligent student of 1980 they are likely to be commonplace. He cannot understand why we experienced difficulties in taking the steps forward that to him now seem obvious if not trivial: *Parturiunt montes et nascitur ridiculus mus.* However, I find solace in the words of SHERRINGTON (1946, p. 142): "To ask something which the time is not yet ripe to answer is of small avail. There must be means for reply and enough collateral knowledge to make the answer worthwhile."

In a way I can comprehend the supposedly prevalent attitude of indifference to things historical, because even for me it is neither easy to recreate the state of ignorance in which one dwelt 60 years ago, nor possible fully to revive the emotional excitement that inspired one's activities at that time. Yet I can wholeheartedly say, quoting RAMÓN Y CAJAL (1937), that "the retina was my fist love."

When I entered university in 1919 my interests were centered on psychology, but an uncle who was a practicing physician convinced me that psychology as a science required a medical degree, or at least a major in zoology with supporting subjects from the natural sciences. At Helsingfors University psychology was subordinated to philosophy, and so I had to take a degree in the humanities before turning to medicine.

B. The Psychophysical Background

At the time the so-called Gestalt psychology was the rising school in German psychological science, my excellent teacher at Helsingfors, the philosopher Eino

Kaila, suggested a stay with Adhemar Gelb in Frankfurt am Main to acquaint me with the leading ideas of that movement. I undertook this in 1922, and found Gelb a highly stimulating and personally attractive man. Six years later I wrote a fictitious discussion with him in Swedish, now also accessible in a German translation by Eberhard Dodt (GRANIT 1974). My psychological articles – the first in 1921 (GRANIT 1921) – all fell within the field of vision, but in the present context they are of little interest. Exposed to the life of a medical student, I gradually realized that physiology would provide a better approach to a science of the eye than Gestalt psychology. There did not seem to be much of a future for labeling observations "Gestalts" without any substrate to support them. My ambitions centered on a desire to be able to put in a brick or two into the grand edifice of natural science – something definite, to put it simply.

I was therefore delighted when, in May 1926, I was appointed demonstrator (assistant) at the Physiological Institute, which was founded by Robert Tigerstedt and then directed by his son, Carl Tigerstedt. Experimentation gave me great pleasure, and I started perfecting my knowledge of the instrumentation and procedures of a physiological laboratory. Circulation and heart were the traditional interests of the Tigerstedts, and I had to do the operative work on rabbits required for the experiments, as well as running the experimental class. I remember taking a childish pride in not breaking the string of the Edelmann string galvanometer more than once.

But now, what about vision? I treasured this secret love from my psychological anacrusis. Once, while I was doing some psychophysical experiments on color, old Robert Tigerstedt (circulation man, polyhistor, and author of a well-known textbook) came round, and seeing that I was interested in colors said: "Everyone who begins studying color vision is lost forever to sensible work in physiology." I then promised myself – and possibly said openly to him – that this should not be my fate. There is a lot more to the eye than colors, and while studying the psychophysics of vision I was thinking of ways and means of finding a worthwhile opening into visual physiology.

Also in those days there were things one definitely had to know. Psychophysics was, and is, an exact science as far as measuring is concerned, and von Helmholtz's three renowned pupils, König, von Kries, and Nagel, had created a body of knowledge that no one could afford to overlook. In retrospect, König (whom the other two were said to look down upon) stands out as by far the greatest experimenter of the three (KÖNIG 1903). VON KRIES (1929) was recognized as the father of the duplicity theory, but his deductions were, after all, based on the earlier realization of the fine anatomist SCHULTZE (1867) that the rods were scotopic and the cones photopic receptors, to use the two terms that were much later introduced by Sir John PARSONS (1927) for vision in the dark and in daylight respectively. PARINAUD (1898) had connected night blindness with a deficiency in the rod mechanism.

Rods, cones, and dark adaptation occupied the center of interest for many years. AUBERT (1865) was the first to measure dark adaptation as a function of time, but BOLL's (1877) discovery of visual purple and his description of its regeneration initiated a line of development of – so it seems – almost permanent actuality. Firstly, it set KÜHNE (1877–1878) on the path of elucidating the properties of this substance, now generally spoken of as rhodopsin. He studied its bleaching and regeneration and located it in the rods. The improved spectral energy control available to König and his pupils KÖTTGEN and ABELSDORFF (1896) made possible the first plotting of the rhodopsin absorption curve, as well as its identification with the human scotopic luminosity curve. HERING (1891) had already shown that a congenitally color-blind observer had a spectral distribution of luminosity similar to that of the scotopic normal.

In psychophysics the rod-free fovea came to occupy a central place in the development of the duplicity theory, clearly because it provided a means of separating rod and cone functions. The German workers (VON KRIES 1929) availed themselves of foveal contra peripheral vision to study adaptation, color vision, the Purkinje shift, etc. KOHLRAUSCH (1922) in Germany and HECHT (1931 a) in the United States around 1920–1922 separated the rod and cone branches of the standard curve for dark adaptation. Flicker fusion had been well known since the last decade of the previous century, and was used to measure photopic luminosity curves. As early as 1902, the flicker phenomenon had been related to adaptation by SCHATERNIKOW (1902).

C. Early Attempts to Develop a Retinal Neurology

Thus for many years the efforts to define the properties of photopic and scotopic vision dominated visual psychophysics. An indirect consequence of this work became a tendency to place the retina and its receptors in the foreground of theoretical thinking about visual problems. The early rhodopsin physiology of KÜHNE (1877–1878) and KÖNIG (1903) added weight to this tendency. An international commission in 1924 devoted itself to establishing the standard photopic and scotopic luminosity curves of man.

However, I did not feel inclined to enter this particular sphere of work. I had, in fact, been very much attracted by the work of Ewald HERING (1925), probably because of Gelb, who was one of his admirers. Hering's ideas concerning two antagonistic nervous processes, anabolism and catabolism, seemed to embody an essential element of truth, but for the time being I was not ripe to handle such problems: I came to them later. But there was one thing I began to understand at a relatively early stage during my learning years, and this was the fact that the retina was, according to RAMÓN Y CAJAL (1894), a "true nervous center." I also noted that this insight played no role whatsoever in contemporary thinking in visual psychophysics. Here seemed to me a line of approach worth taking up in earnest. It thus became my lofty ambition to try to create some kind of retinal neurology.

This general idea was my lodestar during the years that I pursued vision. At the beginning I was reduced to using simple methods. I chose afterimages and proceeded to demonstrate interaction between center and periphery of the field of vision (GRANIT 1927). Having gained my MD by the end of that year (1927), I was faced with a final decision: should I devote myself to physiology or take up a clinical discipline, such as neurology, internal medicine, or ophthalmology? I decided to go on experimenting for five years; if, within that time, I felt that I had succeeded in creating something, I would remain in physiology; in case of failure, I would still be young enough to revert to the physician's honorable life of dedication to others *(vivre pour autrui)*. The clinical years, after all, had not been without their temptations.

Realizing my ignorance of the physiology of the central nervous system, I went to Sir Charles Sherrington in Oxford early in January 1928 and mentioned to him my notion of taking up study of the retina as a nervous center. He replied that I was on the right track and added that he had always wanted someone to do visual work in his laboratory. Having read SHERRINGTON's (1906) *Integrative Action of the Nervous System*, I understood the basis for his appreciation of my program. The book contains a large number of visual analogies, such as "spinal contrast," "immediate spinal induction," and "successive induction," and the statements that the afterdischarge of a reflex "may be considered analogous to a positive afterimage left by a visual stimulus" and that the flexion–extension antagonism" presents obvious analogy to visual contrast." At a much later date Sherrington told me that during his early days at Gonville and Caius College in Cambridge, Hering's ideas of two fundamental opposite processes in the nervous system held a strong position among his contemporaries. He himself looked upon excitation and inhibition in the reflexes as being opposed like black and white in Hering's conceptual world.

At Oxford I thus landed in 1928 in the midst of creative biology. I have described the life I then entered in two publications: in my appraisal of Sherrington (GRANIT 1966) and in *The Neurosciences: Paths of Discovery* (GRANIT 1975). I had a friendly reception from the group of young and well-trained people at that time engaged in work under the direction of Sherrington: Sybil Cooper, Stephen Creed, Derek Denny-Brown, John C. Eccles, and E. G. T. Liddell. In 1928 Creed and I experimented on interaction between center and periphery in afterimages (CREED and GRANIT 1928), but our talks often deviated to our common interest, English literature. Eccles and I worked together and with Sherrington on the spinal cord. There is a lively description of this period by Eccles in ECCLES and GIBSON's (1979) joint biography of Sherrington, which is authoritative, scholarly, and highly readable.

The paper by LIDDELL and SHERRINGTON (1924) on the stretch reflex must have impressed me a great deal, to judge by what I later did during my "motor period." This was also the time when ADRIAN and MATTHEWS (1927 a, b, 1928) at Cambridge published their three exciting papers on the eye and optic nerve of the conger eel, with the first records of the mass discharge from the nerve at "on" and "off". I went to see Adrian, armed with a letter of introduction by Sherrington, and met with a very friendly reception, though I was not yet ripe myself for this kind of work.

It must have been in February or March 1929 that Alan Gregg of the Rockefeller Foundation visited Helsingfors University and called upon me to serve as an interpreter for his visits to the professors of the Medical Faculty, who at that time had German as their first foreign language. The textbooks, too, were in German. Gregg and Sherrington recommended me to D. W. Bronk, who, after spending some time with Adrian, had been appointed head of a brand-new institute, the Eldridge R. Johnson Foundation of the University of Pennsylvania, and needed staff members at the postgraduate level. His first choices were H. K. Hartline, W. A. H. Rushton, and myself, the three of us in due course doing reasonably well in vision and remaining good friends.

Rushton was then successfully engaged in undermining Lapicque's concept of isochronism between muscle and nerve; Hartline, during my first year, was studying in Munich, and during my second year started building apparatus for his excellent work on the eyes of *Limulus, Pecten,* and the frog (HARTLINE 1974). Bronk was similarly engaged in setting up the equipment for his first expert recording of the discharges in single nerve fibers of Pacini bodies and the carotid sinus. This place provided an ideal environment for us young enthusiasts. Nearby was the Physiology Department, headed by H. C. Bazett, an Oxford man, and including Grayson McCouch; these were two keen minds with much to give to a younger colleague. For my wife and myself this was also our wedding trip, often since repeated by ship and air, tying us to friends and experiences in the United States.

Still in the aftermath of psychophysics and psychology, I decided to find out whether the idea of the retina as a nervous center could be promoted by using flicker fusion as an index of level of excitation. This application of the flicker method was suggested by the well-known Ferry-Porter law and its use for the measurement of the spectral luminosity function. There was ADRIAN and MATTHEW's (1928) four-spot experiment, in which it had been shown that the latency of the mass discharge of the eel's eye was shorter when all four were illuminated together compared with the value for each of them illuminated singly, suggesting spatial summation. I showed that the results could be repeated psychophysically with four 1° spots against a background weakly illuminated to counteract stray light. The four had a higher fusion frequency than the singles, all viewed at 10° toward the periphery (GRANIT 1930). From this starting point I went on to systematic work on area and intensity as determinants of fusion frequency in the fovea and at 10° peripheral (GRANIT and HARPER 1930). The influence of area (size of flickering spot) was very much greater in the periphery, as was to be expected from anatomical information on the structure of the retina. With C. H. Graham a split circular field was used, the halves of which could be set at different distances apart and illuminated at different relative intensities, all done in order to demonstrate interaction in terms of excitation and inhibition (GRAHAM and GRANIT 1931; GRANIT 1941).

The impact of that work on contemporary psychophysics and later developments in this field has been well reviewed by BROWN (1965), who was, I believe, a pupil of the late C. H. Graham (who ended up as Professor of Psychology at Columbia University in New York). Some later comments of my own are found in a lecture of 1978 (GRANIT 1978). The papers from the Johnson Foundation were six in number, all concerning various aspects of spatial and temporal summation, and interpreted on the basis of what one knew about nervous processes in the spinal cord. They were published in the *American Journal of Physiology* 1930–1931.

I still think it likely that the findings described had their origin in the retina. Nevertheless, it was obvious that the next thing to do was to go for retinal electrophysiology and valve amplification. Back in Helsingfors after the two profitable years at Penna, I sat down to build a dc amplifier, as one had to do in those days, matching valves to work against one another in a push–pull arrangement. A small permanent magnet string galvanometer was placed in a bridge between the anode circuits and balanced to zero by potentiometers in the grid circuits. This scheme had been suggested by Hartline, and Adrian advised me about suitable valves obtainable in Europe. This simple apparatus was to serve me for many years.

Alan Gregg again came to the rescue and provided me with a Rockefeller fellowship for my second period at Oxford (1932–1933), where my wife and I were warmly welcomed by Sir Charles and Lady Sherrington and by my contemporaries in his team, in particular by those with whom I was privileged to work: Sybil Cooper, Stephen Creed, and J. C. Eccles. I settled for an analysis of the electroretinogram (ERG) into components and of their relation to the discharge in the optic nerve (cat). Creed and I studied ERG flicker and Cooper, Creed, and I recorded each others' ERGs. We had great fun, and in addition to the papers born out of it, this collaboration led to the marriage of Sybil and Stephen Creed. Eccles held me to work on the spinal cord and, with J. Z. Young, to recording impulses from the thick nerve of the earthworm. Impressed by the work of ERLANGER and GASSER (1937), Eccles and I collected a large number of high-tension batteries and rigged up a cathode ray oscillograph to play with. One seemed to have an endless amount of time for everything in those days!

D. Analysis of the Electroretinogram Inhibition

But to return to the retina, my general aim was to find out whether Frithiof Holmgren's old discovery, the ERG, stabilized by amplification, could be made useful for the development of a retinal neurology. I went through the whole literature on the ERG [since summarized in a monograph (GRANIT 1947)], finding it valuable at the descriptive level but not very useful from the point of view of vision. In the best papers component analyses were attempted. Having completed my own analysis of the ERG into the components PI, PII, and PIII, I gave the manuscript to Sherrington and, on recovering it, said: "I am sure there must be inhibition in the retina; after all, there is the off-effect when light is turned off, so strikingly like reflex rebound – and have we ever heard of a nervous center without inhibition? But I cannot see how one will ever be able to prove it." Sherrington's reply was: "Don't you worry! After a couple of years you will prove it yourself." I went away skeptical, but he was right, and this is the way it came about.

On my return to the Physiological Institute in Helsingfors, with an Australian co-worker, H. A. Riddell, I began analyzing the ERG of the frog from various points of view (GRANIT and RIDDELL 1934), and then rediscovered the negative dip in the ERG obtained by a flash on the positive off-effect. This, I then found, had been seen previously by EINTHOVEN and JOLLY (1908). We used it to plot the return to the baseline of the negative PIII by measuring its magnitude at different intervals of reillumination. The obvious question then was: Since the positive off-effect coincided with excitation in the optic nerve, would the negative dip coincide with inhibition? I sat down to build a condenser-coupled amplifier, and with Therman (GRANIT and THERMAN 1934, 1935) started leading off the mass discharge from the optic nerve. And there it was, the inhibition! Thrilled to the core I went on repeating this experiment an endless number of times, anxious not to make a mistake on what I held to be a fundamental issue: (a) Can light inhibit as well as excite? and (b) Are inhibition and excitation associated with opposite changes of potential?

At about that time I was appointed Professor of Physiology with the responsibility of teaching in the Swedish language (as deputy in 1935, permanently from 1937). Several of the young Swedish-speaking medical students willingly turned up to have some experience of laboratory work. Although I had a very good time with them, none of them knew much physiology. I therefore felt lonely, having been spoilt abroad by the company of friends many of whom were in the course of making their mark on science. The trusting Rockefeller Foundation generously gave me a substantial grant, and I certainly had plenty of plans up my sleeve, yet at the same time felt the need for someone critical to consult while proceeding on my lonely path to advance retinal neurology.

E. Dark and Light Adaptation

Dark and light adaptation at the time were thought of merely in terms of regeneration and bleaching of rhodopsin, but I – doubting Thomas – found HECHT's (1931 a) purely photochemical explanation too good to be true. Hecht, of course, was equally skeptical about my line of approach to the retina, and would not admit to any major significance of the retinal nervous center. Once, in 1930, while I was walking with him outside the Columbia University buildings, the talk came round to some experiments on flicker by Frank Allen of Winnipeg, and Hecht said: "The fool, he even thinks there is inhibition in the retina!" My reply then was: "For all we know there may well be." Much later, when I had a chance of studying adaptation at Helsingfors, it became possible to produce clear-cut evidence in favour of nonphotochemical processes involved in sensitizing the eye to light and darkness.

Firstly, the ERG of the thoroughly dark-adapted frog eye left exposed to a bright intermittent light was found to undergo striking transformations (GRANIT and RIDDELL 1934). The eye began by tolerating only very low rates of flicker, to which it responded with b waves. Gradually, its properties altered so that each intermittent flash elicited an increasingly larger negative a wave followed by a small b wave. At the same time the eye started responding with this kind of a–b flicker to increasingly faster rates of intermittent stimulation. This seemed to me inexplicable without assuming that light adaptation produced some kind of redistribution of excitation and inhibition in the retinal nervous center. It now became necessary to take a look at the bleaching and regeneration of rhodopsin.

Dark adaptation of well light-adapted frog eyes was next studied at the Helsingfors Institute by ZEWI (1939). Thus research was based on extracting rhodopsin from batches of frog eyes from animals which had been in the dark for varying lengths of time, making use of the digitonin technique of TANSLEY (1931). Zewi acquired a considerable degree of skill in handling this technique accurately, and so we were able to start comparing size of the ERG b wave with measured densities of rhodopsin. Our first finding was striking (GRANIT et al. 1938); when rhodopsin solutions were exposed in our Tutton monochromator to monochromatic light within a number of physiologically relevant wavelengths, their reduction in density was negligible, averaging 1%, whereas the b wave of the opened frog eyes, exposed to the same stimuli, underwent a large reduction in size. For confirmation with modern techniques, see DONNER and REUTER (1976).

This now forgotten experiment was the first attempt ever to relate retinal processing of a stimulus to an objectively measured photochemical indicator of the same event. It was followed up in a second study (GRANIT et al. 1939) on frog and cat eyes in which, after adaptation to a strong light, regeneration of rhodopsin in the dark was correlated with the growing size of the b wave. It turned out that the b wave did not start to grow in parallel with rhodopsin concentration until the latter had reached about 50% of its maximum. An intermediate process of some kind had to be postulated to explain the delayed rise of the b wave. We suggested alternatives: a reorganization required in the neural layers or the possible need for the rhodopsin molecules to form an excitable structure with the receptor membrane. The experiments with Riddell agreed better with the first alternative.

There have since been many interpretations of "the intermediate processes." I refer to LYTHGOE (1940), RUSHTON (1962), BARTLETT (1965), DOWLING (1977), and VIRSU (1978). For those who believe that everything can now be understood, let me quote Rushton: "[Why is it that] removal of some 10% of the [rhodopsin] molecules will incapacitate rods to the verge of blindness?"

F. Localization of ERG Components

I have no intention of reviewing all the experiments of my visual period. My selection will be restricted to some results and conclusions which, in spite of being rooted in the modes of thinking of that time, nevertheless also opened some forward-looking perspectives. Perhaps this could be said about the attempts to localize the components of the ERG, as finally elaborated in my monograph of 1947. Thus PI was found to have no counterpart in the discharge of impulses in the optic nerve and for several reasons was "localized early in the chain of events initiated by stimulation of rod receptors." The ganglion cells could be excluded from participation in the ERG by backfiring into them without causing any changes in the ERG. The excitatory "PII originates somewhere in the neural pathways between the receptors and the ganglion cells." As to the inhibitory PIII, there was "some reason for placing it in the receptors themselves," but if this was done "we must believe that PIII differs from all the other isolated receptor potentials hitherto discovered with respect to its electrical sign." PIII was found to precede PII and differed from PII in not being obliterated by depolarizing agent. "It is probable that PIII might turn out to be made up of two components, one localized in the neural structures, the other in the receptors."

These quotations are taken from my monograph of 1947, virtually completed in 1943, but delayed in publication by the war. It is hardly necessary for me to review developments in this field, based on intraretinal and intracellular recording, as Tomita, a pioneer in both these techniques, is contributing to this volume.

Despite Tigerstedt's timely warning, an old interest made me take up color vision, at first with the spectrum of the Tutton monochromator, later on with a more elaborate colorimeter designed by my friend W. D. Wright of Imperial College, London. At least at some stage I must have been aware of the risks, as according to RUSHTON (1977): "Long ago Granit warned me "Color is the *femme fatale* of vision. When once seduced, you will never be a free man again." I was indeed seduced ..." Nevertheless, in 1977 he could look back upon highly successful experimental attacks on the trichromatic primaries and on color blindness, two subjects perfectly handled in terms of classic psychophysics by WRIGHT (1929, 1946).

G. The First Microelectrodes: The Response to Spectral Lights

When I took up color reception, HECHT (1931 b) had shown that several well-known properties of color vision could be quantitatively accounted for by assuming the existence of three nearly identical primaries (spectral absorption curves) whose small differences emerged as ripples along their contours. These minor differences sufficed to take care of color specificities. Though stuck together in a most plausible manner, the theory failed to convince. We (GRANIT and WREDE 1937) soon had results with the b wave of the frog's ERG demanding "a minimum of three types of fiber: (I) fibers connected with rods containing visual purple (sc. rhodopsin), (II) rods (or cones) containing a substance absorbing in the blue and violet part of the spectrum, (III) cones." The latter, in strong light adaptation, shifted their maximum toward the red wavelengths. These findings are well understood today (cf. DONNER and REUTER (1976).

Hartline and I had been corresponding after I had left Penna and so, in 1938, I was well aware of his success in isolating single units by dissecting optic nerve fibers radiating into the "blind spot" (HARTLINE 1935, 1938). While greatly admiring his skill, patience, and results, I was not prepared to take up color reception on these terms. Clearly, however, the next step did require high isolation, preferably of both light source and recording. I happened to know that Svaetichin in the nearby anatomy building was engaged in tissue culture work with single cells and intended to record, or possibly had recorded, from them by microelectrodes. These were pulled out in glass tubes provided with a core of silver wire, the two components melting at about the same temperature in the flame.

For microillumination Svaetichin pulled out glass rods into a fine tip and coated the outside with a layer of silver reflecting the light from the Tutton monochromator internally to the tip. Soon specially purified glass was obtained from Zeiss for the rods. The silver coating was covered with a fixative. Armed with these gadgets and two micromanipulators I went to work. The results were published in *Uppsala Läkareförenings Förhandlingar* (GRANIT and SVAETICHIN 1939, pp. 1–4), the journal that had seen Holmgren's first description of the electrical response of the eye to light. As this journal has a small circulation and the results have mostly been quoted and misquoted secondhand, I will at this point deviate from my general plan of avoiding experimental detail and give a description of the actual experiment to show how it differed from its numerous progeny.

The eyes of light-adapted frogs were excised and opened in bright light and placed under the microscope, where they were illuminated till the final arrangements were completed. The sensitivity of the eye in the dark increased rapidly to a semistationary level, so that the initial values had to be discarded. Then followed a period of stationary or slowly increasing sensitivity lasting for some 15 min, during which the experiment had to be run. It proved necessary to exclude incipient dark adaptation by comparing values for a long and a short wavelength. Exposures followed at half-minute intervals. In the fully light-adapted eyes most units discharged at "off." Many units underwent a Purkinje shift during dark adaptation. In a few cases units stayed permanently light-adapted. It proved easy to match the illuminating pipette to a discharging site that was heard rattling in the loudspeaker. This done, the pipette could be stuck into the retina deep enough not to leave any visible halo. The threshold could then be determined by adjusting calibrated wedges until the site became silent. In the light-adapted frog eye the threshold was unexpectedly precise, as since noted by others. We concluded that isolated spikes came from nerve fibers because often there was a considerable distance between the illuminated spot and the site recorded from. A less well isolated discharge was likely by the threshold criterion to be restricted to the most sensitive component.

Later, in Stockholm, when the retina of mammals was studied. Rushton (1949) had evidence for localizing its large well-isolated spike to the large ganglion cells. However, the same electrode gave equally good spikes when applied directly onto the dorsal roots of the spinal cord of the cat (Skoglund 1942; Granit and Skoglund 1943). Which alternative is right for the retina may not be ascertainable.

For details of spectral slit width in relation to energy control, the calibration of the neutral filters in different wavelengths, color temperature of the lamp, and stability of the energy supply from its batteries, I must refer the reader to the original paper.

I was very much intrigued by the results because often the distribution curves of spectral sensitivity were very narrow. Some were provided with two or three narrow peaks. The summits tended to be in three regions, blue, red, and green. Complex curves could, of course, be ascribed to insufficient isolation. Perhaps I should remind the reader of the fact that in 1939 only the rhodopsin absorption curve was known, the recently determined values of which I had obtained in a letter from R. J. Lythgoe. Dartnall's (1953) nomograms for absorption curves arrived 14 years later. However, it became impossible to pursue these experiments. The Russian bombardment of Helsingfors interfered, and even my limited experience as a physician was needed and put to use elsewhere.

In 1940, after the "winter war," I was invited to Harvard and Stockholm, almost simultaneously. At this critical time there were many reasons for choosing Stockholm, where I then remained at Karolinska Institute until my retirement in 1967.

It seemed natural to continue the study of the retinal spikes with the big Wright colorimeter, at least for a while. My first task became to improve the microelectrodes, because the silver-in-glass type was shortlived and often noisy. In Stockholm my standard microelectrode became a 25-µ gauge platinum wire stuck into the capillary end of a glass tube sealed off by heating. The protruding wire was then cut close to the tip and frog eyes were used for selecting the best ones from those of a batch. The electrode was not very "micro" by present standards, but was a serviceable innovation in those days.

The restriction of my experience to frogs was a limitation that had to be overcome, and I therefore started to use whatever animals were available in war time. The major findings of those experiments can be very briefly summarized.

In light-adapted rats it proved possible to demonstrate the existence of two narrow-banded spectral distributions, one in 500-nm green, the other in 600-nm red. Green (1971), studying the rat eye 30 years later, said: "This led [Granit] to the hypothesis that cones filled with visual purple and cones with a long wavelength sensitive pigment were connected to a common channel which mediated the light-adapted response. These notions are consistent with the findings reported here" (by him). In the cone eye of the grass snake (*Tropidonotus*), a 560-nm broad-band response of the type I called "dominator" was described, as also was a quite constant narrow-band 600-nm "modulator" that often occurred together with a green 520-nm hump or peak.

The mixed eye of the frog was taken up again on the basis of a larger material, this time discarding microillumination. The frog's photopic dominator agreed with that of the snake's pure cone eye. Narrow curves of modulator type were obtained in three regions: 500–600 nm, 520–540 nm, and 450–470 nm. The blue modulator band was the most interesting new finding because it had adaptive properties different from those of rhodopsin rods. It dark-adapted at much faster rates, as was shown when it was recorded in parallel with the latter, that is, alternating responses to 450 nm and to 500 nm. With blue sensitivity at its maximum its distribution curve appeared as a large hump on that of its rhodopsin partner. It has since been possible to ascribe this prominent "blue response" to the green rods of Schwalbe (DENTON and WYLLIE 1955; DONNER and RUSHTON 1959), as in fact we had already suggested (GRANIT and MUNSTERHJELM 1937) on the basis of ERG work. Rhodopsin and porphyropsin fish (*Cyprinus, Tinca, Anquilla*) and a tortoise (*Testudo*) were studied, as well as mammals such as rats, guinea pigs, and cats. For details I refer to my monograph (GRANIT 1947).

In the end selective adaptation was used with the eye of the cat (GRANIT 1945), in which it had not been possible to obtain narrow bands merely by isolation of spikes. These always produced the photopic dominator 560 nm, which after dark adaptation became a scotopic dominator 500 nm, showing that in the cat, as in frogs and other animals with mixed retinas, rods, and cones fire through the same ganglion cell. But selective adaptation brought out narrow bands of specific color sensitivity. With the improved microelectrodes of today, SAUNDERS (1977) has isolated units in the optic nerve and geniculate body of the cat, and has found color-sensitive ones with maxima at 470, 570, and 600 nm, while MELLO (1968) has shown in well-designed experiments that the cat can be taught to distinguish colors.

H. Wavelength Analysis by Neural Interaction

The psychophysicists who in those days ruled the field were unwilling to accept the existence of spectral distributions of sensitivity narrower than those determined by their data on color mixing based on KÖNIG's (1903) classic trichromatic curves. They seemed to reason as if the three primaries had to be carried to the cortex and there be delivered solely by their equivalents in the receptors. We know today (see below) from work on man and monkeys that narrow-banded peaks like those I found in frogs and snakes and DONNER (1953) found in pigeons are also seen in cortical records.

My problem at the time was to find a convenient method of attacking the question of possible interactions. I had taken a look at the effects of polarization on the retina of the cat and was – as I recall – much excited by finding two easily identifiable spikes, one large, the other small, picked up by the same electrode, the one firing to the anode and inhibited by the cathode, the other responding in an exactly opposite way. Such changes were seen only in on/off units, not in pure on units. Complex effects on the units could thus be obtained by polarization, necessarily involving other layers than the receptors. By combining polarization with spectral analyses, it proved possible to produce narrow color bands undoubtedly dependent on interaction. Having arrived at this point, I realized that my experimentation with color reception had opened up a field the tilling of which would require several lifetimes.

With the papers on polarization I virtually gave up working on the eye, and wrote a final summary in *Ergebnisse der Physiologie* (GRANIT 1950), stating that "the basic evidence for the existence of a neural process of interaction capable of sharpening the colour bands is now definite enough in some types of the experiments described." I was, to say the least, surprised when DE VALOIS (1973), after having found modulator types of curve in the geniculate body of monkeys, pronounced that I had failed to understand that inhibitory interaction could account for the narrow bands of color sensitivity that I had described!

Today it is well understood that the maxima of pigment distributions of spectral sensitivity in the receptors can undergo considerable shifts when recorded by different methods at the cortical level. Thus Sperling and his co-workers (SIDLEY and SPERLING 1967; SPERLING et al. 1968; SPERLING and HARWERTH 1971) have described four peaks located at 450 nm, 530–540 nm, and 610 nm, with sharp dips in between at 480–490 nm and 570–590 nm. They used trained monkeys rewarded for correct responses. The existence of their spectral peaks and dips has been confirmed by PADMOS and NORREN (1975) recording evoked potentials, and the nature of the interactions involved has been analyzed by Sperling and Harwerth.

J. Generator Potentials: Centrifugal Effects

The color experiments did not wholly succeed in suppressing the earlier interest in the role of slow potentials in the retina. The electrotonic spread of a slow wave of depolarization into the optic nerve was an observation that led to the formulation of the theory of generator potentials capable of initiating a discharge in a sensory nerve, now generally accepted. BERNHARD (1942) studied it in *Dytiscus*, and he and I (BERNHARD and GRANIT 1946) experimented on a model for impulse generation by cooling a nerve segment.

Another line of interest took its origin in the discovery (GRANIT and KAADA 1952) that the muscle spindle could be controlled from various sites in the brain. Since Cajal had asserted that there are efferent fibers in the optic nerve, I stimulated the midbrain of the cat stereotactically, searching for evidence of centrifugal effects on the discharge from large ganglion cells of the retina. I had some evidence for such an effect, but more surprising was the finding that repetitive antidromic stimulation of some of those ganglion cells made them fire repetitively for some time afterward, as if the antidromic spikes had succeeded in entering the retina (GRANIT 1955). This observation has since been confirmed by FUKADA (1971). I reviewed the relevant literature in 1978, pointing out that the ganglion cells responding to the antidromic input were to be found within the group of Y cells discovered in the retina by ENROTH-CUGELL and ROBSON (1966). This was my last experimental paper in retinal physiology, a little afterdischarge long delayed.

K. Giving up Working on Retina

I have often been asked why I gave up retinal work in the 1940s and took to motor problems instead. Perhaps this is the right place for an answer. The motives were complex, but one of the major reasons was certainly that I was bored by the color experiments and was well aware of the fact that a scientist – or at least I – must be excited in order to satisfy a *conditio sine qua non,* (necessary condition), which is that he must think of his experiments also between the acts! An equally important consideration was that I had been given a fine institute and a full-time research position. These were great privileges that made it imperative to do something for neurophysiology in a country that was too small to support retinology on such a scale. To contribute to creating a school of neuroscience in Scandinavia seemed to me a chance of a lifetime.

The retina had served me well. It had taught me something about myself, it had given me a great number of friends in many countries, as well as good co-workers capable of doing excellent work in this field; for me the time had come to break away. An old friend, William Rushton, arrived for a sabbatical year in autumn 1948, like myself looking for a fresh opening, and he wholeheartedly went in for vision.

Invited by the *Annual Review of Physiology* to provide an introduction to its 1972 volume, I chose to discuss "discovery and understanding" (GRANIT 1972), and will now confess that I thought of my own visual era in writing:

Young people are out for themselves, to make discoveries, to see something that others have not seen. They may be satisfied with a modicum of analysis because there is always something round the corner to look at – perhaps something new and unexpected, exciting, and important, at any rate a temptation hard to resist.

However, a more fitting end to these remarks on my personal vision than my comments on the youthful beginners in science is a quotation from Ramón y Cajal's autobiography as slightly shortened and reworded by SHERRINGTON (1937) in his review:

It is certain and even desirable that in the course of time my insignificant personality will be forgotten: with it will doubtless perish many of my ideas. In spite of all the blandishments of self-love, the facts associated at first with the name of a particular man end by being anonymous, lost forever in the ocean of Universal Science. The monograph impregnated with individual human quality becomes incorporated, stripped of sentiments, in the abstract doctrine of the general treatise. To the hot sun of actuality will succeed the cold beams of the history of learning.

References

Names containing *von* are alphabetized in this list under *v*

Adrian ED, Matthews R (1927a) The action of light on the eye, part I. The discharge of impulses in the optic nerve and its relation to the electric change in the retina. J Physiol (Lond) 63:378–414

Adrian ED, Matthews R (1927b) The action of light on the eye, part II. The processes in retinal excitation. J Physiol (Lond) 64:279–301

Adrian ED, Matthews R (1928) The action of light on the eye, part III. The interaction of retinal neurones. J Physiol (Lond) 65:273–298

Aubert H (1865) Physiologie der Netzhaut. Morgenstern, Breslau

Bartlett NR (1965) Dark adaptation and light adaptation. In: Graham CH (ed) Vision and visual perception. Wiley & Sons, New York, pp 185–207

Bernhard CG (1942) Isolation of retinal and optic ganglion response in the eye of *Dytiscus*. J Neurophysiol 5:32–48

Bernhard CG, Granit R (1946) Nerve as model temperature end organ. J Gen Physiol 29:257–265

Boll F (1877) Zur Anatomie und Physiologie der Retina. Arch Anat Physiol (Lpz) pp. 4–35

Brown JL (1965) Flicker and intermittent stimulation. In: Graham CH (ed) Vision and visual perception. Wiley, New York, pp 251–320

Creed RS, Granit R (1928) On the latency of negative after-images following stimulation of different areas of the retina. J Physiol (Lond) 66:281–298

Dartnall HJA (1953) The interpretation of spectral sensitivity curves. Br Med Bull 9:24–30

Denton EJ, Wyllie JH (1955) Study of the photosensitive pigments in the pink and green rods of the frog. J Physiol (Lond) 127:81–89

De Valois RL (1973) Central mechanisms of color vision. In: Jung R (ed) Central processing of visual information. Springer, Berlin Heidelberg New York, pp 209–253 (Handbook of sensory physiology, vol VII/3)

Donner KO (1953) The spectral sensitivity of the pigeon's retinal elements. J Physiol (Lond) 122:524–537

Donner KO, Reuter T (1976) Visual pigments and photoreceptor function. In: Llinás R, Precht W (eds) Frog neurobiology. Springer, Berlin Heidelberg New York, pp 251–277

Donner KO, Rushton WAH (1959) Rod-cone interaction in the frog's retina analyzed by the Stiles-Crawford effect and by dark-adaptation. J Physiol (Lond) 149:303–317

Dowling JE (1977) Receptoral and network mechanisms of visual adaptation. Neurosci Res Program Bull 15:397–407

Eccles JC, Gibson WC (1979) Sherrington. His life and thought. Springer, Berlin Heidelberg New York

Einthoven W, Jolly WA (1908) The form and magnitude of the electrical response of the eye to stimulation by light of various intensities. Q J Exp Physiol 1:373–416

Enroth-Cugell C, Robson JG (1966) The contrast sensitivity of retinal ganglion cells of the cat. J Physiol (Lond) 187:517–552

Erlanger J, Gasser HS (1937) Electrical signs of nervous activity. University of Pennsylvania Press, Philadelphia

Fukada Y (1971) Receptive field organization of cat optic nerve fibres with special reference to conduction velocity. Vision Res 11:209–226

Garten S (1906) Über die Veränderungen des Sehpurpurs durch Licht. Albrecht Von Graefes Arch Ophthalmol 63:112–187

Graham CH, Granit R (1931) Comparative studies on the peripheral and central retina: VI, Inhibition, summation, and synchronization of impulses in the retina. Am J Physiol 98:664–673

Granit R (1921) A study on the perception of form. Br J Psychol 12:223–247

Granit R (1927) Über eine Hemmung der Zapfenfunktion durch Stäbchenerregung beim Bewegungsnachbild. Z Sinnesphysiol 58:95–110

Granit R (1930) Comparative studies on the peripheral and central retina. I. On interaction between distant areas in the human eye. Am J Physiol 94:41–50

Granit R (1945) The colour receptors of the mammalian retina. J Neurophysiol 8:197–210

Granit R (1947) Sensory mechanisms of the retina. Oxford University Press, Oxford

Granit R (1950) The organization of the vertebrate retinal elements. Ergeb Physiol 46:31–70

Granit R (1955) Centrifugal and antidromic effects on ganglion cells of retina. J Neurophysiol 18:388–411

Granit R (1966) Charles Scott Sherrington. An appraisal. Nelson, London

Granit R (1972) Discovery and understanding. Annu Rev Physiol 34:1–12

Granit R (1974) Gespräch mit einem Psychologen. Hess Ärztebl 35:938–942

Granit R (1975) Half a century in the neurosciences: personal comments on choices and decisions. In: Worden FG, Swazey FG, Adelman JP (eds) The neurosciences: paths of discovery. The MIT Press, Cambridge, pp 323–332

Granit R (1978) The significance of antidromic potentiation and induced activity in the retina. Med Biol 56:44–51

Granit R, Harper P (1930) Comparative studies on the peripheral and central retina. Am J Physiol 95:211–228

Granit R, Kaada BR (1952) Influence of stimulation of central nervous structures on muscle spindles in cat. Acta Physiol Scand 27:130–160

Granit R, Munsterhjelm A (1937) The electrical responses of dark-adapted frogs' eyes to monochromatic stimuli. J Physiol (Lond) 88:436–458

Granit R, Riddell LA (1934) The electrical responses of light- and dark-adapted frogs' eyes to rhythmic and continuous stimuli. J Physiol (Lond) 81:1–28

Granit R, Skoglund CR (1943) Accommodation and the autorhythmic mechanism in single sensory fibres. J Neurophysiol 6:337–348

Granit R, Svaetichin G (1939) Principles and technique of the electrophysiological analysis of colour reception with the aid of microelectrodes. Upsala Läkarefören. Förh (Ny följd) 45:161–177

Granit R, Therman PO (1934) Inhibition of the off-effect in the optic nerve and its relation to the equivalent phase of the retinal response. J Physiol (Lond) 81:47P–48P

Granit R, Therman PO (1935) Excitation and inhibition in the retina and in the optic nerve. J Physiol (Lond) 83:359–381

Granit R, Wrede CM (1937) The electrical responses of light-adapted frogs' eyes to monochromatic stimuli. J Physiol (Lond) 89:239–256

Granit R, Holmberg T, Zewi M (1938) On the mode of action of visual purple on the rod cell. J Physiol (Lond) 94:430–440

Granit R, Munsterhjelm A, Zewi M (1939) The relation between concentration of visual purple and the retinal sensitivity to light during dark adaptation. J Physiol (Lond) 96:31–44

Green DG (1971) Light adaptation in the rat retina: evidence for two receptor mechanisms. Science 174:598–600

Hartline HK (1935) Impulses in single optic nerve fibres of the vertebrate retina. Am J Physiol 113:59P

Hartline HK (1938) The response of single optic nerve fibers of the vertebrate eye to illumination of the retina. Am J Physiol 121:400–415

Hartline HK (1974) Studies on excitation and inhibition in the retina. A collection of papers from the laboratories of H. Keffer Hartline. Rockefeller University Press, New York

Hecht S (1931 a) Die physikalische Chemie und die Physiologie des Sehaktes. Ergeb Physiol 32:243–390

Hecht S (1931 b) The interrelation of various aspects of color vision. J Opt Soc Am 21:615–639

Hering E (1891) Untersuchung eines total Farbenblinden. Pflügers Arch Gesamte Physiol 49:563–608

Hering E (1925) Grundzüge der Lehre vom Lichtsinn. Gräfe-Sämisch Handb Gesamte Augenheilk 3(12):1–294

Kohlrausch A (1922) Untersuchungen mit farbigen Schwellenprüflichtern über den Dunkeladaptationsverlauf des normalen Auges. Pflügers Arch Ges Physiol 196:113–117

König A (1903) Gesammelte Abhandlungen zur physiologischen Optik. Barth, Breslau

Köttgen E, Abelsdorff G (1896) Absorption und Zersetzung des Sehpurpurs bei den Wirbeltieren. Z Psychol Physiol Sinnesorg 12:161–184

Kühne W (1877–1878) Zur Photochemie der Netzhaut. Unters Physiol Inst Heidelb 1:1–15

Liddell EGT, Sherrington CS (1924) Reflexes in response to stretch (myotatic reflexes). Proc R Soc Lond [Biol] 96:212–242

Lythgoe RJ (1940) The mechanism of dark adaptation. Br J Ophthalmol 24:21–43

Mello NK (1968) Color generalization in cat following discrimination training on achromatic intensity and on wavelength. Neuropsychol 6:341–354

Padmos P, Norren DV (1975) Increment spectral sensitivity and colour discrimination in the primate, studied by means of grated potentials from the striate cortex: Vision Res 15:1103–1113

Parinaud H (1898) La vision. Étude physiologique. Doin, Paris

Parsons JH (1927) Theory of perception. Cambridge University Press, Cambridge

Ramón y Cajal S (1894) Die Retina der Wirbeltiere. Bergmann, Wiesbaden

Ramón y Cajal S (1937) Recollections of my life. Americian Philosophical Society, Philadelphia

Rushton WAH (1949) The structure responsible for action potential spikes in the cat's retina. Nature 164:743–744

Rushton WAH (1962) Visual pigments in man. Liverpool University Press, Liverpool

Rushton WAH (1977) In: Some memories of visual research in the past 50 years. The pursuit of nature. Informal essays on the history of physiology. Cambridge University Press, Cambridge

Saunders R McD (1977) The spectral responsiveness and the temporal frequency responses (TFR) of cat optic tract and lateral geniculate neurons: sinusoidal stimulation studies. Vision Res 17:285–292

Schaternikow M (1902) Über den Einfluß der Adaptation auf die Erscheinung des Flimmerns. Z Psychol Physiol Sinnesorg 29:241–255

Schultze M (1867) Über Stäbchen und Zapfen in der Retina. Arch Mikr Anat 3:215–247

Sherrington CS (1906) The integrative action of the nervous system. Yale University Press, New Haven

Sherrington CS (1937) Scientific endeavour and inferiority complex. Nature [Suppl] 140:617–619

Sherrington CS (1946) The endeavour of Jean Fernel. Cambridge University Press, Cambridge

Sidley NA, Sperling HG (1967) Photopic spectral sensitivity in the rhesus monkey. J Opt Soc Am 57:816–818

Skoglund CR (1942) The response to linearly increasing currents in mammalian motor and sensory nerves. Acta Physiol Scand 4 [Suppl 12]

Sperling HG, Harwerth RS (1971) Red-green cone interactions in the increment-threshold spectral sensitivity of primates. Science 182:180–184

Sperling HG, Sidley NA, Dockens WS, Jolliffe CL (1968) Increment-threshold spectral sensitivity of the rhesus monkey as a function of the spectral composition of the background field. J Opt Soc Am 58:263–268

Tansley K (1931) The regeneration of visual purple: its relation to dark adaption and night blindness. J Physiol (Lond) 71:442–458

Virsu V (1978) Retinal mechanisms of visual adaptation and afterimages. Med Biol 56:84–96

von Kries J (1929) Zur Theorie des Tages- und Dämmerungssehens. Handb Norm Pathol Physiol 12(1):679–713

Wright WD (1929) A re-determination of the trichromatic mixture data. Spec Rep Ser Med Res Counc Lond 139

Wright WD (1946) Researches on normal and defective colour vision. Kimpton, London

Zewi M (1939) On the regeneration of visual purple. Acta Soc Sci Fenn N.S.B. 2(4)

CHAPTER 11

Taste Electrophysiology, Sensory Coding, and Behavior

CARL PFAFFMANN

A. How I Got Started in Research

As in the case of many other scientists, I can trace the beginnings of my interest and actual laboratory work largely to one individual, the late Leonard Carmichael, who was Professor and Director of the Laboratory of Psychology and Sensory Physiology at Brown University from 1927 to 1936. As an undergraduate at Brown University, the first of my family of any generation to attend a university, I found the academic environment a new and exciting experience. My father, the son of German immigrants, had little formal education, but was moderately successful in business. The prospects of following in his footsteps did not attract me, but he never discouraged me or tried to influence my decision as I became more and more inclined toward an academic career. Midway through my undergraduate period, I decided finally to become a professor and considered majoring in mathematics or possibly American history, the latter largely because of a very stimulating young professor. Then I took Leonard Carmichael's introductory psychology course, and found the subject that really aroused my interest. Psychology at Brown University was treated as a life science in a department with a strong biological approach. The undergraduate courses did include a broad range of psychological topics (mental testing, personality, and abnormal psychology, etc.), but the research emphasis was biological (e.g., sensory processes and psychophysics, the mechanisms of learning and conditioning, brain and behavior interrelations). My undergraduate academic record was quite good, and after I had earned nearly all A's in most introductory and intermediate psychology courses, Carmichael invited me to enroll in the Honors program. This permitted me to participate in graduate seminars while still an undergraduate, and to conduct a number of research projects in addition to that for an Honors thesis. Carmichael personally supervised most of the Honors students, and in discussing a choice of research, he observed that the sensory psychology and physiology of taste was a neglected and almost forgotten field. The basic findings had been made in the classic period of the German psychophysicists, and included subjects such as the distribution of sensitivity across the tongue surface using punctate stimulation; the effect of various blocking agents, such as gymnemic acid, on sweetness; and the analysis of basic taste qualities and their reduction to just four: salt, sour, bitter, and sweet. As late as the 1930s, one notable advance by Helmut Hahn in Germany had been the development of the *Geschmackslupe* (taste microscope), a glass chamber that could be held in place over a circumscribed area on the human tongue. Solutions flowing through a system of tubes provided accurate information on area, time, and temperature of stimulation. His psychophysical studies of adaptation were classic (Hahn 1943, 1949). The anatomists and physiologists had described the taste buds and some of the neural pathways for taste. The zoologist G. H. Parker (1912, 1922), and subsequently Crozier (1934), had studied the sense of taste and the common chemical sense in animals and other lower organisms in an effort to determine the mechanism and kinetics of taste stimulation. C. J. Herrick (1903, 1905) had carried out his epic-making behavioral experiments of taste in fish and described the taste pathways of the fish brain, in particular – not only the primary synaptic relays of the nucleus tractus solitarius of the medulla, but their cephalic projections to the secondary gustatory nucleus in the parabrachial brain stem. From here the major projection is to the ventral diencephalon, the inferior lateral lobe, a homolog of the mammalian hypothalamus. Herrick's classic work was the forerunner of the very contemporary findings in my laboratory on taste brain stem neuroanatomy and physiology of mammals (Norgren and Leonard 1973; Norgren and Pfaffmann 1975). Considerably earlier, after beginning his research with me, Robert Benjamin (Benjamin and Pfaffmann 1955) subsequently worked out the medullary thalamocortical circuitry (reviewed by Burton and Benjamin 1971). Such previous studies relied on procedures that were, in a sense, indirect, depending on behavioral responses of an animal or psychophysical and verbal reports of human subjects. But the new method of sensory electrophysiology had come of age in the 1920s, epitomized by Adrian's (1928) classic, *The Basis of Sensation*. Here at last was a direct method by which one could tap in on the electrical impulse traffic in the sensory nerves from end organs. Adrian (1926, 1927), Adrian and Bronk (1928, 1929), and Adrian and Zotterman (1926a, b) showed that the intensity of sensation and movement was coded in the frequency of discharge in individual afferent and motor nerve fibers. The stronger the stimulus and sensation, the higher the frequency; the quality of sensation was determined by which sense organ, and hence which nerve fiber, had been activated. At about the same time in the United States, Erlanger and Gasser (1937) had recorded the mixed elevations in the nerve trunk action potentials and showed that the different elevations of the compound action potential of a mixed sensory nerve reflected the responses of fibers of different diameters with different conduction velocities. It was presumed that different modalities of cutaneous sensation were mediated by different groups of fibers of different sizes. Thus the quality of sensation appeared specifiable in physiological and anatomical terms. This new technology ultimately provided the means of recording from the sense organs themselves, as well as their afferent nerves and the sensory brain centers.

The first senses to be examined, of course, were vision, hearing, the cutaneous senses, proprioception, and later vestibular apparatus. The chemical senses, however, especially gustation, were not attacked until relatively late. Adrian's (1953) work on the olfactory nerves and the olfactory bulb did not come until the 1950s, and he himself never studied the gustatory apparatus. As a graduate student at Brown, my first research efforts in the sense of taste employed psychophysical methods. My first publication in the *American Journal of Psychology* (PFAFFMANN 1935) was a methodological study of difference thresholds (just-noticeable difference) in taste in humans using the method of single stimuli. This method was developed in the 1930s by a number of investigators, including Glen Wever of Princeton who later achieved fame in the Wever and Bray experiments on electrophysiology of auditory sensation. Lester F. Beck, then a young assistant professor at Brown, suggested I try the new single-stimulus method on taste. There was a pragmatic basis for this research because the method of single stimuli eliminated the so-called standard stimulus for comparison, thus reducing the number of chemical stimuli applied to one-half. I vividly recall presenting my first scientific paper at a New York University meeting of the Eastern Psychological Association in 1935. The well-known psychologist and psychophysicist Samuel Fernberger, of the University of Pennsylvania, was Chairman of the session. At the conclusion of my paper, there was a long, dead silence, whereupon Fernberger undertook a laudatory appreciation of my study and its significance. I was forever grateful to him for his kind words of encouragement at that early stage in my career. My other taste research was stimulated by Leonard Carmichael's ongoing study of the ontogeny of sensory function in fetal and newborn cats. I conceived the idea of determining whether newborn kittens could, in fact, respond differentially to taste stimuli. By fitting a small toy nursing bottle with a hydraulic system to activate a kymograph recording lever, I was able to determine how much normal sucking of dilute milk was disrupted by the injection of acid, bitter, or salt stimuli into the nursing bottle. Sugar solutions facilitated sucking. The newborn kittens' clear differential responses showed taste to be functional at birth (PFAFFMANN 1936).

Also important for my subsequent career was the arrival of Herbert Jasper as a member of the Brown Psychology Department and as Director of the psychology laboratory at the neighboring Bradley Home for disturbed children. Working with Leonard Carmichael, Jasper's main interest was developing methods and procedures for studying human electroencephalograms (EEGs) (JASPER and CARMICHAEL 1935). Berger had just published his epic study of human brain wave recording. Many investigators the world over quickly followed up his amazing finding that human EEGs could be recorded in normal waking subjects merely by electrodes fastened to the outside of the scalp. Here was a noninvasive way of tapping the electrical activity of the human brain. As a graduate student in need of support in the summer months, I worked as an assistant, along with my graduate school roommate Karl U. Smith, helping Jasper develop one of the earliest human EEG laboratories in the United States at Bradley. Having a good alpha rhythm, I often served as a subject.

Jasper's laboratory was also well equipped for general electrophysiology, and he encouraged me to use it after hours to record action potentials in the frog's dorsal cutaneous nerve when chemicals were applied to the frog's skin. ADRIAN et al. (1931) had found two classes of nerve fiber in the dorsal cutaneous nerves: one with a large spike and rapid conduction velocity activated by tactile stimuli, the second of lower spike amplitude with a slower conduction velocity, activated by acetic acid. I examined the response of these nerves to solutions flowing over the skin by means of a *Geschmackslupe* and reported my findings at another Eastern Psychological Meeting. While a student at Brown, I also carried out a number of other research projects; one was on conditioning the knee jerk in psychotic and manic depressive patients under Harold Schlosberg's direction. This was one of the earlier experiments in experimental psychopathology (PFAFFMANN and SCHLOSBERG 1936). We found systematic differences in the conditionability of psychotic patients and other aberrations in their conditioning process upon which subsequent investigators further elaborated. The important point about my undergraduate and master's degree years at Brown was that I lived in a vital, growing Department with young, active faculty and graduate students who were all committed to research. The lights were lit every night; Leonard Carmichael and the other faculty members often joined us in those long exciting days in the laboratory.

The great breakthrough in my academic career came when Carmichael urged me to apply for a Rhodes Scholarship. At that time, there was no formal Psychology Department or psychology instruction at Oxford University except for the Wilde Readership in mental philosophy, a position which enjoined any empirical investigation. However, since I had had little formal training in physiology, it was entirely in keeping with my now established interest in physiological psychology to read for the BA in physiology at Oxford as an undergraduate. I knew that the Rhodes Scholarships could be extended for a third year at Oxford or elsewhere, so I had in mind taking my third year in Adrian's laboratory at Cambridge. My tutor at New College, Oxford was Richard S. Creed, one of the few sensory physiologists of the Sherrington School. He was very helpful, not only as a tutor but in introducing me to Adrian at the appropriate time for his sponsorship of my dissertation research on taste electrophysiology.

B. The Setting for Taste Electrophysiology in 1937

There had been a few beginnings in the electrophysiology of taste by other workers. HOAGLAND (1933) had recorded taste impulses in the barbel nerves of catfish, the external body surface of which is richly endowed with taste buds. The impulses initiated by chemicals were relatively small compared to those aroused by tactile stimulation of the same region. PUMPHREY (1935) had recorded impulses in the nerves from the frog's palate in response to salts and acids. BARRON (1936) had reported similar observations in the cat, and ZOTTERMAN (1935) had recorded the temperature and tactile and other modalities, as well as taste, from the cat chorda tympani and lingual nerves. In the cat, as in catfish, taste impulses were of relatively small size compared to those elicited by touch, thus indicating a specificity of the nerve fiber type carrying taste information. There was thus not much doubt that different sensory modalities, that is, taste versus touch, hearing versus vision, proprioception versus skin sensation, carried impulses specific to their own sensory modality.

The question of receptor specificity and sensations had been dominated by Johannes MÜLLER's (1830) concept of "the specific energies of nerves" *The quality of the perceived sensation resides not in the stimulus but in the nerve stimulated.* Pressure against the skin is felt as touch; pressure against the eyeball is perceived as light. In 1811 Sir Charles Bell, writing about the four kinds of papillae on the tongue, noted:

> Of these, the papillae of one kind form the seat of the sense of taste; the other papillae (more numerous and smaller) resemble the extremities of the nerves in the common skin, and are the organs of touch in the tongue. When I take a sharp steel point and touch one of these papillae, I feel the sharpness. The sense of touch informs me of the shape of the instrument. When I touch a papilla of taste, I have no sensation similar to the former. I do not know that a point touched the tongue, but I am sensible of a metallic taste, and the sensation passes backward on the tongue.
>
> (Bell 1811; cited by CRANEFIELD 1974)

SCHIFF (1867) found that when the epidermis of the tongue had been removed by a blister, the applications of solutions of sugar, quinine sulphate, or citric acid, gave rise to quite different sensations which bore no resemblance to taste.

Beyond the specificity of the different modalities, however, lay the question of whether different qualities of sensation were mediated by specific nerve fibers and sense organs. In fact, Hermann von Helmholtz, the great genius of nineteenth-century German physics, physiology, and psychology of perception, believed that the different qualities of sensation resulted from activities in specifically different receptors and nerves. The Young–Helmholtz theory of vision postulated three different color receptors, red, blue, and green, each sensitive to its particular region of the spectrum. All color experience could be produced by color mixture, i.e., various ratios and combinations of activity of each these three basic color receptors. In hearing, von Helmholtz postulated that different tonal experiences depended on which part of the ear and, therefore, which particular nerve fibers from basilar membrane receptors of the ear were activated, low tones stimulating at the apex and high tones at the base.

Early classification of taste sensations in the eighteenth century tended toward multiplicity. Linnaeus (BORING 1942) enumerated 11 categories: sweet, acid, astringent, sharp, viscous, fatty, bitter, insipid, aqueous, saline, and nauseous. Other equally long lists nearly always agreed with the inclusion of salt, sour, bitter, and sweet. Such other terms as sharp, harsh, pungent, and aromatic were attributed to combinations of pain, touch, or odor. There was more debate about the status of alkaline and metallic. Alkaline, a mixture of bitter, sweet, and general sensibility, was also said to have an odor component. Metallic was attributed to a mixture of sour, bitter, and odor. By 1893, WUNDT in his *Grundzüge der physiologischen Psychologie* called alkaline and metallic doubtful, thus reducing the basic list to four: salt, sour, sweet, and bitter.

A most important finding in support of specificity within the subqualities of taste was the report that masticating the leaves of an Indian herb, *Gymnema sylvestre,* completely abolished perception of sweetness (FALCONER 1847). HOOPER (1887) reported that the sensations of sweet and bitter were entirely removed, but SHORE (1892) reported the action to be more intense for sweet, less for bitter, slight for salt, and nil for acid. More recent studies with gymnemic acid have indicated that the effect is largely upon sweetness; the effect on bitterness is due to adaptation of bitterness by other components in the crude extract. The specific blocking effects of other agents like cocaine, stovaine, and so on, although acting differentially on the different qualities, were not so striking as the case of gymnema, which even to-

Table 1. Responses of 989 gustatory papillae

	Responding	Exclusively
Sour	91	12
Sweet	79	3
Bitter	71	0
Sweet and sour	72	12
Bitter and sour	67	7
Sweet, bitter, and sour	60	0

day remains one of the strongest instances of a differential blockade of a specific taste quality.

SHORE (1892) and KIESOW (1894), by locally stimulating the surface of the tongue, reported that the tip was most sensitive to sweet, the sides to acid, and the base to bitter; sensitivity to salt was more or less equal over the whole surface, while the dorsum was insensitive to all. HÄNIG (1901) more thoroughly examined the areal distribution of taste threshold values along a series of parallel "isochymes" on the tongue surface. Sensitivity to sweet was greatest at the tip of the tongue and least at the base, but also decreased from the edge to the center. Bitter sensitivity is maximal in the region of the circumvallate papillae and minimal at the tip of the tongue. Note that Hänig did not say that the tip of the tongue was insensitive, but that it could in fact detect all four qualities, although the region of maximal sensitivity differed for the different qualities. Taste substances with more than one quality taste differently on different parts of the tongue. For example, bromo-saccharin tastes sweet at the apex and bitter at the base, while sodium sulfate tastes salty on the tip and bitter at the base.

The early histological investigations of LOVÉN (1868) and SCHWALBE (1867) showed that each taste bud in humans consisted of modified epithelial cells clustered together in a pear-shaped organ 70–80 µm in length and 40 µm wide. Two kinds of cell were described: (a) the supporting cells forming a compact layer at the edge of the organ, and (b) the gustatory cells with smaller nuclei, somewhat more slender and slightly longer with a peripheral taste hair (now called microvilli), which projected into the taste pore. Direct contact between solutions and the ends of the taste cells is possible through the taste pore. This anatomical arrangement did not permit stimulation of individual taste receptor cells, but only clusters of them. Since the afferent nerve fibers entering the base of the taste bud branch and entwine around the taste cells, an exact one-to-one relation between a single taste cell and an afferent nerve seemed unlikely. Nevertheless, OEHRWALL's (1891) very important work showed that it was possible to stimulate individually the highly vascularized, bright pink, isolated fungiform papillae on the tip of the tongue. Concentrated solutions of sucrose, tartaric acid, sodium chloride, and hydrochloric acid were applied to single papillae by a fine brush, smaller than the papillae themselves. Oehrwall abandoned the use of sodium chloride because the resulting sensations were not distinct enough for his subjects. Individually stimulating 125 papillae, of which 98 elicited sweet, bitter, and sour sensations, he obtained the results shown in Table 1.

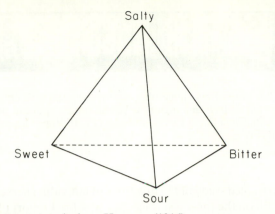

Fig. 1. The Henning taste tetrahedron. HENNING (1916)

KIESOW (1894) extended Oehrwall's work, employing salt solutions as well as the other three, and essentially confirmed Oehrwall's results. Thus some taste papillae react to a single taste, others to two or to three, and still others to all four basic qualities. OEHRWALL (1901) argued that not only were there specifically different receptors for the different basic qualities, these were, in fact, different modalities. Kiesow objected to the interpretation; consequently, a furious academic debate raged between Oehrwall and Kiesow on the nature of the basic taste sensitivities. The demonstration of a number of contrast phenomena across the different qualities led KIESOW (1896) to conclude that the basic tastes were different qualities within a single modality.

HENNING (1916) schematized the relations among taste qualities by a figure (the taste tetrahedron) in which salt, sour, bitter, and sweet appeared as the principal qualities located at the four corners (see Fig. 1). Such tastes as that of potassium iodide lay along the edge between salty and bitter, ammonium chloride between salty and sour. Noting that alkaline lay between sweet and sour, Henning apparently accepted a specificity of taste receptors by attributing this locus to stimulation of both the sweet- and sour-sensing papillae, but he insisted that the result of such stimulation aroused a unified single experience in the taste continuum. Interestingly, modern multidimensional scaling of stimuli traditionally describable by the four basic tastes tends to validate his phenomenological conception. However, the loci of some mixed tastes, such as ammonium chloride and alkaline, do not agree with his original assignment. Alkaline and a number of less familiar amino acids and other nutrients fall outside the tetrahedron, in fact (SCHIFFMAN and ERICKSON 1971). Be that as it may, salt, sour, bitter, and sweet represent important and unique, if not primary, taste sensation qualities for which prototypic stimuli can be found.

C. The Adrian and Bronk Connection

It was against such a background of psychophysical investigations that I embarked on the study of single-unit sensitivities in the cat. My studies during the late 1930s

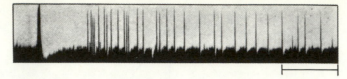

Fig. 2. The first publication of my single-fiber record from the cat's chorda tympani. The large baseline deflection at the beginning of the record signals application of stimulus solution 0.05 N acetic acid. Time line 0.1 s. Pfaffmann (1939). Reproduced by permission of the Cambridge Univ. Press

provided the first detailed study of the functions of individual nerve fibers activated by gustatory stimuli on the tongue surface. My first brief report ("Specific Gustatory Impulses") was presented at a Spring Meeting of the Physiological Society in Oxford, and was based on part of my doctoral dissertation in Adrian's laboratory at Cambridge (1939) (see Fig. 2). Beside studying gustatory afferents from a cat's tongue, I also recorded from the dental nerves of the canine tooth from the upper jaw. These were some of the first recordings from dental nerves. I demonstrated the preparation at a Cambridge meeting of the Physiological Society (1939) and published two papers in the *Journal of Physiology* (Pfaffmann 1939 a, b). A more detailed account of my taste research appeared in the *Journal of Cellular and Comparative Physiology* (Pfaffmann 1941). The chorda tympani nerve of anesthetized cats was exposed by appropriate surgery and single nerve fibers were teased out with needles under a binocular dissecting microscope. I began these studies in order to apply the objective recording procedure to the question of the four basic taste sensitivities for salt, sour, bitter, and sweet. The cat nerve did not respond to sugar, but the response to salt, acid, and bitter proved to be complicated. Acid sensitivity did occur in specific acid-sensitive units (type H) which did not respond to sodium chloride or quinine. However, salt-sensitive units responded both to sodium chloride and acid (type H + N), and quinine-sensitive units responded both to quinine and acid (type H + Q). This was an unexpected finding and led me to conclude that the coding of taste information was not simply due to the activation of one set of specific receptors and their fibers, but involved concomitant activity in the different sets of sensitivities with which the tongue was endowed. Theoretically, sourness could be coded by concurrent activity in all three types of fiber, since acid seemed a common stimulus. Saltiness could be coded by fractional activity of the N + H group only; similarly, bitterness could be coded by the discharge of the Q + H group alone. Thus taste coding was not simply due to specific activity alone, but to the activity of specific groups in relation to the pattern of other fibers concurrently activated. My later studies of gustatory nerve impulses in the rat, cat, and rabbit (Pfaffmann 1955) confirmed these findings and ideas. This led me to formulate what came to be known as the "pattern theory of taste quality," in which a central step was required to decode the total pattern of activity in all active fibers entering the central nervous system in parallel.

I recall that Adrian was very intrigued by these findings. He introduced my dissertation lecture with the observation that such paradoxical findings made my research much more interesting than if they had simply confirmed the earlier classic theories. We shall see that such multiple sensitivity of taste single units has been confirmed by many other investigators, including a number of my students. The latter have extended these ideas significantly, but there still remains a debate within my academic family, so to speak. Some argue that there is more specificity to the basic taste stimuli than first appears on the surface, whereas others argue for an overall pattern theory of sensory coding.

At the time I made these original observations, the classic views in sensory psychology and sensory physiology, especially in audition and cutaneous sensitivity, were under attack. The von Helmholtz theory of auditory perception implied that the specific nerve fibers of different regions of the basilar membrane were tuned to different frequencies, and hence were the mediators of pitch. WEVER and BRAY (1930), however, had made the striking observation that the pattern of electrophysiological discharge in the auditory nerve, fed into a loud speaker, reproduced the auditory signal so well that they could understand what was spoken into the cat's ear. The auditory nerve as a whole seemed capable of conveying the entire range of audible frequencies well up to 20,000 Hz, a frequency far in excess of the frequency-following capability of any one fiber. Their volley principle permitted individual nerve units to fire every other or every third, fourth, etc. cycle as subcomponents of the high frequencies, thus enabling the nerve as a whole to reproduce the entire audible frequency range. Their findings supported the telephone theory of auditory pitch perception (RUTHERFORD 1886), i.e., that the nerve for hearing acted as a telephone cable, the pattern of the nerve response as a whole being necessary for auditory perception. At the same time the sensory psychologist John Paul Nafe was very critical of the classic view that different qualities of cutaneous sensation resulted from activity of specific warm receptors, touch receptors, cold receptors, etc., propounding instead his quantitative theory of feeling. NAFE (1934, p. 1041) wrote:

It is not obviously true that all felt experiences are patterns but psychological analysis has discovered no criterion by which we may always distinguish a complex experience from a simple one. This difficulty has not appeared to be serious because it should be possible by studying the skin and its end organs to determine what types of experiences have separate mechanisms. But this study too has faltered, and after 50 years of investigation, we have no demonstrated correlation between any particular type of sensitivity and the special end organs and fibers that subserve it.

My observations of taste seemed to be in line with these trends. However, with subsequent study, greater technical competence (especially the sophistication of microelectrode unit recording), and better appreciation of the interaction between peripheral and central processes, there has been a swing of the pendulum to a more classic position regarding peripheral specificity and sensory coding in general. For example, GALAMBOS and DAVIS's (1943) tuning curves of individual second-order auditory nerve fibers showed that at lowest threshold intensity each auditory sensory unit responded only to one specific "best frequency," but as stimulus intensity increased, the range of frequencies that could stimulate any one fiber spread both to higher and lower frequencies. However, the best frequency for any particular unit was still apparent by its higher rate of neural discharge, the side bands causing relatively lesser discharges. Yet the work of von BÉKÉSY (1928) showed that at frequencies less than 100 Hz, a wide area of the basilar membrane is involved, so that nearly all nerve fibers will be in synchrony at low pitches. There is the possibility of a dual mechanism, so that at low pitches temporal patterns of auditory discharge may be responsible for discrimination; at higher frequencies specific nerve fibers may be the basis for discriminating different tones. Contemporary theorists of neurobiology (CRICK 1979) have argued more broadly on first principles that in the nervous system as a whole individual sensory channels cannot function in isolation, and that some cross-fiber pattern process must be invoked even in the perception of the simplest sensory quality.

A few personal notes about life in the Cambridge laboratory as a research student might be appropriate at this juncture. In the late 1930 s, graduate students at Cambridge were relatively few in number, the presumption being that an Oxford or Cambridge BA Honors degree would provide a more than ample grounding for most academic disciplines, including physiology. The BA Honors examinations were said to be equivalent to the doctoral preliminary examinations set in American universities. Since Oxford and Cambridge recognized each other's degrees, I was treated as a Cambridge BA, and needed only two years of residence besides research for the thesis. Adrian was still actively engaged in research while serving as Professor of Physiology. Adrian was, for me, mostly a gray streak rushing past my corridor door to and from his laboratory. However, on one occasion he stopped abruptly, because out of the corner of his eye he had seen me fiddling with the Matthews oscillograph. Its optics were such that my photographic records read from right to left instead of left to right, necessitating photographic reversal for publication. I wondered whether this could be corrected, either by mounting the oscillograph upside down or by some other adjustment. I had got only as far as removing the case when I heard a rather anguished "What are you doing? What are you doing? Put it back together." My records continued to read right to left. I think Adrian regarded the Matthews oscillograph with some considerable awe.

Bryan Matthews had designed the oscillograph – a moving iron tongue and mirror – while still a Cambridge undergraduate. Manufactured by the Cambridge Instrument Company, it provided some of the most elegant single unit records published, as in MATTHEWS' (1933) own classic study of muscle afferents. But it was not without its vagaries, especially the sputtering carbon arc light that could go out at some crucial moment in an experiment. Fast photographic emulsions and high actinic cathode ray oscillograph phosphors were to come much later. As Director of Research, Bryan Matthews was most helpful in initiating research students and visiting scientists in the ways of the laboratory. I built my own breadboard single-triode preamplifier from a sketchpad design by Bryan. It had only a slight tendency to self-oscillation, which could be stopped by a well-aimed kick at its shielded celotex box just beneath the recording table. I recall spending nearly four desperate months fruitlessly trying to record taste impulses in the lingual nerve, which remained strangely silent save for tactile or temperature responses. Not until I perfected the surgical approach to the chorda tympani nerve did I begin to have success. It was sink or swim all the way.

Adrian's own laboratory was a very large room across the end of the basement. It contained the most glorious clutter ever seen. For the visitor, Adrian would reach under one of the many tables and bring out some apparatus he and Keith Lucas had used, perhaps a capillary electrometer or an inductorium or rheotome for electrical stimulation. I also recall Adrian's homemade three-dimensional manipulator for frog preparations, essentially a large blob of modeling clay into which glass tubing and silver–silver chloride wire was embedded. The other electrode grounded the preparation. By the time I got there, Adrian's own chicken-wire-screened cage was so riddled with apertures for various mechanical control devices, optical stimulators, camera control handles, etc., that it was almost a non-cage. His moving film camera fed directly into his darkroom, so that by the end of each experiment he had developed the film and frequently made photographic prints of sections of interest. I do not think he pored at length over miles and miles of electrophysiological record, but went right to the heart of the matter, picking out the most interesting and revealing sections. Of course, most of the sense organs which he studied could be stimulated by short bursts of controlled stimulation. In my experiments, the flow of solutions over the tongue tended to give long discharge trains, and I spent many hours laboriously counting single-unit spike records.

In my second year, I was Adrian's assistant in the mammalian physiology course. Only professional licensed scientists were allowed to prepare animals, even for laboratory exercises. My Home Office certification was a most impressive document with a large blue seal and imprimatur. On one occasion, Adrian and I each personally had to prepare a number of spinal animals just before the laboratory period. There were two rows of operating tables; Adrian worked rapidly down one row and I down the other. Although I had a reasonably cordial relationship with Adrian, I did not really get to know him at a very personal level until the later years, when we met from time to time under somewhat more relaxed circumstances: at scientific meetings, at the dedication of the new biophysics laboratory of John Hopkins University, at several International Symposium on Olfaction and Taste meetings, and even at Brown University, which he visited as the leader of a United Kingdom academic delegation. I recall still later the occasion of the celebration of his 70th birthday, a gala gathering of physiologists from all over the world at Cambridge.

During my last year at Cambridge, the clouds of World War II were rapidly gathering. My thesis work was not complete but was well advanced, and I had returned to the United States for the summer of 1938, the summer of the Munich Crisis. I had, in fact, canceled my return steamer reservation until the outcome was clear. "Peace in our time" gave me the opportunity to return for the final year and complete my research and dissertation.

Detlev W. Bronk visited Cambridge during that year. He had worked with Adrian on their classic studies of the single-unit activity in motor nerves, and had elucidated the frequency principle for the control of intensity of muscle contraction, among other things. Adrian introduced me, and in the course of the discussion of my research, Bronk kindly suggested I write to him upon my return to the United States. At that time Bronk was the Director of the Johnson Foundation for Medical Physics at the University of Pennsylvania. Toward the end of the year I wrote to Bronk, and was offered a postdoctoral position. I completed and defended my dissertation in the late spring of 1939, and returned to the United States on the last normal passenger crossing of the French liner *Normandie* before its conversion to wartime service.

The Johnson Foundation was one of the preeminant electrophysiology centers, with Keffer Hartline on vision, Frank Brink on the biophysics of nerve conduction,

Martin Larrabee and Bronk himself on autonomic function and synaptic conduction, plus a host of other up-and-coming younger investigators. I participated in several ongoing projects: one suggested by Frank Brink on conduction in myelinated nerve fibers (PFAFFMANN 1940), another on the effect of pressures and induced pain in peripheral nerves (AIRD and PFAFFMANN 1947), and another on the effect of lead poisoning on nerve function. Thus began my long-term friendship with Bronk and his colleagues, who were later to be my colleagues again at the Rockefeller University when I joined it as a vice-president and professor in 1965.

During the year in Philadelphia, I received several academic offers, including one from Brown University as an instructor in psychology. The distinguished behavioral psychologist Walter S. Hunter, for whom psychology was an objective biological science, was chairman. Though relatively small, the Brown Department under Hunter's leadership was among the distinguished departments of the country. When I went to Brown University in 1940, it was not for long, because World War II had fully burst upon the scene. I joined a volunteer group of psychologists and physiologists on a summer project at the Naval Air Station in Pensacola. Participating were such physiologists as Alexander Forbes, Hallowell Davis, and Hudson Hoagland, who were all interested in the possible correlation of EEG wave patterns with behavior and a possible aid to selecting naval aviators. I worked largely on psychometric and psychophysiological measures. Many of us joined the Naval Reserve. For the years 1942–1945 I became an applied scientist as an aviation psychologist, but I did manage one publishable study on depth perception in flight (PFAFFMANN 1948).

D. 1945 and Beyond

I returned to Brown University in 1945 as an assistant professor and began to pick up the unraveled threads of my teaching and research. A number of my friends and colleagues doing war work had developed a taste for practical work, and had shifted to applied psychology and human engineering. For me, study of the chemical senses still seemed a virgin yet fascinating field, and I decided to return to that enterprise. There was not only the prospect of rounding out knowledge of the electrophysiology of taste, but also the prospect of relating that electrophysiology to behavior (in particular to motivated behavior), and thus fulfilling in some measure the promise of a true physiological psychology.

Taste had interesting significances for ingestive behavior, preference, acceptance, and the pleasures or displeasures of sensation. In the first century BC, Lucretius, in his long didactic poem *De Rerum Natura* (cited by OATES 1940), wrote:

... so you may easily see that the things which are able to affect the senses pleasantly consist of smooth and round elements while all those, on the other hand, that are found to be bitter and harsh are held in connection by particles that are more hooked and for this reason are wont to tear open passages into our senses.

Aristotle observed that the function of the pleasures aroused by taste were nutritive; that is, taste directs the choice of foods and beverages in such a way that pleasant-tasting substances are consumed while unpleasant ones are rejected. Both Aristotle and Plato recognized that some odors appealed because they arise from objects necessary to physiological well-being. Aristotle remarked, "pleasantness and unpleasantness of the odor of food and drink belong to them contingently. These smells are pleasant when we are hungry, but when we are sated and not requiring to eat, they are not pleasant" (Aristotle, cited by Ross 1906). This was one of the earliest statements of what has more recently become a general theory of "alliesthesia," proposed by CABANAC (1971).

Luigi Luciani's book *Human Physiology*, edited by Gordon Holmes, includes the following:

> In daily life we make a distinction between the sapid substances, based on the affective impression they make upon us rather than on the quality of their tastes: thus we discriminate between agreeable, indifferent, insipid, and disagreeable tastes. Agreeable and disagreeable substances excite different expressional movements of the facial muscles; indifferent and insipid substances produce no facial movements, or at most arouse an expression of indifference or slight disgust. These reactions may be considered as instinctive reflexes, because they are involuntary; they were even noted by Sternberg in an anencephalic foetus.
>
> By means of these expressional reactions it is possible even in babies of a few months old and in many animals to distinguish clearly between the sensations aroused by different tastes in the mouth. A sweet taste always gives them a pleasurable sensation, even when it is in excess. Other substances, on the contrary, give a disagreeable sensation in concentrated solutions, or are indifferent if very dilute. In the first case the reaction is a movement of sucking or licking; in the second there are efforts at repulsion and evidences of displeasure or disgust.   (LUCIANI 1917, p. 139)

These comments are striking antecedents of Jakov STEINER's (1973) observations on the gustofacial reflexes of newborn infants so vividly documented by means of modern photography.

Curt P. Richter in his psychobiology laboratory at Johns Hopkins had developed a wide-ranging series of studies on the biology of behavior: animal drives, the effects of hormones on behavior, cyclicity of behavioral phenomena, and most significant for taste, behavioral homeostasis. He showed that Claude Bernard's and Walter B. Cannon's ideas of the constancy of the internal environment as a necessity for the maintenance of life and health depended not only upon internal physiological mechanisms but upon behavioral mechanisms as well. Most dramatic was the description of a specific hunger in a child with an adrenal tumor who displayed an inordinate craving for table salt (WILKINS and RICHTER 1940). In a series of subsequent experiments in rats, in which the adrenal and other glands were removed to induce specific mineral or metabolic deficiencies, the experimental animals were shown to selectively increase the intake of the missing ingredient even when this was presented as a pure chemical in a cafeteria free-choice situation. Richter developed the two-bottle self-selection test, in which the relative intake of a particular substances of nutrient in solution compared to that of water in the other container could index a taste preference and/or aversion. In the white rat, adrenalectomy and the consequent excessive excretion of salt in the urine proved fatal when only plain water and standard chow were available. When salt solution was freely available, the rats increased the intake of salt sufficiently to maintain health and life (RICHTER 1942). In a two-bottle choice test, such animals seemed to detect salt at a lower concentration than did normals. Richter hypothesized that adrenalectomy had lowered the threshold of the salt receptors (RICHTER 1939). Here was a unique problem for which taste electrophysiology was ideally suited.

As I prepared for research at Brown in 1945, among the returning veterans was John K. Bare, who had an interest in this problem. I was very glad to have him as PhD student. He did a series of behavioral preference tests confirming the lowered preference threshold, but also showed that at high concentrations even the adrenalectomized animals showed a relative aversion to salt, albeit much less than that of normals. We did the recording experiment together and found no difference in salt thresholds of adrenalectomized rats and normals. In fact, the electrophysiological thresholds of both were the same and close to the behavioral preference threshold of the salt needy animal (PFAFFMANN and BARE 1950). Apparently, the normal rats could taste the weak salt but did not prefer it, whereas the adrenalectomized did. In some respects I was disappointed with our negative finding, for the question of how the salt deprivation switches on behavior still remained. Subsequent work in my laboratory years later by Robert CONTRERAS (1977) and CONTRERAS and FRANK (1979) showed that there is a change resulting from dietary salt deprivation, but this constitutes a decrease, not an increase, in salt sensitivity. Thresholds were not changed, but there was a reduction in sensory response to the high concentrations. This might facilitate repletion by the deprived animal by reducing the aversiveness of the strong salt solutions. This, however, does not explain the increased motivation to ingest salt, for which more central neural changes seem necessary.

My disproof of one of Curt Richter's well-known theories had a salutory impact on my scientific status at the time but did not impair our mutual scientific respect and subsequent personal relationship. Indeed, we became and remain quite good friends. Richter's work stands out to this day as seminal and significant, and is a source of concepts that challenge simplistic explanations of the determination of behavior. Thus, although the preference for and control of intake of sugars and synthetic sweeteners seemed easily explainable by variations in the magnitude of their chorda tympani sensory discharge, certain discrepancies between physiology and behavior still remain, a case in point being what I like to call the "maltose paradox." Richter showed that maltose is one of the most preferred sugars (RICHTER and CAMPBELL 1940), even when postingestive effects are minimized, as in recent short-exposure tests (DAVIS 1973); yet it is a relatively poor chorda tympani stimulant. The rank order of the rats' sugar preference is maltose > glucose > sucrose > fructose > galactose; the electrophysiological order is sucrose > fructose > glucose > maltose > galactose. The position of maltose is particularly paradoxical.

Species differences in taste sensitivity (PFAFFMANN 1953) and in preference behavior (CARPENTER 1956) are readily demonstrable and must be borne in mind when generalizing from one organism to all organisms. In addition, such preference behavior is usually the composite of both taste and postingestive effects. The latter can be minimized by limiting intake by means of an operantly conditioned task where many bar presses are required for the delivery of a small drop of natural or synthetic sweetener. Both bar pressing and lick rate are sensitive to concentration and to efficacy of the sweetener (see Fig. 3) even in a need-free (undeprived) organism. Indeed, such behavior can be said to be a consequence of the "pleasures of sensation" (PFAFFMANN 1960).

Although Zotterman had recorded taste activity in the chorda tympani in 1935, he had been more actively engaged in the study of touch, pain, and temperature sensitivity and only returned to the study of taste in the late 1940s. One of his first

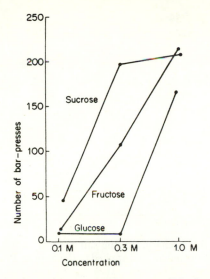

Fig. 3. Bar pressing by squirrel monkey on an operant conditioning schedule that provides a brief sip of sugar after every 30 s of bar pressing. PFAFFMANN (1969)

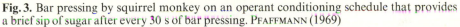

studies then revealed that a number of frog taste fibers in the glossopharyngeal nerve were stimulated by water (ZOTTERMAN 1949). Subsequently, water responses were also found in certain mammals. Zotterman was simply a name to me from his published works until 1951, when I had the opportunity of meeting him personally by way of the International Congress of Psychology held in Stockholm in the summer of that year. My paper at the Congress was entitled "Gustatory Intensity, Its Peripheral, Behavioral, and Psychological Aspects." I wrote to Zotterman telling him of my projected visit and my hope of meeting him. I still have the copy of his gracious reply written from his home at the Experimentalfältet. At that time he was Professor of Physiology at the Royal Veterinary School in Stockholm. Transoceanic air service had not yet been perfected, so my wife and I made the trip to Sweden by boat. I visited Zotterman's laboratory, and we discussed the general problems of taste and sensory physiology and demonstrated each other's operative procedures for exposing the chorda tympani. His lateral approach seemed superior to my ventral approach, and we shifted to his approach in most of our subsequent work.

At this International Congress I also made the personal acquaintance of Zoran Bujas of the University of Zagreb, Yugoslavia. He had been a student of Henri Piéron in Paris. Bujas carried out many of the more recent quantitative psychophysical studies of taste reaction time, rise time of taste sensation, differential sensitivity, adaptation, and the parameters of "electric taste." That summer marked the beginning of long-enjoyable personal and scientifically rewarding friendship with both men.

Bujas and I discovered another common bond, the love of sailing. Indeed, we shared interesting and enjoyable cruises aboard his sloop *Vihor* along the Dalmatian coast to Dubrovnik, and on my *Isis* in New England waters when Bujas spent

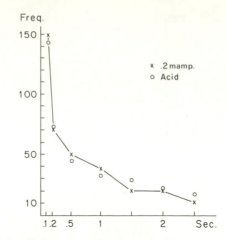

Fig. 4. Comparison of the discharges in the same single chorda tympani unit elicited by 0.2 mA anodal polarization and an acid applied to the tongue. PFAFFMANN (1941)

six months in my laboratory at the Rockefeller University in 1967. Together with Marion Frank, we studied the electrophysiology of electric taste in the rat chorda tympani. In my 1941 paper, I had reported that single taste fibers from salt- or acid-sensitive receptors also responded to weak anodal currents on the tongue surface (see Fig. 4). Cathodal stimulation inhibited resting neural activity but produced a stimulatory effect upon the cathodal break. At much stronger currents, the cathode onset stimulated a discharge with some evidence that this activated sweet-sensitive receptors. In humans, "anode-on" produces a sour taste at the lowest current; "cathode-off" produces a salty-sour taste sensation. "Cathode-on" at higher currents causes a complex bitter-sweet taste. There is thus a seeming parallel between many aspects of electrophysiology and human reports of taste electrical polarization.

The phenomenon of electric taste has been known since the earliest work on electricity. Sulzer (1754, cited by BUJAS 1971) described the induction of taste when two different, interconnected metals touched the tongue, whereas each metal by itself was tasteless; but he did not arrive at the correct explanation. Volta (1792, cited by OETTINGEN 1900 and BUJAS 1971) rediscovered the same effect and correctly attributed it to the "electric fluid" flowing through the tongue from one metal to the other. He carried out numerous experiments using bipolar and monopolar stimulation, finding that the taste quality depended on the particular metal touching the tongue. The positive pole caused sourness; the negative caused a more alkaline, sharp sensation with some bitterness which lasted throughout the duration of current flow.

In general, two opposite hypotheses had been advanced for the mechanism of electrical taste, one electrochemical and the other physical (BUJAS 1971). At the anode, OH^- ions are neutralized, leaving a surplus of hydrogen ions there; at the cathode, H^+ ions are neutralized, causing a consequent surplus of OH^- ions. These changes seem to explain the sour taste at the anode and the indistinct bitter-sweet taste at the cathode. The flow of a cathodal steady current was thought to produce a concentration gradient of ions in the electrolyte, so that at the sudden break of a cathodal current, a diffusion potential of opposite polarity appears which acts as a weak anodal current and sourness is reported. On analogy with the effect of electric current on the nerves, one would expect the opposite from that found for electric taste. Cathodal stimulation is normally the most effective for nerves, whereas anodal polarization can block transmission. Direct electrical stimulation of taste receptor membranes thus seems unlikely. Other evidence supporting the chemical theory is provided by OEHRWALL (1891), who stimulated single papillae with a small brush electrode. All papillae sensitive to acid reacted with a sour taste to the anode; papillae sensitive to bitter and sweet solutions reacted to the "cathode-on" with these latter sensations. On papillae insensitive to taste solutions, the current could not elicit a definite taste. BUJAS and CHWEITZER (1934) also studied the effects of alternating, iterative, or progressively rising electrical currents, and measured the anodal threshold in cases where a constant polarizing current was superimposed on the stimulating pulse in human subjects. The latter showed that "anelectrotonus" slightly decreases the threshold value for a transient stimulation anodal pulse, and "catelectrotonus" considerably increases it. This is in agreement with the enhancing effect of anelectrotonus and suppression of neural activity by the cathode in the chorda recordings. While working in my laboratory, PIERREL (1955) warned that intermittent square wave anodal pulses between 20 and 1,000 Hz could stimulate a cutaneous pulsatile sensation as well as taste, the latter occurring at a lower current level. Taste sensation did not appear to fluctuate.

In 1948, Keffer Hartline, then at Johns Hopkins University, told me of one of his students, Lloyd Beidler, who was interested not in vision but in the chemical senses. Having little experience with mammalian preparations, Keffer asked whether I would demonstrate my rat preparation. Lloyd and his wife, Mary Lou, came to Brown that summer. Lloyd was impressed by the vigor of the rat's chorda tympani response compared with those of the frog and insect preparations which he had been using. On returning to Hopkins, he not only turned to the rat chorda tympani but in due course developed the electronic summator, which provided a quantitative measure of multiunit neural activity and a permanent record when combined with a chart recorder. This great technical advance was immediately adopted by all taste electrophysiologists. Lloyd's first research (BEIDLER 1953), and especially his theory of taste receptor stimulation (BEIDLER 1954), provided a most important and necessary biophysical foundation for the now burgeoning field of taste electrophysiology. From the beginning Lloyd and I hit if off, and we have maintained a firm and deep friendship over the years. Our frequent interchanges at each other's laboratories or homes, or at meetings, are always lively and productive. I recall many a last moment of lively discussion on train platforms, at air terminals, or in driveways.

Yngve Zotterman, Lloyd Beidler, and I had the occasion to meet again in 1960 when Walter Rosenblith organized a symposium on sensory communication at the M.I.T. Endicott House. By then, Zotterman had become more active in taste, recording activity in the chorda tympani in a number of species, including rhesus monkey and humans, in the latter case with Diamant in the course of otological surgery (DIAMANT and ZOTTERMAN 1959). The summator records of human nerve activity were remarkably like those from animals and provided the rare opportunity of correlating individual records with the psychophysical measures of perceived intensity in each patient obtained prior to surgery. Later, they also showed that gymnemic acid brushed onto the tongue obliterated the neural activity to sugar and saccharin but not the response to salt, sour, or bitter stimuli. Beidler (1961) reported on mechanisms of gustatory and olfactory receptor stimulation. With Erickson, Frommer, and Halpern, I reported on gustatory discharges in the rat medulla and thalamus (Pfaffmann et al. 1961).

Following the Boston meeting, Zotterman, Beidler, and I adjourned to my laboratory at Brown University. Besides touring the laboratory and meeting my students, we held the bull session at which we dreamed up the International Symposium on Olfaction and Taste (ISOT). Yngve Zotterman proposed that the first ISOT be held in Stockholm just prior to the 1962 International Congress of Physiology in Holland. He had moved to the Wenner Gren Center, a newly endowed Swedish scientific conference center with international residential facilities for scholars. The first symposium, in 1962 (Zotterman 1963), was a great success; its opening address was given by Adrian. It may be recalled that he had done a number of studies of olfactory function by recording from the olfactory bulb. I quote from Adrian's opening address (Adrian 1963) concerning sensory perception, in which he noted that our recognition of what is happening around us is guided by all the information available, whatever its source.

Olfactory recognition, like visual recognition, need not depend on a single method of sensory analysis, it may depend on several methods taken together. If smells can be separated into five categories by the spatial pattern and five more by the temporal, and another 50 by the specific receptors, the number of different smells that might be distinguished would be very large.

To some degree this statement might also be applicable *now* to the sense of taste, which at first seemed simpler with its fewer major categories of quality: salt, sour, bitter, and sweet. Specificity of electrolyte taste receptors have shown more overlapping sensitivity and seem to form a more continuous distribution than do receptors for sweet stimuli, for example. In addition, many workers have reported a periodic bursting of impulse discharge to stimulation by sweet stimuli, so that such a temporal pattern might be the distinctive coding feature for sweetness. There is still much debate as to the essential sensory code for taste. There may be more than one.

There were just 67 participants at the ISOT (see table of contents reprinted in the Appendix), but nearly all the major problems in chemical senses were at least touched upon or signaled at that meeting. Among those present was Emil von Skramlik, whose *Handbuch der Physiologie der Niederen Sinne* (Physiology of the Lower Senses) (von Skramlik 1926) was one of the most comprehensive, classic summaries of the status of the field when it was published. Von Skramlik, though retired, contributed a paper comparing the relative effects of different anesthetic agents upon taste thresholds. He arranged the susceptibility to most anesthetics as follows: bitter > salty > sour > sweet. This is not the order of sensitivity for taste substances, which (excluding the new synthetic sweet substances) is bitter > sour > salty > sweet. He concluded in a relatively classic vein that the different anesthetic agents can affect the sensation qualities and their substrates relatively independently of each other.

His earlier work, as described in his handbook, was the most serious experimental effort to reconstruct complex tastes of different substances (especially salts) by means of taste mixtures. In his general taste equation:

$$N = xA + yB + zC + vD$$

A, B, C, and D correspond to bitter, salty, sour, and sweet components respectively; x, y, z, and v, the molar concentrations of quinine, sodium chloride, tartaric acid, and sucrose in a mixture to match a particular complex taste. Ammonium chloride, for example, required a mixture of three components (sodium chloride, quinine, and tartaric acid). Other salts might require four components, some only two. Although such taste equations for any one individual were constant from test to test they differed between individuals, unlike the trichromatic mixture equations for color vision, which are very similar for optically normal trichromats. The equations were also specific for concentration and changed as the solutions became diluted, although following dilution the taste components dropped out in the order of their apparent subjective intensity. Von Skramlik concluded that no inorganic salt tastes like another salt, each giving rise to its unique combination of the sweet, sour, salty, and bitter components.

Also present at the first ISOT was my former student Robert Erickson, who in his laboratory at Duke University began to examine and extend the implications of my 1941 and 1955 papers demonstrating the multiple sensitivity of individual taste fibers. At the Symposium he introduced the cross-fiber correlation coefficient as a measure of the degree of relationship between sensitivities of individual fibers. In a sample of neuron records, a high correlation coefficient between unit discharges to two stimuli meant that they fired in the same manner to both; a low correlation signified little relation. A common finding for the rat was a high coefficient between the discharges to sodium and lithium chlorides but a low correlation between sodium and potassium chlorides. This cross-correlation method has since been adopted by a great many investigators as a convenient way of indicating degree of similarity or dissimilarity of receptor sensitivities. Erickson also developed a hypothetical schema of sensitivities assuming taste units to be a continuum, not a clustering into three or four sensitivities as the classic theory had postulated. Over the years he has elaborated this formulation using improved statistical and computer methods applied not only to peripheral units but also to CNS units. His evidence, largely derived from electrolyte-sensitive units, is compatible with the later extensive studies of Japanese investigators, especially SATO et al. (1975), on *Macaca rhesus* chorda. Electrolytes such as sodium chloride, potassium chloride, ammonium chloride, and various acids tend to show multiple overlapping sensitivities, but there is little overlap with such stimuli as sugars and quinine. The rat's anterior tongue is richly endowed with electrolyte sensitivity, less so with sensitivity to sugar and quinine. Sugar-best and quinine-best units in the IX nerve supplying the posterior rat tongue, well documented by Marion FRANK (1975), are specific to quinine and sugar. However, more work remains to be done on such issues.

At the first ISOT, I elaborated on the relationships between taste physiology and preference behavior (PFAFFMANN 1963), reviewing a number of experiments carried out with my colleagues: Marvin Nachman on the chorda tympani response in salt-deprived rats, McBurney on the adaptation of sodium chloride sensitivity in humans, G. L. Fisher on behavioral indices of salt appetite, and Bruce Oakley on the effect of thalamic lesions upon taste preferences. I also reported on brain stem medullary taste relay with Makous, Nord, and Oakley (MAKOUS et al. 1963). I pointed out that the relation between the physiology and behavior was often more complex than would appear at first glance, and required variations upon several different behavioral procedures, including operant conditioning and learned and unlearned preference behavior.

On the occasion of a trip abroad in 1960, I was able to visit Helmut Hahn, the inventor of the "taste microscope," then in retirement at his home. His work represented some of the last in that long and distinguished German tradition of sensory psychophysics. His studies of adaptation, in particular, still stand as one of the best specifications of the adaptive process in human taste. He studied the rise in absolute threshold with time of self-adaptation by the method of constant stimuli. After complete adaptation (i.e., the adapting solution became tasteless), the threshold was raised to a value just above the adapting concentration (HAHN 1934). Cross-adaptation among substances arousing similar qualities occurred only for sour. Two minutes' exposure to an acid raised the threshold for all other acids. For sweet and bitter cross-adaptation was partial, occurring for some but not for others. No cross-adaptation was seen between members of a group of 24 different salts. This latter finding stands in striking contrast to the much later results of my student McBurney and his students (MCBURNEY and LUCAS 1966; SMITH and MCBURNEY 1969), who used magnitude estimation psychophysics with suprathreshold concentrations. Cross-adaptation among salts can be well documented both psychophysically and electrophysiologically (FRANK et al. 1972). In the latter case, the amount of cross-adaptation betwen a particular pair of salts is directly related to the magnitude of the chorda tympani cross-fiber correlation to the same salts. The greater the cross-adaptation, the more similar their afferent neural inputs. Direct magnitude scaling of sensory magnitude was developed in the 1950s by S. S. Stevens and his colleagues because of dissatisfaction with indirect just-noticeable difference steps which did not properly predict perceived intensity. Extending the work of BEEBE-CENTER and WADDELL (1948), the method was first applied to taste (to scale sweetness) in 1953, but was not published until much later in a summary article by S. S. STEVENS (1969).

BARTOSHUK et al. (1964) showed that human threshold measures are often accompanied by the so-called water taste, which is contingent upon taste receptor adaptation. Such effects might have confounded Hahn's experiments. I did appreciate the opportunity of meeting him, albeit toward the end of his career. I treasure the copy of his *Beiträge zur Reizphysiologie* (HAHN 1949) which he personally presented to me and two reprints from *Klinische Wochenschrift* (HAHN 1943) which he inscribed and autographed.

Thus, in concluding my story with Helmut Hahn, I complete my personal history as one who has had the good fortune to have known or worked with some of the major figures in the sensory science of taste: Hahn and von Skramlik of the older tradition of psychophysics; Curt Richter of psychobiology and animal behavior; and Adrian, Bronk, and Zotterman of sensory electrophysiology. My research and conceptual formulations drew from each throughout my career, and I have tried to mold a unified sensory science of gustation combining all three traditions.

E. Postscript

My editorial instructions were not to go much beyond the 1950s in this personal history, since such current controversies as those concerning sensory coding of taste are well documented in more recent literature and reviews. I followed these instructions in most cases except where some closure on an issue in the text seemed necessary. This resulted in omitting reference to the work of some of my many former PhD students or co-workers over the years, who I hope will excuse my apparent neglect of them. None was intended.

Acknowledgements: My doctoral research was carried out under a Rhodes Scholarship for the first year and additional support for the second year from the Theresa Rowden Fund of New College, Oxford and a George Henry Lewes Studentship from Cambridge.

From 1945 onward, my research on taste was supported by grants from the Office of Naval Research and the General Foods Company, and then for a long period by successive grants from the National Science Foundation. The present NSF grant is number BNS 811816. Without such support our research efforts would have been less productive.

F. Appendix

The following is the table of contents of the proceedings of the First International Symposium on Taste and Olfaction (see ZOTTERMAN 1963)

Contents

The Opening Address. LORD ADRIAN
Studies on the Ultrastructure and Histophysiology of Cell Membranes, Nerve Fibers, and Synaptic Junctions in Chemoreceptors. A. J. D. de LORENZO
Odor Specificities of the Frog's Olfactory Receptor. R. C. GESTELAND, J. Y. LETTVIN, W. T. PITTS, and A. ROJAS
Generation and Transmission of Signals in the Olfactory System. D. OTTOSON
Olfactory, Vomeronasal and Trigeminal Receptor Responses to Odorants. D. TUCKER
Electrical Activity in the Olfactory System of Rabbits with Indwelling Electrodes. D. G. MOULTON
Electrophysiological Investigation of Insect Olfaction. D. SCHNEIDER
The Fine Structure of the Olfactory Receptors of the Blowfly. V. D. DETHIER, J. R. LARSEN, and J. R. ADAMS
On the Olfactory Sense of Birds. W. NEUHAUS
The Fundamental Substrates of Taste. E. VON SKRAMLIK
Dynamics of Taste Cells. L. M. BEIDLER
Discussion. H. DAVIS
The Significance of the Terminal Structure of Afferent Nerve Fibers. A. IGGO
The Effects of Temperature Change on the Response of Taste Receptors. M. SATO
Chemical Structure and Stimulation by Carbohydrates. D. R. EVANS
Electrophysiological Responses to Sugars and Their Depression by Salt. H. T. ANDERSEN, M. FUNAKOSHI, and Y. ZOTTERMAN
Electrophysiological Studies on Human Taste Nerves. H. DIAMANT, M. FUNAKOSHI, L. STRÖM, and Y. ZOTTERMAN
Sensory Neural Patterns and Gustation. R. P. ERICKSON
Taste Functions in Fish. J. KONISHI and Y. ZOTTERMAN
Comparative Anatomical and Physiological Studies of Gustatory Mechanisms. R. L. KITCHELL
Taste Stimulation and Preference Behavior. C. PFAFFMANN
Chemical Coding in Taste – Temporal Patterns. B. HALPERN
Comparative Studies on the Sense of Taste. M. R. KARE and M. S. FICKEN
The Variations in Taste Thresholds of Ruminants Associated with Sodium Depletion. F. R. BELL

Some Thalamic and Cortical Mechanisms of Taste. R. M. Benjamin
Natural Conditioned Salivary Reflex of Man alone as well as in a Group. T. Hayashi and
    M. Ararei
The Olfactory Identification of Chemical Units and Mixtures and Its Role in Behaviour. J.
    LeMagnen
The Role of Taste and Smell in the Regulation of Food and Water Intake. P. Teitelbaum
    and A. N. Epstein
The Relationship between Body Temperature and Food and Water Intake. B. Andersson,
    C. C., Gale, and J. W. Sundsten
Patterned Activities from Identifiable "Cold" and "Warm" Giant Neurons (Aplysia). A.
    Arvanitaki and N. Chalazonitis
The Gustatory Relay in the Medulla. W. Makous, S. Nord, B. Oakley and C. Pfaffmann

References

Names containing *von* are alphabetized in this list under *v*

Adrian ED (1926) The impulses produced by sensory nerve endings, part I. J Physiol (Lond)
    61:49
Adrian ED (1927) The impulses produced by sensory nerve endings, part IV. J Physiol
    (Lond) 62:33–51
Adrian ED (1928) The basis of sensation. Christophers, London
Adrian ED (1953) Sensory messages and sensation. The response of the olfactory organ to
    different smells. Acta Physiol Scand 29:5–14
Adrian ED (1963) The opening address. In: Zotterman Y (ed) Olfaction and taste I, Pro-
    ceedings of the first international symposium on taste and olfaction, Stockholm, 1962.
    Pergamon, Oxford, pp. 1–5
Adrian ED, Bronk DW (1928) The discharge of impulses in motor nerves, part I. J Physiol
    (Lond) 66:81
Adrian ED, Bronk DW (1929) The discharge of impulses in motor nerves, part IV. J Physiol
    (Lond) 67:119
Adrian ED, Zotterman Y (1926a) The impulses produced by sensory nerve endings, part II.
    J Physiol (Lond) 61:151–171
Adrian ED, Zotterman Y (1926b) The impulses produced by sensory nerve endings, part
    III. J Physiol (Lond) 61:465–483
Adrian ED, Cattell McK, Hoagland H (1931) Sensory discharges in single cutaneous nerve
    fibers. J Physiol (Lond) 72:377–391
Aird RB, Pfaffmann C (1947) Pressure stimulation of peripheral nerves. Proc Soc Exp Biol
    Med 66:130–132
Barron DH (1936) A note on the course of the proprioceptive fibers from the tongue. Anat
    Rec 66:11
Bartoshuk L, McBurney D, Pfaffmann C (1964) Taste of sodium chloride solutions after
    adaptation to sodium chloride: implications for the "water taste." Science 133:967–968
Beebe-Center JG, Waddell D (1948) A general psychological scale of taste. J Psychol
    26:517–524
Beidler LM (1953) Properties of chemoreceptors of tongue of rat. J Neurophysiol 16:595–
    607
Beidler LM (1954) A theory of taste stimulation. J Gen Physiol 38:133–139
Beidler LM (1961) Mechanisms of gustatory and olfactory receptor stimulation. In: Rosen-
    blith WA (ed) Sensory communication. Wiley, New York, pp 143–157
Benjamin RM, Pfaffmann C (1955) Cortical localization of taste in albino rat. J Neuro-
    physiol 18:56–64
Boring EG (1942) Sensation and perception in the history of experimental psychology. Ap-
    pleton-Century, New York, pp 437–462
Bujas Z (1971) Electrical taste. In: Beidler LM (ed) The chemical senses 2, taste. Springer,
    Berlin Heidelberg New York, pp 180–199 (Handbook of sensory physiology, vol 4)
Bujas Z, Chweitzer A (1934) Contribution à l'étude du goût dit électrique. Annee Psychol
    35:147–157

Burton H, Benjamin RM (1971) Central projections of the gustatory system. In: Beidler LM
    (ed) The chemical senses 2, taste. Springer, Berlin Heidelberg New York, pp 148–164
    (Handbook of sensory physiology, vol 4)
Cabanac M (1971) Physiological role of pleasure. Science 173:1103–1107
Carpenter JA (1956) Species differences in taste preferences. J Comp Physiol Psychol
    49:139–144
Contreras RJ (1977) Changes in gustatory nerve discharges with sodium deficiency: a single
    unit analysis. Brain Res 121:373–378
Contreras RJ, Frank M (1979) Sodium deprivation alters neural responses to gustatory
    stimuli. J Gen Physiol 73:569–594
Cranefield PF (ed) The way in and the way out. Futura, Mt Kisco, NY, pp 9–10
Crick FHC (1979) Thinking about the brain. Sci Am 241:219–232
Crozier WJ (1934) Chemoreception. In: Murchison C (ed) A handbook of general ex-
    perimental psychology. Clark University Press, Worcester, pp 1005–1036
Davis JD (1973) The effectiveness of some sugars in stimulating licking behavior in the rat.
    Physiol Behav 11:39–45
Diamant H, Zotterman Y (1959) Has water a specific taste? Nature 183:191–192
Erlanger J, Gasser HS (1937) Electrical signs of nervous activity. University of Pennsylvania
    Press, Philadelphia
Falconer (1847) Über eine merkwürdige Eigenschaft einer indischen Pflanze (*Gymnema syl-
    vestre*). Pharm J Trans 7:551–552
Frank M (1975) Response patterns of rat glossopharyngeal taste neurons. In: Denton D,
    Coghlan JP (eds) Olfaction and taste V. Academic, New York, pp 59–64
Frank M, Smith DV, Pfaffmann C (1972) Cross-adaptation between salts in the rat's chorda
    tympani response. In: Zotterman Y (ed) Oral physiology. Pergamon, Oxford, pp 227–
    237
Galambos R, Davis H (1943) The response of single auditory-nerve fibers to acoustic stimu-
    lation. J Neurophysiol 6:39–57
Hahn H (1934) Die Adaptation des Geschmackssinnes. Z Sinnesphysiol 65:105–145
Hahn H (1943) Geschmackssinnes- und Permeabilitätsforschung I und II. Klin Wochenschr
    22:245–249, 269–272
Hahn H (1949) Beiträge zur Reizphysiologie. Scherer, Heidelberg, S. 125–229
Hänig DP (1901) Zur Psychophysik des Geschmackssinnes. Philos Studien 17:576–623
Henning H (1916) Die Qualitätsreihe des Geschmacks. Z Psychol 74:203–219
Herrick CJ (1903) The organ and sense of taste in fishes. Bull US Fish Com 22:237–272
Herrick CJ (1905) The central gustatory paths in the brains of bony fishes. J Comp Neurol
    Psychol 15:375–456
Hoagland H (1933) Specific nerve impulses from gustatory and tactile receptors in catfish.
    J Gen Physiol 16:685–693
Hooper D (1887) An examination of the leaves of *Gymnema sylvestre*. Nature 35:565–567
Jasper HH, Carmichael L (1935) Electrical potentials from the intact human brain. Science
    81:51–53
Kiesow F (1894) Beiträge zur physiologischen Psychologie des Geschmackssinnes. Philos
    Studien 10:329–368, 523–561
Kiesow F (1896) Beiträge zur physiologischen Psychologie des Geschmackssinnes. Philos
    Studien 12:255–278, 464–473
Lovén C (1868) Bidrog till kännedomen am tungans smakpapiller. Contribution to the
    structure of taste buds on the tongue. Medicinskt Archiv 3:1–14
Luciani L (1917) Human physiology, vol 4. The sense organs. Macmillan, London, pp 126–
    159
Makous W, Nord S, Oakley B, Pfaffmann C (1963) The gustatory relay in the medulla. In:
    Zotterman Y (ed) Olfaction and taste I. Proceedings of the first international sym-
    posium on taste and olfaction, Stockholm, 1962. Pergamon, Oxford, pp 381–393
Matthews BHC (1933) Nerve endings in mammalian muscle. J Physiol 78:1–53
McBurney DH, Lucas JA (1966) Gustatory cross-adaptation between salts. Psychon Sci
    4:301–302
Müller J (1830) Handbuch der Physiologie des Menschen für Vorlesungen, vol I und II.
    Holscher, Coblenz

Nafe JP (1934) The pressure, pain, and temperature senses. In: Murchison C (ed) Handbook of general experimental psychology. Clark University Press, Worcester, pp 1037–1087

Norgren R, Leonard CM (1973) Ascending central gustatory pathways. J Comp Neurol 150:217–238

Norgren R, Pfaffmann C (1975) The pontine taste area in the rat. Brain Res 91:99–117

Oakes WJ (ed) (1940) The stoic and epicurean philosophers: the complete exrant writings of Epicurus, Epictetus, Lucretius, and Marcus Aurelius. Random House, New York, pp 69–219

Oehrwall H (1891) Untersuchungen über den Geschmackssinn. Scand Arch Physiol 2:1–69

Oehrwall H (1901) Die Modalitäts- und Qualitätsbegriffe in der Sinnesphysiologie und deren Bedeutung. Scand Arch Physiol 11:245–277

Oettingen AJ (ed) (1900) Ostwalds Klassiker der exakten Wissenschaften. Engelmann, Leipzig

Parker GH (1912) The relation of smell, taste, and the common chemical sense in vertebrates. J Natl Acad Sci 15:221–234

Parker GH (1922) Smell, taste, and allied senses in the vertebrates. Lippincott, Philadelphia

Pfaffmann C (1935) An experimental comparison of the method of single stimuli and the method of constant stimuli in gustation. Am J Psychol 48:470–476

Pfaffmann C (1936) Differential responses of the newborn cat to gustatory stimuli. J Genet Psychol 49:61–67

Pfaffmann C (1939a) Afferent impulses from the teeth. J Physiol 95:1–2

Pfaffmann C (1939b) Specific gustatory impulses. J Physiol 96:41–42

Pfaffmann C (1940) Potentials in the isolated medullated axon. J Cell Comp Physiol 16:1–4

Pfaffmann C (1941) Gustatory afferent impulses. J Cell Comp Physiol 17:243–258

Pfaffmann C (1948) Aircraft landing without binocular cues: a study based upon observations made in flight. Am J Psychol 61:323–334

Pfaffmann C (1953) Species differences in taste sensitivity. Science 117:470

Pfaffmann C (1955 Gustatory nerve impulses in rat, cat, and rabbit. J Neurophysiol 18:429–440

Pfaffmann C (1960) The pleasures of sensation. Psychol Rev 67:253–269

Pfaffmann C (1963) Taste stimulation and preference behavior. In: Zotterman Y (ed) Olfaction and taste I. Proceedings of the first international symposium on taste and olfaction, Stockholm, 1962. Pergamon, Oxford, pp 257–273

Pfaffmann C (1969) Taste preference and reinforcement. In: Tapp J (ed) Reinforcement and behavior. Academic, New York, pp 215–441

Pfaffmann C, Bare JK (1950) Gustatory nerve discharges in normal and adrenalectomized rats. J Comp Physiol Psychol 43:320–324

Pfaffmann C, Schlosberg H (1936) The conditioned knee jerk in psychotic and normal individuals. J Psychol 1:201–206

Pfaffmann C, Erickson R, Frommer G, Halpern B (1961) Gustatory discharges in the rat medulla and thalamus. In: Rosenblith WA (ed) Sensory communication. Wiley, New York, pp 455–473

Pierrel R (1955) Taste effects resulting from intermittent electrical stimulation of the tongue. J Exp Psychol 49:374–380

Pumphrey RJ (1935) Nerve impulses from receptors in the mouth of the frog. J Cell Comp Physiol 6:457–467

Richter CP (1939) Salt taste thresholds of normal and adrenalectomized rats. Endocrinology 24:367–371

Richter CP (1942) Total self-regulatory functions in animals and human beings. Harvey Lect 38:63–103

Richter CP, Campbell KH (1940) Taste thresholds and taste preferences of rats for five common sugars. J Nutr 20:31–46

Ross GRT (ed) (1906) Aristotle: De sensu and de memoria. Cambridge University Press, Cambridge, pp 41–99

Rutherford W (1886) The sense of hearing. J Anat Physiol 21:166–168

Sato M, Ogawa H, Yamashita S (1975) Response properties of macaque monkey chorda tympani fibers. J Gen Physiol 66:781–810

Schiff M (1867) Du sens du goût. Leçons sur la physiologie de la digestion, I. Loescher, Florence, pp 78–124

Schiffman SS, Erickson RP (1971) A psychophysical model for gustatory quality. Physiol Behav 7:617–633

Schwalbe G (1867) Das Epithel der Papillae vallata. Arch Mikrosk Anat 3:504–508

Shore LE (1892) A contribution to our knowledge of taste sensations. J Physiol 13:191–217

Smith DV, McBurney DH (1969) Gustatory cross-adaptation: does a single mechanism code the salty taste? J Exp Psychol 80:101–105

Steiner JE (1973) The gusto-facial response: observation on normal and anencephalic newborn infants. In: Bosmas JF (ed) Fourth symposium on oral sensation and perception. Superintendent of Documents, U.S. Government Printing Office 1973, Washington DC, pp 254–278

Stevens SS (1969) Sensory scales of taste intensity. Percept Psychophys 6:302–308

von Békésy G (1928) Zur Theorie des Hörens: Die Schwingungsform der Basilarmembran. Phys Z 29:793–810

von Skramlik E (1926) Handbuch der Physiologie der niederen Sinne, I. Die Physiologie des Geschmackssinnes. Thieme, Leipzig, S. 346–520

Wever EG, Bray CW (1930) Action currents in the auditory nerve in response to acoustical stimulation. Proc Natl Acad Sci 16:344–350

Wilkins L, Richter CP (1940) A great craving for salt by a child with corticoadrenal insufficiency. JAMA 114:866–868

Wundt W (1893) Grundzüge der physiologischen Psychologie, 4th edn. Engelmann, Leizpig, S. 438–441

Zotterman Y (1935) Action potentials in the glossopharyngeal nerve and in the chorda tympani. Scand Arch Physiol 72:73–77

Zotterman Y (1949) The response of the frog's taste fibers to the application of pure water. Acta Physiol Scand 18:181–189

Zotterman Y (ed) (1963) Olfaction and taste I. Proceedings of the first international symposium on taste and olfaction, Stockholm, 1962. Pergamon, Oxford

CHAPTER 12

A Personalized History of Taste Biophysics

LLOYD M. BEIDLER

A. Description of Taste Structures

Accumulation of knowledge concerning the basis of taste paralleled the historical development of science itself. The perfection of the compound microscope allowed scientists to observe the gross anatomical structures of the tongue surface associated with taste sensation. In 1662, Malpighi, the founder of microscopic anatomy, published a manuscript, *Epistolae Anatomicae,* in which he described the tongue's surface and related taste to observed tongue papillae (MALPIGHI and FRACASSATI 1662). This description was carried further in Laurentium BELLINI'S (1666) book *Gustus Organum.* The book review in the *Philosophical Transactions of the Royal Society of London* (1666) stated: "this author [is] proposing to himself to discover both the principal Organ of the Taste, and the nature of its object." Bellini described "little Risings called Papillares," which were the taste organs. He demonstrated that only the areas of the tongue containing these structures will bring forth taste sensations when stimulated with salt.

VAN LEEUWENHOEK (1708) improved the optics of the microscope. His description of the tongue and the structures associated with taste did not differ very much from those of Bellini. Little additional information was afforded until better histological techniques were developed many years later.

A flurry of anatomical descriptions of taste structures occurred during the latter half of the nineteenth century. Taste organs were first described in fish (carp) by WEBER in 1827. In 1863, SCHULZE detailed their fine structure. It was not until

1867 that taste buds were described in mammals, including man. A personal controversy immediately developed between Lovén, a Swede, and Schwalbe, a German. Both claimed the distinction of being the discoverer of human taste buds as the organs of taste. The argument arose because Lovén's (1867) paper was the first to be published but was relatively unknown since it appeared in a Swedish journal. The following year (1868) the two researchers published in the same volume. Lovén added the following paragraph to his manuscript:

The preceding article, the experiments for which were completed in mid-June this year, is the translation of a communication in Swedish which published in September. Later I had the opportunity of seeing a preliminary communication on the same topic by Dr. G. Schwalbe of the Anatomical Institute at Bonn, and am pleased to find that this researcher has obtained essentially the same results.

M. Schultze followed the above paragraph with his own observation:

In support of the completely simultaneous nature of the experiments of Dr. Lovén and Dr. G. Schwalbe and their mutual independence, I note here that the offprints of the Swedish article by Dr. Lovén were dispatched to Bonn after the preliminary communication of Dr. Schwalbe, which was printed in mid-October 1967, had already been sent off and was in the hands of Prof. Axel Key in Stockholm. Previously we had no knowledge whatsoever of the work of Dr. Lovén. Dr. Schwalbe's detailed treatment will appear in the next issue of this journal.

Personal controversies often occur between two scientists, who then analyze each other's publications in detail. In 1960, von Békésy commented on such rivalries. He said:

An enemy is willing to devote a vast amount of time and brain power ferreting out errors both large and small, and this without any compensation. The trouble is that really capable enemies are scarce; most of them are only ordinary. Another trouble with enemies is that they sometimes develop into friends and lose a good deal of their zeal. It was in this way that the writer lost his three best enemies.

A letter to Tuckerman in 1892 (Fig. 1) suggests that Lovén and Schwalbe did indeed become friends after many years had passed.

After the discovery of taste buds, numerous anatomical and histological studies were undertaken. There were great similarities in the morphologies of the taste buds of fish and mammals. The cells within the buds varied in their ability to accept the stain. On this basis as well as that of their shapes, histologists partitioned the cells into two groups, the supporting and the sensory. Within the taste pore, the cell projections were described as taste hairs.

There were numerous discussions of the taste bud innervation. A nerve plexus was observed beneath the buds and fine nerve endings emerged to enter the bud. Did the nerves enter the cells or not? This was difficult to ascertain until years later, when electron microscopy allowed a closer examination. It is known that the cell membranes wrap themselves around the nerve ending, which never enters the taste cells or comes in contact with their cytoplasm. In most mammals, classic synaptic formations are seldom observed.

Species differences in the spatial distribution of both circumvallate and fungiform papillae were noted well before the nineteenth century. Very detailed studies were conducted in the early twentieth century. Evolutionary and environmental factors were sought but few were found. One of the most prolific writers in this area of research was Tuckerman (1892) in the United States. He wrote to many researchers, including Lovén and Schwalbe, to obtain tongues from unusual species.

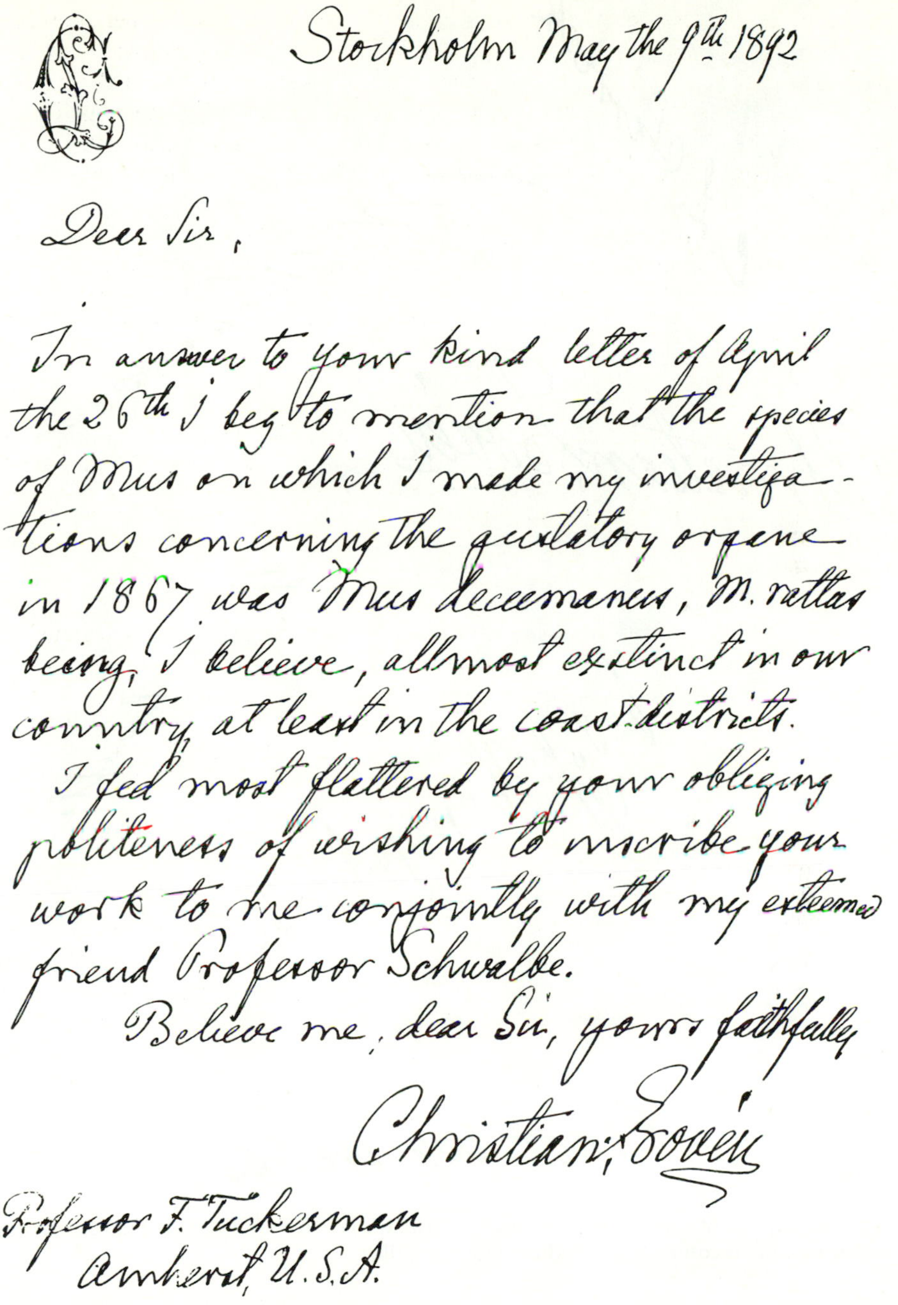

Stockholm May the 9th 1892

Dear Sir,

In answer to your kind letter of April the 26th I beg to mention that the species of Mus on which I made my investigations concerning the gustatory organe in 1867 was Mus decemanus, M. rattus being, I believe, allmost extinct in our country, at least in the coast districts.

I fed most flattered by your obliging politeness of wishing to inscribe your work to me conjointly with my esteemed friend Professor Schwalbe.

Believe me, dear Sir, yours faithfully

Christian Lovén

Professor F. Tuckerman
Amherst, U.S.A.

Fig. 1. Letter from Christian Lovén, a discoverer of human taste buds, to F. Tuckerman concerning the species of rat used in his famous 1867 research. Note reference to his "esteemed friend Professor Schwalbe"

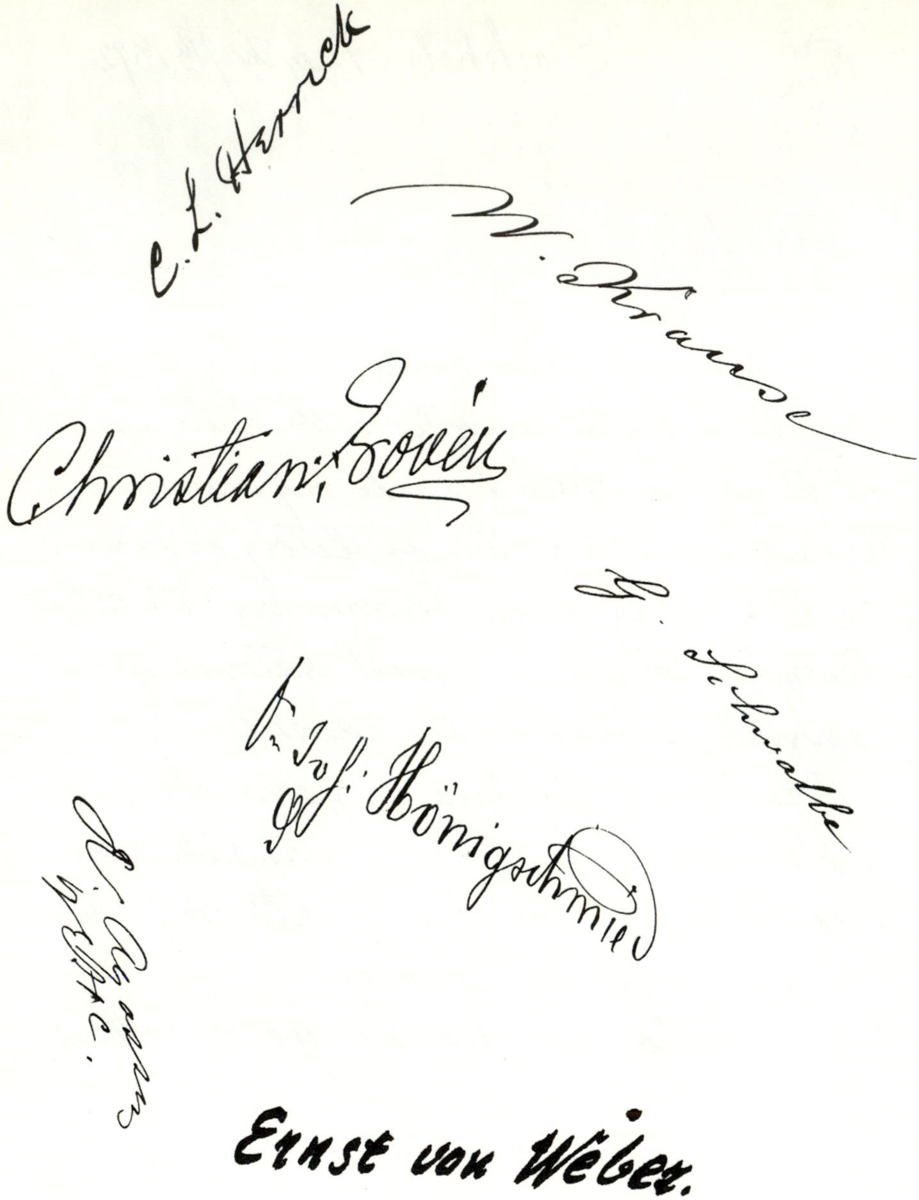

Fig. 2. Signatures of some of the famous scientists who corresponded with Tuckerman during the time of his comparative studies of taste papillae

His letters and laboratory records form one of the few historical collections from this period of taste research (Fig. 2).

It is of interest to note that not all microscopic studies of taste cells were based upon examination of tissue sections. Frequently, the cells were dispersed with chromic acid and the individual cells examined. Perhaps this practice was a natural extension of the separation of the epidermis from the attached connective tissue. WALLER (1849) noted "By the application of a minute quantity of solution of potash over a fungiform papilla, we sometimes observe a curious appearance. The external zone becomes separated from the central area by a deep fissure, and forms a kind of cup containing the blood-vessel ..." FISH et al. (1944) used a similar technique to separate the dorsal epithelium from the remainder of the rat tongue. After discussing this technique with Curt Richter while I was at Johns Hopkins, I decided to try less drastic chemical procedures. I finally found collagenase to be very effective; it was used many years later by MISTRETTA (1971) to study chemical penetration of the epithelium.

B. Early Electrical Experiments in Taste

The discovery in about 1740 of the Leyden jar as a means of storing electricity greatly increased public interest in electrical experimentation. A Leyden jar consists of a corked glass jar partly filled with water, with a wire or nail inserted through the cork into the water. The jar is grasped with the hand and the free end of the wire moved close to an electric machine. The Leyden jar stores the electricity so that it can be used to shock people at a later time.

A large number of electrical phenomena were shown to the public by lecturers throughout populated America and Europe. Demonstrations involving electrical shocks were particularly well received. Men of distinction, such as John Wesley, founder of Methodism, wrote books on electrical phenomena. Benjamin Franklin also became interested. He demonstrated the identity of lightning with electricity and proved it scientifically. His first book on electricity (FRANKLIN 1751) presented the one-fluid theory of electricity, which was well accepted in Europe and became the basis for understanding electricity. He first used the words "positive" and "negative," and thought the electrical fluid always flowed from the positive to the negative.

During the latter half of the eighteenth century, most electrical experiments were performed with animals. The ability of some fish to generate large electrical shocks was well known. Animal electricity was widely studied, and GALVANI (1953) demonstrated sources of electricity in nerve and muscle. However, a major argument between Galvani of Bologna and Volta of nearby Pavia developed over the source of electricity in many animal experiments.

Volta showed that two dissimilar metals were a source of electricity that could be used to stimulate tissue. Sulzer had earlier observed taste sensations when two different metals were applied to this tongue. Volta repeated these experiments and developed many more. He often published in English journals, and therefore descriptions of his experiments on electrical taste are readily available to all students.

Volta used the one-fluid theory of Franklin and showed that anodal stimulation is necessary for taste. In a letter to Covallo, VOLTA (1793 b) states: "I have varied, in many ways, the experiments respecting the taste excited upon the tongue, by the application of the two metals, Tin and Silver. I found that the acid taste is excited when the electric current comes against the point of the tongue (when the fluid enters it)". He concluded that "this is a mere artificial Electricity, induced by an external cause ... and the animal organs, the nerves and the muscles, are merely passive, though easily thrown into action ..." Is stimulation due to the particles of the metal dissolving in saliva? Volta's new experiment was described by Galvani's nephew, Giovanni ALDINI (1792).

> ... he immersed the tip of the tongue into a level of water, in which he had placed a scrap either of tin or of paper covered with tin: when a metal arc was carried from the middle of the tongue to the tin layer, the sensation of an acid taste was excited, which continued to be felt, as long as the contact lasted ... Hence it seems that it can be inferred that the tongue perceives the taste not of dissolved metal but of the electricity running out through it.

Better understanding of electrical taste did not appear for over 100 years after Volta died. The ionic nature of electrolytes was only described at the end of the nineteenth century. Thereafter, an ionic basis of electrical taste was considered in a number of papers, but no completely satisfactory explanation appeared. The psychophysical properties associated with electrical taste were also described, but a physicochemical basis has not yet been published.

C. Early Theories on Taste Cell Stimulation

Development of taste theories paralleled the development of the disciplines of chemistry and biology. In the seventeenth century, molecules were described in terms of their conceived shapes. BELLINI (1666) stated "that the particles of Salt passing through those pores, which pierce the Papillaryi Eminences, and penetrating as far as the nerves, that meet them there, do by means of their small points prick them; which pricking is called the taste."

The distinction between the tastes of salt and sugar was based upon the contours of the two substances. Sugar was thought to be smooth and soft on the tongue, affecting it with pleasure. Salt was described as small rigid particles that pricked the tongue, although not so stiff as to wound it. This concept was nicely illustrated by VAN LEEUWENHOEK (1674) when he wrote:

> I shall here speak of the difference of the taste between Salt and Sugar. The grain of Sugar then consists of divers pointed and angular small Figures; and yet how angular and pointed soever these Figures are, they would not, if they remained entire, cause any taste upon our Tongue, forasmuch as (with submission to better Judgment,) their angles and points are big, each point or angle of these grains of Sugar not touching one or two globuls of our Tongue, but comprizing a great number of them; and that the rather, because I take it for granted, that a single globul, (of which bodies the pointed protuberances of our Tongue are made up,) is many thousand times smaller than a common grain of Sand, and therefore can produce no taste. For, take a polisht pointed Diamond, of an ordinary bigness, and put it on the back of your hand with the point downward, and press it upon your hand with the force of a pound weight; this pressure will cause but little smart to the hand, in regard that the pressure or force, put to the Diamond, doth not only touch the extream point of a Diamond, but many other points, forasmuch as our skin, being soft and pliable, will, where that extream point comes to touch, sink a little inward, and so, according to the bigness of the Diamond, will close about the whole, or the greatest part of the same; whereby the skin will be toucht, as was said, not in one only point, but in many, though indeed most of all by that which is the sharp end of the Diamond. Now this seems to be the reason, why Sugar, if it were so hard and rigid as not to be dissolved in water, or warmth, would be insipid, forasmuch as it would not cause any pungency upon the globuls of the Tongue, when the Sugar-grains lye thereon, by reason of the small pressure made by the Tongue against the roof of the mouth. But then, if we should suppose, that a Diamond were thousands of

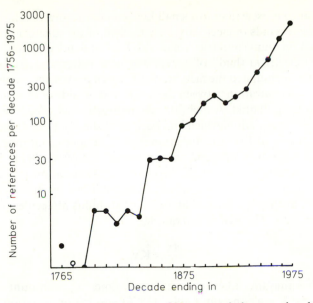

Fig. 3. Number of references to taste cited over a 200-year period accumulated by Beidler

times less, and were put upon our hand with the pressure of one pound weight, it would then not only cause smart, but doubtless, if no bones did hinder, run through the whole hand.

Just so, if the small grains of Sugar were thousands of times less than they are, and rigid withal, then their points would not touch many globuls at once, but only one globul, and so would produce no pleasure but pain, for with their sharp angles they would wound the globuls of our Tongue. But, Sugar is a body dissoluble in water, and that the more readily if warmth do accompany it. Wherefore that substance, when put upon the Tongue, is dissolved by the moisture and warmth it meets with there, and unites with the Saliva of the mouth, and so proves even smooth and soft upon the Tongue, affecting it with pleasure. But Salt, on the contrary, though it dissolves in water as to its great parts, yet doth it retain some rigid small particles, which by warmth, when they are taken upon the Tongue, grow yet more rigid, and are so subtile, that they prick the globuls of our Tongue, though not so stiff, that they wound them.

The properties of salts and acids were studied during the next 200 years, but many, such as osmotic pressure and electrical conduction, were not well understood. Understanding leaped forward when a Swedish student, ARRHENIUS, presented his dissertation in 1884. He developed the thesis that salts and acids dissociate when placed in water and their individual ions act rather independently (ARRHENIUS 1887).

The concept was so daring that his professors were slow to accept it. In fact, he was awarded the lowest mark that could be given without a refusal of the doctoral degree. Subsequent development of his dissertation led to the award of the Nobel Prize. Within about five years of his dissertation defense, a series of papers written by well-known chemists appeared, in which they tried to explain sour and salty taste on the properties of the ions in solution.

It is interesting to remember that Galvani had said: "It would perhaps be a not inept hypothesis and conjecture, not altogether deviating from the truth, which should compare a muscle fiber to a small Leyden jar, or other similar electric body, charged with two kinds of electricity." By the end of the nineteenth century, Galvani's research on animal electricity had also been expanded by numerous investigations. The "electrical fluid" of nerves was now better understood. Indeed, in 1902 BERNSTEIN formulated the membrane theory of nerves and implicated the difference in K^+ concentration between the inside and outside of the cell as the source of the membrane potential. A quantitative treatment was applied with the aid of the famous Nernst equation, which had been published in 1892. In addition, Donnan had recognized in 1911 the importance of the impermeant ions, such as proteins, in the development of membrane potentials (DONNAN 1911). Such was the state of science when the first general theory of taste stimulation appeared.

The first comprehensive theory of taste was published by RENQUIST in 1919. He proposed that, at threshold, equal amounts of stimulus molecules or ions are adsorbed per unit time. The adsorption rate is:

$$\frac{dx}{dt} = Kx_\infty,\tag{1}$$

where: dx/dt = amount adsorbed per unit time, x_∞ = amount adsorbed at equilibrium, and K = a constant. Gibbs' (1876) adsorption equation relates x_∞ to the stimulus concentration, C, and the surface tension, σ:

$$x_\infty = \frac{C}{RT}\frac{d\sigma}{dc}\tag{2}$$

With additional considerations, the adsorption rate is:

$$\frac{dx}{dt} = k^{l/m} D\alpha C^{l/m}\tag{3}$$

where k, m, and α are constant for neutral salts and D is the diffusion coefficient. If it is assumed that dx/dt has the same value for all salts at threshold, $DC_t = a$ constant (GIBBS 1948). Thus threshold is inversely proportional to the diffusion velocity.

Renquist also applied his adsorption theory to thresholds of organic molecules, duration of taste sensation, Weber's law of just-noticeable differences, and taste qualities. Taste cell excitation was related to electrical potentials across the cell membrane derived from different diffusion rates of ions.

Other taste theories were quickly presented. LASAREFF (1922) assumed the taste stimulus enters the cell and interacts with a specific protein. The latter breaks down to ionized products, which initiates the cell's response. Proof given for this theory was based upon adaptation rates. Others related sour thresholds to lipid permeability. All the theories lacked quantitative and objective data with which they might be adequately tested.

D. The Rise of Taste Electrophysiology

Although Galvani is primarily remembered for his experiments with animal electricity, he was an excellent anatomist by profession. He examined the human ear in detail and discovered the chorda tympani taste nerve where it passed through the middle ear. It was not until 1850 that electrical stimulation of this taste nerve was accomplished. DUCHENNE (1850) described his experiments in the article "Recherches Électro-physiologiques et Pathologiques sur les Propriétés et les Usages de la Corde du Tympan." He partly filled the external ear canal with water and inserted an electrode into it. The other side of the head rested on a moist sponge with another wire attached. When galvanic current was sent through the wires, a metallic taste sensation was experienced. It appeared to arise from the front of the tongue.

Many years passed before nerve impulses were recorded from taste nerves. In the meantime, compound action potentials were recorded from slow-acting nerves with the capillary electrometer. With the advent of fast-acting string galvanometers, precise recordings could be made from most nerve bundles. However, information about sensory cells could best be obtained from the fine single fibers that innervated them. The first single-fiber recording was to be later obtained by a young Swedish postdoctoral student, Yngve Zotterman (Fig. 4), in Adrian's laboratory in Cambridge in 1926 (ADRIAN and ZOTTERMAN (1926). Another postdoctoral student, Detlev Bronk, also recorded from single motor fibers the following year (ADRIAN and BRONK 1928). These studies led to the development of Adrian's law, which states that the intensity of a sensory stimulus is coded by the nerves in terms of the frequency of electrical nerve impulses over each nerve fiber as well as the number of fibers active. This was to be the basis for the quantitative study of many sense organs.

E. My Early Life

Such was the state of the art in the field of the chemical senses when I was born in 1922. The proof that electric charges consisted of discrete particles called electrons had just been presented. The triode electron tube had been invented by DeForest in 1906 and the first vacuum tube amplifier introduced a short time later. Commercial sound broadcasting was just beginning in 1922. Airplanes were seldom seen in the skies and Lindbergh had not yet flown over the Atlantic.

I was born and raised in a small rural community near Allentown, Pennsylvania. My mother's family was of German origin, recently migrated. My father's descendants were Mennonites from south Germany and Switzerland. There they were severely persecuted because of their religious beliefs. They were simple, hardworking people with the belief that war is wrong and that government authority should not interfere with their religion. They migrated to Holland and left Rotterdam by ship to arrive in Philadelphia. They then settled in 1740 about 25 miles north of the city, shortly before Franklin began his electrical experiments nearby. The Beidlers purchased their land from William Penn's family in 1789.

The Beidlers remained in the same area for over 150 years. My grandfather moved north about 15 miles to the city of Allentown when my father was quite young. Although my mother and both grandmothers had high school educations, none of their husbands went beyond the 8th grade. My father became a railroad clerk. He was self-educated and a prolific reader. My two older sisters and I were raised in a small house in a small rural community north of Allentown. There was no bathroom or running water until I was a teenager.

My first six years of schooling were obtained about half a mile away in a two-room schoolhouse with an outhouse nearby. Since the four grades were in one room and with one teacher, self-discipline was a necessity. My later schooling was received in a rather new consolidated school to which several hundred students were bussed from a rather great distance. Only two curricula were available in high school, commercial and academic. I chose the latter and developed an interest in science. Fortunately, all students had to take courses in music, art and shop every year from grades 7 to 12. My experience in electric, wood, and metal shop was to become of great importance to me in later years.

The great depression had a great influence on me during my early life. However, I had a large advantage over many of my fellow students. We lived within several hundred yards of an abandoned iron mine, which became a city dump. This was a treasure of old parts of automobiles, bicycles, radios, etc. Here I learned to collect the parts necessary to make my first bicycle. All kinds of electronic components were available for the many simple radios and other gadgets that I made. Indeed, it was a true learning laboratory. I would never overcome the urge to build things!

Throughout high school I maintained an interest in science. The teacher and principal allowed me to build things in the physics and chemistry laboratory while I was supposed to be in study hall. I did not think of a college education, probably because few of the high school graduates ever went to college. One day, however, the principal took me out of class and said we were going to visit Muhlenberg College. The visit resulted in a scholarship and a different direction in life.

I decided to major in physics. The Head of the Department, Zartman, had been a National Research Council fellow and was the first to measure the velocities of molecules. He graduated during the depression and the only position he could get was at the small Lutheran College, Muhlenberg. The curriculum was excellent, with about six majors. We had much independence and were very close to the young professors.

One Sunday, while I was studying for an examination in atomic physics, the radio announced the attack on Pearl Harbor. This was during my junior year. The war accelerated our interest in physics and electronics and I graduated the following year. At this time, there was a great need for physicists with graduate training. Zartman, who several years earlier had gone to Johns Hopkins to do Naval research, helped me to obtain a junior instructorship in physics at Johns Hopkins.

For about 18 months I studied physics, and then the war effort resulted in a change of plans. I moved one floor down and worked for the Navy as a civilian to develop electronic proximity fuses. These fuses were attached to antiaircraft shells and shot toward airplanes. They contained small radio transmitters and receivers that measured the amount of waves reflected from the airplanes. Since this quantity was dependent upon the distance between the shell and airplane, the fuse controlled the time of explosion for maximum damage. There were a number of physicists working on this secret project, and it was here I met Mary Lou. She had just graduated from Goucher College as a physics major and had come to work on the Navy project.

When the war was over, I decided to study biophysics at the Johnson Foundation for Medical Physics at the University of Pennsylvania. This was really a research institute where a few students studied almost as apprentices. Detlev Bronk had developed excellent laboratories that attracted scientists from all over the world. Since I had only one freshman biology course, all my biological education was obtained at the University of Pennsylvania.

During my first year at the Johnson Foundation, Mary Lou and I married. She studied graduate physics and assisted in the laboratory at Bryn Mawr. Her research was in X-ray diffraction with a well-known professor, A. L. Patterson. She later worked at the Franklin Institute in Philadelphia. We often studied together and the knowledge I gained concerning X-ray diffraction proved valuable a few years later.

I worked closely with Frank Brink. His interest was in neurophysiology, as most research at the Foundation was in this area. I slowly became involved in such studies, but not with too much enthusiasm. By the time I was to start a dissertation, I thought that I could best use my previous study of molecular structure, quantum mechanics, and physical chemistry in the study of olfaction.

The students at the Johnson Foundation received wonderful opportunities. Most of the professors came to work around 10:30 a.m. The students worked closely with them. Everyone brought their lunches and ate together in the library. Usually visitors from other areas of the medical school also appeared. Frequently we would also eat dinner together and then work until 11:00 p.m. In addition, there were excellent electronic and machine shops where the students could obtain individual attention.

One day Bronk announced that he was to be President of Johns Hopkins University. Many of the faculty and students were to move to Hopkins to form a new Department of Biophysics. Keffer Hartline asked if I would like to do my dissertation in chemoreception, since Vincent Dethier at Hopkins was an expert in the chemical senses of insects. My working near him would help form a needed relationship with the Department of Biology. Of course, Keffer knew that I was interested, and I was forever grateful to him for the opportunity.

Mary Lou and I were delighted to return to Johns Hopkins. She worked in a visual laboratory in the Wilmer Institute of Ophthalmology at the medical school, across the hall from the laboratories of Steve Kuffler.

Since Dethier had detailed information on blowfly preference thresholds to chemicals, I decided to try to record from the blowfly. A tarsus was dissected free and the nerve isolated. Chemicals were applied to one end of the tarsus while recordings were made from the nerve at the other end. This was a very small preparation for me, and I worked for about a year without much success. Hartline, who was now Chairman of the Biophysics Department, encouraged me and told me not to despair. In the meantime I became a good friend of Dethier. We had many discussions, particularly about the suitability of an electrophysiological approach compared to a behavioral approach in the study of chemoreception. A close friendship also developed with Elliot Stellar of the Psychology Department, who was interested in food intake of animals. Curt Richter was studying preference thresholds of rats with particular reference to diet selection. He later became a member of my examining committee.

My insect research was progressing slowly. At that time it was not certain that the insect taste nerves utilized action potentials to communicate, since the distances were so small. The first action potential recording from insect taste nerves was to be performed a few years later by Ned Hodgson, who was a graduate student with Dethier while I was at Hopkins.

At this time (1948) I heard that Carl Pfaffmann at Brown University was successfully recording from the rat taste nerve. Although I disliked working with mammals, I decided to visit his laboratory. Mary Lou and I planned to include a hike through the White Mountains. After making an appointment, we took a bus to Providence. On our arrival, our luggage was missing. This presented a real problem to me as all our good clothing was in the luggage and we were wearing old hiking clothes. Should I buy a new suit to meet the Professor? As a student, I had little money. I decided to take a chance and visit in the clothes I had already been wearing for several days. Upon meeting Pfaffmann, I soon learned that my clothes didn't matter. He and his wife, Louise, were most gracious and our visit started a friendship that grew with the years.

We had an exciting time in the laboratory. The surgery needed to expose the chorda tympani was studied in detail. The response to salt was vigorous, not like my recordings from the frog sciatic nerve or the blowfly. The remainder of the day we talked about taste. His (PFAFFMANN 1941) paper on single-fiber recordings was well known to me. I also learned that he had studied at the Johnson Foundation and that we knew many of the same people. This day was to become one of the most important in my scientific career.

Upon returning to Hopkins, I ordered a few rats and tried to repeat the experiment seen at Brown. After many disappointing attempts, I finally obtained a preparation that responded. For some reason, 0.1 M HCl was used as a stimulus and my amplifier was turned up rather high. What a magnificient response! The sound was so loud that the amplifier reverberated. Immediately, I wondered if the response could be quantified. It was late at night and no sound-measuring equipment was available. What was I to do? Finally, it was decided to measure the voltage across the loudspeaker. The preparation lasted for about an hour and every chemical solution at hand was tried. This was the beginning of my quantitative studies.

The next morning I showed the results to another student, Ted MacNichol, and he suggested summing the nerve impulses electronically. What should be used as a measure of neural response magnitude? Adrian's law indicates that nerve impulse frequency signals the stimulus magnitude delivered by the sense organs. If this is true, then the activity of the sensory system can be adequately measured by counting the total number of nerve impulses per unit time. This is easily accomplished with single-fiber preparations. However, nerve impulses may overlap in multifiber preparations and thus cause errors in interpretation. Also, the heights of the impulses are dependent upon the electrical coupling between the single fiber within the nerve bundle and the recording electrode. Thus the spike heights vary. Additionally, the magnitude of spike height is related to the nerve fiber diameter. In a mixed nerve, fiber of many diameters is present. Fortunately, one can stimulate the tongue chemically and activate only the taste fibers (about 4 μm in diameter) without affecting other sensory fibers within the chorda tympani nerve bundle.

The first recorder of the nerve message is the synapse. It has the characteristic of low pass filtration as well as rectification. Since precise measurement of total nerve impulse frequency per unit time is difficult, why not use a simple integrator and rectifier? Only a rectifier tube, capacitor, and several resistors are needed. Its output is a running average of the rectified activity, which may be a better index of neural response than impulse frequency. It worked like magic. The use of the integrated circuit quantified the taste response and was a huge step forward. Since calibration of the circuit was difficult and since the value of the integrated response is dependent upon the recording conditions, all measures were related to some controlled response, such as that to 0.1 M NaCl. Fortunately, a good rat preparation may produce a 0.1 M NaCl response that is constant in magnitude to within 10% for over 12 h. Since one may apply a 10-s stimulus every minute if high concentrations are not used, over 700 quantified responses can be obtained with one animal.

Up to this time, no oscilloscope or electric recorder was available. All recordings were made with a Cambridge camera, consisting of a string galvanometer with mirror located 1 m from an electric carbon arc. The arc light was focused to the mirror and then to a moving photographic paper camera located 1 m away. One day, however, Brink received an electronic oscilloscope and, since he was not ready to use it, suggested that I try it. This luxury, together with a recorder and the new summator, was available to me for three or four months before having to be returned. I had never worked so hard. Quantitative measurements were made using large numbers of taste stimuli. In order to keep the area of stimulation constant, a flow chamber was made that fitted over the front of the rat's tongue.

It should be remembered that at this time no one published summated sensory activity. Many would frown at such results, and only original nerve recordings were accepted. For this reason, I never intended to use the summated responses in my dissertation. They were to be used only to determine the type of stimuli and concentrations to be used in short-term single-fiber experiments.

Single-fiber preparations came slowly for me and they did not last very long. A 45-min preparation was thought to be excellent. One day, Brink suggested that I should discuss my results with Keffer Hartline. We had had only limited contact, since he was Head of the Department and was interested in vision. Although we all worked in the same room and I was close to his graduate students and research associates, we seldom talked. One Saturday morning I decided to show him my progress. That morning was not to be forgotten. He postponed his experiments and spent the entire day showing me how to make finer dissecting tools and how to get single nerve fibers. The fact that a scientist of his stature would take that much time with a graduate student was very impressive. From that time on, there was much interaction and our relationship became closer.

One day it was announced that it was my time to give a seminar to the biophysics group. I was frantic, since only about two dozen single-taste-fiber preparations had been obtained. I decided to expand my talk to the allotted time by introducing my summated results for background purposes. Bronk, who was then President of Johns Hopkins, attended the seminar. The seminar went better than expected. Afterward, Hartline informed me that there were enough data for a dissertation and that I should finish up and get a job. I was stunned! No thought had been given to looking for a position. How did one get a teaching post? I went to Hartline for advice, but he said that he had never had this problem before. I was his first student. He did suggest that he could help me get a good job if given more time. I broke the news to Mary Lou and discussed it with Brink the next day.

Hartline sugested we make a joint proposal to the Sugar Research Foundation (there was no National Science Foundation or National Institutes of Health at this time) for a grant to study single-taste-fiber responses to sugars. Thus I would be able to stay at Hopkins for another year. Unfortunately, the application was turned down! This was my first experience of grant failure.

In the meantime, I wrote to a Chicago employment office. Several weeks later, as I was finishing my research, I received a telephone call from Ed Walker, Dean of Arts and Sciences at Florida State University; he wanted me to have dinner with him that evening in Washington. After running home and getting into my best clothes, I was off to Washington. Dean Walker was charming, and invited Mary Lou and me to visit the University in Tallahassee. Neither of us had ever been in the deep south and we thought it might be fun. This trip led to an offer. Upon my discussing the opportunity with Brink and Hartline, they suggested that I might go to Tallahassee for a year and gain teaching experience in physiology. I took a driving course the week before it was time to leave and bought a second-hand Kaiser car.

I left Hopkins in the fall of 1950 without taking my final examination. At Florida State I prepared lectures and laboratory sessions for courses in general physiology, human physiology, and sensory biophysics. In the evenings and on weekends I built equipment for my research. More equipment was needed, so I thought of writing to Bell Laboratories to see if they had any electronic instruments that they were ready to discard. To my surprise, they sent a large box full of electronics!

In May of 1951, Mary Lou, my five-month-old son Allan, and I traveled back to Hopkins to defend my dissertation. During the long trip I constantly worried about losing my job if I failed. The examination started poorly but ended quite well. We quickly returned to Tallahassee, greatly relieved.

Shortly afterward I wrote my first paper, which was published in the *Journal of Neurophysiology* (BEIDLER 1953). I was to write many more, but a remark by Frank Brink was never forgotten. He said if a scientist writes but one outstanding paper every ten years, this is more than most scientists ever accomplish. Looking back over my career, I find I have published several papers each year, but only a few per decade were really outstanding.

I soon started experiments but more equipment was needed. Since the Office of Naval Research (ONR) was the major source of research support, I wrote my second grant proposal. This effort proved successful. However, another learning experience was on the horizon. The ONR required quarterly research reports. When the first was due, there were no data available from my initial experiments. What was I to do? I telephoned Hartline and he suggested that I forget writing research reports. He said it would take too much of my time, someone in Washington might feel obligated to read the report, and some clerk would have to file it. Thus it wasted the time of everyone. For six years I sent no reports. One day I received a very apologetic letter stating that ONR had lost all my reports. Would I send a one-page summary of my six years of research! From that time on, I always wondered what happened to all the reports tens of thousands of researchers sent to Washington every year.

F. A Theory of Taste Receptor Stimulation

The quantification of the neural activity from the taste cell population led to my correlation of stimulus magnitude and receptor response. Although sugars, acids, and salts were considered, most attention was devoted to the salts.

Initially, thermodynamic activity was used as a measure of the stimulus intensity. However, lectures and discussions soon convinced me that the use of activities in my publications would result in little understanding of my message. For this reason, I correlated molar concentration of the stimulus to taste response magnitude. Although a sizable error in stimulus intensity was involved, it was not reflected in a large change in the magnitude of stimulus binding to the receptor at high concentration.

The simple mass action law was applied to the binding of the stimulus to the receptor, resulting in a hyperbolic relationship between the stimulus concentration and the taste response. This adsorption theory of taste was simple and well received. Its application was broadened to a variety of stimuli, and a detailed account of acid stimulation was presented.

The simple adsorption theory said nothing about all the transductive events that must exist between the time the stimulus is adsorbed and the time the taste cell is depolarized. MORITA (1969) was one of the few who were concerned with this problem and suggested modifications. However, since such modifications made the theory more complicated, few researchers utilized them.

Our concept that the taste stimulus is weakly bound (1–2 kcal/mol) to a receptor site later led SHALLENBERGER (1963) and others to develop precise molecular descriptions of the binding process. It was also an important element in the development of methods to isolate the receptor protein itself.

Serious challenges to the completeness of the adsorption theory were not provided until several decades later. Interestingly, the two major groups of Kurihara (Japan) and DeSimone (United States) once again placed emphasis on surface potentials, as biologists had 80 years previously.

G. The Question of Chemical Specificity

Nerves, like all other cells, are electrically charged. Their membrane potentials can be changed by various kinds of stimuli and elicit action potentials; we thus refer to the nerve's "general irritability." Indeed, under appropriate conditions, any peripheral nerve can mimic the responses of many sense organs. For example, it is well known that if the nerve is stained with eosin, it will respond to light. Similarly, mechanical pressure will also stimulate the nerve. The ability of all nerves to respond to a variety of chemicals was widely known at the beginning of the twentieth century. The exact mechanism was not known, although changes in osmotic pressure were suspected. Most responses to chemical stimulation were irreversible. In addition, specific chemicals such as sodium citrate were used to stimulate the nerve reversibly. In this case the citrate chelates the calcium ions, lowers the free Ca^{2+} concentration, and increases the nerve's excitability. This may result in spontaneous neural activity.

Since all cells, and nerves in particular, respond to chemical stimuli, how are these responses differentiated from those of specialized chemoreceptors? There are several characteristics that may be considered. First, the chemoreceptors respond to a wider variety of chemicals at lower concentrations. Secondly, the chemoreceptors respond quickly and reversibly. Other cells are often slow to respond and may be injured in the process. Thirdly, chemoreceptors are thought to respond specifically to chemicals and differentiate between closely related structures such as *d*- and *l*-forms. Finally, the response profiles of single chemoreceptors may be placed in groups loosely related to the primary tastes or odors.

My first research in chemical stimulation utilized the isolated frog sciatic nerve. Placing one end in high acid or salt concentration elicited electrical nerve impulses. If the experiment was repeated, the nerve had to be placed more deeply in the stimulus solution. Thus the stimulation involved injury. I decided that a better comparison between stimulation of nerves and taste cells could be made by simultaneously recording from the taste cells innervated by the chorda tympani and the tongue's free nerve endings innervated by the lingual nerve. Again, the taste cells responded more quickly, were more sensitive, responded to a wider variety of stimuli, and responded reversibly.

My interest in the response of free nerve endings was sustained over many years. When Don Tucker joined our technical staff, I discovered that he was interested in biology as well as electronics. It was suggested that he remove the sheet of olfactory tissue from the nasal turbinates of the opossum. The tissue was densely innervated and a fine nerve twig contained six to ten active C fibers. To our amazement, each fiber exhibited a different response profile to odors. For this reason we thought that these were olfactory fibers. It was not until several years later that we were convinced that they were indeed trigeminal fibers.

Why should free nerve endings show specificity for certain chemicals, and why should each fiber have a different response profile? My only conclusion is that the odor stimulation injured the fiber endings to a different extent and that the ability to respond to a given chemical depends upon the previous history of the stimulated fiber. Another possibility, however, is that not all the free endings are identical or that the tissue around them may alter their irritability.

It is well known that people shed tears while peeling onions. How sensitive to odors are the free nerve endings of the cornea? A postdoctoral student, Bill Dawson (1962), investigated the response to the odors amyl acetate and phenyl ethyl alcohol. The amyl acetate threshold was higher than that reported by Tucker for the rabbit nasal trigeminal nerve, but it did indeed stimulate the corneal nerves. Again, this demonstrates the general irritability of nerve cells.

All of the above examples of chemical stimulation emphasize the fact that the nerve and its environment determine the ability of the nerve to respond to chemical stimuli. In some areas of the body, such as the nose, chemical stimulation of the nerve endings results in reflexive action and can control important body functions, such as respiratory and cardiovascular activity. Although the majority of chemoreceptor studies are related to sensory functions and perception, the related motor functions may be of equal importance. Perhaps in the near future there will be a shift of emphasis from psychology to physiology in the study of chemoreceptors. Certainly, the oral and nasal chemoreceptors can monitor the chemical input to the body. They presumably could also initiate actions that would serve to regulate body functions in response to changes in chemical input.

H. Species Differences

RENQUIST'S (1919) correlation of human taste thresholds for salts to their mobility or diffusion velocity in aqueous medium was accepted for many years. Since mobility of a specific ion in an aqueous solution is a constant for a given concentration and temperature, all animal species should display the same sequence of cations if arranged according to threshold. A quarter of a century later, Hubert FRINGS (1946) measured taste thresholds for several insects. He concluded that "the other modalities perceived by man seem for the roach, and possibly for caterpillars and the honey-bee, to fall into a series which can be defined in terms of thresholds or stimulative efficiencies." He also stated that "the order of stimulative efficiency for inorganic salts and acids is possibly the same for man as for species from three orders of insects. ... The cation arrangement in such a series is that of mobilities." Thus, since many species appeared to respond to salts in a similar manner, there was little interest in looking at species differences when the number of electrophysiological studies dramatically increased in the early 1950s.

Differences in the responses of mammals to a given series of salts was observed quite unexpectedly. We had a cat that was used for the study of cochlear microphonis. One evening, since it was still in good shape, I suggested that a graduate student, Clarence Hardiman, record from the chorda tympani in the middle ear. We were surprised that the response to NaCl was very poor compared to that of the rat, while the potassium response was quite good! This discovery led to experiments by Hardiman, Fishman, and me with a variety of species, including wild animals (BEIDLER et al. 1955). We were quite excited. Shortly afterward, I related our results to Pfaffmann, and was quite surprised when he said he was also looking at different species and had come to the same conclusions concerning response differences. We agreed to publish simultaneously but in different journals. This was not to be the last time our laboratory was to discover something new and to find later that another laboratory was working on the same problem.

Tallahassee is surrounded by a national forest and many unsettled areas, and wild animals are relatively easy to obtain. We studied raccoon, skunk, possum, fox, etc., as well as large domesticated animals, such as calves, sheep, and goats. NH_4Cl was a good stimulus for all of these animals, as was KCL. NaCl, on the other hand, produced large responses in rats, mice, etc., but small responses in cats, dogs, etc. All the carnivores responded poorly to Na^+ as compared to K^+, whereas the rodents responded very well to Na^+. These observations reminded me of the relative concentrations of the same ions in red cells that I had read about in graduate school. Was there a causal relationship?

At the time we were working on this problem, I attended a lecture on red cells at Woods Hole. I learned of the individual differences of the Na^+/K^+ ratio in red cells in sheep and goats. Some individuals had high red cell K^+ content and others low. Was there also a variation in taste response to Na^+ and K^+ in these individuals? We rented a truck and drove to the middle of Georgia to buy a dozen sheep. After we returned, the chorda tympani responses to NaCl and KCl were measured on each sheep and the content in red cells was also determined. All the sheep gave the same Na^+/K^+ taste response ratio even though both high and low red cell K^+ content animals were in the group. Thus there appears to be a high relation between the red cell Na^+ and K^+ content and the taste response to these ions in many species, but no such relationship exists between individuals of a species including high K^+ and low K^+ animals.

It is interesting to note that the level of K^+ in red cells is correlated to the amount of adenosine triphosphatase (ATPase) in the red cells. Is there a relationship between taste cell ATPase concentration and the ability of the taste cell to respond to Na^+ and K^+ ions? We do not yet know.

Studies reveal that different single taste nerve fibers in the same animal do not necessarily show the same stimulative efficiency for a series of cations. In fact, it is difficult to find two single fibers that show an identical order of response magnitudes to a reasonably large series of taste stimuli. Although the individual taste nerve fibers may vary greatly in response profiles, the population as a whole responds in a predictable manner and is very similar from animal to animal of the same species.

Studies of species differences, as well as single-fiber studies, have great implications for theories of taste mechanisms. Their results imply that no taste theory can be based solely upon properties of the stimuli in aqueous solution, such as diffusion rates, cation size, and polarity. What is at least equally important is the nature of the membrane with which the stimulus reacts. Apparently, the membrane has many different places where the stimulus can react and the membrane properties also differ slightly from one cell to another and from one species to another. Only this can explain why different taste cells respond differently to a series of chemical stimuli.

J. Response of a Single Taste Cell

The classic single-fiber study of PFAFFMANN (1941) demonstrated that a single taste fiber can respond to stimuli associated with several taste qualities. However, each single fiber innervates many taste cells. The question remains, can a single taste cell respond to taste substances associated with more than one quality?

LING and GERARD (1949) introduced microelectrode techniques to the study of the nervous system. Can they be applied to the recording from the narrow taste cells of the living tongue? This procedure requires much patience and manual dexterity.

One of my first research associates was Katsumi Kimura of Japan. I suggested that he try such microelectrode techniques. The rat and hamster were selected, since they were well studied using whole taste nerve recordings. They showed good responses to sugars and other natural stimuli that might not be very effective with the more easily penetrated frog taste cells. Kimura found that taste cells can respond to a variety of stimuli not solely associated with one taste quality (KIMURA and BEIDLER 1956, 1961). Furthermore, the sensitivity and response profile varied from one cell to another. Tateda (TATEDA and BEIDLER 1964) repeated the study and also measured the magnitude of responses as the membrane potential was altered with $FeCl_3$ or cocaine. The responses to chemical stimulation appeared to approach an equilibrium potential regardless of whether the taste cell was depolarized or hyperpolarized before stimulation. Proof that all recordings were from microelectrodes in the taste bud was afforded by the use of iron stains.

The above studies set the stage for a series of more sophisticated researches on the response of taste cells. OZEKI's (1971) group in Japan and T. SATO (1973, 1975) in my laboratory not only measured membrane potential changes to a variety of stimuli, but also studied the accompanying changes in membrane resistance.

The mature mammalian sensory taste cell, as distinguished from other cells of the taste bud, has never been undisputedly characterized using histological methods. On the other hand, the frog taste cell was well differentiated from supporting cells of the frog fungiform papillae by GRAZIADEI and DE HAHN in 1971. This research suggested that T. Sato should use intracellular stains to identify the type of cell of the frog taste bud into which he thrust his microelectrode. Since it was known that all cells are electrically charged and that the magnitude of charge can be changed by the application of some chemicals, it was necessary to compare responses from sensory taste cells to those of supporting cells. This was accomplished by T. Sato with the frog, using the intracellular stains.

The early single taste cell recordings were criticized because the observed latency of the receptor potentials was large when chemical stimuli were used. The experimenters replied that this was a reflection of the slow transport of the stimulus to the taste buds. This argument was concluded when SATO (1976) was able to place the chemical stimulus within 100–400 μm of the recording taste cell. The latency dropped to a predictable value of 50 ms, in agreement with the values of latency as measured by single-fiber recordings.

K. Life Span of Taste Cells

The classification of cell types within the taste bud became almost a pastime for histologists at the beginning of the twentieth century. Each histologist had his own classification. This changed rather quickly in 1910 when Kolmer stated that cell types were merely transitions in the growth stage of taste cells. This conclusion was supported by suggestions of HERMANN (1888) and RETZIUS (1912) that mitotic figures are occasionally seen in the taste bud. However, others regarded these as foreign invading cells, and leukocytes were often observed. OLMSTEDT (1920) stated: "I have never observed a case of mitosis in a normal taste bud, though it is not a rare occurrence in the germinative layer of the epidermis."

The need for taste cell renewal within the taste bud was recognized and clearly stated by KOLMER in 1927. He wrote:

It is no easy matter to prove that taste bud cells die and are replaced by new ones in the course of life. However, in view of the extraordinary degree of wear and tear to which the lining of the oral cavity is subjected as a result of chemical, mechanical, and – in man – thermal factors, it must be assumed that the continual death and replacement of degenerate cells takes place here, as in the rest of the oral epithelium.

This statement proved to be prophetic.

The concept of taste cell renewal was disregarded by most students of taste physiology of later years. Even the electron microscopists returned to the arguments over taste cell classification. More direct experiments on taste cell turnover were needed. I decided to see whether disruption of cell division altered taste function. Two methods were used, colchicine injection and tongue X-irradiation. Rats irradiated for different time periods were used in electrophysiological experiments. No obvious differences in responses to taste stimuli were noted. Colchicine injections did change the magnitude of taste responses, and they often completely disappeared within 10 h. Unfortunately, colchicine not only inhibits mitosis but has many other effects. One of these is the rapid degeneration of the endings of the taste nerve beneath the taste bud.

We decided to inject colchicine and then look for cells with mitotic figures in the tongue epithelium. No such cells were observed within the taste bud, but the epithelial cells surrounding the bud were affected. At this time I became familiar with the use of tritiated thymidine for cell tagging. After a short visit to Quastler's laboratory at Brookhaven Laboratory by Ron Smallman and me, successful experiments were conducted. We determined (BEIDLER and SMALLMAN 1965) that the epithelial cells surrounding the taste bud undergo division. The daughter cell may enter the bud, differentiate, and live for an average of about 10 days. The determination that taste cells are continually replaced had a great effect on histologists and electron microscopists who studied taste bud structure.

The taste bud was the first sensory cell known to be replaced by mitotic division. When this was first reported, resistance to the concept was widespread. However, it was of immediate interest to those who studied turnover of epithelial cells. Bertlanfy, an anatomist specializing in cell renewal processes, wrote to me in 1963 and stated:

I cannot conceal my great surprise about the rapid turnover of sensory taste bud cells in rodents. It is the general consensus that neural elements, including sensory cells of olfactory epithelium, taste buds, and retina, are not replaced if lost by trauma or otherwise. I have never heard anybody propose that these cells would undergo renewal. The reason for this presumably is that until now nobody took the trouble to find out. I believe that your finding is of greatest significance inasmuch as it is the first to show turnover of neuroepithelial elements.

After a few years passed, the concept of taste cell replacement was generally accepted and even expected, since the cells were neuroepithelial and not neural. However, we began to wonder whether olfactory sensory cells were also replaced when injured. One of our graduates, Dick Jackson, did some preliminary experiments. Dave Moulton went one step further and tagged the cells with tritiated thymidine some time after he left Tallahassee. Pasquale Graziadei became interested in the problem after he arrived in Tallahassee, and performed a series of well-designed experiments to prove to his satisfaction and that of others that olfactory receptors indeed are replaced. This led to his general interest in the degeneration and regeneration of olfactory receptors and their nerve processes. Again, many anatomists were slow in accepting the idea that these neural cells are indeed continually replaced. Many laboratories have now studied these processes, and turnover of taste and olfactory cells is now accepted by all.

If taste cells are continually renewed, what effect does this have on the ability of individual taste cells to discriminate taste stimuli? Does innervation of a given taste cell also change with time? I suggested the possibility that taste cell sensitivity might depend upon taste cell age. That is, the younger cells are those just entering the taste bud and presumably are innervated by those nerve endings in that region. As new taste cells arise, the same nerves in the periphery of the bud would innervate them. Thus a given nerve would always innervate taste cells of a given age.

The concept of continuous nerve turnover of taste cells was intriguing to Hallowell Davis when it was presented at the First International Symposium held in Stockholm in 1962. However, he was concerned with the maintenance of neural specificity as related to the taste qualities if the synaptic connections with the individual taste cells change. He proposed a model based upon a quasi-random distribution of connections of the afferent neurons on the taste cells. Noting that most taste cells respond to stimuli associated with several taste qualities, he introduced the concept of mutual inhibitory action found in other sensory systems to reject unwanted activity and thus peak the response to one quality. In this manner he explained specific chemical sensitivity even though afferent connections are quasi-random. He concluded, "An interesting feature of this model is its statistical character, which makes the overall action independent of the details of the connections of individual afferent neurons or of the exact patterns of sensitivity found for individual neurons." His insight into neural taste coding is as worthy of consideration today as it was 20 years ago.

L. A Diversion – The United States Science Exhibit

Research quickly becomes a consuming passion. It is often difficult to balance it against teaching and service, the two other areas of faculty concern. Seldom do other activities command attention. In my case, however, an incident arose that developed into an interest I never suspected. I received a telephone call from a good friend, Leroy Augustine. He asked me to come to Washington, D.C. for a day to give some advice on plans for the United States Science Exhibit to be held at the Seattle World's Fair. Congress gave 10 million dollars to display science to the general public.

We had a good day, and about an hour before my plane was to depart, the Associate Commissioner asked me to spend a year coordinating all the science matters needed for designers to produce exhibits. I was amazed and not immediately interested. To make the decision negative, I asked for a salary I was sure they would not consider. To my surprise they agreed to the salary. All the way home I wondered how I would explain this abrupt change in plans to my family and colleagues.

A leave of absence was granted and I left for Washington. About a dozen science writers were assigned to me and we went about the job of obtaining science material. Most of my time was spent jointly with a designer whose responsibility was to oversee all exhibit design. This meant much traveling to see scientists, designers, and producers of motion pictures. After three or four months, I shifted my office from Washington, D.C. to a design firm on Madison Avenue in New York.

Shortly before the Fair was to open, my family and I moved to Seattle. The job was made much more interesting by the creativity of the Commissioner, Athelstan Spillhaus. I decided to employ 40 young women to serve as intermediaries with the public. To train them I selected my former graduate student, Ron Smallman.

After the Fair opened, my work changed. Television interviews were given with almost no notice. Dignitaries and scientists from around the world visited the Exhibit and had to be greeted. These ranged from Prince Philip to the Shah of Iran, Vice President Johnson to Governor Rockefeller, and John Glenn to John Wayne. These experiences have proved beneficial throughout the remainder of my career.

While I was on leave of absence, four days a month were allowed for my return to the laboratory in Tallahassee. Research continuity was made much easier by my research associates, Dave Moulton and Don Tucker. I suspect their research as well as that of the graduate students was more independent and therefore of greater training value during my absence. From this time on, all the students and postdoctoral students were given a tremendous amount of research freedom and advice was only given when thought needed. Frequently, this strategy seemed time-consuming for the students, but the confidence and laboratory competence they gained proved beneficial when they assumed their first faculty positions. It was also decided that they should each attend at least one international meeting where they could meet other scientists. In addition, when outstanding scientists visited our laboratory, the graduate students were asked to have lunch with them without any faculty participation. They soon learned that a scientist's personality plays a great role in the acceptance of his research.

M. Attempts to Record from Man's Chorda Tympani

In 1952, Samuel L. Rosen, an otolaryngologist of New York, published a paper on stimulation of the human chorda tympani in the middle ear. Of interest to me was the fact that the chorda tympani taste nerve in the middle ear was cut to give an unobstructed view of the stapes. Could one record from the human taste nerve? Since only local anesthetics were used, perhaps a verbal response could also be obtained, since the other chorda tympani was intact. I wrote to Rosen in 1954 and outlined what I wanted to do. He replied on 26 August 1954:

Your letter and reprint interested me very much. Experiments similar to the ones you describe were performed by Dr. Puharich and myself in his laboratory at the Round Table Forum. We were concerned however with stimulating the tongue with sound to see if we could then pick it up in the chorda tympani. We thought we had done this accurately until we submitted our tracings to Dr. Grundfest at Columbia. He thought the work should be repeated, as he felt that some of the tracings might be artifacts.

At any rate, your letter sounds very inviting. I will be willing to cooperate since I have ample human material with which to make these important measurements. We could set up the experiments in the operating room of Mount Sinai Hospital in New York, if you could bring your equipment there. We could make at least one experiment every day of the week. In this way I think very important data might be found which would throw light not only on the physiology of taste, but the physiology of hearing and equilibrium as well, both of which I believe are tied up with the chorda tympani nerve.

Will you therefore let me know how you propose to set up your experiments so I can give it consideration.

At this time my research was supported by ONR. On being advised that I wanted to record from the chorda tympani with Samuel Rosen, they suggested I first discuss the problem with Glen Wever of Princeton University. A visit proved that he was quite sympathetic with the plans. I gathered that ONR questioned my research plans because Rosen's stapes mobilization procedure for patients with otosclerosis was not yet accepted.

My equipment was taken to New York, including a special device to hold an electrode with the ear speculum. In the middle of stapes mobilization surgery, the nerve was placed onto the electrodes. Experiments were tried for several weeks during each of two summers. Hardiman, a graduate student, helped during one of the summers. Unfortunately, the local anesthetic was applied near the eardrum and anesthetized the chorda tympani shortly after the surgery began. Thus our experiments were always short-lived and not conclusive.

Although we failed, researchers in Sweden were quite successful. I first learned of this research in 1957 from William Miller, a student of vision who was working with Hartline at Rockefeller Institute for Medical Research. He wrote:

You are probably aware of Zotterman's recent work; however, some of it is so close to what you have been doing that I thought I would drop you a line and risk repetition. Zotterman gave a lecture on Taste yesterday afternoon at P and S. Like you, he is recording from the human chorda tympani during ear operations. He has met with some success. In two cases he has recorded activity, getting the strongest response to sucrose (if I understood him rightly). These experiments are just getting up steam and apparently he hadn't any more than this to say on the subject.

An otolaryngologist, Diamant, performed stapes mobilization with patients under general anesthesia. He had an interest in salivation and thus was quite familiar with the functions of the chorda tympani. He teamed up with his friend Yngve Zotterman to try to record from the chorda tympani. Their experiments were most successful and showed that the responses of human taste receptors are very similar to those of laboratory animals. In addition, together with their colleagues they measured subjective responses from the patients before surgery. Thus they could compare human psychophysical data with electrophysiological recordings from the same subjects (DIAMANT et al. 1963).

Today, surgeons who operate for otosclerosis do not routinely cut the chorda tympani. Thus it is difficult to record from human taste nerves. It is unfortunate that more research on the human chorda tympani has not been carried out by taste researchers located near medical centers. A wealth of information is waiting to be discovered.

Although our experiments on human taste nerves were unsuccessful, much experience was gained and insight into the medical arena was received. When I first met Rosen, his stapes mobilization surgery for otosclerosis was greeted with suspicion by many of his colleagues. The second year many otolaryngologists came to him to observe the surgery. The third year his new surgical technique was accepted around the world. He was a very active and inventive otolaryngologist.

N. An Interlude by von Békésy

Laboratory visits by scientists in other sensory areas are most helpful. Von Békésy visited Tallahassee each year for about six years. He was a rather shy individual but with definite ideas as to how experiments should be designed. During the first two visits he emphasized the need for better stimulus control. At this time I was using an automated taste solution dispenser to study taste in children. He was most interested, but suggested a more sophisticated method of stimulus application similar in principle to that used in audition. He viewed olfactory research as very primitive and suggested that no fundamental discoveries would be made until more attention was given to the manner in which odors are transported to the mucosa. At no time did he reveal that he was thinking of contributing to the study of chemoreceptors.

One day he sent me a manuscript on chemical stimulation of single papillae for comments. I was amazed that this great student of audition had now designed taste experiments. I read the manuscript and sent back several pages of suggestions. He was most grateful and accepted many of them. His terminology had confused taste buds with papillae. This was corrected. However, he said nothing about criticism of his method of papilla stimulation and in particular, the diagram of a fungiform papilla which he used. It contained taste buds only on the walls and none on the dorsal surface. A confusion with the circumvallate papilla appeared to be the problem. I later discovered that such a confusion was common with students of sensory systems other than taste.

The experiments of von Békésy, including those on electrical stimulation of taste buds, suggested that taste receptors may initiate but one taste quality. This was contrary to the current thought based primarily upon single-fiber experiments. It was, however, consistent with earlier views and was accepted by many students of other sensory systems. One such senior investigator reviewed the paper of von Békésy and stated that the well-designed experiments of von Békésy conclusively demonstrated that a single taste bud elicits but one taste sensation, although taste researchers would probably not take kindly to this concept. He was correct that taste scientists would not easily accept these conclusions! Many papers later appeared with conclusions opposite to those of von Békésy. The fact that he stimulated the walls of the fungiform papilla which contain no taste buds made acceptance of his paper on chemical stimulation most difficult.

Today we are reasonably certain that a single human taste bud may elicit the perception of several taste qualities. A single human fungiform papilla may have no taste bud or as many as seven or more. Thus it is difficult to stimulate but one taste bud and determine the subject's perception of taste quality. However, ARVIDSON and FRIBERG (1980) successfully stimulated single human fungiform papillae, noted the subject's taste sensation, and then excised the papilla and counted the number of taste buds. They concluded that a single taste bud can initiate a taste response of several taste qualities.

Both single taste cells and single taste nerve fibers of many animals respond to a variety of taste stimuli that man perceives as initiating different taste qualities. On the other hand, each taste bud contains up to 50 taste cells and each bud is innervated by an average of only about two fibers of the taste nerve. Thus there may be a great amount of interaction between the signals from the individual taste cells. Indeed, MILLER (1971, 1974) demonstrated such interactions between cells of two different taste buds innervated by the same single nerve fiber! It is apparent that we know little of the amount of information processing that may occur at the level of an individual taste bud or between taste buds. The fact that a single taste cell or a single taste fiber can respond to many stimuli may have no bearing on the question of whether a single taste bud or papilla can produce more than one quality of sensation.

Von Békésy was greatly interested in the interaction between receptors. I believe that this was his motivation for his study of taste. Hartline had studied lateral inhibition in the visual system and showed its importance in visual perceptions. Von Békésy accepted similar interactions in audition and then designed beautiful experiments to show such interactions when the skin of the arm is stimulated. Perhaps the lack of complete acceptance of his first series of taste experiments truncated a continued interest in chemoreception.

During one of his last visits he indicated a lack of interest in remaining at Harvard. As he related it, Harvard would not buy him a comfortable chair and the National Institutes of Health did not allow such purchases on their grants. Perhaps he overstated his position, but it was evident that he was disturbed. He also indicated interest in moving to Tallahassee, so Florida State University quickly made an offer. He initially accepted but later became concerned with the pension plan. Eventually, he moved to Hawaii and never returned to his studies on taste. I often wonder how different the fields of taste and olfaction would be if von Békésy had continued his studies and brought his unusual originality, insight, and expertise in instrument design to this field.

O. Taste Modification

Knowledge of taste and the ability to manipulate it has been noted throughout man's history. Perhaps one of the earliest accounts of taste modification is found in the book of Exodus. After Moses led the Israelites from the Red Sea, they went three days without water. When they found water, it was bitter and they could not drink it. Moses "cried to the Lord; and the Lord showed him a tree, and he threw it into the water, and the water became sweet." On a visit to Israel, I inquired about the source of this plant. No information could be given.

Several other plants that modify taste sensation have been described in the literature. The most studied is *Gymnema sylvestre* from India. Its sweet-inhibition properties have been studied in several laboratories. I suggested that Yoshie Kurihara study the active molecule in our laboratory. She was particularly interested in the acids that esterified the molecule. Throughout my career I have learned much from research associates such as the Kuriharas.

Miracle fruit from the shrub *Synsepalum dulcificum* makes sour things taste sweet. This characteristic was noted by visitors to Nigeria and Ghana at the turn of the century. However, the active ingredient is inactivated within a few days, so that shipping quantities of fruit to the United States is pointless. George INGLETT (1965) made preliminary investigations using solvents common for organic separation. I decided to buy a number of small plants and grow them in our greenhouse.

After several years, we also tried organic solvents without success. I decided to make an artificial saliva and see whether the active ingredient would be soluble. It was! Then I decided to make a bicarbonate buffer and try it. This procedure succeeded.

At this time, Kenzo Kurihara, a physical biochemist, joined our laboratory for several years. His investigation resulted in the isolation, purification, and partial characterization of the active ingredient (KURIHARA and BEIDLER 1965). To our surprise it was a glycoprotein of molecular weight of about 44,000. This was the first protein known to possess either a taste or ability to modify a taste. It was such an unexpected result that we were wary of publication! Today, a number of proteins are known to stimulate taste receptors of man and other animals.

Bob Harvey, a student of Linda Bartoshuk, studied the effects of miracle fruit on taste using electrophysiological techniques. One day he asked if he could have some of our plants. At the time, we had hundreds growing in our greenhouse. He took a group of them back to Boston and continued his research on their fruit. He soon started a small company in 1968 to develop products using miracle fruit. At about this time I had a telephone call from someone at Reynolds Metal Company. They wondered whether the miracle fruit plants could be grown on their strip-mined land in Jamaica. I referred them to Bob and this led to a close relationship between Reynolds Metal and Harvey's company, Mirlin Inc. During the next few years, over 6 million dollars were spent on research and development by the company. Tablets, menus, and associated foods were sold. Legal counsel suggested in 1973 that extracts of miracle fruit were not food additives and thus could obtain GRAS (generally regarded as safe) status. Ultimately, the Food and Drug Administration (FDA) requested additional information on miracle fruit. For example, they had been informed by others that miracle fruit glycoprotein molecules might pass directly from the oral cavity to the brain and thus modify the response of its taste centers! However, it had already been shown by Zotterman's human electrophysiological experiments that miracle fruit merely altered the response of acids applied to the tongue. Thus its action was on the taste buds. Soon thereafter, the FDA required tests on three animal species in addition to those already performed by Mirlin. These tests were expected to cost several million dollars and led to the ultimate dissolution of the company. It was not until several years later that the FDA formally replied to Mirlin's initial request for approval to distribute a product containing miracle fruit extract. When the FDA's action was finally registered, they banned all interstate selling of miracle fruit itself, as well as any products arising from it.

When we published the research on miracle fruit, I used the phrase "taste modification." This referred to the ability to change a sour sensation to one of sweetness. We did not mean to imply that any modification of the taste receptors were involved. In fact, we suggested the glycoprotein merely reacts with the conventional sugar receptor sites when they are exposed to low pH's. Unfortunately, the phrase "taste modification" implied to some that the glycoprotein actually modifies the taste receptors. Thus one must be most careful when choosing words or phrases to describe physiological processes.

In 1968, M. Nejad, a former student of mine, sent me a copy of a page from a Persian manuscript handwritten in the seventeenth century. The author was court physician to Shah Soleiman Safari. It translated as "... its leaves cause the perception of taste be changed, it is so that food cannot be differentiated." I traveled to Tehran and Nejad took me to the shores of the Caspian Sea. After a few days, we found a tree called "onab," which produced the described leaf. We collected and dried several bushels of leaves and then shipped them to my laboratory in Tallahassee. The leaves inhibited sweetness and our investigations showed that the active ingredient was identical to one of the forms of gymnemic acid.

In the meantime, KENNEDY and HALPERN (1980) investigated the leaves of the plant, *Ziziphus jujuba*. They concluded that the active ingredient was not gymnemic acid, although some of the taste attributes were similar. We were surprised to learn that our onab plant from Iran was actually *Ziziphus jujuba!* The difference in chemical description of the active ingredient by the two laboratories is still not resolved.

P. Finale

The study of taste has attracted researchers from many disciplines over the years. The history of taste research is thus flavored with the history of chemistry, anatomy, electricity, physiology, psychology, and electronics. What I have written in this chapter is just a concise and personalized history of a selection of taste topics.

Each of us contains reflections of those with whom he has come in contact. The list includes not only teachers but also graduate students and research associates. Tallahassee is a small and isolated community; Florida State University is a growing university with many of the flavors of a small college. As a consequence, a very independent research atmosphere was created and one could dare to initiate any type of experiment without criticism. Most of the experiments I personally initiated failed. A few opened new frontiers in the science of chemoreception. Students were encouraged to develop their own little areas of science where they were their own masters, and which they could continue to develop in their subsequent positions. They were also encouraged to read the old literature and to keep their own research in proper perspective.

During the course of training graduate and postdoctoral students, we were most fortunate to have a number of our colleagues visit Tallahassee for various periods. Perhaps the most colorful and knowledgeable was Yngve Zotterman. He had a wealth of experience with many receptor systems. His life also spanned the complete period of single-nerve-fiber recording. Most of all, he brought to the laboratory a great interest in students and a childlike curiosity that immediately stimulated all those around him. All of us were grateful for each visit.

A close relationship with Carl Pfaffmann was formed from the first time we met. This was often extended to our students. He was trained in both physiology and psychology. He, more than any other, made us aware of the possible behavioral implications of our biophysical and physiological researchers. Gradually, my students became more interested in the contributions of the experimental psychologists in our own university. Pfaffmann trained a large number of students of taste and olfaction who, over the years, have had a dominant influence on the course of research in taste and olfaction.

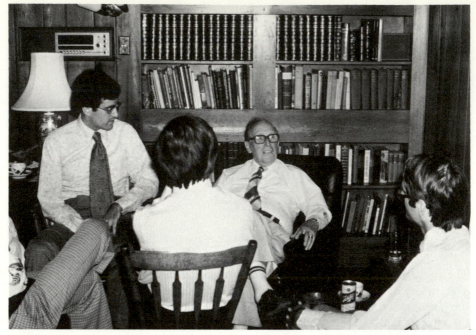

Fig. 4. Yngve Zotterman in 1977 discussing taste physiology with three postdoctoral students while visiting Tallahassee

Scientific research is often portrayed as a very rational and objective search for truth. This is, of course, quite true. However, a great portion is also a result of the personalities of the researchers themselves. In writing this personalized sketch of the history of taste biophysics, I placed stress on the people involved rather than merely their contributions.

References

Names containing *von* are alphabetized in this list under *v*

Adrian ED, Bronk DW (1928) The discharge of impulses in motor nerve fibres, part I. Impulses in single fibers of the phrenic nerve. J Physiol 66–81
Adrian ED, Zotterman Y (1926) The impulses produced by sensory nerve endings, part II. J Physiol 61:151–171
Aldini G (1953) Dissertation on the origin and development of the theory of animal electricity (1792). In: Green R (ed) A translation of Luigi Galvani's De viribus electricitatis. Waverly, Baltimore
Arrhenius S (1887) Über die Dissoziation der in Wasser gelösten Stoffe. Z Physikal Chemie 1:631–648
Arvidson K (1979) Location and variation in number of taste buds in human fungiform papillae. Scand J Dent Res 87:435–442
Arvidson K, Friberg U (1980) Human taste: response and taste bud number in fungiform papillae. Science 209:807–808
Beidler LM (1953) Properties of chemoreceptors of tongue of rat. J Neurophysiol 16:595–607
Beidler LM (1954) A theory of taste stimulation. J Gen Physiol 3:133–139

Beidler LM, Smallman RL (1965) Renewal of cells within taste buds. J Cell Biol 27:263–272

Beidler LM, Fishman IY, Hardiman CW (1955) Species differences in taste responses. Am J Physiol 181:235–239

Bellini L (1666) Gustus organum. Philos Trans R Soc Lond [Biol] 1:366–367

Bernstein J (1902) Untersuchungen zur Thermodynamik der bioelektrischen Ströme. Pflügers Arch 92:521–562

Davis H (1969) Discussion of dynamics of taste cells. In: Pfaffmann C (ed) Olfaction and taste. Rockefeller University Press

Dawson W (1962) Chemical stimulation of the peripheral trigeminal nerve. Nature 169:341–345

Diamant H, Funakoshi M, Strom L, Zotterman Y (1963) Electrophysiological studies on human taste nerves. In: Zotterman Y (ed) Olfaction and taste I. Pergamon, Oxford

Donnan F (1911) Theorie der Membrangleichgewichte und Membranpotentiale bei Vorhandensein von nicht dialysierenden Elektrolyten. Ges Eelektrochem 17:572–581

Duchene (1850) Recherches électro-physiologiques et pathologiques sur les propriétes et les usages de la corde du tympan. Arch Gen Med 24:385–412

Fish HS, Malone PP, Richter CP (1944) The anatomy of the tongue of the domestic Norway rat. I. The skin of the tongue; the various papillae; their number and distribution. Anat Rec 89:429–441

Franklin B (1751–1754) Experiments and observations on electricity. London

Frings H (1946) Gustatory thresholds for sucrose and electrolytes for the cockroach, *Periplaneta americana* (Linn.). J Exp Zool 102:23–50

Galvani L (1953) De viribus electricitatis in moto musculari commentarius. Waverly, Baltimore

Gibbs JW (1948) Collected works, vol I. Yale University Press, New Haven

Graziadei P, DeHan R (1971) The ultrastructure of frog's taste organs. Acta Anat 80:563–603

Harvey R (1970) Gustatory studies relating to *Synsephalum dulcificum* (miracle fruit) and neural coding. PhD dissertation, Worcester Polytechnic Institute

Hermann F (1888) Studien über den feineren Bau des Geschmacksorgans. 18:277–318

Ingelett G, Dowling J, Albrecht J, Hodge F (1965) Taste-modifying properties of miraclefruit (*S. dulcificum*). J Agric Food Chem 13:284–287

Kennedy L, Halpern B (1980) Extraction, purification and characterization of a sweetnessmodifying component from *Ziziphus jujuba*. Chem Senses Flavor 5:123–143

Kimura K, Beidler LM (1956) Microelectrode study of taste bud of the rat. Am J Physiol 187:610–611

Kimura K, Beidler LM (1961) Microelectrode study of taste receptors of rat and hamster. J Cell Comp Physiol 58:131–140

Kolmer W (1910) Über Strukturen im Epithel der Sinnesorgane. Anat Anz 36:281–299

Kolmer W (1927) Geschmacksorgan. Hand Mik Anat Mem 3:54–96

Kurihara K, Beidler LM (1968) Taste-modifying protein from miracle fruit. Science 161:1241–1243

Lasareff P (1922) Untersuchungen über die Ionentheorie der Reizung. III. Ionentheorie der Geschmacks-Reizung. Arch Ges Physiol Mens Tiere 194:293–297

Ling G, Gerard R (1949) The normal membrane potential of frog sartorius fibers. JCCP 34:383–396

Loven C (1867) Bidrag till kannedomen om tungans smakpapiller. (Contribution on the knowledge of tongues' taste papillae) Medicinskt Arch 3:1–14

Loven C (1868) Beiträge zur Kenntnis vom Bau der Geschmackswärzchen der Zunge. Arch Mikrosk Anat 4:98–110

Malpighi M, Fracassati C (1662) Epistolae anatomicae.

Miller I (1971) Peripheral interactions among single papilla inputs to gustatory nerve fibers. J Gen Physiol 57:1–25

Miller I (1974) Branched chorda tympani neurons and interactions among taste receptors. J Comp Neurol 158:155–166

Mistretta C (1971) Permeability of tongue epithelium and its relation to taste. Am J Physiol 5:1162–1167

Morita H (1969) Electrical signs of taste receptor activity. In: Pfaffmann C (ed) Olfaction and taste. Rockefeller University Press, New York

Olmsted J (1920) The results of cutting the seventh cranial nerve in amiurus nebulosus (Lesueur). J Exp Zool 31:369–401

Ozeki M (1941) Conductance change associated with receptor potentials of gustatory cells in rat. J Gen Physiol 58:688–699

Pfaffmann C (1941) Gustatory afferent impulses. J Cell Comp Physiol 17:243–258

Renquist Y (1919) Über den Geschmack. Skand Arch Physiol 38:97–201

Retzius G (1912) Zur Kenntnis des Geschmacksorgans beim Kaninchen. Biol Unters NF 17:72–80

Rosen S (1952) Effect of stimulation and section of the chorda tympani nerve. Neurology 2:244–247

Sato T (1975) Membrane resistance change of the frog taste cells in response to water and NaCl. J Gen Physiol 66:735–763

Sato T (1976) Does an initial phasic response exist in the receptor potential of taste cells? Experimentia 32:1426–1428

Schulze FE (1863) Über die becherförmigen Organe der Fische. Z Wissensch Zool 12:218–222

Schwalbe G (1868) Über die Geschmacksorgane der Säugethiere und des Menschen. Arch Mikrosk Anat 4:154–187

Shallenberger RS (1963) Hydrogen bonding and the varying sweetness of the sugars. J Food Sci 28:584–589

Sulzer J (1953) New theory of the pleasures. In: Galvani L (ed) De viribus electricitatis in moto musculari commentarius. Waverly, Baltimore

Tateda H, Beidler LM (1964) The receptor potential of the taste cell of the rat. J Gen Physiol 47:479–486

Tuckerman F (1892) Further observations on the gustatory organs of the mammalia. J Morphol 7:69–94

Van Leeuwenhoek A (1674) Other microscopical observations, made by the same, about the texture of the blood, the sap of some plants, the figure of sugar and salt, and the probable cause of the difference in their taste. Philos Trans R Soc Lond [Biol] 9:380–385

Van Leeuwenhoek A (1708) Microscopical observations upon the tongue. Philos Trans R Soc Lond [Biol] 26:111–123

Volta A (1793 a) Account of some discoveries made by Mr. Galvani of Bologna; with experiments and observations on them. Philos Trans R Soc Lond [Biol] 83:10–44

Volta A (1793 b) Estratta della lettera a Tiberio Cavallo. Account of some discoveries. 203–208 Sequito

von Békésy G (1960) Experiments in hearing. McGraw-Hill, New York

von Békésy G (1964) Sweetness produced electrically on the tongue and its relation to taste theories. JAPY 19:1105–1113

von Békésy G (1964) Duplexity theory of taste. Science 145:834–835

von Békésy G (1966) Taste theories and the chemical stimulation of single papillae. JAPY 21:1–9

Waller A (1849) Minute structure of the papillae and nerves of the tongue of the frog and toad. Philos Trans R Soc Lond [Biol] 139–150

Weber E (1827) Über das Geschmacksorgan der Karpfen. Merkels Arch Anat 2:309–315

CHAPTER 13

Insect Olfaction – Our Research Endeavor

DIETRICH SCHNEIDER

A. How to Become Addicted to This Field

In the early 1950s I was studying morphogenetic processes in invertebrates, and in parallel did some follow-up studies of my 1949 thesis on nerve fiber function in the frog. It then happened that one of my neighbors in the hall of residence at Tübingen University, the biochemist Peter Karlson, told me of some rather advanced attempts to isolate and identify one of the "magic" odor compounds. This was the female sexual attractant of the silkworm moth *Bombyx mori*. It had been reported in the work of FABRE (1879), FOREL (1910), and others (see GÖTZ 1951) that females of wild moth species are able to lure their males over long distances (Fig. 1). The effect seemed to be so powerful that some of the observers could not believe this to be an odorous stimulus but rather some mysterious radiation (FABRE 1879).

The chemical work my friend told me of was initiated in the 1930s by Adolf Butenandt, who was at that time Director of the Kaiser-Wilhelm-Institut für Biochemie (now the Max-Planck-Institut für Biochemie). Butenandt's interest in such analytical work derived on one hand from his experience with biologically active secretions (notably the sexual hormones of the vertebrates) and on the other hand

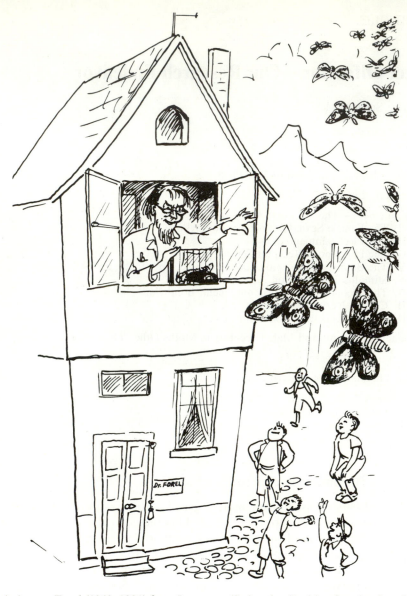

Fig. 1. August Forel (1848–1931) from Lausanne (Switzerland) with a female of a wild silk-moth (*Saturnia caprini*) in his studio while numbers of males approach her to the amazement of all the neighborhood boys. Forel described this in his 1910 book *Das Sinnesleben der Insekten,* and points out that these magnificent diurnal moths are normally not seen in towns and must have come from the country over some distance. Forel was a keen insect observer as a boy; later he became a well-known professor of psychiatry, but retired early to come back to his insect studies. He observed the behavior of insects, found new functions and structures, and described 3,500 new species of ant. I am grateful to my former Tübingen laboratory colleague Albrecht Egelhaaf (now at Cologne) for the sketch

from the hope among entomologists that agricultural pest moths might be trapped using the chemically pure female attractant.

This first contact with the *Bombyx* work struck a chord with me. Although I had not worked on sensory functions personally, I had – after all – come from Hansjochem Autrum's school at Göttingen University (see Autrum's chapter in this volume; SCHNEIDER 1977), where mechanoreceptors and auditory and visual receptors were studied, and I knew that among the sensory modalities, olfaction was one of the least understood. Here in the moth – I suspected – one has an extremely effective odor on the stimulus side, and on the receiving side in the olfactory organ, namely the male moth antenna, very probably a large number of highly specialized receptors. Whether it would ever be possible to record single receptor cell responses was, of course, still an open question, but I hoped to be able at least to record summed generator potentials from the moth antenna, provided the chemists could supply me with enriched extracts of female moths' lure glands. At this time, I did not hope to see a response when stimulating the male moth's "nose" directly with the excretion from the female gland, because I assumed this stimulus to be much too weak for an electrophysiological experiment. When I thought of generator potential recordings, I was influenced by Ragnar GRANIT's (1947, 1955) writings and of the (at that time) quite established concept that "slow" electrical responses (the generator potentials) in the periphery of receptor organs are the first detectable electrical signs of excitation, which elicit the "fast" sensory nerve impulses by which the message is carried to the higher centers.

Contacts with the analytical chemists, particularly Erich Hecker, were soon established. I received from this colleague enriched lure gland extracts, blew the odor of this onto an isolated male moth antenna, which was mounted between electrodes, and saw a significant response. Later we called this deflection of the oscilloscope beam the "electroantennogram" (EAG) on the analogy of the well-known electroretinogram (ERG). Interestingly, the analogous response of the vertebrate olfactory mucosa, the electroolfactogram (EOG), was found at about the same time (OTTOSON 1956, 1971). That was nearly 30 years ago, and the first reports on my findings were published in 1955 and 1956. Insect olfactory research and related studies have been my major occupation ever since.

B. The Main Lines of Our Work

In the following sections I will describe how our research projects on insect olfaction fared. More and more fellow workers joined me after I had moved in 1958 from Tübingen to Munich, and in 1966 to Seewiesen. In 1968 one of my associates, J. Boeckh, left the group to move first to Frankfurt and from there to the newly founded University of Regensburg. K.-D. Ernst and U. Waldow followed him later; all three continued to work on insect olfaction and related problems.

Since my contribution to this volume is not meant to be a scientifically complete report on our results or even one on the state of art, but rather an autobiographical sketch, I shall proceed by giving examples. This can best be done by highlighting what I think were particularly interesting or even blind alleys. I am aware of my bias and may not treat the contributions of all my partners equally.

While the study of the male *Bombyx* receptors for the female attractant (later to be called "pheromone") was in its infancy, other parallel research was soon undertaken. One may ask: Was all this the result of straightforward planning, and what and where is the clue to our work?

The objectives of our research were in the initial phase quite clear and simple. After the "discovery" of the EAG as an overall antennal reaction, our goal became the identification of the relevant morphological type of sensillum with its odor receptor cells. To approach this, the antennal structures had to be studied next, first using standard light microscopic techniques. In the course of the years, these morphological investigations of the receptor system became more and more refined as a result of the availability and development of new techniques. Sometimes an interesting interplay between the morphologists and the physiologists took place when one group had seen something "ahead" of the other. When, for example, the physiologist suggested that the lumen of the thick-walled sensory hairs on the antenna of the male moth is innervated by receptor dendrites, the histologist needed to verify this with his electron microscope. Even more importantly, the structure of the hair wall was found to be penetrated by pores and pore tubules, as was predicted from the thin-walled sensilla. In general, I may say that structural findings, particularly those which differ from expectations, greatly stimulated the development of functional hypotheses.

Even before we knew of the ultrastructure of the odor receptor hair, we succeeded in recording from its sensory cells. This was essentially an approach to single-cell specificities, and thus opened the way to a number of projects. In its most advanced form, this method led to stimulus transduction studies, which now even include the recording of elementary receptor potentials. But also in the more general studies of species-specific communicative odors or of general odors of food, prey, or the environment, this technique was essential. The EAG still remains useful, particularly for screening experiments or with large populations of uniformly responding receptors, but details of these reactions are only revealed by direct recordings from the sensillum.

Over the years, a number of research directions were developed by my senior associates, notably odor stimulus transduction (K.-E. Kaissling), comparative physiology of female moth attractants (E. Priesner), odor molecule structure and "odor generalist" receptor cells (W. A. Kafka), pheromone metabolism (G. Kasang), structure of antennal sensilla and nerves (R. A. Steinbrecht), and odor orientation (E. Kramer). When doctoral students joined the group, they were put on a path which seemed to me to be interesting and promising. Visiting scientists usually wanted to learn our methods and often brought their own experimental insects with them, thus stimulating and enlightening the group.

My personal interest still lies in the understanding of principles of chemical communication in our model moth *Bombyx,* but my daily activities have shifted to the study of other moths and also butterflies, where male pheromones and plant-derived pheromone precursors form a fascinating ecophysiological complex.

In summary, our interests now range from a selective analysis of fine structure and a variety of odor-producing and odor-perceiving functions all the way to chemistry, orientation, and insect–plant interrelationship. Although this may seem to be too wide an array of fields, it is the diversity of this powerful sensory system

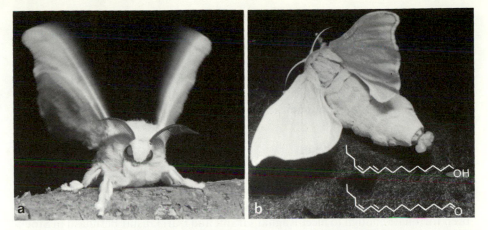

Fig. 2 a, b. The Chinese silkworm moth *Bombyx mori* (wingspan 4.5 cm) is flightless and is said to have been in human culture for 3,000 years or more. **a** male moth in full excitement after smelling the female's attractant bombykol; **b** female moth in the process of "calling" with fully expanded abdominal luring glands (sacculi laterales). These glands produce as major components two substances (*inset*): bombykol and bombykal in a 10:1 ratio. The alcohol stimulates the male to search for his female. The role of the geometrically identical aldehyde is not fully understood yet. Added in higher than natural concentrations, it depresses the male's tendency to search for the female

which deserves and even necessitates such an approach. As physiologists we try to understand the processes taking place on each level, and as biologists we are curious about how this all works together. Such a deeper understanding of one of the key communication systems of insects may even introduce new thinking on biological control measures against pest species.

C. *Bombyx mori* – The Silkworm Moth

I. The Female Sexual Attractant: Bombykol

Isolation of the attractant was begun in the 1930s by A. Butenandt in Berlin-Dahlem, but progress was slow because of the analytical procedures available at that time, and later also because of the war. Interestingly, as early as 1950 it was suspected that the attractant was an alcohol (BUTENANDT 1955 a, b).

At this time, and indeed up until the last decade of analytical work, the different fractions of the eluted female glands were tested in a behavioral bioassay. Eventually, the attractant was identified as E-10,Z-12-hexadecadien-1-ol and named "bombykol" (Fig. 2; BUTENANDT et al. 1959, 1961 a, b). Soon after this, synthetic bombykol and its three geometrical isomers became available for physiological research (see SCHNEIDER 1963 a, b). Years before this date, I had been fortunate enough to be allowed to use enriched gland extracts, but had myself already found that – unexpectedly – fresh female glands are powerful stimuli in EAG recordings. The bombykol identification was based on the extraction of a few milligrams of the attractant from nearly 0.5 million female glands. In our own work, we later determined the bombykol content of the gland of one female to be between 1.0 and 0.1 µg. Part of this alcohol seems to be stored, possibly in ester form, in lipophilic vacuoles of the glandular cells (BUTENANDT and HECKER 1961; STEINBRECHT 1964 a, b; SCHNEIDER 1965; KARLSON and SCHNEIDER 1973).

At the time of the identification of bombykol, KARLSON and LÜSCHER (1959) proposed the term "pheromone" for exocrine glandular products which serve the purpose of intraspecific communication.

II. The Electroantennogram

My thinking on how to record electrical responses from the antenna of *Bombyx* was strongly influenced by ERG studies (cf. GRANIT 1933, 1947, 1955; BERNHARD 1942; AUTRUM 1950; and others). I should not forget to mention here that I had been fortunate enough to meet Ragnar Granit and Carl Gustaf Bernhard in Stockholm in 1950 (see Sect. G), and had even been with Granit for a few weeks while he was working on the stretch receptors of the cat, which was after he had already discontinued his retina research. I also knew that ERGs could easily be recorded even from the eye of an isolated head of a fly. Since the insect's "nose" was definitely shown to be the antenna (VON FRISCH 1921), I tried the analogous recording from the isolated *Bombyx* antenna mounted between Ag-AgCl needle electrodes connected to a dc or to a long-time-constant ac amplifier (Fig. 3). Stimulation was done either by sending a puff of air over a glass rod which had been dipped into the test solution, or by air blown over the expanded lure gland of a female *Bombyx* (Fig. 3a). Ten years later, we improved the stimulating methods by the use of exchangeable glass cartridges holding the test odor papers (Fig. 3b). An even more refined olfactometer was designed later by KAFKA (1970).

Since it was clear to me from the beginning that it was most important to ascertain the biological nature of such "slow" receptor organ reactions, I planned control experiments. The danger was that the higher the resistance of the electrode and of the preparation, the more likely it was that a strong odor stimulus would elicit "artificial" electrochemical potentials, which would also be recorded and might in critical situations simulate a receptor potential. In *Bombyx*, the requested proof of the bioelectrical nature of the reaction was easily found. The most impressive sign for this came from the sexual specificities of the antennae. While the pectinate male and female antennae are morphologically very similar, only the male antenna shows an EAG when stimulated with the female odor; antennae of both sexes, however, respond equally to some general odors. Furthermore, the antennae of both sexes can be reversibly narcotized with ether or chloroform and show complex EAGs during this process. Antennae of insects which have been irreversibly narcotized (killed) by ether or cyanide may still "respond" with non-biological, artificial electrode potentials to strong vapors, but never to bombykol or other relevant odors (Fig. 4).

This was and is for me the necessary and sufficient proof that the EAG is an odor-elicited generator potential; but in 1956 these facts were not sufficiently persuasive for the peers of the Tübingen University Faculty of Sciences, who refused to accept my application for membership as a lecturer *(Privatdozent)*, based on the *Bombyx* antennal morphology and EAG studies.

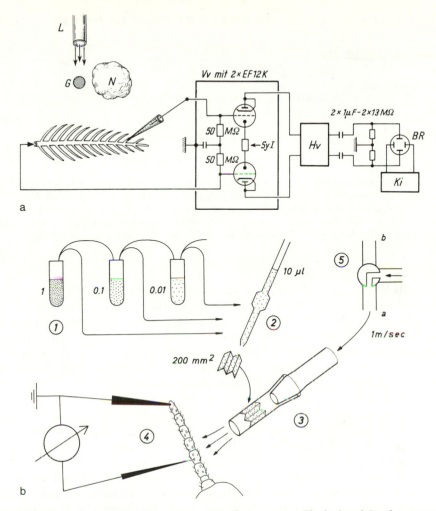

Fig. 3a, b. Electroantennogram recording and olfactometry. **a** The isolated *Bombyx* antenna is mounted between capillary electrodes which lead to the input stage of the push–pull preamplifier (*Vv*), and from here to the main amplifier (*Hv*) and the Braun tube (*BR*) of the oscilloscope. This electronic equipment was made by my fellow doctoral student F. W. Schlote after an earlier design by H. Autrum. *Ki,* horizontal sweep.

The stimulating air current (*L*) can be directed over the tip of a glass rod (*G*) contaminated with lure gland extract, thus producing an odor current. *N*, cotton impregnated with narcotic such as chloroform. Schneider (1957a). **b** Advanced experimental procedure in the 1960s. (*1*) Dilution of the odorant in $\log_{10}$ concentration steps; (*2*) application of a known amount of the odorant to a piece of fluted filter paper, from which the solvent evaporates rapidly while the compound to be tested evaporates slowly; (*3*) transfer of the filter paper (odor source) to a glass cartridge which can be stored in the cold or mounted on a ground glass outlet tube of the air current system in front of the preparation; (*4*) antenna of a living insect mechanically fixed with electrodes; (*5*) two-way air system with an electric valve to give puffs of air: normally the air leaves via (*b*) but can be directed to the cartridge via (*a*) without building up pressure. Boeckh et al. (1965)

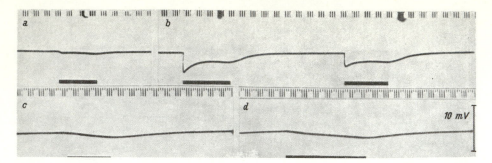

Fig. 4a–d. Electroantennogram recordings from isolated antenna of male *Bombyx* (cf. Fig. 3a). **a** pure air control stimulus; clean glass rod, one air puff, indicated by *black bar* under the record; **b** glass rod with female gland extract, two air puffs; **c** other antenna of the same male, which had now been killed by ether vapor: stimulus as in **b**; one air puff; **d** same antenna as in **c**: one pure air puff. *Time marks* 0.1 Hz. Schneider and Hecker (1956)

In the later phase of the work, when pure bombykol was available, the EAG response was quantified and the expected exponential stimulus–response function found (Schneider et al. 1967). Particularly interesting was the comparison of the effectiveness of all the four hexadecadienol stereoisomers. The "wrongly" shaped molecules were between 100 and 1,000 times less effective than bombykol (Fig. 5).

The determination of the bombykol EAG threshold was a difficult task. We prepared bombykol stimuli by decadic dilution steps from 1 µg/ml of the solvent down to less than 10^{-10} µg/ml. From these solutions we loaded the odor sources, which were pieces of paper with the corresponding amounts in µg of bombykol (Fig. 3b). Unfortunately, it took us years before we eventually found that the odor sources holding 10^{-3} or 10^{-4} µg bombykol were not significantly "better" than a paper holding only the solvent – which means that this was the electrophysiological threshold range under the given conditions (Schneider 1963a; Boeckh et al. 1965; Schneider et al. 1967). In the earlier phase of these experiments we thought that the EAG threshold would be much lower. In fact, we encountered similar problems to those of the chemists who, during their behavioral biotests, at one time assumed that they would be able to stimulate the male moth with the tip of a glass rod dipped into a solvent which (they thought) contained only 10^{-12} µg (1,000 molecules) bombykol per milliliter (Butenandt et al. 1961a). After we had found that the EAG threshold is close to 10^{-4} µg bombykol on the odor source, while the behavior threshold is much lower, we left the delicate problem of the true bombykol threshold alone until radiolabeled pheromone was available (see Sect. C.IV).

One psychological difficulty with respect to the preparation of the pheromone odor stimulus must now be mentioned: bombykol is odorless to the human nose! It is over and again striking that the female *Bombyx* lure gland has no odor for us, while its emanation activates the male moth; the EAG shows us why. Preparing a dilution series of such "odorants" is like working in the dark or with ultraviolet light, or ultrasound receptor systems. In the meantime we have learned more of this in our studies of other insect pheromones, of which many are odorless to us, particularly the female moth attractants.

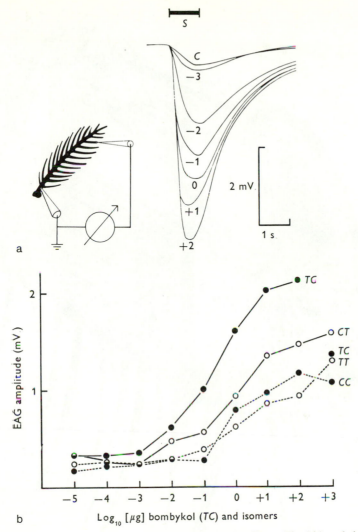

Fig. 5 a, b. Male *Bombyx mori.* **a** recording scheme (for details see Fig. 3 b) and electroantennogram (*EAG*) response to a control paper (*C*) holding only the bombykol solvent and to a series of papers holding bombykol of increasing concentration (log$_{10}$ values in μg). *S*, duration of stimulus, **b** EAG amplitudes at different concentrations of bombykol and its isomers. Mean amplitudes of between 30 and 200 recordings. *TC*, hexadeca-10-*trans*,12-*cis*-dien-1-ol (bombykol); *CT, CC, TT*, curves of the corresponding *cis-trans, cis-cis*, and *trans-trans* isomers, respectively. After BOECKH et al. (1965), (see also SCHNEIDER 1965; SCHNEIDER et al. 1967)

III. The Pheromone Receptor Sensilla

My first inspection of the *Bombyx* antenna showed me that it was doubly comb-shaped, had many segments, and was covered with a variety of hairs and pegs which seemed to be sensilla serving several sensory modalities. Since at this time only rather general descriptions of the antennae of distant relatives of *Bombyx* ex-

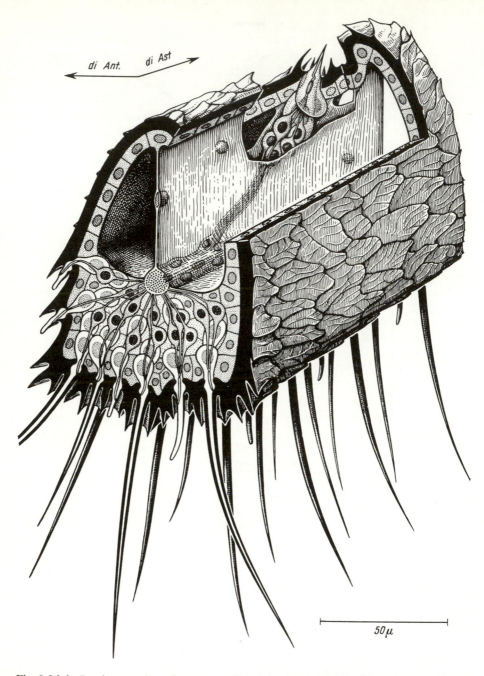

Fig. 6. Male *Bombyx:* section of an antennal branch with cuticle (*black*), sensory epithelium, and hemolymph space. The *arrows* point to the distal (*Ast*) end of the antennal branch and distal (*Ant*) outer end of the antenna. The lymph space is divided by a septum. Here, a sensillum coeloconicum with five receptor cells (*dark nuclei*) and two bigger cells (tormogen and trichogen cell) are shown. The dendrites reach to the tip of the cone. On the other side, the long, thick-walled sensilla trichodea are prominent. They are innervated by one or two odor

isted in the literature, the only way out of this dilemma was to study this structure in my laboratory (SCHNEIDER and KAISSLING 1956, 1957, 1959).

We found on the antennal flagellum two types of thin-walled sensilla (sensilla coeloconica and sensilla basiconica), and among the thick-walled sensilla with potential olfactorial function the sensilla trichodea (Fig. 6). While earlier work had shown the insect antenna to be the major odor-perceiving part of the insect, no proof that any particular sensillum type served this function was available. For the honeybee, VON FRISCH (1921) had by a process of exclusion claimed the pore plates to be the odor-receptive sensilla, but even there the final proof was missing.

After completion of the assessment of the morphological types and average numbers of the antennal sensilla, I attempted to correlate the olfactory function (as seen in the EAG) to one of the sensillum types (SCHNEIDER 1957a, b). Candidates were the thin-walled sensilla basiconica (presumed to be olfactory sensilla because they could be stained through the wall of the hair (SLIFER 1961; RICHTER 1962; SCHNEIDER 1964; SCHNEIDER and STEINBRECHT 1968), the sensilla coeloconica, and the sensilla trichodea. Because of their thick wall and because it was not then possible to see the dendrite in the hair, I discounted the more than 15,000 sensilla trichodea along with their 30,000 receptor cells from possibly responding to the sex attractant and even to any odor. The sensilla basiconica (approximately 5,000 with 10,000 cells) I considered – wrongly – to be the best candidates for producing the bombykol EAG (SCHNEIDER 1957a). The sensilla coeloconica were in my opinion also candidates, although their number was rather small.

The matter stood like this until we learned how to record from single sensilla by penetrating the cuticle near the base of a sensillum basiconicum (BOECKH 1962; SCHNEIDER and BOECKH 1962) in a beetle and a sphingid moth. In the case of *Bombyx*, this technique proved the sensilla trichodea (in spite of their thick wall) to be the bombykol receptor organs (Fig. 7; PRIESNER, cit. BOECKH et al. 1965; KAISSLING and PRIESNER 1970). This method was a great improvement over my earlier attempts to record unit cell responses from the inside of an antennal branch (Fig. 8), where recordings were barely reproducible and the identification of the activated sensilla often impossible (SCHNEIDER 1955a).

For good reasons, single-cell recordings were and still are "magic goals" of neurobiologists; in the case of our work, this needs no special explanation. Historically, the first successful recordings ever done of "impulses produced by sensory nerve endings" are described in three papers by ADRIAN (1926) and ADRIAN and ZOTTERMAN (1926) on a new three-stage electron tube amplifier and the responses of vertebrate mechanoreceptors. These two authors later also did pioneer work on vertebrate olfaction and taste (see Pfaffmann's and Beidler's chapters in this volume). With respect to our work, it may be of interest to record that my first attempts to register odor receptor responses under optical control from single sensilla of insects were not particularly successful. While I was visiting the University of

receptor cells which were later found to respond to bombykol and bombykal, respectively. Between the long hairs and on the side we found thin-walled sensilla basiconica innervated by one to three odor receptor cells for general odorants. When this light microscopic study was made, we did not know that the dendrites of the odor receptor cells reached into the hair lumen, nor were we aware that the walls of these hairs were penetrated by a multitude of pores. SCHNEIDER and KAISSLING (1959)

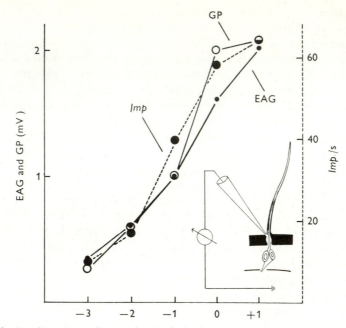

Fig. 7. Male *Bombyx mori*. Comparison of the bombykol electroantennogram reaction (from Fig. 5) with the generator potential (*GP, left-hand ordinate*) and the mean impulse frequency (*Imp, right-hand ordinate*) during the first 500 ms of the response. *Abscissa:* bombykol concentration. The GP and Imp values are averages of between three and six measurements. *Inset:* recording scheme for extracellular activities of individual olfactory cells (sensillum trichodeum). Priesner, 1965, in Schneider (1965)

California in Los Angeles in 1959–1960, I occasionally recorded odor receptor impulses from sensilla basiconica of a skipper butterfly antenna. During my stay in the United States, my colleague Jerry Lettvin (Massachusetts Institute of Technology) showed me one Sunday morning how two of his BSc candidates recorded odor spikes from the antenna of a cockroach mounted on the stage of a compound microscope in his laboratory.

Our first histological study (Schneider and Kaissling 1957) of the antennal sensilla was done with light microscopic techniques. The methylene blue which we used did not stain the receptor cell processes within the hairs. We thought at this time that the sensilla trichodea were empty, and assumed that the dendrite of the receptor cell did not extend into the hair lumen. In the 1960s we became able to check on these problems using electron microscopic techniques, and found that the walls of the sensilla trichodea (as well as the walls of the sensilla basiconica) are actually penetrated by pores and pore tubules (Schneider 1964; Schneider and Steinbrecht 1968). We now know that the sensilla trichodea (of rather similar structure in many male lepidoptera) are the receptor organs for the female sexual attractants. The first report of this was given by Steinbrecht (cit. Schneider et al. 1964) with reference to pheromone receptors in the wild silkmoth *Antheraea pernyi*.

Thorough morphological studies of olfactory sensilla were later done by Ernst (1969) on a sensillum basiconicum of the beetle *Necrophorus*, and by Steinbrecht

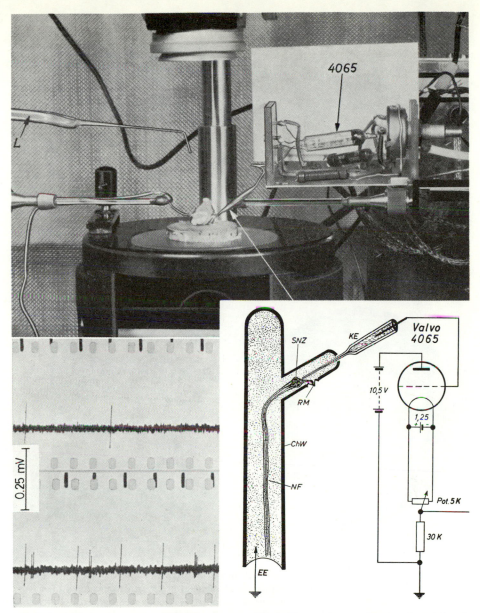

Fig. 8. Unit for extracellular odor impulse recordings. *Upper picture:* the experimental animal (e.g., *Bombyx*) or its isolated antenna is mounted on the stage of a dissecting microscope. The odor stimulus can be given by a puff of odor (*L*) from a fine tube or by placing the odor source near the antenna. The rod of the left micromanipulator holds the indifferent (reference) electrode. The rod of the right manipulator holds a hand-pulled recording capillary electrode. On the right manipulator (and thus moving with its electrode-holding rod) is a miniature input stage amplifier (opened for the photo) to insure a short, low-capacitance grid lead. *Lower right:* scheme of the cathode follower amplifier. The essential element of this homemade instrument is the miniature electrometer triode (Philips Valvo 4065). The recording capillary electrode (*K*) is slipped into an opened antennal branch until spontaneous impulses of sensory cells (*SNZ*) are observed (*left, upper trace*). The cells might respond to an odor stimulus (here cycloheptanone, *lower left trace*) or not. *RM*, peg of a sensillum coeloconicum (see Fig. 6); *ChW*, antennal wall; *NF*, nerve fibers leading the impulse directly to the brain; *EE*, reference electrode. After SCHNEIDER (1955a)

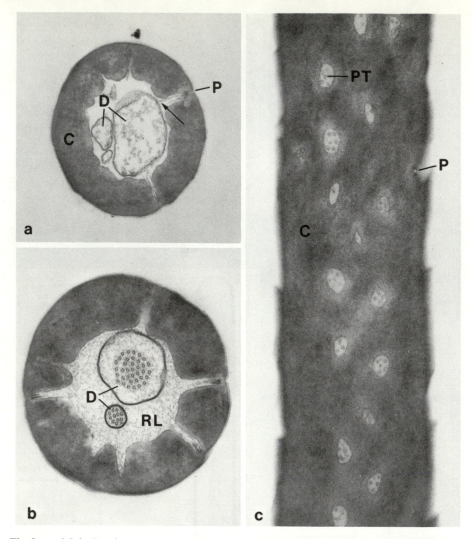

Fig. 9 a–c. Male *Bombyx mori*. **a, b** Cross section through sensory hair of a pheromone-sensitive sensillum trichodeum. Two receptor dendrites (*D*) are seen in the hair lumen, surrounded by receptor lymph (*RL*). The cuticular wall (*C*) is perforated by pores (*P*) leading into four to six pore tubules. The pore tubules are delicate structures and difficult to preserve in their full length during specimen preparation for electron microscopy. After fixation with a mixture of osmium tetroxide and potassium dichromate (**a**), some pore tubules are seen to end in contact with the receptor membrane (*arrow*), but the dendrites are severely swollen. The dendrites, on the other hand, are preserved best by cryofixation and freeze substitution (**b**), which damages the pore tubules. × 30,000 (Steinbrecht 1980). **c** Tangential section through the hair wall showing pores (*P*) and pore tubules (*PT*) in cross section. × 50,000 (Steinbrecht 1973)

(1970, 1973) on *Bombyx*. Pores and tubules as the connecting system between the outer world and the dendritic membrane (see also Fig. 10) were discussed in a comparative article by STEINBRECHT (1969) and recently summarized by ALTNER and PRILLINGER (1980). A sensillum is defined as a sense organ composed of a group of receptor cells, formative cells, and auxiliary cells. Some of these cells are intimately connected with specialized cuticle structures, and this makes the appropriate fixation procedures "tricky" for the histologists. Our attempts to improve on the available methods to reach a minimum of tissue distortion still continue. Recently, cryofixation, freeze substitution, and freeze etching have given us surprising new views of the shape of the cellular elements, dendrites, membrane surfaces, and neurotubules and pore tubules (Fig. 9; STEINBRECHT 1980).

IV. The Bombykol Receptor Cell: Threshold, Specificity, and Adaptation

After tritiation of bombykol by KASANG (1968), it was possible to handle the threshold problem properly (KAISSLING and PRIESNER 1970). We will here distinguish between the behavior threshold of the male moth and the receptor cell threshold. An airstream containing approximately 1,000 bombykol molecules per cubic centimeter sufficed to elicit the typical wing fluttering of the male moth. Measurements of adsorption of bombykol onto the antenna and onto the receptor hairs led to the estimate that several hundred sense hairs receive one molecular hit each per second. Since double hits are too rare in this situation, the receptor cell responds to single molecule hits, and a few hundred hits per antenna are then the behavior threshold (KAISSLING and PRIESNER 1970). This, of course, is only true for the fully receptive or "dark-adapted" receptors.

In sensory physiology a "threshold" is the level between a sub- and a suprathreshold amount of stimulus units. But the threshold concept is not applicable if – as in our case with single receptor cells – a subthreshold stimulus is not possible. One bombykol molecule is an "olfactory quantum," on the analogy of the light quantum, which is the minimum stimulus to the most sensitive visual receptor cells (KAISSLING and PRIESNER 1970).

The behavior-controlling system of the male moth responds only if a few hundred receptor cells are hit in the course of about 1s and react with one impulse each. This number is just enough to overcome the spontaneous firing rate, the "noise" of the receptor cells.

The specificity of the bombykol receptor cells was found to be identical with the EAG responses, which again showed us that the EAG is an overall expression of the receptor potentials. Derivatives of bombykol are less effective stimuli. Some interesting relationships between molecular shape and responses appeared later in these studies (KAISSLING 1974).

Adaptation and deadaptation were to some extent studied in the honeybee (VARESCHI 1971) and in *Bombyx* (KAISSLING 1971), and systematically in two saturniid moths. After a strong stimulus, the receptor cell needs more than 10 min for a 50% and more than 20 min for a 100% recovery to the earlier sensitivity (ZACK 1979).

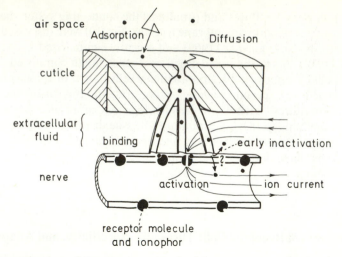

Fig. 10. Schematic view of the structures involved in sensory transduction in an olfactory hair in a male *Bombyx mori*. It may be possible for the odor molecules to reach the nerve membrane without leaving the lipophilic phase, which could be continued from the outer surface via the pore tubules. The early inactivation might be a diffusion into the extracellular receptor lymph. The picture shows 11 molecules (*black dots*) adsorbed per three pore tubules. This would correspond to a stimulus of 1 s using about 3 μg bombykol on the odor source. Nothing is known so far about the nature, number, and distribution of receptor molecules and about the ion-gating mechanism and its connection with the receptor molecules. In this scheme, the pore tubules are depicted as reaching directly onto the dendritic (nerve) membrane. Whether this is always the case is still an open question (see also Fig. 9). KAISSLING (1974)

V. Stimulus Transduction

Transduction is here understood to comprise all the processes from the capture of the molecule on the surface of the olfactory hair to the elicitation of a dendritic receptor potential (generator potential) and the subsequent impulses. KAISSLING (1974) described steps of the transduction processes – such as adsorption, diffusion, binding and activation, conductance changes, inactivation, receptor potential, and nerve impulse elicitation – which could either be observed directly or indirectly (Fig. 10; SCHNEIDER 1969, 1971, 1980).

The highly radiolabeled bombykol was truly essential to our work, but even this tool failed with lower stimulus intensities; we therefore had to extrapolate from our measurements at higher bombykol concentrations. Furthermore, the bombykol can only be "seen" when it diffuses on the hair surface, and later it is found inside the hair and the antenna, where it is rather slowly metabolized (STEINBRECHT and KASANG 1972; KASANG and KAISSLING 1972). In and on these structures, bombykol is metabolized with a half-time of 4 min. This is too long for the postulated inactivation (acceptor clearance), but might be an important process for preventing a bombykol "pollution" on and in the moth. Even the bombykol on the scales undergoes this cleaning process (KASANG 1971, 1974).

Detailed studies of the transduction mechanism by KAISSLING (1974, 1979) were only possible after he developed a method of recording from the opened tip

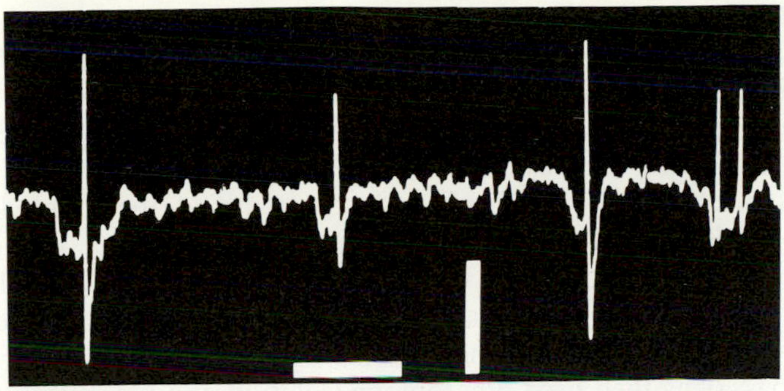

Fig. 11. Extracellular recording from an antennal pheromone receptor hair in a male *Bombyx mori*. Reference electrode on the tip of a clipped sensillum trichodeum. Two receptor cells are active: the bombykol receptor (*large impulse*) and the bombykal receptor (*small impulse*). The impulses are preceded by elementary receptor potentials (*bumps*). Weak pheromone stimulus containing both components. Calibration 100 ms; 0.5 mV. Courtesy K.-E. KAISSLING (1981)

of the receptor hair. He could now see and study discrete elementary receptor potentials of about 0.3 mV (like the "bumps" of the visual receptors), which are understood as signs of membrane channel openings due to the binding of stimulating molecules (Fig. 11). These bumps differ in size depending upon the stimulus compound, and they sum up to form the receptor potential (KAISSLING 1974, 1979; KAISSLING and THORSON 1980). Recently, biochemical studies of the receptor hairs have also been initiated (KLEIN 1980).

VI. The Second Pheromone Component: Bombykal

Bombykol was identified in 1959. Since the extracts of the *Bombyx* lure gland showed only this one component which attracted male moths, one thought that this would be the normal case. Consequently, it was assumed that different species – at least the sympatrically living ones – must use different female attracting substances in order to avoid confusion and interbreeding. Observed cases of such cross-matings (PRIESNER 1973) were thought to be accidents occurring either because the neighboring species had a rather similar attractant, or because ecologically separated species (by space, or daily rhythm, or other means) sporting the same attractant had just met by chance.

But the nice scheme "one species – one pheromone substance" collapsed when more and more cases of two, three, or more attractant pheromone components became known for a given species. In the years after the bombykol work, many laboratories launched large-scale analytical work on pheromones, particularly on the attractants of pests, such as moths and barkbeetles (PRIESNER 1973, 1977; BRAND et al. 1979; SILVERSTEIN 1981).

When K.-E. Kaissling recorded from single sensilla trichodea in *Bombyx*, he always noticed that pure bombykol only elicited the response of one large impulse type, while with the odor of the female gland he saw in addition the response of a second cell of which the impulse amplitude was smaller. In the course of this work it appeared that this second cell was sensitive to unsaturated aldehydes, which had approximately the same carbon atom chain length as bombykol. Then an aldehyde which was geometrically identical to bombykol was synthesized and found to be most effective as a stimulus for the second cell, but not for the bombykol receptor cell with the bigger impulse (Fig. 11). Now it was only a matter of time before this aldehyde – later called "bombykal" – was found in the female glands (Fig. 2). The bombykal content of the gland was only one-tenth of the bombykol content (KAISSLING et al. 1978; KASANG et al. 1978). These two female lure gland components are "served" by one male receptor cell each (Figs. 6, 7, and 11), both of them neighbors in one sensillum trichodeum. Ironically, bombykal escaped the analytical chemists of the Butenandt team since it would not show with the behavioral bioassay as then used. Pheromone isolation and identification is now a routine, particularly with the use of an electroantennogram detector (EAD), where the EAG is used as a highly specific and sensitive detector at the output of a gas chromatograph (see MOORHOUSE et al. 1969; ROELOFS et al. 1971; ARN et al. 1975).

Over 20 years have now passed since bombykol became known. Hundreds of female moth sexual attractants have been identified since, mostly from pest species. Even phylogenetic relationships can now be considered on the basis of the attractants in a taxonomic group. The adaptive significance of these substances is obvious, because a female moth without her attractant will never mate and have offspring. Speciation in most cases seems only possible if the female pheromone composition is changed in some way (MINKS et al. 1973; for additional examples see PRIESNER 1973, 1977, 1980; SCHNEIDER 1980).

A case like *Bombyx* with one attractant (bombykol) and one "behavior-inhibiting" substance (bombykal) is exceptional. Often, the attractant pheromone components are synergists, usually with fixed quantitative relations. Related species sometimes differ only in the proportions of otherwise identical components of the female attractant pheromone.

VII. Central Nervous Responses

Studies of the central olfactory system in insects are only now making a slow start, 20 years after our first successful single sensillum recordings. At the same time, investigations on the processing of visual and mechanoreceptor messages in insects have been quite successful (see ZETTLER and WEILER 1976; HUBER 1978, 1980). My plans to study the corresponding function as elicited by sensory odor input to the insect brain date back to the 1960s, but until recently we were not too successful, either in olfactory brain histology (although see PARETO 1972) or physiology. Recent unpublished work by M. Koontz, R. Olberg, and D. Light on *Bombyx* shows that bombykol and bombykal receptor messages are first processed in the macroglomerular complex of the male moth's deutocerebrum. This observation fits in nicely with work on other moths (BOECKH and BOECKH 1979; HILDEBRAND et al. 1980; MATSUMOTO and HILDEBRAND 1981; TOLBERT and HILDEBRAND 1981) and the cockroach (BOECKH et al. 1977; ERNST et al. 1977). R. OLBERG (1983) also found bombykol-related responses in descending interneurons of the thoracal nervecord which might directly influence the wing and leg motoneurons.

All this is only a beginning, but it seems as if in *Bombyx* the study of the system processing the pheromone message might eventually lead to some understanding of at least one specialized type of odor response, based on the two components bombykol and bombykal. This, of course, does not really enlighten us in our ignorance of how a great number of odors are discriminated. This ignorance is sometimes called the "odor problem" (see also Sect. E). But there is hope, again from research on insects. Our Regensburg colleagues, working on the cockroach, have undertaken to unravel the puzzle of how the messages of a set of antennal receptor cells sensitive for food odors are treated in the brain (BOECKH 1974, 1980; BOECKH et al. 1976; see also Figs. 13–15).

VIII. Pheromone-Elicited Behavior

The female *Bombyx* moth (and most other moths in an analogous manner) exposes her lure gland, the sacculi laterales, some time after she emerges from the pupa. The male *Bombyx,* which is flightless due to domestication, becomes very active when he scents his female. In still air he is now more or less turning on the spot, but his march becomes directional when there is a wind which carries the bombykol message to him (SCHWINCK 1954, 1955; SCHNEIDER 1957 a, 1974, 1975; KAISSLING and PRIESNER 1970). The female odor actually distributes downwind in a so-called odor plume, of which the boundaries are defined as the range where the bombykol concentration is approaching the behavior threshold of the male. Walking insects, for obvious reasons, have no difficulty in identifying the direction of the wind. *Bombyx* males now exercise an extremely efficient orienting behavior after they are alerted by bombykol. They cruise in a zigzag manner upwind, like a sailing boat with an individually rather constant angle of 30°–50° (KRAMER 1975). This behavior is called an "alternating anemomenotaxis." Turns to the opposite side become more probable when the concentration of the bombykol signal is reduced, as is the case near the border of the plume. By this mechanism, males reach a female promptly because the plume becomes narrower closer to the female. If the odor disappears either when it is switched off or if the male loses the plume, he circles. He also circles on the spot if the wind drops but there is still bombykol in the air (KRAMER 1975). Even blinded males find their mate, but at least one antenna is essential. Some other insects which normally walk behave similarly (KRAMER 1978). Gypsy moth males (when walking with clipped wings), however, can be put under the *Bombyx* scheme of anemomenotaxis only with difficulty (PREISS 1980).

With flying moths (and many other insects in general) the odor-searching upwind flight seems to be similar to the march of *Bombyx,* although the cruising angle in relation to the wind direction may even approach 90° and is also dependent upon the wind speed. Experimentally, changes of the visually detectable ground pattern or the influence of head or tail wind can be simulated by the movement of a carpet-like floor of the wind tunnel (KENNEDY and MARSH 1974; KENNEDY 1977; DAVID et al. 1982). We now began to study details of this complicated optical control system in the tethered gypsy moth. It flew on a circular path over a controlled ground pattern and showed several reaction types: fixating the pattern ("landing reaction"), speeding up, slowing down, or keeping constant speed. Some of these reactions will help to understand how the central nervous system of this insect controls a flight with or without wind under natural conditions (PREISS 1980; PREISS and KRAMER 1983 b). The essential problem in keeping a course is for any actively flying "thing" to track the underground pattern and to notice how its own efforts are changed by the wind. The pheromone is – as we recently saw – not only the "command" to fly upwind, but also to keep the moth's height above the ground stable. In the case of the gypsy moth, only (+)-disparlure has an effect on its orientation (Preiss and Kramer 1983 a).

D. Female Attractants and Male Receptors in Moths Other Than *Bombyx*

Soon after my first *Bombyx* research phase, I used the opportunity as a visiting researcher and teacher in California to study with the EAG technique the extent of stimulatory cross-effects in related species. The moth family Saturniidae appeared to be suited for such an approach. After all, some of the famous earlier observations (Fabre 1879; Forel 1910; Mell 1922) had been made with species of this family, and we had already studied the morphology of the saturniid antenna in some examples (Boeckh et al. 1960). In this first attempt with "cross-stimuli" of female glands, I found that of seven saturniid species, some male antennae also responded to the odor of the gland of the female of other species (Schneider 1962). Similar results were later obtained by Priesner (1968, 1969) in a much more detailed study. But it became quite clear that the EAG is not the appropriate technique in such comparative studies, since related species appear to share some components of their pheromone (see Kochansky et al. 1975; Kaissling 1980; Priesner 1977, 1979, 1980 and references therein). Obviously, the receptor cell recordings were needed to clarify the situation.

From *Bombyx* and from the saturniids we learned the close correspondence of the number of pheromone components and of the respective receptor cells in the sensilla trichodea. In those cases where up to five components were found, one doubts that this still holds true (Priesner 1979).

In spite of intensive search, so far only one active substance was found in the lure gland of some species. One particularly interesting example is the gypsy moth (*Lymantria dispar*). We had already in the earlier phase of work been invited by chemists to try our methods on this moth. A first proposal for the chemical composition of the pheromone was found to be incorrect and a later one to be correct (cf. Schneider 1963 a, in contrast to Bierl et al. 1970, and Schneider et al. 1974, 1977). The naive physiologist is, of course, helpless if the real content of an odor-containing vial is not identical with its label (see an additional case of this from a study of the cockroach pheromone: Boeckh et al. 1963; cf. Boeckh et al. 1977).

The finally identified gypsy moth pheromone (Z-7,8-epoxy-2-methyl-octadecane = disparlure; Bierl et al. 1970) is an interesting compound which was later also found to be the only active substance of the closely related nun moth, *L. monacha* (Bierl et al. 1975). In spite of considerable efforts, the behavioral principle of the reproductive isolation of these two species – which in some areas occur sympatrically – was not found until recently (Schröter 1976; Schneider et al. 1974, 1977; Schneider 1980). One possibility (as expressed in some of the quoted papers) was that the two species use different optical isomers (enantiomers) of the same compound as attractants (see also Vité et al. 1976). The thought of a discrimination of odorous optical isomers was not surprising in our laboratory (see KAFKA et al. 1973). Unfortunately, the optical properties of the natural pheromones were and are not known, but optically rather pure synthetic enantiomers of disparlure were available.

Some time ago, we had already found specific responses of single receptor cells on the antennae of males of both *Lymantria* species when stimulated with these enantiomers (Schneider and Boppré, unpublished work). Recently, HANSEN et al. (1983) took this work up and found: on the male *L. dispar* antenna, equal numbers of receptor cells for (+)- and (−)-disparlure; on the male *L. monacha* antenna, however, only receptor cells for (+)-disparlure. Deductions from a comparison of the responses when the cells were either stimulated with the synthetic enantiomers or with the gland extracts of both species allow the following prediction: the *L. monacha* female produces 90% (−)- and 10% (+)-disparlure; the *L. dispar* female produces only (+)-disparlure. This now explains why the nun moth female is not approached by gypsy moth males, who shy away from the (−)-disparlure, but the nun moth male, which can only smell the 10% (+)-disparlure, comes to her. So far, we do not fully understand how the gypsy moth female "avoids" luring nun moth males, since the diel activity rhythms of the two species overlap somewhat (SCHRÖTER 1976).

E. Receptors for General Odors

So far, I have described what we found out about the pheromone biology and pheromone odor perception in the Lepidoptera. But what about other insects and their pheromones; what about insect olfaction of substances which are not pheromones but "general" odors of the surroundings?

A case of particular biological interest was the carrion beetle *Necrophorus*. The antenna of this insect is supplied with sensilla basiconica which respond to a variety of compounds, many of which signify decaying meat (BOECKH 1962). These recordings were, in fact, the first ones wherever single olfactory receptor cells were studied in detail. It was furthermore the first case where it clearly appeared that EAGs or slow receptor potentials of a polarity opposite to the usually observed one blocked an excitatory or spontaneous impulse volley. Here, the analogy between the odor receptor neuron and a central neuron with excitatory and inhibitory synapses is obvious, but after all, both cells are chemoreceptors (Fig. 12). In this and in later studies by this author on other beetles, the flesh fly, and the migratory locust, a pattern of response of a set of olfactory receptors (excitation, inhibition, no response, Fig. 13) became visible (BOECKH 1962, 1967 a, b; see also SCHNEIDER et al. 1964). On the basis of such a pattern, we thought, the brain would be able to discriminate quite a number of odors. This work was then supplemented by a histological study which was the first complete reconstruction of an odor-receptive sensillum on the basis of ultrastructure (ERNST 1969). In a following investigation, ERNST (1972) even succeeded in proving the cuticular nature of the pore tubules, which were previously thought to be dendritic outgrowths. This then – contrary to earlier claims – made clear that the dendrites of the odor receptor cells have no fine processes which are directly in contact with the air (see SCHNEIDER 1964; SCHNEIDER and STEINBRECHT 1968).

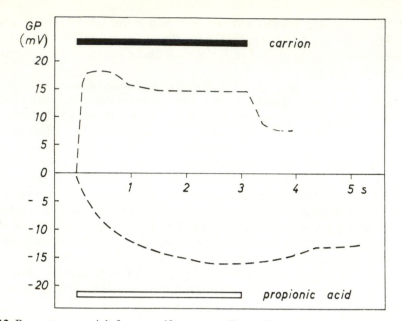

Fig. 12. Receptor potentials from an olfactory sensillum of a carrion beetle. Stimulation with carrion odor (*black bar*) and propionic acid (*white bar*). The excitatory (depolarizing) potential is depicted upwards, the inhibitory potential downwards. BOECKH (1967a)

The study of the locust olfactory system was later continued by KAFKA (1970), who assessed details of the "reaction spectra" of receptor cells of the pit sensillum (sensillum coeloconicum). The organ was stimulated by related chemicals with variations in their functional group, shape, etc. The conclusion of this work was that the binding forces between the odor molecule and the receptor (acceptor) are weak (noncovalent), such as dispersion bonds, dipole properties, hydrogen, and polarization bonds (KAFKA 1974).

Another insect which we intensively investigated during these years was the honeybee. In the first phase of this research, LACHER (1964) found that the pore plate sensilla are in fact – as predicted by VON FRISCH (1921) – the olfactory organs. Extracellular single-cell recordings were possible, although each sensillum has many receptor cells, of which only some show up. These experiments indicated that each of the receptor cells possesses its "private" reaction spectrum to a series of odors, including fatty acids. Lacher's study, together with another one on the non-pheromone receptors in the sensilla basiconica of the saturniid moth *Antheraea pernyi* (SCHNEIDER et al. 1964; Figs. 14 and 15), led us to name such cells "odor generalists" in contrast to the "odor specialists" (see also below). The latter, including the bombykol receptor, reacted identically to the pheromone and in a graded manner to other compounds; they were very sensitive to the major stimulus and were found in great numbers on the antenna. The generalists did not respond to the pheromone and were not as sensitive, and, more importantly, their specificity varied from cell to cell with a considerable overlap of the reaction spectra. Here it should be mentioned that in consideration of the complex taste and odor spec-

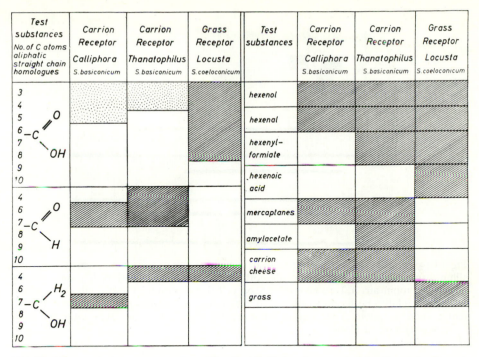

Fig. 13. Odor receptor responses in a blowfly (*Calliphora*), a carrion beetle, and a locust. Reaction spectra of specialized food odor receptors. Fatty acid, aldehyde, and alcohol stimuli on the *left-hand side,* all from a homologous series of saturated, unbranched hydrocarbon derivatives. The *right-hand part* shows reactions to the vital odors of these animals and to other compounds. *Hatched areas* indicate excitatory responses, *dotted areas* inhibition, *white areas* no response. BOECKH (1967 a)

ificities in vertebrate sensory fibers, a "cross-fiber pattern," concept was developed to interpret such phenomena (see Pfaffmann's chapter in this volume). This compares well to some of our thoughts and is, of course, a kind of "Gestalt" of the chemical environment.

This was the situation for several years, until new recordings from the honeybee and some other insects showed us that some of the receptor cells which we had before classified as generalists could be grouped according to common specificities. In the bee, VARESCHI (1971) found seven or more major reaction groups as defined by the substances to which they responded. None of these groups fitted the earlier generalist concept because there was no overlap between the spectra of effective stimuli of the respective groups, although the cells of one group were not equally sensitive to all the compounds in their spectrum. Cells of the fatty acid reaction group also responded to the queen substance (a pheromone) in high dilution (Fig. 16). One might, therefore, call this group the queen substance "receptor." But the group differs from a typical specialist like the bombykol receptor because of the uneven sensitivities of its cells to the less effective members of its spectrum. For example, cell 1 responds to substance $a \gg b > c$, cell 2 to substance $a \gg c > b$, and so on.

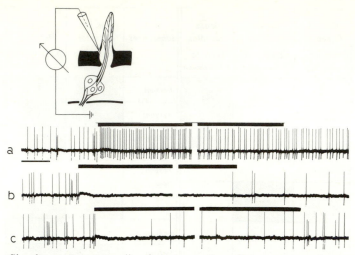

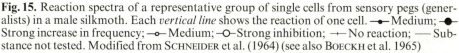

Fig. 14 a–c. Simultaneous ac-recording from two active cells in an antennal sensory peg (sensillum basiconicum) in a male wild silkmoth (*Antheraea pernyi*). Both cells show a resting activity in room air. **a** Terpineol excites on cell (large impulses) and inhibits the other; **b** Geraniol inhibits both cells to a large extent; **c** Isosafrole inhibits both cells to a minor extent. **c** *Antheraea pernyi*. Time marker below **a**, 300 ms. *Black bars* indicate stimuli. Modified from SCHNEIDER et al. (1964)

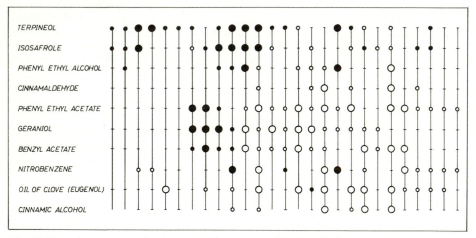

Fig. 15. Reaction spectra of a representative group of single cells from sensory pegs (generalists) in a male silkmoth. Each *vertical line* shows the reaction of one cell. ─•─ Medium; ─●─ Strong increase in frequency; ─○─ Medium; ─O─ Strong inhibition; ─┼─ No reaction; ── Substance not tested. Modified from SCHNEIDER et al. (1964) (see also BOECKH et al. 1965)

    In the behavior part of his bee study, VARESCHI (1971) saw that the discrimination of a given odor (to which the insect was conditioned) from other odors was best when the respective stimuli belonged to different electrophysiologically determined reaction groups. We thought that the discriminatory power of the bee could be explained on the basis of the reactivities of its receptor cells. The honeybee's ca-

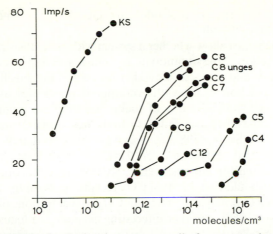

Fig. 16. Impulse response of a single odor receptor cell of an antennal pore plate sensillum in a honeybee drone. This cell belongs to the fatty acid reaction group. The responses are plotted as functions of the stimulus intensity (in molecules per cubic centimeter air). This set of curves characterizes the specificity of this cell. The C_4–C_{12} curves relate to saturated fatty acids; C_8 *unges* relates to an unsaturated compound. Note the high sensitivity of this cell to the queen substance (*KS*, 9-oxo-decenoic acid). Vareschi (1971)

pacity to discriminate, learn, and remember odors was a striking experience for the observer. In some cases not only a given odor but also its concentration was remembered (Vareschi 1971).

We then extended our investigations to another hymenopteron, an ant, to clarify the effects of alkane alarm pheromones. Dumpert (1972) found highly specifically reacting receptor cells for undecane, decane and dodecane being more than 100 times less effective. Since alarm substances of other ants acted on other receptor cell types, this author warns that receptor properties should be deduced from behavior reactions alone, as was done by Amoore et al. (1969).

On the basis of his study, Vareschi (1971) defined the following terms:

The *reaction spectrum* of an odor receptor cell comprises all those substances which are effective excitatory or inhibitory stimuli in a physiological concentration range.

The *specificity* of such a cell is expressed by the whole set of stimulus–response characteristics (Fig. 16).

Odor specialists are a population of cells with identical specificities.

Odor generalists are a population of cells with significantly different but partly overlapping specificities. The odor-discriminating function of the generalists as a system is probably based on the similarities (overlap) and differences of their specificities.

During the years when these experiments were being carried out, my laboratory group met frequently for work sessions. Hot debates on topics like specificity, binding, specialists, and generalists lasted for hours. We all felt the excitement of dealing with new observations, but we also realized the complexity of our field of research and the limitations of our analytical technique. Quite naturally, scientific debates tend to extend with the complexity of the matter. One example makes this clear: compared to specificities in visual or auditory receptors, odor receptor specificity is not easily determined and defined. A visual or an auditory stimulus spectrum is finite; not so a spectrum of odorants. Quantification and timing of odor stimuli is particularly difficult.

Future research must show whether a system with generalists really exists in insects. A reinvestigation of the situation in *Antheraea* with improved recording techniques is under way, and seems to show that the cells of the sensilla basiconica can be separated into reaction groups with overlapping specificities, as in the honeybee (Kafka, unpublished work). Studies of cockroach and flesh fly odor receptors by our Regensburg colleagues also failed to find "real" generalists (BOECKH 1974; KAIB 1974; SASS 1976; SELZER 1981). A weevil and bark beetles also have no typical odor generalist cells (MUSTAPARTA 1975, 1977).

Finally, our search for antennal odor receptors revealed organs with special properties. Here I should first mention CO_2 receptor cells on the honeybee antenna, which are tuned to biologically relevant CO_2 concentrations of between 0.03% and 100% (LACHER 1964). Another interesting example is a locust sensillum with a triad of receptor cells tuned respectively for temperature, moisture, and dryness (WALDOW 1970). Even the "classic" question of the sense of smell under water was examined in an amphibian beetle. It was found that the odor receptor cells respond equally well to the same substances in air and under water (BEHREND 1971).

F. Male Pheromones of Butterflies and Moths

The female sexual pheromones of the mainly nocturnal moths are attractants which bring the male to her by means of anemotaxis. In most of the sympatrically living moths, the species-specific blend of the pheromone components suffices (together with differences in the activity rhythm and male pheromones in some cases) for sexual isolation. In the diurnal butterflies, however, visual cues of the female are the distance signals for the males, which then locate and pursue their females.

With butterflies, identification problems seem to be greater than with the moths. In many cases, the males follow anything looking even vaguely similar to their females. Males of the same species are also tracked but then abandoned like the "wrong" females. What then are the recognition signals involved? To date, we can answer this question only in a few cases. Specific behavior combined with short-distance chemical signals by the males (rarely also by the females) are essential. Male chemical recognition signals are not restricted to the butterflies, but are also used by many male moths as a chemical "identity card" (aphrodisiac) to seduce their females (BUTLER 1967).

This introductory description incorporates quite a lot of information gained after Butler's definition, at least with respect to the Lepidoptera. What I would like to describe now is how I became interested in this branch of pheromone biology in general, and even more how it happened that we are now also trying to unravel ecophysiological interactions where pheromones and odor receptors are only part of a chain of causal events. Major elements of this network are secondary substances of the larval food plants, and of certain dry plants which are visited by the imagines. Here pheromone production, chemical defence, and mimicry come into play.

In 1965, my Cornell University colleague Thomas Eisner persuaded me to try electrophysiological methods on the male butterfly pheromones found in the subfamily Danainae (the monarchs). This proposal was consonant with my own interest, because I had often wondered about the role of chemical signals in butterfly communication. One famous case was the grayling *Hipparchia (Eumenis) semele* (TINBERGEN et al. 1942), and in Tübingen I had seen D. B. E. MAGNUS (1950, 1958) carrying out his well-known experiments on the silver-washed fritillary *Argynnis paphia*. Here visual female signals attract the male, but later chemicals come into effect at close range.

The males of the monarchs possess elaborate pheromone-producing abdominal hair pencils, which they quickly expand close to their females during courtship (Fig. 17). BROWER et al. (1965) had made key studies of this behavior. In the Trinidad species *Lycorea ceres* and the Florida queen (*Danaus gilippus*), the Cornell group then found a heterocyclic substance – pyrrolizinone – to be the major volatile component of the hair pencils (MEINWALD et al. 1966, 1969). This substance was later called "danaidone" (Fig. 17), and was found to be widespread in this group of butterflies (MEINWALD et al. 1971). PLISKE and EISNER (1969) then found in the queen butterfly that males raised indoors do not have this hair pencil component and have a very low courtship success rate. This was clear evidence that danaidone was a pheromone. When we started EAG recordings from this butterfly, we saw that the antennae of both sexes responded to the male pheromone (SCHNEIDER and SEIBT 1969). This was surprising in a sex pheromone because nearly all the female attractants of moths are only perceived by the respective males and not by the pheromone-producing females themselves.

One interesting analogy between danaidone and human perfume application should be mentioned here. Many of these butterflies use a particularly sophisticated method of applying their odor to the female antennae: when the hair pencils are opened during courtship, pheromone transfer particles are set free and some of them adhere to the female antennal structures, including the odor-sensitive pegs (PLISKE and EISNER 1969; BOPPRÉ 1979). In the Florida queen those particles were found to contain longer-chain alcohols in addition to danaidone (MEINWALD et al. 1969). These alcohols serve as fixative in a double sense: (a) as "solvents" for the danaidone, and (b) as glue for the particles.

The danaidone deficiency remained a puzzle for some time, in spite of the prediction by MEINWALD et al. (1969) that the insects might not be able to synthesize this pheromone de novo and that some plant alkaloids were its potential precursors. Eventually, after field observations of the African monarch on dry *Heliotropium* plants, imbibing the alkaloid, EDGAR et al. (1973) and EDGAR (1975), as well as my group (SCHNEIDER et al. 1975), were able to explain this as the necessary first step of the biosynthesis (Fig. 17). We then later found a second step, which is also essential, namely contact between the hair pencils and the glandular wing pouches (BOPPRÉ et al. 1978).

Studies of male moth pheromones revealed in some cases an aphrodisiac function, while in other cases the function still remains a puzzle (see the reviews by PRIESNER 1973; BIRCH 1970, 1974; TAMAKI 1977; SCHNEIDER 1980). Particularly interesting for us was that the males of an arctiid moth of the genus *Utetheisa* produce hydroxydanaidal (see Fig. 17) in their hair pencils (CULVENOR and EDGAR

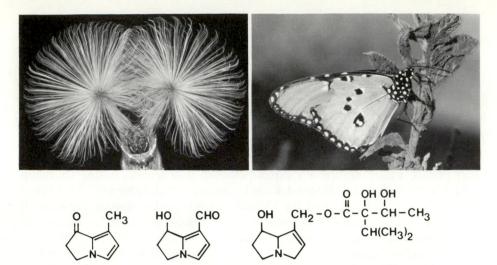

Fig. 17. *Danaus chrysippus* (African monarch butterfly). *Upper right:* male sitting on a dry part of a *Heliotropium* plant (field photo from East Africa). The insect ejects fluid through its proboscis onto the plant surface, which contains a pyrrolizidine alkaloid (*lower right* formula). The insect finds the plant by the alkaloid odor, it reimbibes the juice and eventually transforms the alkaloid into the pyrrolizine (danaidone, *lower left formula*). The danaidone odor acts as aphrodisiac during the mating behavior and is emitted from the expanded abdominal hair pencils of the male (*upper left*). Other danaines and some arctiid moths transform such alkaloids into hydroxydanaidal (*middle formula*). [Original photograph shown on the left by M. Boppré]

1972). Later it was found that this product is an effective aphrodisiac and again depends upon the uptake of pyrrolizidine alkaloids from the larval food plants of the genus *Crotalaria,* Fabaceae (Conner et al. 1980, 1981).

At present, we are studying rather bizarre male odor-producing organs in arctiid moths of the genus *Creatonotos* from southeast Asia. Males of these species have big pneumatic brushorgans which also contain hydroxydanaidal (Schneider et al. 1982; see also Willis and Birch 1982). The novel observation here in these species is that the males also lure the females, although the females still use their powerful attractants. In *Creatonotos,* even morphogenetic effects come into play, since lack of male pheromone precursors in the larval diet leads to minute brushes. This work is a combined project between Cornell University (J. Meinwald and associates), the University of Regensburg (M. Boppré), the University of Cologne (A. Egelhaaf), and Seewiesen (myself, H. Wunderer, and K. Hansen).

G. Retrospect

It is now over 30 years since I first became engaged in biological research, always with the privilege of the free choice of the field. During this time my curiosity has led me to try quite a number of different projects in animal physiology and the complementing morphology. I would like briefly to mention four fields in which

I have worked for a few years, and of which the last three relate directly to sensory inputs.

For my doctoral thesis project, I was asked to check on the question of saltatory conduction in myelinated nerve fibers. At this time (1947), Germany had opened up to scientific exchange again, and my *Doktorvater* (supvervisor), H. Autrum, had heard of the fascinating and, of course, evolutionarily most striking "jumping" nerve impulse. He asked me to learn the dissecting technique which G. Kato (1934) and later I. Tasaki (1939) had developed, and which was now also in use by A. von Muralt and R. Stämpfli in Switzerland (cit. VON MURALT 1946). After quite a number of months, I was able to isolate functional single A-α fibers from the frog sciatic nerve. My experimental technique for determining the function was to stimulate the proximal nerve, which was then farther distally "thinned" to a single fiber, and then to observe the passage of the impulse in the nerve fiber by the appearance of the muscle twitch. For stimulation, a galvanic couple or an induction coil sufficed, and the "yes" or "no" of the response was clear. I then tried to interfere reversibly with the impulse transfer by means of local cooling of the internodal segment or pressure at the same place. Since this was possible, I developed a "tunnel" hypothesis, which meant that conduction was by local miniature currents (*Strömchen*) over the nerve fiber membrane but under the myelin (SCHNEIDER 1950). This interpretation was, of course, in direct contradiction of recent experiments by HUXLEY and STÄMPFLI (1949), who had no doubt about the jumping impulse. Since no experimental control of the electrical status of the nodal membranes of the blocked fiber was possible for me at this time, I had to leave it like this until I met B. Frankenhäuser in Stockholm in 1950.

Just before I obtained my doctorate it so happened that the Rector of Göttingen University selected me for a three-month scholarship to Sweden, which allowed me to visit the Nobel Institute for Neurophysiology, of which Granit was the Director. After a seminar talk on my thesis work, Frankenhäuser expressed skepticism, and this led to two months of joint intensive experimentation on these nerve fibers, but now using all the sophisticated electronic equipment of which I had previously dreamed. We repeated my experiments, but now found that the effects of my tricks of impulse blockage were not restricted to the internodal area but also blocked the nodal membrane, which meant that I had to abandon the tunnel concept (FRANKENHÄUSER and SCHNEIDER 1951). This was altogether an impressive experience for me, and taught me to remain critical and always ready to question model concepts which are only crude approximations to the real processes. My nerve fiber research phase ended with one more paper on nerve fiber stretching (SCHNEIDER 1952) and another on the effect of saponine and electrolytes on the internode and the conduction. This was a joint work with M. Sato, whom I persuaded to visit me for a few weeks at Tübingen in 1953 while he was working on Pacinian corpuscles with J. A. E. Gray in London (SATO and SCHNEIDER 1954). At this time I was already the lucky owner of an oscilloscope, and had myself built amplifiers, which I used mainly for the just-emerging research on olfactory receptors (see Fig. 8).

The second field I should like to mention is the visual guidance of prey orientation and prey-catching in frogs and toads, which started from field observations. In order to do the nerve fiber experiments which I just described, I spent quite some time outdoors catching the animals. I lured them with decoys, a trick well known to every countryboy. I succeeded in improving the decoys (which, in the language of ethology, were close to being definable as the releasing stimulus). Since only part of what I saw was covered in the literature, I extended my observations by laboratory studies (SCHNEIDER 1954a). Before a frog can approach a prey, he has to see it. I wondered about the visual fields of these animals, and found interesting differences among the species (SCHNEIDER 1954b, 1957c, d). The biological relevance of these differences is still not entirely understood. This approach has never been my major occupation, but it is fascinating for me to see how others have chosen amphibia as model animals to study the sensory and neural basis of prey orientation and catching (EWERT 1980).

The third study was on light-directed (phototropic) growth in marine Bryozoa, the moss animals. Since even some zoologists barely know this group of coelomatic, colonial animals, one may wonder how I started it. It was at the time when I took up my first appointment, and the director of the institute, Alfred Kühn, asked me to test the effects of physical factors such as electricity on morphogenetic processes, for instance on wing pattern determination in a moth. I was familiar with problems of morphogenesis from the Zoological Institute at the University of Göttingen, where we physiologists of the Autrum group learned much from the group under Karl Henke, which was studying developmental processes in insects. Henke, then Professor of Zoology there, was a former student of Kühn and now his successor to the Göttingen Chair. When I considered how to approach the problem of the wing pattern of the moth, I thought this to be too complex a structure for such an attempt and wanted to do it with a budding hydroid. These proved not to be available, but I could "borrow" the bryozoan *Bugula* from a nearby colleague. Although I was unable to influence the growth of the buds of this animal by electricity, I found them to react properly to the direction of the light (SCHNEIDER 1955b, 1959, 1963b). Interestingly, the action spectrum indicated that the basis of this phototropism is a rhodopsin-like photopigment (KAISSLING 1963), and that the discrimination of the direction of the light is a process of differentiation between several inputs, as in several other sensory functions in fungi and mammals (SCHNEIDER and KAISSLING 1964). It should be mentioned that the fossil forms of these attractive animals are well studied by paleontologists, but recent species receive very little attention, especially from physiologists. The time spent with *Bugula* made me aware of what it means to be nearly alone with an experimental animal and the phenomena one is observing. If neither the organism nor the topic fits into the scientific trends which are then in fashion, one finds little resonance and reassurance in the daily work. Although the Bryozoa turned out to be a good model system for the study of a number of basic biological phenomena, such as morphogenetic processes, primitive light sense, etc., I abandoned them later when I needed all my resources to concentrate on the olfaction projects.

The fourth field I became interested in was insect olfaction. I have already described my start in the introductory section. A number of circumstances contributed to my involvement in this field and encouraged me to continue. With only a knowledge of the *Bombyx* chemistry work but without the readiness of the local chemists to supply me with the gland extracts, I would never have tried to record from the antenna. The early success induced me to continue the work which has been described in this chapter. The development of many aspects of our work along different lines was dictated by our daily progress, and was not without logic, but one might wonder why I myself eventually became so interested in the comparative aspects of male pheromones and even the plant–insect interrelationships (see Sect. F). To explain this, I ought to mention that when I returned to university in 1947, I wanted to do my doctoral thesis on an ecophysiological project, but could not find a professor guiding work in what we would now call "sensory ecology." I therefore returned to H. Autrum, at this time one of the few sensory physiologists in Germany who used modern methods. He was now in Göttingen, and I knew him from my prewar zoology studies at Berlin University.

Looking back, I must say that ethoecology, which was a daydream at the beginning of my scientific career, has become a fact in recent years. My steady interest in sensory ecology found a basis in plant–insect relationships, for which functional understanding of several subsystems is required. As an example, people who may be called pure physiologists study receptor processes and are satisfied if they know *how* this organ works. They are satisfied with their success perhaps even independently of the general biological relevance. I agree that it is exciting and essential to learn these facts, but even more exciting for me is also to ask the "why" question. Let me give another example. Why do the males of some moths have large pectinate antennae with long olfactory sensilla? After many years of systematic analytical work on a number of species, we may say that such antennae provide the male in those species (where the females produce the attractant in amounts smaller than a microgram) with an almost perfect odor-receiving organ. Such questions, of course, lead to evolutionary problems of high complexity, and it is here that comparative work may provide some understanding. In returning to our example and by considering the comparative aspect, we can go even further. While all male moths have long sensilla with which to catch the female odor molecules, only some groups, such as *Bombyx,* saturniids, and lymantriids, have these huge antennae. But many others have only whip-like antennae, which are much less effective molecule-catching devices (see KAISSLING 1971). Do the females of these species with whip antennae produce more of the attractant to compensate for the less effective male antennae? Since this has never been found to be the case, the males must find behavioral ways of overcoming what we naive observers think of as a weakness in the sensory system. This brings us to the trivial statement that any organism is the result of evolutionary processes and, therefore, a compromise. These processes cannot, of course, be observed directly, and can at the very best be deduced from comparative "how" studies. But it gives me, and I am sure also many other biologists, great pleasure if one at least understands here or there a little of the "why!"

References

Names containing *von* are alphabetized in this list under *v*

Adrian ED (1926) The impulses produced by sensory nerve endings, part I. J Physiol 61:49–72

Adrian ED, Zotterman Y (1926) The impulses produced by sensory nerve endings, parts II and III. J Physiol 61:151–171, 465–483

Altner H, Prillinger L (1980) Ultrastructure of invertebrate chemo-, thermo-, and hygrore-ceptors and its functional significance. Int Rev Cytol 67:69–139

Amoore JE, Palmieri G, Wanke E, Blum MS (1969) Ant alarm pheromone activity: correla-tion with molecular shape by scanning computer. Science 165:1266–1269

Arn H, Städler E, Rauscher S (1975) The electroantennographic detector – a selective and sensitive tool in the gas chromatographic analysis of insect pheromones. Z Naturforsch [c] 30:722–725

Autrum H (1950) Belichtungspotentiale and das Sehen der Insekten (Untersuchungen an *Calliphora* and *Dixippus*). J Comp Physiol 32:176–227

Behrend K (1971) Riechen in Wasser und in der Luft bei *Dytiscus marginalis* L. J Comp Phy-siol 75:108–122

Bernhard CG (1942) Isolation of retinal and optic ganglion response in the eye of *Dytiscus*. J Neurophysiol 5:32–48

Bierl BA, Beroza M, Collier CW (1970) Potent sex attractant of the gypsy moth: its isola-tion, identification, and synthesis. Science 170:87–89

Bierl BA, Beroza M, Adler VE, Kasang G, Schröter H, Schneider D (1975) The presence of disparlure, the sex pheromone of the gypsy moth in the female nun moth. Z Natur-forsch [c] 30:672–675

Birch MC (1970) Pre-courtship use of abdominal brushes by males of the nocturnal moth, *Phlogophora meticulosa* (Lepidoptera: Noctuidae). Anim Behav 18:310–316

Birch MC (ed) (1974) Pheromones. North Holland, Amsterdam

Boeckh J (1962) Electrophysiologische Untersuchungen an einzelnen Geruchsrezeptoren auf den Antennen des Totengräbers (*Necrophorus*, Coleoptera). Z Vergl Physiol 46:212–248

Boeckh J (1967 a) Inhibition and excitation of single insect olfactory receptors, and their role as a primary sensory code. In: Hayashi T (ed) Olfaction and taste II. Pergamon, Oxford, pp 721–735

Boeckh J (1967 b) Reaktionsschwelle, Arbeitsbereich und Spezifität eines Geruchsrezeptors auf der Heuschreckenantenne. Z Vergl Physiol 55:378–406

Boeckh J (1974) Die Reaktionen olfaktorischer Neurone im Deutocerebrum von Insekten im Vergleich zu Antwortmustern der Geruchssinneszelle. J Comp Physiol 90:183–205

Boeckh J (1980) Neural basis of coding of chemosensory quality at the receptor cell level. In: Starre H (ed) Olfaction and taste VII. I.R.L. London, pp 113–122

Boeckh J, Boeckh V (1979) Threshold and odor specificity of pheromone-sensitive neurons in the deutocerebrum of *Antheraea pernyi* and *A. polyphemus* (Saturniidae). J Comp Physiol 132:235–242

Boeckh J, Kaissling K-E, Schneider D (1960) Sensillen und Bau der Antennengeißel von *Te-lea polyphemus* (Vergleiche mit weiteren Saturniiden: *Antheraea, Platysamia* und *Philo-samia*). Zool Jahrb (Anat) 78:559–584

Boeckh J, Priesner E, Schneider D, Jacobson M (1963) Olfactory receptor response to the cockroach sexual attractant. Science 141:716–717

Boeckh J, Kaissling K-E, Schneider D (1965) Insect olfactory receptors. Cold Spring Har-bor Symp Quant Biol 30:263–280

Boeckh J, Ernst K-D, Sass H, Waldow U (1976) Zur nervösen Organisation antennaler Sin-neseingänge bei Insekten unter besonderer Berücksichtigung der Riechbahn. Verh Dtsch Zool Ges. Fischer, Stuttgart, pp 123–139

Boeckh J, Boeckh V, Kühn A (1977) Further data on the topography and physiology of cen-tral olfactory neurons in insects. In: LeMagnen J, MacLeod P (eds) Olfaction and taste VI. I.R.L., London, pp 315–321

Boppré M (1979) Untersuchungen zur Pheromonbiologie bei Monarchfaltern (Danaidae). Diss Fak Biol, Univ München

Boppré M, Petty RL, Schneider D, Meinwald J (1976) Behaviorally mediated contacts be-tween scent organs: another prerequisite for pheromone production in *Danaus chrysip-pus* males (Lepidoptera). J Comp Physiol 126:97–103

Brand JM, Young JC, Silverstein RM (1979) Insect pheromones: a critical review of recent advances in their chemistry, biology, and application. Fortschr Chem Organ Naturst 37:1–190

Brower LP, Van Zandt Brower J, Cranston FP (1965) Courtship behavior of the queen butterfly, *Danaus gilippus berenice* (Cramer). Zoologica (New York) 50:1–39

Butenandt A (1955a) Wirkstoffe des Insektenreiches. Nova Acta Leopoldina (Halle). N.F. 17:445–471

Butenandt A (1955b) Über Wirkstoffe des Insektenreiches. II. Zur Kenntnis der Sexual-Lockstoffe. Naturwissenschaften Rundschau 8:457–464

Butenandt A, Hecker E (1961) Synthese des Bombykols des Sexual-Lockstoffes des Seidenspinners und seiner geometrischen Isomeren. Angew Chem 73:349–358

Butenandt A, Beckmann R, Stamm D, Hecker E (1959) Über den Sexuallockstoff des Seidenspinners *Bombyx mori*. Reindarstellung und Konstitution. Z Naturforsch 14b:283–284

Butenandt A, Beckmann R, Hecker E (1961a) Über den Sexuallockstoff des Seidenspinners. I. Der biologische Test und die Isolierung des reinen Sexuallockstoffes Bombykol. Hoppe-Seylers Z Physiol Chem 324:71–83

Butenandt A, Beckmann R, Stamm D (1961b) Über den Sexuallockstoff des Seidenspinners. II. Konstitution und Konfiguration des Bombykols. Hoppe Seylers Z Physiol Chem 324:84–87

Butler CG (1967) Insect pheromones. Biol Rev 42:42–87

Conner WE, Eisner T, Vander Meer RK, Guerrero A, Ghiringelli D, Meinwald J (1980) Sex attractant of an arctiid moth (*Utetheisa ornatrix*): a pulsed chemical signal. Behav Ecol Sociobiol 7:55–63

Conner WE, Eisner T, Vander Meer RK, Guerrero A, Meinwald J (1981) Precopulatory sexual interaction in an arctiid moth (*Utetheisa ornatrix*): role of a pheromone derived from dietary alkaloids. Behav Ecol Sociobiol 9:227–235

Culvenor CCJ, Edgar JA (1972) Dihydropyrrolizidine secretion associated with coremata of *Utetheisa* moths (family Arctiidae). Experientia 28:627–628

David CT, Kennedy JS, Ludlow AR, Terry JN, Wall C (1982) A reappraisal of insect flight towards distant point source of wind-born odor. Chem Ecol 8:1207–1215

Dumpert K (1972) Alarmstoffrezeptoren auf der Antenne von *Lasius fuliginosus* (Latr.) (Hymenoptera, Formicidae). Z Vergl Physiol 76:403–425

Edgar JA (1975) Danainae (Lep.) and 1,2-dehydropyrrolizidine alkaloid-containing plants – with reference to observations made in the New Hebrides. Philos Trans R Soc Lond [Biol] 272:467–476

Edgar JA, Culvenor CCJ, Robinson GS (1973) Hairpencil dihydropyrrolizidines of Danainae from the New Hebrides. J Aust Ent Soc 12:144–150

Ernst KD (1969) Die Feinstruktur von Riechsensillen auf der Antenne des Aaskäfers *Necrophorus*. Z Zellforsch 94:72–102

Ernst KD (1972) Die Ontogenie der basiconischen Riechsensillen auf der Antenne von *Necrophorus*. Z Zellforsch 132:95–106

Ernst KD, Boeckh J, Boeckh V (1977) A neuroanatomical study on the organization of the antennal pathway in insects. Cell Tiss Res 176:285–308

Ewert J-P (1980) Neuroethology. Springer, Berlin

Fabre JH (1879) Souvenirs entomologiques. Delagrave, Paris

Forel A (1910) Das Sinnesleben der Insekten. Reinhardt, München

Frankenhäuser B, Schneider D (1951) Some electrophysiological observations on isolated single myelinated nerve fibres (saltatory conduction). J Physiol 115:177–185

Götz B (1951) Die Sexualduftstoffe an Lepidopteren. Experientia 7:406–418

Granit R (1933) The composition of the retinal action potentials and their relation to the discharge of the optic nerve. J Physiol 77:207–240

Granit R (1947) Sensory mechanism of the retina. Oxford University Press, London

Granit R (1955) Receptors and sensory perception. Yale University Press, New Haven

Hansen K, Schneider D, Boppré M (1983) Chiral pheromone and reproductive isolation between the gypsy- and nun moth. Naturwissenschaften 70:466–467

Hildebrand JG, Matsumoto S, Camazine SM, Tolbert LP, Blank S, Ferguson H, Ecker V (1980) Organization and physiology of antennal centers in the brain of the moth *Manduca sexta*. In: Insect neurobiology and pesticide action (Neurotox 79). Society of Chemical Industry London, pp 375–382

Huber F (1978) The insect nervous system and insect behaviour. The Nico Tinbergen Lecture 1977. Animal Behav 26:969–981

Huber F (1980) Zoologische Grundlagenforschung aus der Sicht eines Insektenbiologen. Verh Dtsch Zool Ges. Fischer, Stuttgart, pp 12–37

Huxley AF, Stämpfli R (1949) Evidence for saltatory conduction in peripheral myelinated nerve fibres. J Physiol 108:315–339

Kafka WA (1970) Molekulare Wechselwirkungen bei der Erregung einzelner Riechzellen. Z Vergl Physiol 70:105–143

Kafka WA (1974) Physicochemical aspects of odor reception in insects. Ann NY Acad Sci 237:115–128

Kafka WA, Ohloff G, Schneider D, Vareschi E (1973) Olfactory discrimination of two enantiomers of 4-methyl-hexanoic acid by the migratory locust and the honeybee. J Comp Physiol 87:277–284

Kaib M (1974) Die Fleisch- und Blumenduftrezeptoren auf der Antenne der Schmeißfliege *Calliphora vicina*. J Comp Physiol 95:105–121

Kaissling K-E (1963) Die phototropische Reaktion der Zoide von *Bugula avicularia* L. Z Vergl Physiol 46:541–594

Kaissling K-E (1971) Insect olfaction. In: Beidler L (ed) Handbook of sensory physiology, vol IV, Chemical senses, part I. Olfaction. Springer, Berlin, pp 351–431

Kaissling K-E (1974) Sensory transduction in insect olfactory receptors. In: Jaenicke L (ed) Biochemistry of sensory functions 25. Moosbacher Coll Ges Biol Chem. Springer, Berlin, pp. 243–273

Kaissling K-E (1979) Recognition of pheromones by moths, especially in saturniids and *Bombyx mori*. In: Ritter FJ (ed) Chemical ecology: odour communication in animals. Elsevier/North Holland Biomedical, Amsterdam, pp. 43–56

Kaissling K-E (1980) Studies on the functional organization of insect olfactory sensilla (*Antheraea polyphemus* and *A. pernyi*). In: Starre H (ed) Olfaction and taste VII. IRL, London, p 81

Kaissling K-E, Priesner E (1970) Die Riechschwelle des Seidenspinners. Naturwissenschaften 57:23–28

Kaissling K-E, Thorson J (1980) Insect olfactory sensilla: structural, chemical, and electrical aspects of the functional organization. In: Satelle DB, Hall LM, Hildebrand JG (eds) Receptors for neurotransmitters, hormones, and pheromones in insects. Elsevier/North Holland Biomedical, Amsterdam, pp 261–282

Kaissling K-E, Kasang G, Bestmann HJ, Stransky W, Vostrowsky O (1978) A new pheromone of the silkworm moth *Bombyx mori*. Sensory pathway and behavioral effect. Naturwissenschaften 65:382–384

Karlson P, Lüscher M (1959) "Pheromones": a new term for a class of biologically active substances. Nature 183:55–56

Karlson P, Schneider D (1973) Sexualpheromone der Schmetterlinge als Modelle chemischer Kommunikation. Naturwissenschaften 60:113–121

Kasang G (1968) Tritium-Markierung des Sexuallockstoffes Bombykol. Z Naturforsch 23b:1331–1335

Kasang G (1971) Bombykol reception and metabolism on the antennae of the silkmoth *Bombyx mori*. In: Ohloff G, Thomas AF (eds) Gustation and olfaction. Academic, London, pp 245–250

Kasang G (1974) Uptake of the sex pheromone ^3H-bombykol and related compounds by male and female *Bombyx* antennae. J Insect Physiol 20:2407–2422

Kasang G, Kaissling K-E (1972) Specificity of primary and secondary olfactory processes in *Bombyx* antennae. In: Schneider D (ed) Olfaction and taste IV. Wissenschaftliche Verlagsgesellschaft, Stuttgart, pp 200–206

Kasang G, Kaissling K-E, Vostrowsky O, Bestmann HJ (1978) Bombykal, eine zweite Pheromonkomponente des Seidenspinners *Bombyx mori*. Angew Chem 90:74–75

Kennedy JS (1977) Olfactory responses to distant plants and other odor sources. In: Shorey HH, McKelvey JJ Jr (eds). Wiley Interscience, New York, pp 67–91

Kennedy JS, Marsh D (1974) Pheromone-regulated anemotaxis in flying moths. Science 184:999–1001

Klein U (1980) Investigations of proteins from isolated insect olfactory hairs. In: Starre H (ed) Olfaction and taste VII. IRL, London, p 89

Kochansky J, Tette J, Taschenberg EF, Cardé RT, Kaissling K-E, Roelofs WL (1975) Sex pheromone of the moth *Antheraea polyphemus*. J Insect Physiol 21:1977–1983

Kramer E (1975) Orientation of the male silkmoth to the sex attractant bombykol. In: Denton DA, Coghlan JP (eds) Olfaction and taste V. Academic, New York, pp 329–335

Kramer E (1978) Insect pheromones. In: Hazelbauer GL (ed) Taxis and behaviour (receptors and recognition) Series B. vol 5. Chapman and Hall, London, pp 206–229

Lacher V (1964) Elektrophysiologische Untersuchungen an einzelnen Rezeptoren für Geruch, Kohlendioxyd, Luftfeuchtigkeit und Temperatur auf den Antennen der Arbeitsbiene und der Drohne (*Apis mellifica* L.). Z Vergl Physiol 48:587–623

Magnus DBE (1950) Beobachtungen zur Balz und Eiablage des Kaisermantels, *Argynnis paphia* L. Z Tierpsychol 7:435–449

Magnus DBE (1958) Experimentelle Untersuchungen zur Bionomie und Ethologie des Kaisermantels *Argynnis paphia* L. Z Tierpsychol 15:397–426

Matsumoto SG, Hildebrand JG (1981) Olfactory mechanism in the moth *Manduca sexta:* response characteristics and morphology of central neurons in the antennal lobes. Proc R Soc Lond [Biol] 213:249–277

Meinwald J, Meinwald YC, Wheeler JW, Eisner T, Brower LP (1966) Major component in the exocrine secretion of a male butterfly (*Lycorea*). Science 151:583–585

Meinwald J, Meinwald YC, Mazzocchi PH (1969) Sex pheromone of the queen butterfly: chemistry. Science 164:1174–1175

Meinwald J, Thompson WR, Eisner T, Owen DF (1971) Pheromones VII. African monarch: major components of hairpencil secretion. Tetrahedron Letters 38:3485–3488

Mell R (1922) Biologie und Systematik der südchinesischen Sphingiden. Friedländer, Berlin

Minks AK, Roelofs WL, Ritter FJ, Persoons CJ (1973) Reproductive isolation of two tortricid moth species by different ratios of a two-component sex attractant. Science 180:1073–1074

Moorhouse TE, Yeadon R, Beevor PS, Nesbitt BF (1969) Method for use in studies of insect chemical communication. Nature 223:1174–1175

Mustaparta H (1975) Responses of single olfactory cells in the pine weevil *Hylobius abietis* L. (Col.: Cucurlionidae). J Comp Physiol 97:271–290

Mustaparta H (1977) Responses of single receptor cells in the pine engraver beetle, *Ips pini* (Say) (Coleoptera: Scolitidae) to its aggregation pheromone, ipsdienol, and the aggregation inhibitor, ipsenol. J Comp Physiol 121:343–347

Olberg R (1983) Pheromone sensitive neuronal flip-flop underlying the female-locating behavior of the male silk moth. J Comp Physiol 157:297–307

Ottoson D (1956) Analysis of the electrical activity of the olfactory epithelium. Acta Physiol Scand [Suppl] 35:1–83

Ottoson D (1971) The electro-olfactogram. In: Beidler LM (ed) Handbook of sensory physiology, vol IV. Chemical senses, part I. Olfaction. Springer, Berlin, pp 95–131

Pareto A (1972) Die zentrale Verteilung der Fühlerafferenz bei Arbeiterinnen der Honigbiene, *Apis mellifera* L. Z Zellforsch 131:109–140

Pliske TE, Eisner T (1969) Sex pheromone of the queen butterfly: biology. Science 164:1170–1172

Preiss R (1980) Anemotaxis in Lauf und Flug beim Schwammspinner. Versuche zur Aufklärung des Wirkungsgefüges. Diss Fak Biol Univ München

Preiss R, Kramer E (1983a) Stabilization of altitude and speed in tethered flying gypsy moth males: influence of (+) and (−)-disparlure. Physiol Entomol 8:55–68

Preiss R, Kramer E (1983b) Control of flight speed by minimization of the apparent ground-pattern movement. In: Varju D and Schnitzler H-U (eds) (in press) Localization and orientation in biology and engineering. Springer Series: Proceedings in Life Sciences

Priesner E (1968) Die interspezifischen Wirkungen der Sexuallockstoffe der Saturniidae (Lepidoptera). Z Vergl Physiol 61:263–297

Priesner E (1969) A new approach to insect pheromone specificity. In: Pfaffmann C (ed) Olfaction and taste III. Rockefeller University Press, New York, pp. 235–240

Priesner E (1973) Artspezifität und Funktion einiger Insektenpheromone. Fortschr Zool 22:49–135

Priesner E (1977) Evolutionary potential of specialized olfaction receptors. In: Le Magnen J, MacLeod P (eds) Olfaction and taste VI. IRL, London, pp 333–341

Priesner E (1979) Specificity studies on pheromone receptors of noctuid and tortricid lepidoptera. In: Ritter FJ (ed) Chemical ecology. Elsevier/North Holland Biomedical, Amsterdam, pp 57–71

Priesner E (1980) Sensory encoding of pheromone signals and related stimuli in male moths. In: Insect neurobiology and insecticide action (Neurotox 1979). Society of Chemical Industry, London, pp 359–366

Richter S (1962) Unmittelbarer Kontakt der Sinneszellen cuticularer Sinnesorgane mit der Außenwelt. Eine licht- und elektronenmikroskopische Untersuchung der chemorezeptorischen Antennensinnesorgane der *Calliphora*-Larven. Z Morph Ökol Tiere 52:171–196

Roelofs WL, Comeau A, Hill A, Milicevic G (1971) Sex attractant of the codling moth: characterization with electroantennogram technique. Science 174:297–299

Sass H (1976) Zur nervösen Codierung von Geruchsreizen bei *Periplaneta americana*. J Comp Physiol 107:49–65

Sato M, Schneider D (1954) Mikroskopisch-elektrophysiologische Untersuchung des Internodiums der markhaltigen Nervenfaser unter Einwirkung von Saponin und Elektrolyten. Z Naturforsch 9b:644–655

Schneider D (1950) Die lokale Reizung und Blockierung im Internodium der isolierten markhaltigen Nervenfaser des Frosches. Z Vergl Physiol 32:507–529

Schneider D (1952) Die Dehnbarkeit der markhaltigen Nervenfaser des Frosches in Abhängigkeit von Funktion und Struktur. Z Naturforsch 7b:38–48

Schneider D (1954a) Das Gesichtsfeld und der Fixiervorgang bei einheimischen Anuren. Z Vergl Physiol 36:147–164

Schneider D (1954b) Beitrag zu einer Analyse des Beute- und Fluchtverhaltens einheimischer Anuren. Biol Zentralbl 73:225–282

Schneider D (1955a) Mikro-Elektroden registrieren die elektrischen Impulse einzelner Sinnesnervenzellen der Schmetterlingsantenne. Industrie-Elektronik (Hamburg) 3:3–7

Schneider D (1955b) Phototropisches Wachstum der Zoide von *Bugula avicularia*. Naturwissenschaften 42:48–49

Schneider D (1957a) Elektrophysiologische Untersuchungen von Chemo- und Mechanorezeptoren der Antenne des Seidenspinners *Bombyx mori* L. Z Vergl Physiol 40:8–41

Schneider D (1957b) Electrophysiological investigation on the antennal receptors of the silk moth during chemical and mechanical stimulation. Experientia 13:89–91

Schneider D (1957c) Die Biologie der Wirbeltieraugen. Studium Generale 10:214–230

Schneider D (1957d) Die Gesichtsfelder von *Bombina variegata, Discoglossus pictus,* und *Xenopus laevis*. Z Vergl Physiol 39:524–530

Schneider D (1959) Über den Mechanismus des phototropischen Knospenwachstums bei marinen Bryozoen. Verh Dtsch Zool Ges. Fischer, Stuttgart, pp 239–247

Schneider D (1962) Electrophysiological investigation on the olfactory specificity of sexual attracting substances in different species of moths. J Insect Physiol 8:15–30

Schneider D (1963a) Electrophysiological investigation of insect olfaction. In: Zotterman Y (ed) Olfaction and taste I. Pergamon, Oxford, pp 85–103

Schneider D (1963b) Normal and phototropic growth reaction in the marine bryozoan *Bugula avicularia*. In: Dougherty EC et al. (eds) The lower metazoa. University of California, Berkeley, pp 357–371

Schneider D (1964) Insect antennae. Ann Rev Entomol 9:103–122

Schneider D (1965) Chemical sense communication in insects. Symp Soc Exp Biol 20:273–297

Schneider D (1969) Insect olfaction: deciphering system for chemical messages. Science 163:1031–1037

Schneider D (1971) Molekulare Grundlagen der chemischen Sinne bei Insekten. Naturwissenschaften 58:194–200

Schneider D (1974) The sex-attractant receptor of moths. Sci Am 231(1):28–35

Schneider D (1975) Pheromone communication in moths and butterflies. In: Galun R et al. (eds) Sensory physiology and behavior. Plenum, New York, pp 173–193

Schneider D (1977) H. Autrum – a chapter in comparative physiology. J Comp Physiol 120:1–10

Schneider D (1980) Pheromone von Insekten: Produktion-Rezeption-Inaktivierung. Nova Acta Leopoldina, N.F. 51:249–278

Schneider D, Boeckh J (1962) Rezeptorpotential und Nervenimpulse einzelner olfaktorischer Sensillen der Insektenantenne. Z Vergl Physiol 45:405–412

Schneider D, Hecker E (1956) Zur Elektronenphysiologie der Antenne des Seidenspinners *Bombyx mori* bei Reizung mit angereicherten Extrakten des Sexuallockstoffes. Z Naturforsch 11b:121–124

Schneider D, Kaissling K-E (1956) (1957) (1959) Der Bau der Antenne des Seidenspinners *Bombyx mori* L. Zool Jahrb (Anat) 75:287–310; 76:223–250; 77:111–132

Schneider D, Kaissling K-E (1964) Wachstum und Phototropismus bei Moostieren. Naturwissenschaften 51:127–134

Schneider D, Seibt U (1969) Sex pheromone of the the queen butterfly: electroantennogram responses. Science 164:1173–1174

Schneider D, Steinbrecht RA (1968) Checklist of insect olfactory sensilla. Symp Zool Soc (Lond) 23:279–297

Schneider D, Lacher V, Kaissling K-E (1964) Die Reaktionsweise und das Reaktionsspektrum von Riechzellen bei *Antheraea pernyi* (Lepidoptera, Saturniidae). Z Vergl Physiol 48:632–662

Schneider D, Block BC, Boeckh J, Priesner E (1967) Die Reaktion der männlichen Seidenspinner auf Bombykol und seine Isomeren: Elektroantennogramm und Verhalten. Z Vergl Physiol 54:192–209

Schneider D, Lange R, Schwarz F, Beroza M, Bierl BA (1974) Attraction of male gypsy and nun moths to disparlure and some of its chemical analogues. Oecologia (Berlin) 14:19–36

Schneider D, Boppré M, Schneider H, Thompson WR, Boriack CJ, Petty RL, Meinwald J (1975) A pheromone precursor and its uptake in male *Danaus* butterflies. J Comp Physiol 97:245–256

Schneider D, Kafka WA, Beroza M, Bierl BA (1977) Odor receptor responses of male gypsy and nun moths (Lepidoptera, Lymantriidae) to disparlure and its analogues. J Comp Physiol 113:1–15

Schneider D, Boppré M, Zweig J, Horsley SB, Bell TW, Meinwald J (1982) Scent organ development in *Creatonotos* moths: regulation by pyrrolizidine alkaloids. Science 215:1264–1265

Schröter H (1976) *Lymantria (Porthetria):* Isolationsmechanismen im Paarungsverhalten von Nonne und Schwammspinner. Diss Forstwiss Fak University Freiburg i. Br.

Schwinck I (1954) Experimentelle Untersuchungen über Geruchssinn und Strömungswahrnehmung in der Orientierung bei Nachtschmetterlingen. Z Vergl Physiol 37:19–56

Schwinck I (1955) Weitere Untersuchungen zur Frage der Geruchsorientierung der Nachtschmetterlinge: partielle Fühleramputation bei Spinnermännchen, insbesondere am Seidenspinner *Bombyx mori* L. Z Vergl Physiol 37:439–458

Selzer R (1981) The processing of a complex food odor by antennal olfactory receptors of *Periplaneta americana*. J Comp Physiol 144:509–519

Silverstein RM (1981) Pheromones: background and potential use in insect pest control. Science 213:1326–1332

Slifer EH (1961) The fine structure of insect sense organs. Int Rev Cytol 11:125–159

Steinbrecht RA (1964a) Feinstruktur und Histochemie der Sexualduftdrüse des Seidenspinners *Bombyx mori* L. Z Zellforsch 64:227–261

Steinbrecht RA (1964b) Die Abhängigkeit der Lockwirkung des Sexualduftorgans weiblicher Seidenspinner (*Bombyx mori*) von Alter und Kopulation. Z Vergl Physiol 48:341–356

Steinbrecht RA (1969) Comparative morphology of olfactory receptors. In: Pfaffmann C (ed) Olfaction and taste III. Rockefeller University Press, New York, pp 3–21

Steinbrecht RA (1970) Zur Morphometrie der Antennen des Seidenspinner *Bombyx mori* L.: Zahl und Verteilung der Riechsensillen (Insecta, Lepidoptera). Z Morph Tiere 68:93–126

Steinbrecht RA (1973) Der Feinbau olfaktorischer Sensillen des Seidenspinner (Insecta, Lepidoptera). Z Zellforsch 139:533–565

Steinbrecht RA (1980) Cryofixation without cryoprotectants. Freeze substitution and freeze etching of an insect olfactory receptor. Tissue Cell 12:73–100

Steinbrecht RA, Kasang G (1972) Capture and conveyance of odour molecules in an insect olfactory receptor. In: Schneider D (ed) Olfaction and taste IV. Wiss, Stuttgart, pp 193–199

Tinbergen N, Meeuse BJD, Boerema LK, Varussieau WW (1942) Die Balz des Samtfalters, *Eumenis* (= *Satyrus*) *semele* (L.). Z Tierpsychol 5:182–226

Tolbert LP, Hildebrand JG (1981) Organization and synaptic ultrastructure of glomeruli in the antennal lobes of the moth *Manduca sexta:* a study using thin sections and freeze-fracture. Proc R Soc Lond [Biol] 213:279–301

Vareschi E (1971) Duftunterscheidung bei der Honigbiene – Einzelzell-Ableitungen und Verhaltensreaktionen. Z Vergl Physiol 75:143–173

Vité JP, Kliemetze KD, Loskant G, Hedden R, Mori K (1976) Chirality of insect pheromones: response interruption by inactive antipodes. Naturwissenschaften 63:582–583

von Frisch K (1921) Über den Sitz des Geruchssinnes bei Insekten. Zool Jahrb Zool Physiol 38:1–68

von Muralt A (1946) Die Signalübermittlung im Nerven. Birkhäuser, Basel

Waldow U (1970) Elektrophysiologische Untersuchungen an Feuchte-, Trocken- und Kälterezeptoren auf der Antenne der Wanderheuschrecke *Locusta*. Z Vergl Physiol 69:249–283

Willis MA, Birch MC (1982) Male-lekking and female calling in the same population of the arctiid moth *Estigmene acraea*. Science 218:168–170

Zack C (1979) Sensory adaptation in the sex pheromone receptor cells of saturniid moths. Diss Fak Biol Univ München

Zettler F, Weiler R (eds) (1976) Neural principles of vision. Springer, Berlin Heidelberg New York

CHAPTER 14

Cutaneous Temperature Sensitivity[*]

Dan R. Kenshalo Sr.

A. Introduction

In the spring of 1947 I entered the last semester of my Bachelor of Science degree course at Washington University, St. Louis. At that time I had an established major in zoology and had even applied to several graduate programs to study entomology. In order to complete the second of two minors required for graduation, I needed one more course in psychology. In looking over the course schedule I

[*] Preparation of this chapter was assisted by USPHS grant NS-02992

found one entitled "physiological psychology." The name implied potentially more appealing material for me than another course in learning, child psychology, or statistics. I had no idea of the course content or who was to teach it, but I soon found out. On the first day of class, John Paul Nafe entered the classroom declaring that he was the instructor. Nafe had taught a section of introductory psychology in which I had been enrolled several years before. At that time I had not been particularly impressed by the subject matter – but what sophomore knows what is impressive?

Nafe had a rather large file folder with him, which was full of yellow sheets of paper from which he began to read. (It became clear later that this was a draft of a manuscript for a book on physiological psychology that he was preparing). We heard such words as "superior colliculus," "inferior olive," "medial geniculate," "the tract Lissauer," and "sensory filet." I knew what filet mignon and a fish filet were, but a sensory filet? At this point in my academic career I had not had a course in neuroanatomy or neurophysiology. I remember thinking at the time, "Kenshalo, you'd better get it in gear or you are in deep trouble."

As the semester moved along, we heard a great deal more about the neuroanatomy and neurophysiology of the somatosensory system. Much time was spent on the variables of single nerve fibers (frequency and latency) and of nerve bundles (threshold and conduction velocity). Taken together, according to Nafe, they provided the spatial and temporal patterns of activity conveyed to the central nervous system, where the information about qualities and intensities of stimulation was sorted out and interpreted: "the neural correlates of sensation."

By the end of the semester we had all learned a lot, not only about somatic sensitivity, but also about general neuroanatomy and neurophysiology. John Paul Nafe was an inspiring and challenging teacher. By the end of that semester I had come to appreciate how individual, almost heretical, his views about somatosensory processes were compared to those espoused by the authors of the then current texts of neuroanatomy and neurophysiology. To say the least, I was fascinated.

One day toward the end of the semester, I gathered all my courage and asked, "Dr. Nafe, if there is so much evidence opposing the specificity theory [von Frey's] and so little direct evidence in support of it, why do the textbook authors keep perpetuating it without acknowledging its negative or unsupported tenents?" His reply was, "Textbook authors seldom read primary sources. They simply repeat what other textbook authors have said. Over the years the theory has become etched in stone as though it were the 11th commandment, handed down from Mt. Sinai." Later I came across a similar statement by Karl DALLENBACH (1927), so I am not sure of the statement's author, but it sounds more like Paul because of his deep interest in the study of Bible history. One cannot be certain of that, though, because Paul and Karl enjoyed a close friendship that dated back to the early 1920s, when both were at the Cornell laboratory with E. B. Titchener.

At the end of the semester I proudly received an "A" in the course and forthwith determined that my future should be in psychology; in particular, that I would study in more detail the ideas to which I had just been exposed. I would like to describe the field of somesthesis (with special emphasis on thermal sensitivity) as I saw it when I embarked on its study, and then recount the nature and extent of the progress that has been made in the last 30 years or so.

B. Cutaneous Sensitivity Before ca. 1950

I. The Beginnings of Neurophysiology and Sensation

More than 2000 years ago Aristotle spoke of five senses: sight, hearing, taste, smell, and feeling (as in touch). This last category of sensations later became known as "common sensitivity" or *Gemeingefühl*. In the centuries that followed, primary concern was devoted to the ways in which human organisms obtained accurate information about their environment and how that information was conveyed to the sensorium (consciousness center). In this philosophical period, during the development of the sciences of physiology and psychology, it was generally held that pictures or images – *eidola* – of objects were conveyed to the brain by way of the nerves (BORING 1942).

The image theory of sensation persisted until the turn of the nineteenth century. Then, in 1826, and again in 1840, at the very beginning of the experimental investigations of the nervous system functions, the great German physiologist Johannes MÜLLER (1840) proposed the theory that has become known as the "doctrine of specific nerve energies" (DENNIS 1948). John LOCKE (1690) anticipated many of these ideas 136 years earlier, but it remained for Müller to express them as a series of succinctly stated, general laws. Müller proposed that the brain is directly aware of the activity of the sensory nerves, not the objects that excite them, and that sensory nerves convey nerve impulse to the brain (which are not in themselves different in their ability to produce specific sensations). Different sensations arise because each sensory nerve has its characteristic type of activity. Thus optic nerve activity signals light and color, auditory nerve activity signals sounds, olfactory nerve activity signals odors, and so on. The theory is vividly expressed by the statement that, if the auditory nerve and the visual nerves were crossed, we could see thunder and hear lightning. The experiment is impractical, of course, but there are other ways of identifying the site of this specificity. When, for example, the same stimulus (say electric current) is applied to different nerves, or if different stimuli (say mechanical, chemical, electrical, and so on) are applied to the same nerve, sensations are produced according to the special properties of the nerves stimulated. Müller proposed that these special properties might be in the central part of the nerves themselves or in the part of the brain to which they are connected. There is currently considerable evidence to support this latter view. A blow on the back of the head, over the occipital lobe of the brain where visual pathways terminate, makes one see a flash of light. This atypical form of stimulation has been called "inadequate stimulation." Thus for the sense of sight the adequate stimulus is light, but inadequate ones, including electric current passed through the eyeball, mechanical pressure upon the eyeball, or even a beam of X-ray passed through the eyeball, result in visual sensations.

1. Sensory Modalities

In common conversation we speak of humans as possessing five senses, and when one mentions a "sixth" sense it is common knowledge that the reference is made to the person's intuition. When one begins to examine the question of the number of sensory modalities, in the light of present knowledge of the senses, one finds that the basic five can be divided into many more, depending on the definition that one applies.

Why is sight one sense and hearing another? There are at least five criteria that set them apart as separate or primary sensory modalities (NEFF 1960). Different primary sensory modalities have (1) markedly different receptive organs, which (2) respond to characteristic stimuli. Each set of receptors has its own (3) nerve, which goes to (4) a different part of the brain, and the (5) sensations are different. With these criteria we can identify 9 or perhaps 11 different senses. However, if it be insisted that all of the criteria be fulfilled in each case, our knowledge of the structure and function of several senses disqualifies them as primary sensory modalities. For example, we do not yet know the receptive organs for temperature sensitivity or for pain, nor can specific parts of the brain be identified for each of them.

The obvious confusion may arise from the systematist's assumption of a one-to-one correlation between elementary psychological primary qualities of sensation and elementary physiological or morphological properties of receptors (MELZACK and WALL 1962).

2. Doctrine of Specific Nerve Energies

The doctrine of specific nerve energies was a theory of how an organism can differentiate between the five traditional primary sensory modalities. Müller sought to explain how stimulus objects that become encoded into nerve impulses are represented to the brain so that they yield sensations that are clearly different in their essential nature. He maintained that certain features of nervous activity remain in constant relationship to specific characteristics of the stimulating event. Müller's theory was effective, for it successfully combated the earlier notion that pictures of stimulus objects were conveyed to the brain by the nerves. The doctrine was important for a second reason, as well. It represented a clear exposition of several general laws which were important for the infant field of neurophysiology.

3. Extensions of the Doctrine of Specific Nerve Energies

It is clear that within each of the primary sense modalities there occur different qualities of sensation that must also be taken into account. If differences between visual and auditory sensations are accounted for by specialization of the central part of the nerve or by the part of the brain in which the nerves terminate, how are differences between red and green or between various pitches to be explained? The doctrine was extended to accommodate these.

Extension of the doctrine to account for qualities of sensation within the primary modalities first began in 1860, when von Helmholtz accepted YOUNG'S (1802) trichromatic theory of color vision. VON HELMHOLTZ (1860) knew that any pure spectral hue could be matched by mixing any other three spectral hues, provided they were widely separated on the spectrum. On this basis he proposed that there are red-, green-, and violet-sensitive nerves, which when differentially stimulated could account for all of the discriminatively different hues of the entire visible light spectrum. We now know, of course, from the work of MARKS et al. (1964) and BROWN and WALD (1964) that there are indeed three kinds of cones in the retina.

Each kind shows a different sensitivity to light wavelengths, just as von Helmholtz proposed more than 100 years earlier.

VON HELMHOLTZ (1863) performed a similar service for audition when he suggested that different pitches result from different parts of the cochlea resonating in response to the frequency of the stimulating tone. As we know today, pitch differentiation is not that simple. The basilar membrane does appear to be frequency-tuned, as von Helmholtz proposed, but many other interactions enter into its function to account for pitch differentiation.

The latter half of the nineteenth century saw a great deal of effort devoted to identifying the primary elements of each of the other sensory modalities. The results were at times confusing. As already noted, von Helmholtz started with the known physics of light-mixing when he revived the trichromatic theory of color vision. HERING (1874), on the other hand, started with a knowledge of the psychological primary hues–red, yellow, green, and blue. He proposed two reversible chemical reactions to account for color vision.

Some 30 years after von Helmholtz's extension of the doctrine of specific nerve energies to account for different qualities of visual sensation, Magnus BLIX (1882) took up the matter of feel in order to determine how well founded was the apparent contradiction that earlier work on this sense offered to the doctrine. Until this time the view of WEBER (1846), that there was only one nervous mechanism to mediate tactile and temperature sensations, prevailed. This was based mainly on Weber's failure to find separate spots on the skin from which different sensations could be aroused, and on the fact that a cold object was judged heavier and a warm one lighter than when the objects were at skin temperature. Further support for Weber's position comes from WUNDERLI's (1860) observation that at some points on the skin of the back, the sensation from a brush with cotton wool was sometimes confused with that from a warm object approaching the skin.

In contradiction of Weber's view, it had long been known that tactile and temperature sensations did not vary equally or in concert. For example, cutaneous sensory dissociation was also known to occur. When a limb was made ischemic, tactile sensibility disappeared first, followed by pain and cold sensibility. Other observations had been published to show that the tactile and temperature senses were frequently affected unequally by central nervous system damage. One might entirely disappear and the other remain intact (BROWN-SEQUARD 1855).

By mild electrical stimulation, Blix produced a pain sensation at one spot on the skin, touch at another, cold at a third, and warm at a fourth. These spots were well localized and, except on rare occasions, were not superimposed. Blix concluded from this series of observations that there must be separate nerves for touch, warm, cold, and pain, and that these have distinct terminations in the skin.

Two years later, GOLDSCHEIDER (1884) confirmed Blix's findings and added that the number and sensitivity of the warm and cold spots were related to the general sensitivity of the skin to warm and cold stimuli. A year after that, DONALDSON (1885) reported similar observations concerning the existence of discrete warm and cold spots. He extended the work by excising and examining, histologically, some of the spots on his own skin. The results were completely negative. No unique morphological structures could be identified beneath either the warm or the cold spots.

It is not surprising that the modality of feel was subjected to such an intensive examination for its concordance with the doctrine of specific nerve energies. What is surprising is that its inclusion took so long after von Helmholtz first extended the doctrine. Even more surprising is that within the space of three years three independent investigators, each unknown to the others, published almost identical accounts of the detailed explorations of the skin sense – feel.

In 1885, then, the case for the primary elements of feel was fairly substantial. It was another ten years, 1895, before a serious attempt was made to identify the receptors that might be responsible for these uniquely different sensations. Von Frey extended Müller's doctrine of specific nerve energies to the periphery by proposing particular types of receptor element for each of the four elementary cutaneous sensations. His proposition was simple. He proposed certain structures in the skin with sensory nerves attached to be uniquely sensitive to specific forms of stimulation. Their stimulation resulted in the unique sensations found in the sensory mapping experiments of Blix, Goldscheider, and Donaldson.

The correlations between structure and sensation that he drew were that Meissner's corpuscles in hairless skin and hair follicle receptors in hairy skin signaled touch, Krause's bulbs signaled cold, and Ruffini's cylinders signaled warm, but that only the free nerve endings of the dermal nerve net were widely enough distributed to account for pain. Added to this was the observation that he could only elicit pain where he touched the cornea with his finest boar's bristle. (The cornea is known to be innervated only by "free" nerve endings.) Other cutaneous sensations, such as wetness, oiliness, tickle, roughness, and later, heat, were held to be compounds of the four elementary qualities of feel.

II. Specific Receptor Theories

1. Structure

Three major methods have been employed to attack the problem of the morphological basis of feel. The first approach involved careful sensory testing and permanent marking of the points on the skin that were sensitive to thermal and/or tactile stimulation. After sensory testing and marking, bits of the tissue containing the spots were removed and examined histologically. The second approach involved the determination of the number and types of the sensory spots found in a specific area of skin followed by a histological examination of similarly located tissue, usually obtained from cadavers. The number and types of cutaneous nerve end organs were then related to the number and type of sensory spots. No attempt was made to draw a close relationship between a spot and a particular end organ, as in the first approach. The third approach only described the general location and distribution of various kinds of end organ (KENSHALO and NAFE 1962).

Investigations of the first type have been carried out at least nine times since the first negative report by DONALDSON (1885). With the exception of the study reported by BELONOSCHKIN (1933), these investigations have been conducted only on hairy skin. With one exception [WEDDELL (1941a, b) reported a Krause's bulb beneath a cold spot located on the forearm], the investigators failed to find nerve end organs of any special description beneath the sensitive spots.

Investigations of the second type were conducted primarily on specialized tissues, such as in the conjunctiva, the prepuce, and the palmar side of the fingers. While there is no direct correlation between a sensitive spot and the type of ending beneath it, in general these investigators concluded that the number and type of encapsulated endings corresponded rather well with the number and type of sensory spots reported in those tissues. The list of investigations of the third type, included here, is by no means exhaustive. They are included on the basis of their interest for cutaneous sensation. Again with one exception, when specimens of skin were removed from hairy regions of the body, no apparently specialized encapsulated endings were found, whereas when specimens of skin were obtained from nonhairy portions of the body, encapsulated endings were prevalent. In the list of some 26 morphological investigations using the three different approaches to the relationship between morphology and sensations, there are three exceptions to the general conclusion that apparently specialized encapsulated nerve endings do not occur in hairy skin.

The conclusion was inescapable in the late 1940s and early 1950s. Specialized encapsulated nerve endings do not occur in hairy skin. They exist only in specialized skin areas such as the conjunctiva of the eye, some mucous membranes, the palmar surface of the fingers and the palms, the soles of the feet, and the genitalia. In general, afferent nerves terminate as bare filaments in relation to three types of structures found in the hairy skin (WEDDELL et al. 1955). These are: (a) among the cells of the stratum granulosum of the epidermis and the cells of the dermis; (b) in relation to hair follicles, as filaments entwined about the hair shaft; and (c) in relation to smooth muscle cells of the cutaneous blood vessels.

2. Theories of Stimulation

Attempts to identify the specific characteristic of a cutaneous thermal event that results in a warm or cool sensation has a long history. According to BORING (1942) it started in 1690, when John Locke touched on the problem in his famous *Essay*. He had observed that water at the same temperature may feel warm to one hand and cold to the other. He reasoned that sensations of warm and cold must depend on the "increase or diminution of motions of minute parts of our body, caused by the corpuscles of any other body." Thus, if the hand is immersed in water that diminishes motion of the particles, the hand will feel cooler, and in the same way, if the other hand is immersed in water of such a temperature that the motion is increased, the hand will feel warmer. Locke's theory then means that the hand feels warm when it is being warmed and cool when it is being cooled.

WEBER (1846) accepted Locke's theory, saying that "when the temperature rises, one perceives warmth; when it falls, one perceives cold." However, VIERORDT (1871) faulted Weber's notion, stating that there could well be thermal sensations without a change of cutaneous temperature. As an illustration, he cited the persisting cold sensation that occurs after a very cold object has been removed from the skin. He suggested that cold is experienced when the flow of heat is outward, and warm when the flow of heat is inward.

There were some difficulties with Vierordt's theory. HERING (1879) pointed out that since the blood is warmer than the skin there is a continual outward flow of heat that is not sensed as cold. As a matter of fact, no thermal sensation is experienced at all. A change in skin temperature changes the inward or outward flow of heat. Positive conduction sets up an end organ process which he named "dissimilation" (warm), while negative conduction established a reverse process which he called "assimilation" (cold). According to Hering, both processes are probably going on simultaneously, and what is specified by dissimilation and assimilation is the predominance of one process over the other.

Changes in the intracutaneous spatial thermal gradients have also been proposed as the necessary conditions for the arousal of thermal sensations that are induced in a limb on release of circulatory stasis (EBBECKE 1917). He concluded that sensations of both warm and cold depend on spatial thermal gradients of varying intensity established at different depths as warm blood enters cool skin or vice versa.

BAZETT and McGLONE (1932a) accepted Ebbecke's theory of thermal stimulation as that best fitting the data from stimulation of warm and cold spots on the prepuce from both sides of the skin fold. This particular experiment received considerable notoriety because of the Spartan attitude that their subjects must have developed in allowing their foreskins to be suspended on "dulled" fishhooks during the course of thermal stimulation. [A detailed description of the gradient theory can be found in BAZETT (1941).] Even though Bazett and his collaborators accepted changes in the spatial thermal gradient as the necessary condition for arousal of thermal sensations, they found it necessary to modify Ebbecke's theory somewhat in order to account for the results of the circulatory stasis experiments that they reported (BAZETT and McGLONE 1932b). They proposed a chemical intermediary, perhaps a change in blood pH associated with deoxygenation of the blood supply to the limb, that might account for receptor depolarization. The chemical reaction was proposed as an intermediate step between alteration of the spatial thermal gradient in the skin and the excitation of nerve impulses by the receptor.

JENKINS (1941b) proposed a different form of specific receptor theory and theory of stimulation, in which free nerve endings functionally (but somehow not necessarily morphologically) differed so that some responded only to increases and others to decreases in skin temperature. It has been called the "concentration theory."

Two principal results from his seriatim mapping technique seem to have prompted Jenkins to propose the theory. First, when two adjacent spots ($1–4 \text{ mm}^2$), one of high and the other of low sensitivity were simultaneously stimulated, the two spots gave an intensity score about equal to the average of the scores obtained when the spots were stimulated individually. The encapsulated ending theory predicted that the score should have been at least as high or higher than that of the more sensitive spot stimulated alone (JENKINS 1941b). A second finding not predicted by the encapsulated ending theory was that as stimulus intensity increased, sensation intensity failed to increase in a similar manner.

In order to account for these and similar, apparently contradictory, findings JENKINS (1941a) proposed the receptor concentration theory. Instead of a few more or less isolated warm and cold spots, he proposed hundreds of receptors of varying sensitivity. The sensation intensity from a given stimulation depended on a concentration of active receptors.

The concentration theory offers no receptor structure to mediate warm and cold sensations except free nerve endings, which are also thought to mediate pain and possibly touch as well. Perhaps, as JENKINS (1951) suggested, free nerve endings possess subtle differences, not yet revealed by presently available histological methods, that make some sensitive only to thermal stimulation. Of these, some are uniquely sensitive to increase and others to decrease in skin temperature.

Jenkins also formulated a theory of thermal stimulation, not unlike HERING'S (1877), in which a "pseudoreversible reaction" occurred upon stimulation and a catalyzer reversed the reaction.

3. Paradoxical Thermal Sensations and Heat

VON FREY (1895) reported that some cold spots, identified by previous mapping, gave rise to cold sensations when stimulated by a hot stimulator (45 °C). Thinking this a paradox, he labeled the phenomenon "paradoxical cold." Immediately, investigators began the search for paradoxical warm – the arousal of a warm sensation from stimulation of a warm spot by a cold probe. However, the necessary and sufficient conditions for arousal of paradoxical warm have so far eluded clear-cut identification. Its existence as a bona fide phenomenon of temperature sensitivity is open to question, although JENKINS and KARR (1957) seemed to think it occurs when repeated stimulation of a warm spot by warm stimuli has preceded the application of the cold stimulus.

In early research on somesthesis, the sensation of heat was held to be uniquely different in quality from those of warm and pain. The uniqueness of the heat sensation, as compared to intense warm, apparently lies in the addition of a slight stinging sensation which soon adapts.

Two theories, one that the heat sensation is a compound of the elementary sensations of warm and cold, the other that there are specific heat receptors, have been proposed. The compound theory (ALRUTZ 1898) suggests that the heat sensation is synthesized by simultaneous stimulation of warm and cold receptors. The second (HERGET and HARDY 1942) maintains that the unique quality of the heat sensation that differentiates it from warm – the adapting sting – is mediated by its own receptor type.

The basis of the Alrutz theory was that a warm stimulator (42°–43 °C) aroused a warm sensation and paradoxically aroused a simultaneous cold sensation. The compounding of the heat sensation should also be possible by simultaneously stimulating warm spots and cold spots with warm stimuli. One of the clearer demonstrations of "compounded heat" is that produced by the Cutolo heat grill (CUTOLO 1918). The grill consists of alternate warm and cold tubes arranged in a plane. When the palm of the hand or the volar forearm is first placed on the grill, the immediate reaction is one of withdrawal and the subject's description of the sensation is that he felt he was going to be burned. The initial sensation is short-lived, however, and soon reduces to alternating warm and cool sensations (BURNETT and DALLENBACH 1927).

Evidence favoring the second theory, that heat has its own receptor mechanism, arose as a result of the study of spatial summation of warm, cold, and heat sensations (HERGET and HARDY 1942). Herget and Hardy found that there was less spatial summation for heat than for either suprathreshold warm or cool sensations. Were warm and cold receptors synthesizing the sensation of heat, they reasoned, the rate of spatial summation for heat should lie between those for warm and cool; heat showed less dependence on area than either warm or cool sensations. Because spatial summation of the heat sensation appeared to follow a different course from those of warm and cool sensations, they proposed a third thermal receptor – a heat receptor.

4. Spatial Summation

It has long been known that the size of the area of skin stimulated had a strong influence on the intensity of the thermal sensation and on thermal adaptation (WEBER 1846). However, apparently due to inadequate instrumentation, very little quantitative information was available on the relationship between the area stimulated and sensation intensity. It was not until the early 1930s that BAZETT and MCGLONE (1932a) and BOHNENKAMP and PASQUAI (1932) reported quantitative measures of the relationships between area and threshold warm sensations. The former reported the threshold for a single warm spot to be 0.3 °C when the rate of temperature increase was 0.2 °C/s. When the whole arm was exposed to a warm stimulus, they estimated the threshold to be 0.1 °C when the rate of skin temperature increase was 0.005 °C/s. BOHNENKAMP and PASQUAI reported that the threshold was 0.8 °C for a single warm spot and 0.4 °C for a group of six warm spots. The expression relating threshold to the number of spots stimulated could readily be described by an exponential curve.

The investigations by HARDY and OPPEL (1937, 1938) using radiant heat and "radiant" cold (heat absorption by block of solid carbon dioxide) and the observations of GEBLEWICZ (1940), HERGET et al. (1941), and HERGET and HARDY (1942) all led to the same general result, namely a lowering of the threshold or an increase in sensation intensity above threshold, when the area stimulated was increased. The functions were found to be well fitted by a power function of the form:

$$I = kAb + C \qquad (1)$$

where I is intensity, k is a scaling constant, A is area, b is the rate of decrease in threshold as area is increased, and C is the threshold for large areas. For warm stimuli, area and intensity trade about equally at threshold, so that the exponent b approached -1.0. However, area does not play so prominent a role in the spatial summation for threshold cool stimuli, where b was found to be approximately 0.5 (HARDY and OPPEL 1937, 1938).

There also appeared to be a limit to the area over which full spatial summation occurs at threshold levels. HARDY and OPPEL (1937) found this to be approximately 200 mm² for radiant heat applied to the face. Larger areas including the neck and chest as well as the face showed little additional spatial summation (HARDY and OPPEL 1938).

Area was also known to have a marked effect on the limits to which complete thermal adaptation can occur. With very small stimulators complete thermal adaptation was achieved within a range from 20° to 42 °C. On the other hand, when the whole body was exposed to changes in environmental temperature, the range over which complete adaptation occurred became quite small. When the whole body was exposed to an increase in temperature in a climate chamber, the upper limit for complete adaptation was found to be as low as 34.5 °C when the rate of increase in temperature of the climate chamber was of the order of 0.0015 °C/s (MARÉCHAUX and SCHÄFER 1949).

III. Pattern Theories

Proponents of pattern theories were unimpressed by the evidence marshaled to support the existence of specialized receptors and attached primary afferents that reacted specifically to certain energy forms. As Nafe once told me, "I cannot imagine such inefficiency of design as a pain receptor located, for example, in the viscera, waiting around for all of the life of the organism to be stimulated, but never getting 'the call!'" What did seem to impress the pattern theorists was the richness of adjectives that describe feelings engendered by cutaneous stimulation. DALLENBACH (1939), for example, compiled a list of 44 adjectives that describe painful sensations alone. Specificity theorists maintained that such sensations as heat, wetness, oiliness, or stickiness, to name but a few, were products of "mental chemistry" – combinations of the elementary qualities of sensation. Pattern theorists countered that the work of Adrian and his colleagues on the primary afferent nerves, while extremely important, was misinterpreted in the sense that it was held to support the premise of specifically sensitive cutaneous receptors. According to pattern proponents, Adrian's work showed that single fibers demonstrated variations in: (a) frequency of impulses; (b) duration of the impulse train; (c) area over which impulses arose (receptive field size); and (d) relative number of fibers activated within such an area (NAFE 1929), all of which provided a rich neural language for appropriate interpretation.[1]

1. The Quantitative Theory of Feeling

The principal part of Nafe's scientific life and endeavor was devoted to feeling, not as an affective element of consciousness but as a sensation. He redefined feeling as an all-inclusive term for sensations other than those derived from stimulation of the special senses (vision, audition, olfaction, and gustation) and perhaps the inner ear labyrinth, which has to do with equilibrium. Two influences appear to have merged at this time (the latter part of the 1920s) to determine the future course of Nafe's research. He was quick to see the importance of ADRIAN's (1926) application of the new electronics to the recording of sensory nerve impulses, and was particularly impressed by ADRIAN and ZOTTERMAN's (1926) report on the dimensions of activity in single sensory nerve fibers. Nafe saw in these critical works an opportunity to correlate stimulus variables with changes in afferent nerve activity, and

---

1 Of course, others such as conduction, velocity and latency can now be added. Thus a given stimulus-initiated temporal and spatial pattern of activity in the primary nerve bundle provided a picture of the peripheral event. The pattern could vary almost infinitely with varying conditions of stimulation. The task, according to Nafe, was to identify which variations in the neural response corresponded to variations in sensations – identification of the neural correlates of sensation

these in turn with sensations. His pioneer study of the "neural correlates of sensations" first appeared in his "Quantitative Theory of Feeling" (Nafe 1929). He maintained a marked air of independent thought in not accepting the then current theory of specificity of afferent neural activity. He did not accept all of Müller's doctrine of specific nerve energies. He rejected completely von Frey's correlation between morphologically distinguishable skin structures and sensations, and was critical of Adrian and Zotterman's interpretation of their own findings in terms of specificity of peripheral nerve function. He felt that these neural theories were qualitative in nature, while he preferred a quantitative analysis.

The second major influence was that he was greatly impressed by Gestalt theory. He first met Köhler at Clark University in 1925, and was so impressed by his interpretation of Gestalt theory that he later (1930) accepted an opportunity to work with him in Berlin for a year. From these seemingly incompatible influences Nafe was able to integrate the neural and Gestalt viewpoints into a pattern theory to account for qualitative differences in sensation. His pattern theory emphasized the temporal and spatial relationships between peripheral nerve activity and sensations. In addition to generating much research, the pattern served to make sensory psychology acceptable to the physiologists, and it also preserved the study of sensory processes as a proper psychological endeavor.

Specifically, the theory was called "quantitative" to distinguish it from all other theories that maintained that differences in sensory experience were due to qualities, different receptors, modalities, nerves, or cortical areas, none of which were amenable to quantification (Nafe 1934). On the other hand, he proposed that different patterns of stimulation (and hence activities of primary afferent nerves) resulted in different sensations. After all, he argued, if all pains were alike or all pressures were alike we could deal with specific fibers (receptors); but no two pains are alike, nor are two pressures alike, so even if we grant specificity, patterns must still be invoked to account for these differences in experience. Hence "feeling" must result from a specificity of the neural activity pattern and the quality of experience depends upon changes in the tissues in which these patterns originate. A wave of muscular contraction in the stomach, from the cardiac to the pyloric valves, was said to correlate with hunger pangs, while muscular contraction waves in the reverse direction correlated with the experience of nausea. Have we specific receptors for hunger and others for nausea, or are specific patterns of activity in the same nerves responsible for the different experiences of hunger and nausea?

In the first pronouncement of the "quantitative theory of feeling" (Nafe 1929), very little of a specific nature was said about how these patterns of activity might arise in a reliable fashion from cutaneous stimulation. In the second pronouncement of the theory (Nafe 1934) is to be found the first statement of the vascular theory of warm and cold experiences. Nafe was very candid about the origin of that theory, stating on repeated occasions that he was struck by the close correlation between the thermally induced activity of smooth muscle of the arterioles and perhaps venules as listed in Starling's (1930) *Principles of Human Physiology* and the experiences of warm, cold, heat, and pain. According to Starling, warming the skin above 33 °C produces a relaxation in vascular smooth muscle. When the intensity of warming reaches approximately 45 °C, constricting elements can be observed in a generally dilating muscle, and at 52 °C there is overall spastic constriction and the experience is that of pain. On the other hand, when the tissue is cooled, there is a general contraction of the smooth muscle elements, which increases in severity at approximately 12 °C; some muscle elements show severe muscle constrictions in a generally contracted system, and at less than 3 °C smooth muscle elements contract spastically and the experience is that of pain.

In its third enunciation, the theory contained another important advance (NAFE 1942). He and Wagoner (NAFE and WAGONER 1941 a, b) had completed their studies on the nature of pressure adaptation, the major conclusion from which was that the only "adequate stimulus" to excite cutaneous receptors is movement – movement of the terminal upon itself or in relation to the surrounding tissue. Thus the sensation of pressure applied to the skin does not adapt because the terminal becomes fatigued or accustomed to the pressure, but because the stimulus is no longer adequate – it no longer moves the tissue that contains the afferent terminal. This is a condition of equilibrium between the force exerted and resistance encountered, not a case of fatigue. Applied to temperature sensitivity, as long as the cutaneous blood vessels move in response to a temperature change, the movement so induced will excite the afferent terminals within the vessel walls, and as the response slows the neural activity will reflect the degree of decrease in the sensation. Differences between sensations are represented by corresponding differences between patterns of neural activity, and are perhaps the best description of changes in sensation. So long as a mechanical event at the skin surface produces movement of the terminal and its surrounding tissue, activity will result in the primary afferent fibers and a sensation will be experienced.

For Nafe there was no need for receptive elements that showed marked differences in their response to various energy forms – specific receptors – in order to account for different qualities of cutaneous sensation. Patterns of movement aroused corresponding patterns of nerve discharge and the correlated sensations varied if the patterns varied. Quality, for warm, cool, and touch, refers to differing patterns of neural activity.

Pain sensations were handled in much the same manner by the theory. Basically, patterns of neural activity yielded pain sensations that differed from those that yielded pressure sensations only in the number of impulses aroused per unit time (frequency) and the number per unit area (density). When a human nerve was directly stimulated by an electrical shock, a single shock, regardless of its intensity, did not produce pain. If, on the other hand, the electrical pulses continued at greater than a minimum rate, intense pain was aroused (HEINBECKER et al. 1933). For Nafe, pain was a matter of patterns, painful ones showing higher frequencies and greater densities of neural activity than nonpainful ones. This is not to say that he considered pain to be the same as intense pressure or thermal sensations. He pointed out that introspectively, pain and intense pressure share very little in regard to their sensations. He simply saw no need to invent specifically sensitive pain receptors at that point in time.

2. The Thermopile Theory

As a result of the observations of WEDDELL and ZANDER (1950, 1951) on the morphology of the cornea of the eye, and of WEDDELL and PALLIE (1954) and WEDDELL et al. (1954) on the morphology of mammalian skin in general, the Oxford group was "forced to the conclusion that there are no histological grounds on which such [specific receptor] theories can be based" (WEDDELL et al. 1955, p. 187). Furthermore, the results of SINCLAIR et al. (1952) and HAGEN et al. (1953) demonstrate that responses to warm and cool stimuli may be evoked as readily from the greater part of the body surface, where encapsulated nerve endings are absent, as from the palms of the hand or the soles of the feet, where encapsulated endings abound. In both hairy and glabrous skin, myelinated axons arising from the cutaneous nerve plexus give rise to a series of fine, naked, axoplasmic filaments that appear to terminate at all levels of the skin (from the stratum granulosum to the junction of the dermis with the subcutis). The question is, how do apparently undifferentiated axoplasmic filaments respond differentially to an increase or decrease in skin temperature?

Impulses can be evoked in a nerve trunk when one section of the sciatic nerve is warmed or cooled relative to an adjacent part (BERNHARD and GRANIT, 1946; VON EULER 1947). LELE et al. (1954) proposed a modified version of EBBECKE's (1917) spatial, thermal gradient theory, in which the effective stimulus was a temperature difference between the stem axons and their terminals. Stem axons, for example, that terminate just beneath the basement membrane of the epidermis give rise to arborizations of naked axoplasmic filaments that pass toward the skin surface. Under normal conditions the deeper parts of such terminals are warmer (they are closer to the cutaneus vascular plexus) than their filaments. Action potentials are evoked as a result of this temperature difference. When this difference is increased, as when the skin surface is cooled, the discharge will increase. If the surface is warmed the discharge will decrease.

In contrast, stem fibers that terminate in the dermis arborize; the axoplasmic filaments pass toward the cutaneous vascular plexus and terminate. Under normal conditions the parts of such terminals closest to the blood vessels will be warmer than the parts adjacent to the cutaneous nerve plexus. Action potentials will be evoked as a consequence of this temperature difference. As a result of skin surface warming, the filaments adjacent to the blood vessels will become relatively warmer than those more deeply situated, and their discharge will increase. Surface cooling will result in a decrease in the discharge.

LELE et al. (1954) suggest that the encapsulated nerves in the skin, when suitably stimulated, give rise to a wide range of sensations, including cold, touch, warm, prick, itch, and sharp pain, according to the temporal and spatial patterns of impulses evoked in the primary afferent fibers. Cold is reported when nerve fibers situated in or close to epidermis discharge and those situated more deeply are inhibited. Warm is reported when those endings situated relatively deeply in the skin discharge while those with superficial terminals are inhibited.

C. Thermal Sensitivity Since 1950

An important and exciting event for me ushered in this era. It was the extension of electrophysiological methods to the study of cutaneous thermal receptors by Herbert Hensel, working with Yngve Zotterman. Here was the method by which one might hope to identify changes in the neural events in primary afferents associated with changes in the thermal stimulating events presented to the skin. All that remained was to describe the changes in sensation that resulted from these same changes in the thermal stimulating events. "All that remained ...?" More than 30 years later the work of a number of laboratories, including our own, has yet to establish unequivocally the primary afferent code that represents the amount by which skin temperature has been changed on the one hand and the intensity of the thermal sensation on the other.

I. Models of the Human Temperature-Sensing System

We believed that it was necessary to establish, early on, an adequate subhuman model for the human temperature-sensing system. The utility of such a model lies in the fact that one can do electrophysiological experiments on the model with the expectation that the nervous system of the model will function as a human nervous system would function under similar circumstances of stimulation. There is now a limited alternative to this approach, human microneurography, pioneered by HAGBARTH and VALLBO (1967). This method has the advantage of comparing, within the same species, primary afferent nerve activity and the sensations that result from stimuli. It has the limitation that such comparisons can only be made between primary afferent activity and sensation. Comparisons between neural activity in higher nervous centers and sensation are, to date, not possible in humans. The only method available to us was to find a subhuman species whose behavioral responses to temperature and changes in temperature matched those of humans or were sufficiently similar for any differences to be quantitatively described.

1. Cats

Since cats were the favored preparation for electrophysiological studies, we chose cats as our subjects and avoidance conditioning as the method of measuring their sensitivity to thermal stimuli. In order to immobilize the cats as much as possible during the measurements, Chuck Rice and I fitted them with plaster body casts, put their heads in a stock, and tied three of their four legs firmly to the floor of the support frame (see Fig. 1). The fourth leg, the right hind leg, was tied to a lever that contained electric shock electrodes applied to the leg. The response to be conditioned was flexing that leg, thereby moving the lever. We had a device to measure the intensity of radiation, so with radiant energy as the conditioned stimulus, electric shock as the unconditioned stimulus, and a leg lift as the conditioned response we commenced our investigation of the warm sensitivity of the cat's back. LIPKIN and HARDY (1954) had published a formula estimating the final skin temperature on the basis of radiation intensity and the duration of exposure. After transforming the radiation data to elevation in skin temperature, we found that we achieved conditioning only after we had raised the skin temperature to between 51° and 54 °C. Similar measurements on the backs of humans yielded response thresholds of 44°–44.7 °C, and the humans reported pain (RICE and KENSHALO 1962).

    The next step in our search for an animal model for the human temperature-sensing system was to measure the sensitivity of the cat to changes in temperature

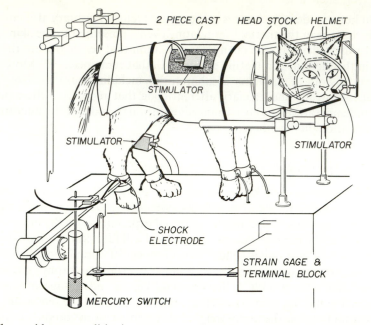

Fig. 1. The avoidance-conditioning apparatus. Cats were completely restrained by a body cast, leg straps, head stock, and metal plates on either side of the head and beneath the chin, except for the right hind leg, which was strapped to the response lever. Stimulators are shown in place in the various areas of the cat's body that were tested for thermal sensitivity, except the left hind footpad. Measurements of temperature sensitivity were made consecutively at these several areas. The stimulator on the upper lip was held in place on the shaved skin by a leaf spring attached to a close-fitting leather helmet. Brearley and Kenshalo (1970)

as a function of the temperature to which the shaved skin of the back was adapted (hereafter called the adapting temperature).[2]

Temperature increases and decreases were applied to the shaved skin of the backs, inner thighs and footpads of cats after the skin had been adapted to temperatures between 28° and 40 °C. We found that the cats could use temperature increases as cues to avoid electric shock only after the skin temperature was raised to about 49°–50 °C, regardless of the adapting temperature. Human warm thresholds on the forearm, however, are about 1 °C at a 28 °C adapting temperature and decrease to about 0.1 °C at a 40 °C adapting temperature. The cats' avoidance thresholds for temperature decreases were about 2.5 °C larger than human cool thresholds. We concluded from these observations that cats were unable to sense mild (short of noxious) increases in temperature on their furred skin and footpad, but did show a reduced sensitivity to temperature decreases in those areas (Kenshalo 1964).

---

2 We had discovered and successfully adapted the Peltier thermal module so that it would maintain a preset temperature and produce changes in that temperature of predetermined direction, intensity, and rate. This was accomplished by control of the direction and intensity of direct current passed through the module (Kenshalo and Bergen 1975)

Casual observation of cat behavior, however, suggested that they can make relatively fine discriminations of warmth, as shown by their ability to choose warmer areas as basking sites, e.g., before a fire, in a sunny window, or on an electric heating pad. Dennis Duncan, Carolyn Weymark, and I set out to find a skin site of sufficient sensitivity to increases in temperature to account for the observations concerning the basking behavior (KENSHALO et al. 1967b). Infrared radiation was used for thermal stimulation. When the whole face was exposed to the radiation, an avoidance threshold was obtained after a 0.2 °C increase in skin temperature. When the area of exposure was limited to 4 cm^2 around the nose, the avoidance threshold increased to about a 1 °C increase in skin temperature.

So the face was the place! But infrared radiation provides only one controllable variable: its intensity. We needed to be able to present temperature decrease and to have a controllable parameter (adapting temperature) as well. The Peltier stimulators used on other areas of the cat were much too large to be fitted to the contours of the cat's face. Beth Brearley and I devised a new Peltier stimulator that had an area of only 1.7 cm^2 (BREARLEY and KENSHALO 1970). We fitted the cat with a leather helmet that held a leaf spring to which the stimulator was attached, and the whole ensemble held the Peltier stimulator against the shaved upper lip of the cat, as shown in Fig. 1. Using the avoidance-conditioning method to measure thermal thresholds of the skin of the cat's upper lip as a function of the adapting temperature, thresholds of response to temperature increases as small as 1 °C and to decreases as small as 0.5 °C were obtained. Thresholds of response to increases in temperature increased when the adapting temperatures were lower than 33 °C, while thresholds to decreases in temperature increased when the adapting temperatures were higher than 33 °C. When compared to human thresholds, the cats were generally less sensitive, but the shapes of the curves as functions of the adapting temperatures were similar. It appeared that this part of a cat's body might serve as a useful model for measurements of neural activity in the trigeminal nerve resulting from changes in skin temperature.

Concurrently with the behavioral measurements, Beth Brearley and I recorded the integrated neural activity in few fiber preparations made from the infraorbital nerve of cats in response to temperature changes when the skin of the upper lip had been adapted to temperatures between 21° and 43 °C (KENSHALO and BREARLEY 1970). Measurements of the steady state activity in these integrated records formed a bell-shaped curve very similar in shape to that obtained from 26 single-unit preparations of myelinated, infraorbital, specifically sensitive cold fibers obtained by Hensel and myself (HENSEL and KENSHALO 1969) and HENSEL and WURSTER (1970). The height of the integrated response to changes in temperature, as functions of adapting temperature, very closely approximated the behavioral thresholds measured by the conditioned avoidance technique; this was further evidence that the trigeminal nerve of cats might serve as an adequate neural model, as well as an adequate behavioral model for human temperature sensitivity.

The principal difficulty with the cat model was that comparisons of measurements were made between species widely separated on the phylogenetic scale and obtained by a different methodology. We considered such a comparison tenuous, at best. A second difficulty was that cats do not seem to have a sensitivity to temperature and temperature changes anywhere on their body except in that region innervated by the trigeminal nerve.

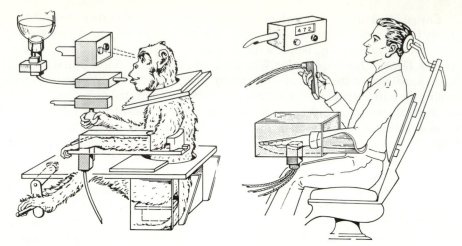

Fig. 2. The experimental arrangements for measurement of detectability of temperature increases and decreases in humans and monkeys. Individual trials were initiated by the subject by pulling a lever or pushing a button. Correct identification of the presence of a change of temperature was rewarded by money (human) or a squirt of apple juice (monkey). Incorrect identification resulted in a 15-s time-out. Kenshalo et al. (1980)

2. Primates

We determined at this point to switch to a species more closely related to humans, the rhesus monkey, to see if we could find a more sensitive measure of threshold than avoidance conditioning. Conditioned suppression was in wide use in various laboratories of our group, and seemed to yield extremely good results in behavioral studies of olfactory thresholds. Conditioned suppression is a technique in which the animal is trained to press a lever at a regular rate. During the lever presses the stimulus to be detected (CS) is presented and its termination is coincident with a brief electric shock (UCS). Within 10 to 20 pairings of the CS and UCS, the animals began to show a decrease in the rate of lever pressing during the CS in comparison to the rate of lever pressing for a similar period just prior to the CS.

Clarice Hall and I found that thresholds to temperature increases decreased from 0.14° to 0.02 °C, while thresholds to temperature decreases increased from 0.05° to 0.28 °C as the adapting temperature was increased from 28° to 40 °C (Kenshalo and Hall 1974). In comparison to humans, the rhesus monkeys were much more sensitive to changes in temperature at all adapting temperatures except to temperature decreases at a 40 °C adapting temperature. From this we inferred that rhesus monkeys were better able to detect increases and decreases in temperature applied to the inner thigh than were human subjects when the human measurements were made by 14.4 cm^2 Peltier on the shaved skin of the right forearm. Comparisons of measurements were made, this time between species closely related on the phylogenetic scale, but still by completely different methods.

We wondered if we might not be able to make our correlations more convincing if we used the same method of threshold measurement on the monkeys and humans. Signal detection seemed to be the most likely candidate. Helen Molinari, Andrew Rożsa, and Joel Greenspan were associated with the project at various times,

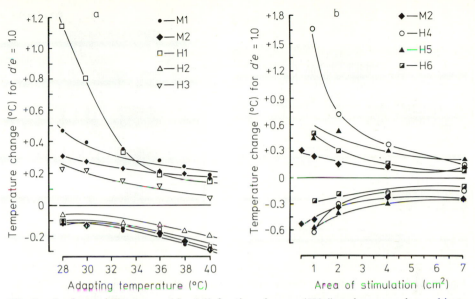

Fig. 3. a Isodetectability curves ($d' = 1.0$) for three human (*H1-3*) and two monkey subjects (*M1, M2*) as functions of the adapting temperature used. **b** Isodetectability curves for three humans and one monkey as functions of the area of stimulation on the palm of the hands. The adapting temperature was 32 °C

as well as I (MOLINARI et al. 1976; RóżSA et al., to be published; GREENSPAN et al., to be published; KENSHALO et al. 1980). Seven years, four monkeys, and over a million trials later we completed our measurements.

We chose the "yes–no" signal detection paradigm because theorists assert that this method of measurement of sensitivity is bias-free and not influenced by variations in the subject criterion, motivation, or a whole host of other variables that might influence the final outcome of sensitivity measurements.

As can be seen from Fig. 3 a, measurements of sensitivity to decreases in skin temperature as a function of the adapting temperature vary in the monkey in a manner similar to the variation found in the human subjects. The detectability of decreases in temperature was greater at low than at high adapting temperatures. Variability between subjects of detectability of increases in temperature was much larger. But the same general conclusion can be reached, however, because the variability between subjects of the same species appeared to be as large as the variability between subjects of different species.

A comparison of the way in which area of stimulation interacts with ability to detect temperature increases and decreases in rhesus and humans is shown in Fig. 3 b. Both species showed an increase in ability as the area of stimulation increased. However, the rhesus showed greater ability to detect thermal stimuli applied to small areas on the palm of the hand.

It seems clear from these results that the rhesus monkey can act as an adequate model for the human temperature-sensing system. Greater confidence can be placed in the assumption that the sensory measurements on humans result from the same set of neural events as are observed in primates.

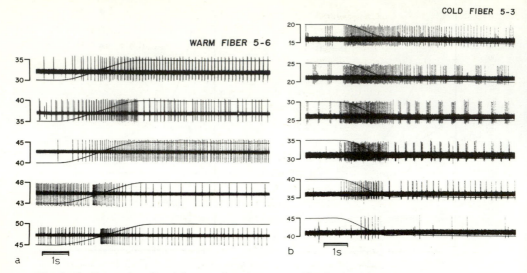

Fig. 4 a, b. Examples of activity seen in primary specifically sensitive **a** warm and **b** cold fibers in the rhesus monkey. The dynamic responses are to 5 °C intensity changes presented at a rate of change of 2 °C/s. KENSHALO (1976)

II. Correlations Between Thermal Sensations and Primary Afferent Activity

1. Quality of the Sensations

In the realm of thermal sensation, there are two and possibly three qualities of thermal sensation of graded intensity – warm, cold, and possibly, heat. Two classes of specifically sensitive thermal afferents innervating the skin have been identified (DODT and ZOTTERMAN 1952a; HENSEL and ZOTTERMAN 1951 a, b, c, d, e). Examples are shown in Fig. 4. As a convenient shorthand they have been labeled "warm" and "cold" fibers. The response characteristics of warm fibers are that they show steady state activity at maintained skin temperature between about 30° and 50 °C, with a static maximum at about 43 °C. Warm fibers show a phasic increase in activity in response to skin warming and a phasic decrease in activity in response to skin cooling, and they are refractory to other forms of stimulation short of injury. Cold fibers also show steady state activity, but only when skin temperature is maintained at between about 10° and 40 °C, with a static maximum at about 29 °C. In contrast to warm fibers, cold fibers show a phasic increase in activity in response to skin cooling and a phasic decrease in activity to skin warming, and like warm fibers are refractory to other forms of stimulation short of injury.

Little is known of the heat receptors postulated by HERGET and HARDY (1942) except that there are some primary afferents that begin to respond when the temperature of the skin is increased to approximately 40°–43 °C (SUMINO et al. 1973).

Certain other receptors respond much like cold fibers to thermal stimuli, but they also show a considerable sensitivity to mechanical stimuli. These are usually classed as slowly adapting mechanoreceptors, for they respond at least as well to mechanical as to thermal stimuli (BURTON et al. 1972; CHAMBERS et al. 1972; DU-CLAUX and KENSHALO 1972; IGGO and MUIR 1969; TAPPER 1965). The possible contribution of these thermally sensitive, slowly adapting mechanoreceptors (types SAI, SAII) to thermal sensation is not clear. It has been maintained that activity of the SAI type does not affect thermal sensations (HARRINGTON and MERZENICH 1970), that they have insufficient channel capacity in response to thermal stimulation to account for thermal sensation (JOHNSON et al. 1973), and their change in sensitivity as a function of adapting temperature is contrary to what would be expected of receptors involved in thermal sensitivity (DUCLAUX and KENSHALO 1972). The thermal sensitivity of the SAII mechanoreceptors has not been extensively investigated (BURTON et al. 1972; CHAMBERS et al. 1972).

There is no direct evidence at this time that the activity in specifically sensitive thermal fibers is a necessary condition for thermal sensations (MELZACK and WALL 1962). Nor is there evidence that it is not. At this point, it seems parsimonious to conclude that activity in afferents specifically sensitive to thermal stimulation conveys information to the central nervous system about the cutaneous skin temperature and that the absence of their activity would be accompanied by an absence of thermal sensations. Thus the temperature-sensing system is considered to be a "labeled line" system in the sense in which POGGIO and MOUNTCASTLE (1963) used the term. The two systems may interact, although evidence of this is scarce.

There are, of course, other alternatives. Bimodal receptors may contribute to thermal sensations and the activity of the thermal modality may converge with that from other (particularly the tactile) modalities at higher-order centers. Other means of encoding quality are also possible, such as the "across fiber pattern" theory (ERICKSON 1973; ERICKSON and POULOS 1973).

2. Responses to Temperature

Thermal sensations can be regarded as static or dynamic depending on whether the thermal sensations arise from a maintained skin temperature or from changes in skin temperature. Under the heading of responses to static temperature, candidate codes are considered for sensations that occur when the skin is maintained at a static temperature within the range of physiological zero, where, given time, thermal sensations may adapt completely; the persisting warm and cool sensations that occur when the skin temperature is maintained outside of the zone of physiological zero; and the temporal course of thermal adaptation.

Responses to changes in temperature include the influence of the adapted skin temperature on warm and cool thresholds, the effect of rate of skin temperature change on threshold and suprathreshold sensations, and the effect of area (spatial summation) on threshold and suprathreshold warm and cool sensations.

a) Static Temperature

As shown in Fig. 5, physiological zero is a range through which skin temperature may be changed, if done sufficiently slowly (0.007 °C/s), without producing a thermal sensation (HENSEL 1950). The upper and lower temperature limits of physiological zero are approximately 36° and 30 °C for an area of stimulation of approximately 15 cm². The range is narrowed when larger areas of skin, such as the whole

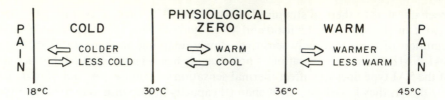

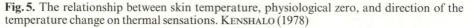

Fig. 5. The relationship between skin temperature, physiological zero, and direction of the temperature change on thermal sensations. Kenshalo (1978)

body, are exposed. Within the zone of physiological zero, thermal sensations adapt completely, and a relatively rapid increase in skin temperature results in a sensation of warmth while a decrease in skin temperature results in a sensation of cool.

When the skin temperature is maintained above or below these limits, sensations of warm or cool persist no matter how long the particular temperature is maintained. When the adapting temperature is below the lower limit of physiological zero, a small decrease in skin temperature will result in a *cooler* sensation, while an increase in skin temperature will result in a *less cool, not* a warm, sensation. In the same way, when the temperature of the skin is maintained above the upper limit of physiological zero, a warm sensation persists. A small increase in skin temperature will result in a *warmer* sensation, while a moderate decrease in skin temperature will result in a *less warm, not* a cool, sensation.

α) *Persisting Thermal Sensations.* As shown in Fig. 6, primate warm and cold fibers show steady state discharges that vary in frequency as functions of the adapting temperature. At low adapting temperatures (10°–15 °C), cold fibers become active; they reach a maximum activity at about 29 °C and then activity diminishes to a minimum at 40°–45 °C (Dodt and Zotterman 1952b; Dykes 1975; Hensel and Wurster 1970; Hensel and Zotterman 1951 a, b, e; Kenshalo and Duclaux 1977; Poulos and Lende 1970a).

There appear to be two types of warm fiber, as far as the steady state discharges are concerned. Most warm fibers show little or no activity at an adapting temperature of 30 °C, reach a maximum at about 43 °C, and again return to a minimum

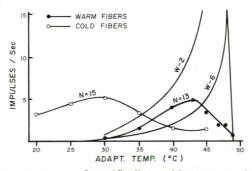

Fig. 6. Mean steady state responses of specifically sensitive warm and cold fibers found in primate skin. There appear to be two types of warm fiber steady state responses. Two fibers in this population (W-2 and W-6) were markedly different from the majority of the others. *Adapt. temp.,* adaptating temperature. Kenshalo (1976)

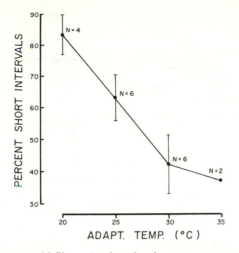

Fig. 7. Bursting in primate cold fibers. As the adapting temperature decreased, the proportion of short intervals compared to long intervals increased markedly, until at an adapting temperature of 20 °C almost 85% of the intervals were intraburst intervals compared to interburst intervals. *Brackets* show the SD of each point except at the 35 °C adapting temperature, where the *n* was too small to provide a variance estimate. *Adapt. temp.,* adapting temperature

at about 49°–50 °C. A few also commence steady state activity at about 30 °C, then rise rapidly to a maximum that varies from 45° to 47 °C adapting temperature. A further small increment in adapting temperature results in a complete cessation of activity. This is not due to injury. The event can be repeated (DODT and ZOTTERMAN 1952a; DUCLAUX and KENSHALO 1980; HENSEL and IGGO 1971; KONIETZNY and HENSEL 1979).

If thermal sensations are the result of activity in warm and cold primary afferents, how then can adaptation become complete at static temperatures in the vicinity of 33 °C? As shown in Fig. 6, there is considerable steady state activity at these skin temperatures in both warm and cold fibers. One way in which this may be correlated with sensations is to assume that low levels of activity in warm and cold fibers do not result in thermal sensations. Rather, such activity must reach a certain level before a thermal sensation occurs. As HENSEL (1952) expressed it, there is a central threshold that must be exceeded before thermal sensations can occur. Another way of expressing it is that the primary thermal afferent activity is integrated by some central mechanism(s), and that sensations result from the integrated level of activity in the center(s). It may be further assumed that the integrator is not a linear operator: it must have some finite time constant. Some notion of its characteristics may be deduced by comparing primary nerve activity with the occurrence of sensation.

A candidate neural code for the persisting warm sensation may be an increased steady state activity of warm fibers and, even though steady state activity may begin to decrease above a 43 °C adapting temperature in most warm fibers, there are still those fibers that show continued high levels of activity at up to approximately

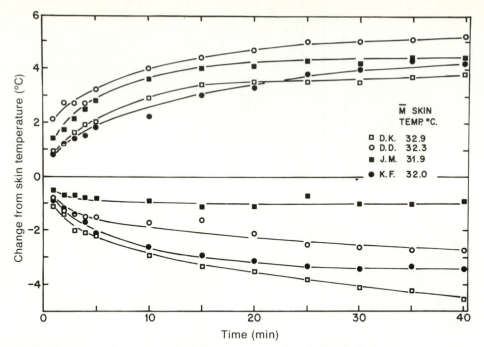

Fig. 8. The temporal course of adaptation to warm and cool stimuli. *Each point on the curves* represents the mean of four observations (taken at the times indicated) of the amount by which the subject had changed the temperature of the stimulator from the initial skin temperature in order to maintain a just-detectable sensation. Also shown are the means of eight measurements of skin temperature just prior to the adaptation measurements for each of four subjects. KENSHALO and SCOTT (1966)

48°–49 °C before they become silent. At these temperatures the nociceptors begin to discharge and the sensation is shifted from one of heat to one of pain.

The situation is different for cold fibers. Steady state cold fiber activity, on average, reaches a peak at about 29 °C. At lower skin temperatures the average frequency of activity decreases until finally, at 5°–10 °C, it is abolished altogether. The question is, how can cool sensations feel more intense at a 20 °C skin temperature than at a 29 °C skin temperature, in the face of a declining level of activity in the primary cold fibers? One possibility is that the bursting nature of the discharge characteristic of many cold fibers in primates may inflate the effect of the neural activity on the integrator at low skin temperatures. As shown in Fig. 7, as the adapting temperature decreases the number of intraburst intervals increases sharply. While bursting does not increase the average frequency of steady state activity, it does provide a sort of temporal code that could remove the ambiguity as to which side of the bell-shaped steady state response curve the skin temperature is maintained (DYKES 1975; HENSEL 1973). It might also raise the level of activity in the central integrator, and hence increase sensation intensity.

On the other hand, bursting may have no significance. There are several reasons: (a) in humans only a few cold fibers burst; (b) neither the average frequency nor the burst parameters of monkey cold fibers correlate well with temperature

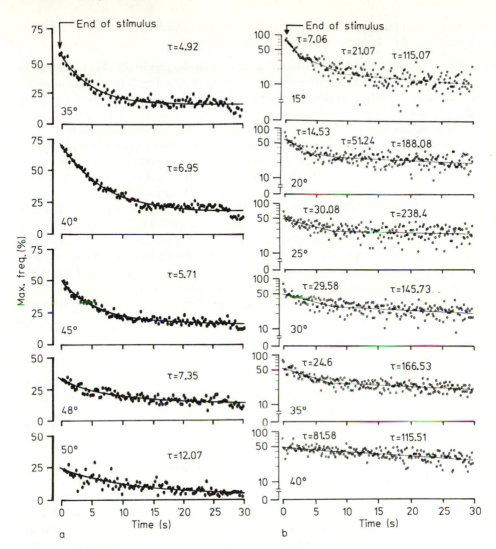

Fig. 9. a Time constants (in seconds) for adaptation of specifically sensitive warm fibers to final temperature levels. In all instances adaptation to the final temperature level commenced at the end of the 5 °C temperature increase delivered at a rate 2 °C/s. Each point represents the mean of the impulse content of the 125-ms bins of the individual peristimulus time (PST) histograms for the 15 warm units. There appears to be a systematic decline in the discharge between 25 and 30 s that does not fit the analytical functions. This resulted from the inclusion of the first 2–3 s response to cooling when the temperature was returned to adapting temperature, and should therefore be disregarded DUCLAUX and KENSHALO (1980). **b** Time constants in seconds, not corrected for interactions for adaptation of specifically sensitive cold fibers to a new temperature level. In all instances adaptation to the new temperature level commenced at the end of 5 °C decreases in temperature at a rate of 2 °C/s from several adapting temperatures. Each point represents the content of the 125 ms bins of the individual PST histograms for the 15 cold units. KENSHALO and DUCLAUX (1977)

sensations of human subjects; and (c) there is no evidence that the burst parameters are conveyed to second-order neurons (Hensel 1981).

β) Temporal Course of Adaptation. Adaptation to changes in the skin temperature is slow within the zone of physiological zero. As seen in Fig. 8, tens of minutes are required in order for the subjects to reach the upper and lower limits of complete adaptation.

The neural analog for sensory adaptation in primary warm and cold fibers may be the establishment of a new steady state response following a change in temperature. Stimulation of warm or cold units by a 5 °C temperature change (increase or decrease) produces a phasic increase in frequency, rapidly followed by a new steady state, as shown in Fig. 9. The time constants for establishing a new steady state in warm units range from 5 to 12 s. Thus one may assume that the new steady state level reaches asymptote in warm units within 20–50 s. The time constant is somewhat longer for cold units but is still a matter of minutes rather than tens of minutes, as indicated by the psychophysical data shown in Fig. 8. But it is not so simple. Cold units show variations in their steady state activity depending on the history of their stimulation. The effect is analogous to hysteresis, in that steady state activity is greater during ascending than during the descending changes in static temperature (Poulos and Lende 1970 a, b).

b) Changes in Temperature

Three principal stimulus variables influence the sensitivity of the organism to changes in skin temperature. These are the static skin temperature at which the temperature change starts (i.e., the adapting temperature), the rate of the temperature change, and the area to which the temperature change is applied (Hensel 1950).

α) Skin Temperature. As seen in Fig. 10, when the skin has been adapted to 28 °C a decrease in temperature of approximately 0.15 °C produces a detectable increase in the cool sensation. As the adapting temperature is increased, the cool threshold remains relatively constant at 0.15 °C, up to an adapting temperature of 35 °C. It then begins to increase rapidly to a point where, at a 40 °C adapting temperature, a 1 °C decrease in skin temperature is required to produce a threshold cool sensation. Warm thresholds, unlike cool thresholds, are large at low adapting temperatures and decrease as the adapting temperature is increased.

The activity of primary warm and cold units at low and at high adapting temperatures is shown in Fig. 11. Warm units were found to be 15 times more active (activity index is impulses during 4 s following onset of the temperature change) at high adapting temperatures (40 °C) than at low (25 °C) adapting temperatures, and cold units were approximately nine times more active at low adapting temperatures (25 °C) than at high (40 °C) adapting temperatures. The form of the curves depicting changes in sensitivity of warm and cold units as functions of the adapting temperature are similar in shape to the psychophysically measured warm and cool threshold sensations shown in Fig. 10.

Figure 10 shows the same series of events described by Fig. 5 in a different way. In Fig. 10, the amounts by which the temperature must be increased in order to de-

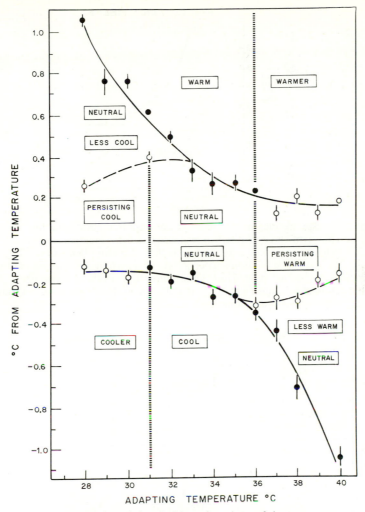

Fig. 10. Changes in warm and cool thresholds as functions of the temperature to which the skin of the forearm was adapted. Warm and cool absolute thresholds are shown by the *filled circles*. The *open circles* show differential "change" thresholds. When the adapting temperature of the stimulator was low, the subject experienced a persisting cool sensation. A detectably cooler sensation occurred when the temperature of the stimulator was lowered by 0.15 °C. When the stimulator was warmed in order to measure warm thresholds from a low adapting temperature, there was first a detectable decrease in persisting cool sensation, then thermal neutrality, and finally a warm sensation. A similar series of sensations occurred when the skin had been adapted to higher temperatures and measurements of the cool thresholds were made. KENSHALO (1972)

tect a decrease in the persisting warm sensation and by which it must be increased in order to detect a change in the persisting cool sensation are shown by the open circles and broken lines. This has been called the "changes threshold."

At adapting temperatures of 40 °C and above, there is little steady state activity in primary cold fibers, and their sensitivity to decreases in temperature is reduced.

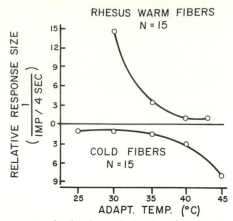

Fig. 11. Relative response magnitudes (cumulative impulses during the first 4 s following stimulus onset) of warm and cold fibers in response to a 0.5 °C temperature change at a rate of 2 °C/s. The reference response magnitude was that of warm fibers at the 43 °C adapting temperature. The reciprocal of impulses per second was used in order to present the *vertical axis* in a more conventional style. Thus the response magnitude of warm fibers at a 43 °C adapting temperature is 15 times greater than that at a 30 °C adapting temperature. *Adapt. temp.*, adapting temperature; *imp.* impulses

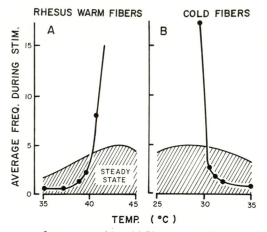

Fig. 12a, b. The responses of **a** warm and **b** cold fibers to cooling and warming respectively. The points above the steady state level on both **a** and **b** represent the responses of warm and cold fibers to a 0.5 °C increase and decrease in temperature respectively. Points below the upper limit of the steady state activity level represent suppression of that activity by temperature decreases applied to warm fibers from a 40 °C adapting temperature (**a**) and suppression of the steady state activity by temperature increases applied to cold fibers from a 30 °C adapting temperature (**b**). These latter temperature changes were of 0.5°, 1°, 2°, and 5 °C intensity. *Freq.*, frequency; *stim.*, stimulus. KENSHALO (1976)

However, in primary warm fibers at high adapting temperatures there is considerable steady state activity. They respond with a suppression of this steady state activity when cooled by a few tenths of a degree, as shown in Fig. 12 a.

At adapting temperatures of 30 °C and below, there is little to no steady state activity in primary warm fibers and their sensitivity to increases in temperature is

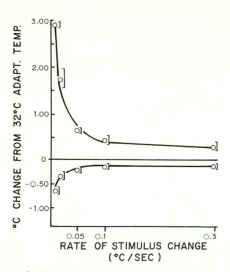

Fig. 13. Effect of the rate of stimulus temperature change on warm and cool thresholds. *Adapt. temp.,* adapting temperature. KENSHALO et al. (1968)

reduced. Cold fibers show a considerable steady state response, as well as bursting at low adapting temperatures. They respond with suppression of this steady state activity when warmed by a few tenths of a degree, as shown in Fig. 12 b.

A candidate code for the change threshold is a reduction in the frequency of activity of warm fibers at high adapting temperatures and in cold fibers at low adapting temperatures.

β) *Rate of Temperature Change.* Figure 13 shows that the rate at which the temperature is changed in measuring a warm or cool threshold has little effect upon the size of the threshold until the rate becomes less than about 0.1 °C/s. At slower rates the threshold increases rapidly.

Rate of suprathreshold temperature change is also without effect on the estimated intensities of warm and cool sensations. As shown in Fig. 14, when estimates of the magnitude of warm and cool sensations produced by 1°, 2°, and 5 °C changes presented at rates of 0.4°, 1°, and 2 °C, from several adapting temperatures, subjects estimated sensations the more intense, the larger the temperature changes, but the rate of change at which they were presented was without effect.

In general, as shown in Fig. 15, the effect of an increase in the rate of temperature change on the responses of primary thermal afferents is to increase the magnitude of dynamic responses at all adapting temperatures. The effect is larger at higher intensities of stimulation than at intensities of 0.5° and 1 °C.

The effect of rate of temperature change on the psychophysical measures of warm and cool sensations and the index of the dynamic response of primary thermal afferents do not correlate well. Rate of warming or cooling was without effect on magnitude estimates of warm and cool sensations, yet both faster rate and greater intensity of temperature change increased the response magnitude of primary afferents.

The concept of a central integrator may be able to accommodate this apparent discrepancy if it is stipulated that the integrator has a long time constant. Slow

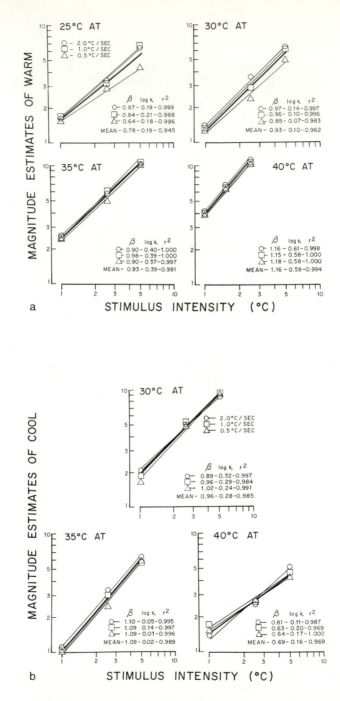

Fig. 14 a, b. Magnitude estimates of **a** warm and **b** cool sensations as functions of stimulus intensity. The best-fitting linear regression lines for the data at each adapting temperature (*AT*) are shown as *thickened lines*. The *mean curves* were calculated by fitting a linear regression line to all nine data points at each adapting temperature. Molinari et al. (1977)

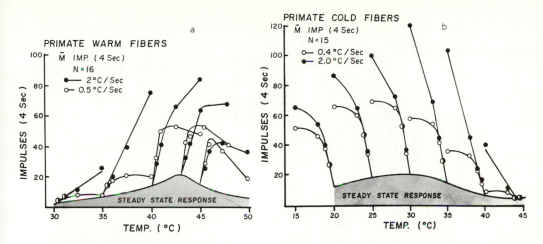

Fig. 15 a, b. The dynamic responses of **a** warm and **b** cool fibers to 0.5°, 1°, 2°, and 5 °C intensities of temperature change at rates of 0.5° and 2 °C/s. **a** DUCLAUX and KENSHALO (1980), **b** KENSHALO and DUCLAUX (1977)

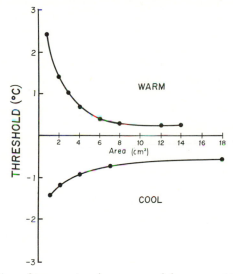

Fig. 16. Areal summation of temperature increases and decreases at threshold. (Warm summation from KENSHALO et al. 1967a; cold summation from BERG 1978)

rates of change require longer time periods to accomplish a given intensity of temperature change than do fast rates of change. For an integrator with a long time constant the rate of input assumes less significance.

γ) *Spatial Summation.* At threshold, area and intensity trade approximately equally for temperature increases, as shown in Fig. 16. This means that if one doubles the area over which a temperature increase is applied to the skin, threshold will decrease by one-half. The trading function can be expressed as $I = kA^{-1} + C$. Area

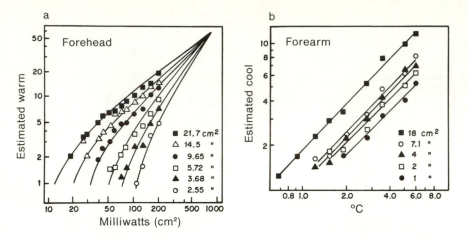

Fig. 17 a, b. Magnitude estimates of **a** warm and **b** cool sensations as functions of the area of stimulation. (Warm data from STEVENS and MARKS 1971; cold data from BERG 1978)

does not seem to play such a prominent role in spatial summation of temperature decreases, as seen in Fig. 16. Here the trading function is expressed as $I = kA^{0.5} + C$.

As suprathreshold intensities of temperature increase the slopes of magnitude estimates of the sensation intensity vary inversely with the area over which the stimulus is applied, as seen in Fig. 17a. One interesting thing about these magnitude estimates is that the functions converge at about the intensity of temperature increase that would produce pain.

Magnitude estimates of cool sensations from several intensities of temperature decrease appear to be more straight-forward. Cooling magnitude estimates for several areas of stimulation are parallel with slopes of approximately 0.5, as shown in Fig. 17b. Area retained its importance at suprathreshold intensities as well as at near-threshold intensities of temperature decrease.

The concept of a central integrator that integrates over space as well as time can account for the effect of the area of stimulation upon thermal sensation. Other characteristics of the central integrator can be inferred from the psychophysical studies of spatial summation. Thermal stimuli applied to symmetrically located body sites show spatial summation (HARDY and OPPEL 1937; ROŻSA and KENSHALO 1977). Thermal stimuli applied to both the forearms result in a much more intense sensation than that produced by either one alone. This suggests that information from the thermal sensing system also summates across the body midline, so that one would expect, as HELLON and MISRA (1973) described, that there would be bilateral representation of the information in the nervous system.

There have been few electrophysiological studies describing the neural mechanisms involved in spatial summation of thermal stimuli. On the basis of psychophysical evidence, HERGET et al. (1941) proposed two mechanisms to account for spatial summation. The first, for areas smaller than 4 cm², was thought to be served by endings whose branches converged near the periphery. The second, for areas larger than 4 cm², was thought to be served by individual primary afferent fibers that converged on common synaptic pools in the central nervous system. Af-

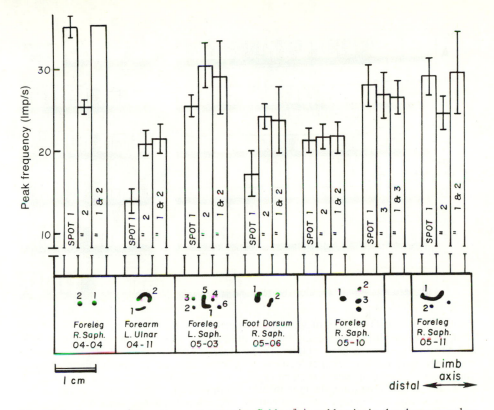

Fig. 18. Scale maps of the cutaneous receptive fields of six cold units in the rhesus monkey are shown at the *bottom of the figure*. The *bar graphs* above each receptive field represent the mean peak frequencies of activity in response to five or ten presentations of a 5 °C decrease in temperature at one, the other, and then both spots. The *brackets* show the size of the standard deviations except for unit 04-04. There both spots were simultaneously decreased in temperature, and their peak frequencies of activity were the same for all five stimulations. The peak frequency of activity when the temperature of two spots was simultaneously decreased was not statistically different from the peak frequency of activity for one or the other spot. For unit 05-10, interactions between spots 1 and 2 were studied first, then the stimulators were moved to study interactions between spots 1 and 3. The difference between the peak frequencies of activity from spot 1 in these two series is attributed to a slightly different position of the stimulator on spot 1 during the second measurement series. *Saph,* saphenous nerve. DUCLAUX and KENSHALO (1973)

ter observing (see Fig. 18) that single primary cold afferent fibers may innervate up to eight individual small areas or spots of skin, Roland Duclaux and I (DUCLAUX and KENSHALO 1973) decided to investigate the proposition that the discharge frequency obtained by stimulating first one and then another spot might be less than the discharge frequency when both spots were stimulated simultaneously. We found no evidence of summation on the response index used, as shown in Fig. 18. Spatial summation of cool stimuli appears to occur as a result of convergence of primary thermal afferents on second- and higher-order neurons in the dorsal horn, the thalamic nuclei, and perhaps higher centers.

Rhesus cold unit 2–9

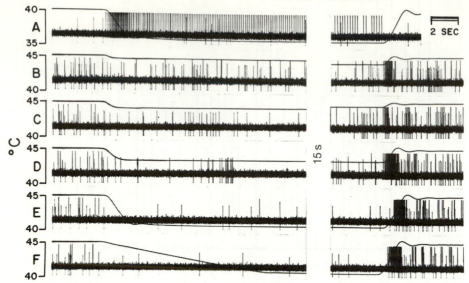

Fig. 19. Paradoxical responses of cold fibers to decreases and increases in skin temperature. Unit *A* showed a phasic increase in frequency in response to temperature reductions of 5 °C at a rate of 2 °C/s from a 40 °C adapting temperature. On rewarming to 40 °C, the discharge was suppressed. Activity from at least one additional unit can be seen in this spike train, but the unit does not appear to respond to the temperature changes. In spike train *B*, at the 45 °C adapting temperature, the monophasic action potentials of the cold unit can be differentiated from the biphasic action potentials. Decreasing the temperature of the receptive field by 0.5°, 1°, 2°, and 5 °C at a rate of 2 °C/s suppressed activity of the cold units shown in spike trains *B, C, D,* and *E*. The decrease in activity was in proportion to the intensity of temperature decrease. When the temperature was increased to a 45 °C adapting temperature, the cold units showed a phasic high-frequency burst of activity. A similar response, spike train *F,* was obtained by a decrease in temperature of 5 °C at a rate of 0.4 °C/s. Kenshalo and Duclaux (1977)

δ) *Paradoxical Responses.* In 1895, von Frey reported the singular discovery that some cold spots not only gave rise to sensations of cool and cold but gave similar sensations when touched by a very warm (45°–50 °C) stimulator. He labeled this a paradoxical cold sensation.

An electrophysiological study by Dodt and Zotterman (1952b) described what appears to be the neural analog of the paradoxical cold sensation. Increasing the temperature of the receptive field of a single cold afferent resulted in suppression of its steady state activity until the temperature was increased beyond 45°–50 °C.

Some primate cold fibers also show dynamic responses to high temperatures. These behaved like typical cold units when cooled from 40° to 35 °C, as illustrated in Fig. 19a. In Fig. 16b–f, when the temperature of the unit was decreased by various intensities from a 45 °C adapting temperature, there was a complete suppression of the activity following the temperature reduction, but a phasic discharge appeared when the temperature was returned to 45 °C. The response process of the receptor appears to have been reversed. The fiber now acts more like a warm fiber than a cold fiber. Paradoxical responses of primate cold fibers correlate well with the paradoxical sensations produced by heating human cold spots.

III. Other Issues

1. Structure and Function of Thermal Receptors

There is now general agreement among histologists that the innervation of hairy skin differs from that of glabrous skin. In hairy skin, nerves end in relation to three principal structures. These are the hair follicles, the Merkel's disks that lie deep in the epidermis close to the basement membrane (IGGO and MUIR 1969), and those that end free of any organized structure other than partial investment by Schwann cells, the dermal nerve net. Pacinian corpuscles are located close to bones, in joint ligaments, and around the joints themselves.

In glabrous skin some nerve terminals form a dermal nerve net and others end in relation to Merkel's disks. In addition, there is an elaboration of organized endings, whose structure seems to contribute to the characteristics of their discharge pattern. The Meissner's corpuscles, located high in the dermal ridges, are presumed to be rapidly adapting mechanoreceptors, responding exclusively to movement of tissue. Ruffini's cylinders, once thought to be warm receptors, have been shown to be slowly adapting mechanoreceptors that respond primarily to shearing force applied to the skin (CHAMBERS et al. 1972). Krause's bulbs, once thought to be cold receptors, have now been shown to be rapidly adapting mechanoreceptors (IGGO and OGAWA 1977). Pacinian corpuscles, located deep in the dermis and at the margin of the dermis and the subcutis, are also rapidly adapting mechanoreceptors capable of responding to high frequencies of skin indentation.

No obviously unique structures of skin have been identified, by modern histological methods, that could conceivably function as thermal receptors. However, by means of a combination of electrophysiological and electron microscopic methods, HENSEL et al. (1974) described cold receptors located beneath cold spots on the cat's nose. They consisted of bundles of nonmyelinated nerve branches with receptor axons in the top of the dermal papillae. Here the receptors branched, left their Schwann's cell envelopes, and penetrated the basal cell laminae of the epithelium, and their tips invaginated the cytoplasm of the basal epithelium. Their results suggest that the properties responsible for the unique responses to temperature and temperature changes seen in specifically sensitive cold fibers reside within the neural terminal membranes, and not in any nonneural elaborations that surround the terminal.

The cornea of the eye provides a structure that might be suitable to test the proposition that free nerve endings differ in their responses to stimulation. It has long been known that the cornea is innervated only by free nerve endings and at a density considerably greater than that of ordinary skin (WEDDELL and ZANDER 1950; ZANDER and WEDDELL 1951).

The cornea has been reported to yield only pain sensations, but reports of contact as well as pain have also been obtained, although thermal stimuli were ineffective in producing sensations (NAFE and WAGONER 1936, 1937). LELE and WEDDELL (1956) also reported contact as well as painful sensations from mechanical stimulation of the cornea. In addition, their subjects reported warm and cool sensations resulting from increase and decrease in corneal temperature. However, when the senior author acted as a subject, it became obvious to him that the qualities of the sensations resulting from corneal thermal stimulation were markedly different from those produced by thermal stimuli applied elsewhere on the skin. In order to emphasize the possible qualitative differences between corneal and cutaneous sensations, we determined to compare thermal thresholds of the cornea, conjuctiva, lip, and forehead. Although no thermal sensations were obtained from the cornea thermal stimuli ranging from 20° to 55 °C, all observers reported changes in sensation at certain temperatures on the scale. These were described in terms of irritation, whereas similar temperatures applied to other sites felt cool, warm, or hot (KENSHALO 1960). BEUERMAN and TANELIAN (1979) have reported similar findings.

The question of corneal sensitivity has also been investigated electrophysiologically. LELE and WEDDELL (1959) reported that the frequency and duration of activity in the primary afferents were related to the mode of stimulation. Mechanical stimuli evoked an immediate high-frequency burst of impulses in three to six individual units. Thermal stimulation, however, produced activity after a latency that varied inversely with stimulus intensity. Individual units responded to both mechanical and thermal stimulation.

Bill DAWSON (1963), in our laboratory, became interested in the apparent lack of specificity of the corneal afferents. He found that some corneal afferents could be stimulated by temperature changes. Furthermore, the activity initiated by an increase or a decrease in temperature never arose from the same axon.

The issue as to whether there are specifically sensitive thermal units in the cornea is by no means resolved, although Dawson's results seem to indicate that specificity is a distinct possibility. The psychophysical studies, however, suggest that if there are such specifically sensitive thermal afferents in the cornea they do not convey their information to the brain in such a manner that it is interpreted as warm or cool sensations.

2. Stimulation of Thermal Receptors

Since the time of Ebbecke, the establishment or alteration of spatial temperature gradients in the skin has been a favored notion about how activity is initiated and altered in thermal afferents. Two lines of evidence weigh heavily against spatial thermal gradients, or their alteration, as a necessary condition for stimulation of thermal receptors. First, VENDRIK and VOS (1958) compared the effectiveness of infrared (gradient-producing) and microwave (nongradient) heating to produce threshold warm sensations. They found the two methods were comparable in terms of the energies required to produce threshold warm sensations. Although HENDLER and HARDY (1960) disagreed with Vendrik and Vos on certain aspects of the experiment, they concurred that changing spatial temperature gradients do not act to initiate activity in thermal afferents or produce warm sensations.

The second line of evidence opposed to spatial temperature gradients as the immediate precursor to thermal receptor stimulation was derived from electrophysiological investigations of temperature-sensitive receptors in the cat's tongue. HENSEL and ZOTTERMAN (1951 e) and later HENSEL and WITT (1959) recorded activity from single cold units supplying the upper surface of cat's tongue. The stimulator was then placed on the underside of the tongue and the measurements were repeated. Cooling either surface led to an uninterrupted increase in the frequency of discharge of the same single cold units. Hensel and Witt concluded that stimulation of these cold units did not depend on either the slope or the direction of the intracutaneous spatial temperature gradient. If these units in the cat's tongue act in the same way as those responsible for human thermal sensations, there is little evidence to support the requirement of spatial temperature gradients as a necessary condition for stimulation of thermal receptors.

A more viable hypothesis of thermal stimulation is one that assumes that the terminals of warm and cold units are inherently unstable – unstable in the sense that within most of the physiological temperature range their metabolism is such that they show continuous activity. The energy for the activity is derived from the terminal itself. Temperature, or changes in temperature, merely modulate the frequency of such activity (HENSEL 1973).

3. The Vascular Theory

From 1947, when I first heard about Nafe's vascular theory of thermal reception, I racked my brain to devise the "crucial" experiment to test it. Everything I thought of was flawed in one way or another. The final test, at least as far as I am concerned, occurred quite serendipitously.

Paul Nafe, Barbara Brooks, and I were measuring the effect of adapting temperature on threshold warm and cool sensations (KENSHALO et al. 1961). The warm thresholds of male and female subjects agreed, with thresholds increasing as adapting temperature decreased. We were surprised, however, to find that the male subjects showed considerably less sensitivity than the female subjects to temperature decreases at high adapting temperatures (above 37 °C). After much puzzling, we decided that the only significant difference that might occur between males and females was due to the female's menstrual cycle. We ran a series of cool threshold measurements on three female subjects after the skin of their forearms had been adapted to 40 °C (KENSHALO 1966). In each of the three there was a marked increase in the cool threshold at the onset of menses and a decrease in the cool threshold at the time of ovulation, as indicated by a change in basal body temperature. In the preovulatory period the cool threshold was about -1.2 °C, but this promptly decreased to about -0.6 °C at the occurrence of ovulation and remained small throughout the postovulatory period. The relationship between the phase of the menstrual cycle and changes in cool threshold after the skin had been adapted to 40 °C was unmistakable. The odds, we calculated, were only about 1 in 10,000 that these changes in cool threshold could have occurred by chance. A change in the cool threshold associated with ovulation appeared to be related to the release of progesterone with the rupture of the Graafian follicle. The next step was to see if we could modulate the female cool threshold by oral contraceptives. The cool thresholds during the 1 st through the 5 th days of the menstrual cycle were as large as they had been during a preovulatory phase of the normal cycle. Upon administration of progesterone on the 5 th and following days, the cool thresholds decreased as though ovulation had occurred.

It is well known that during the postovulatory phase of the menstrual cycle, especially as the onset of menses approaches, the female becomes somewhat edematous (HARTMAN 1962). Other observations suggested that there was a general state of cutaneous vasodilation during the postovulatory phase of the cycle. In order to measure these changes, if they occurred, the thermal stimulator was modified to include a photoelectric plethysmograph in its center. Measurements of the cutaneous blood flow (volume pulse) showed that there was a greater vasodilation during the postovulatory phase of the menstrual cycle than during the preovulatory phase, and thresholds measured simultaneously with the volume pulse showed that the females were more sensitive to cool stimuli when the skin was adapted to 40 °C during the postovulatory phase of their cycle. If there is a cause–effect relationship between progesterone-induced vasodilation and increased sensitivity to cool stimuli at high adapting temperatures, we reasoned, then cutaneous vasoconstriction should produce a reduced sensitivity to cool stimuli at higher adapting temperatures. In order to test the hypothesis, epinephrine was iontophoresed into the forearm skin of two male subjects, and cool thresholds and volume pulse amplitudes were compared to those obtained when iontophoresis was performed without epinephrine in the solution (Kenshalo, unpublished work). Cool thresholds, after the skin had been adapted to temperatures between 36° and 38 °C, were considerably elevated after epinephrine iontophoresis as compared to iontophoresis without epinephrine. Volume pulse measures showed that epinephrine iontophoresis had markedly constricted the cutaneous vessels as compared to that measured under the control condition. It was also clear that sensitivity to cool stimuli was not affected by epinephrine iontophoresis when adapting temperatures of 34 °C and below were used.

At this point Bill DAWSON (1964) published some data from his own laboratory confirming the effect of epinephrine iontophoresis upon the cool threshold after the skin had been adapted to high temperatures. He extended the results to include observations of the effects on warm thresholds. At high adapting temperatures (greater than 35 °C), epinephrine iontophoresis was without effect on warm thresholds; but at lower adapting temperatures (less than 34 °C), warm thresholds increased markedly.

The failure to find any marked influence of manipulation of the cutaneous vascular system on warm and cool sensitivity suggests that there are factors other than movement in vascular walls that influence thermal sensitivity. While there does appear to be an effect of vasoconstriction on the cool threshold at high adapting temperatures and on warm threshold at low adapting temperatures, one would expect that if the receptor was movement in the smooth muscle elements of the cutaneous vessels the effect of manipulating them would be much more profound than we have been able to demonstrate so far.

D. Summary and Conclusion

The principal concepts derived from the early research (up to ca. 1950) are reviewed and examined in the light of more recent evidence. As a first approximation to identification of the neural correlates of thermal sensation, comparisons have been made between psychophysical measurements of thermal threshold and supra-threshold sensations and electrophysiologically measured activity in specifically sensitive (to temperature) primary afferent nerve fibers. The objective is to determine the extent to which variations in activity of these primary afferent fibers are able to account for variations in thermal sensations, given similar conditions of thermal stimulation.

One of the principal concepts derived from the early research was the necessity to account for the different sensations experienced when the skin was exposed to different energy forms. The punctate sensitivity of the skin suggested different receptors uniquely sensitive to only one particular form of energy. When von Frey proposed morphologically discrete innervated cutaneous structures (different types of encapsulated nerve ending) for each, the specific receptor theory emerged. Others, however, maintained that temporal and spatial patterns of neural activity accounted for the unique cutaneous sensations. This formed the basis for Nafe's quantitative theory of feeling.

More recent evidence shows that the encapsulated nerve endings are not distributed throughout the skin of the body to coincide with the bodily distributions of the unique sensitivities. Furthermore, where encapsulations exist, they only modify the response of the nerve ending, e.g., act as a filter for the energy form to which the ending is uniquely sensitive.

There is little doubt that there is response specificity in primary afferent fibers; some show activity in response to the application of mechanical stimulus, others to skin warming, others to skin cooling, and still others only to intense stimulation (for reviews see BURGESS and PERL 1973; CASEY 1978; HENSEL 1981). No anatomical or physiological substrait has, as yet, been identified to account for these relatively specific responses, recorded electrophysiologically, in the primary afferent fibers ending in the skin.

Patterns of neural activity are also of considerable importance. Although it appears likely that the qualities of cutaneous sensation (touch, warm, cold, or pain) are encoded by activity in primary afferents uniquely sensitive to one or two of the several forms of stimulation, cutaneous sensations have other attributes as well. A cutaneous sensation of a given quality may vary in intensity and in spatial and temporal extent. It is for these attributes that patterns of neural activity in the primary afferent fibers, and hence in the central nervous system, vary to allow discriminations between sensations that are basically of the same quality, e.g., roughness, smoothness, sharpenss, bluntness, softness. It is also likely that the neural codes of two or more qualities that differ in other attributes interact to form complex sensations, e.g., wetness, oiliness. Response specificity and spatial and temporal patterns of activity are equally important attributes of the neural correlates (codes) of cutaneous sensation.

The stimulus characteristic critical to arousing thermal sensations was another important concept in the early literature. Temperature changes in cutaneous tissue, reversible chemical reactions, chemical precursors, vascular activity, and thermal spatial gradients have all been proposed as the necessary and sufficient conditions to arouse thermal sensations. All have failed in critical tests of their correctness.

The fact that thermal fibers show activity when tissue temperature is static indicates that no thermal energy is transferred between the environment and the thermal nerve terminal. Presently available evidence indicates that this steady state activity results from an instability inherent in the terminal. Tissue temperature or changes in tissue temperature modulate this instability (HENSEL 1981).

The search for a subhuman model for the human temperature-sensing mechanism led to the conclusion that the cat's face, but not its furred body, possessed sensitivity to thermal stimuli to which responses could be conditioned. In primates (specifically the rhesus monkey), however, thermal sensitivity and primary thermal afferents were found to be generally distributed throughout the body. Comparisons of the thermal sensitivity of the cat's face and the rhesus inner thigh and palmar hand as functions of the temperature to which the skin has been adapted compare favorably with those obtained from humans under similar conditions of measurement.

At least two considerations make the rhesus the species of choice as a model for the human temperature-sensing system. First, the area innervated by the trigeminal nerve, or possibly the trigeminal afferent system itself, seems to be different from the somatic spinal afferent system for at least two reasons:

1. The cat's specifically sensitive thermal afferent fibers and the cat's thermal sensitivity are confined to the distributions of the afferent trigeminal nerve.
2. In the rhesus, warm fibers of the trigeminal nerve are predominantly of the A group, whereas in the somatic spinal afferent system they are predominantly of the C group.

Secondly the irregular contour of the cat's face makes it extremely difficult to place a thermode of any reasonable size on the skin with approximately equal pressure throughout its area.

Comparisons were made between activity in the primary thermal afferents of the rhesus and psychophysically measured thermal sensations in humans produced by similar (as nearly identical as possible) stimulus conditions. These comparisons suggest that the persisting warm sensation at skin temperatures above the zone of physiological zero can be accounted for by the steady state activity in primary warm afferent fibers. However, the persisting cool sensation at skin temperature below the zone of physiological zero does not correlate with the steady state activity in primary cold afferent fibers.

New steady state levels of activity following changes in skin temperature were established in less than 1 min in primary warm and cold afferent fibers. The temporal course of complete thermal adaptation to similar temperature changes within the zone of physiological zero requires as much as 40 min.

The phasic response magnitudes of primary warm and cold afferent fibers, as indicated by several measures of phasic activity, show changes as functions of the temperature to which their receptive fields have been adapted. Warm fibers show low sensitivity at low adapting temperatures (28°–30 °C) and cold fibers show low sensitivity at high adapting temperatures (38°–50 °C). Similar changes occur in absolute thresholds for warm and cool stimuli. Absolute warm thresholds are considerably larger when the skin has been adapted to a low temperature (28 °C) than when it has been adapted to a high temperature (40 °C), whereas cool absolute thresholds are considerably larger when the skin has been adapted to a high as compared to a low temperature.

Suppression of the steady state activity by cooling the receptive field of primary warm afferent fibers or warming those of cold afferents correlates well with psychophysical measurements of the change threshold following adaptation to temperature outside the zone of physiological zero.

The rate of temperature change was directly related to the magnitude of the phasic response of both primary warm and cool afferent fibers. However, rate of temperature change, except at very slow rates, was without effect on either the absolute warm and cool threshold or the magnitudes of suprathreshold warm and cool sensations.

Except for the work of Hellon and his collaborators, little work of an electrophysiological nature has been done on the spatial summation of thermal stimuli. Psychophysical measurements, however, show that both warm and cold sensations summate extravagantly over space at near-threshold intensities, and that spatial summation for warmth, but not for cold, decrease as the stimulus intensity increases. Furthermore, spatial summation occurs bilaterally.

Paradoxical cold sensations can frequently be aroused when a cold spot is touched with a very warm stimulus probe. Approximately 30% of a small population of primary cold afferent fibers showed a phasic increase in activity when their receptive fields were warmed from about 40 °C to 41°–45 °C. This change in response may well be the neural substrate of paradoxical cold sensations.

A central threshold or integrator is proposed to accommodate the apparent differences between the electrophysiological and psychophysical measurements of the steady state activity of cold fibers and the persisting cool sensations below physiological zero. Such a concept also accommodates the differences in the time constants to establish a new steady state and the time required to adapt completely to temperature changes. It may account, as well, for the profound effect of rate of temperature change on the magnitude of the phasic responses in primary thermal afferents and its complete lack of effect on thermal thresholds and magnitudes (except at extremely slow rates), and the strong spatial summation characteristic of the thermal sense.

Evidence in support of the existence of such an integrator is scarce. Electrophysiological information is necessary from second- and higher-order thermal pathways, the existence of which in the lower spinal cord has not been demonstrated. To date the only successful electrophysiological recordings from centrally located thermal afferents are some that have been made in the higher centers of the trigeminal nerve of cats and monkeys and those of Hellon et al. in the spinal cord of the rat. These show no evidence that might have resulted from the operation of such an integrating mechanism. However, neither the conditions of stimulation nor the data analysis were optimal to reveal it, if it exists. Others (primarily Iggo and PERL, personal communication) have searched the spinal cords of primates for thermally active second- or higher-order units, but the yield has been disappointingly small.

Yet it appears that the next important step in understanding the neural substrate of the thermal sensing system is a description of the anatomy and physiology of the central pathways, how they interact with each other and with other cutaneous systems, and how they contribute to the thermoregulatory process.

References

Names containing *von* are alphabetized in this list under *v*

Adrian ED (1926) The impulses produced by sensory nerve-endings: IV. Impulses from pain receptors. J Physiol (Lond) 62:33–51

Adrian ED, Zotterman Y (1926) The impulses produced by sensory nerve-endings: II. The response of a single end-organ. J Physiol (Lond) 61:151–171

Alrutz S (1898) On the temperature senses: II. The sensation "hot." Mind 7:140–144

Bazett HC (1941) Temperature sense in man. In: Temperature, its measurement and control in science and industry. Reinhold, New York, pp 489–501

Bazett HC, McGlone B (1932a) Studies in sensation. II. The mode of stimulation of cutaneous sensations of cold and warmth. Arch Neurol Psychiat 27:1031–1069

Bazett HC, McGlone B (1932b) Studies in sensation. III. Chemical factor in the stimulation of end-organ giving temperature sensations. Arch Neurol Psychiat 28:71–91

Belonoschkin B (1933) Über die Kaltreceptoren der Haut. Z Biol 93:487–489

Berg SL (1978) Magnitude estimates of spatial summation for conducted cool stimuli along with thermal fractionation and a case of secondary hyperalgesia. Doctoral dissertation, Florida State University

Bernhard CG, Granit R (1946) Nerve as model temperature end-organ. J Gen Physiol 29:257–265

Beuerman RW, Tanelian DL (1979) Corneal pain evoked by thermal stimulation. Pain 7:1–14

Blix M (1882) Experimentela bidrag till losning af frogan om hudnervanas specifika energi I (Experimental contribution to the question of the specific energy of the cutaneous nerves). Upsala Lak-Foren Forh 18:87–102

Bohnenkamp H, Pasquai W (1932) Das Verstärkungsgesetz: seine Beziehungen zum Mach-schen Kontrastgesetz. Dtsch Z Nervenheilk 126:138

Boring EG (1942) Sensation and perception in the history of experimental psychology. Appleton-Century-Croft, New York

Brearley EA, Kenshalo DR (1970) Behavioral measurements of the sensitivity of cat's upper lip to warm and cool stimuli. J Comp Physiol Psychol 70:1–4

Brown PK, Wald G (1964) Visual pigments in single rods and cones of the human retina. Science 144:45–52

Brown-Sequard CE (1855) Experimental and clinical research on the physiology and pathology of the spinal cord. Colin and Norvlan, Richmond

Burgess PR, Perl ER (1973) Cutaneous mechanoreceptors and nociceptors. In: Iggo A (ed) Somatosensory system. Springer, Berlin Heidelberg New York, pp 29–78 (Handbook of sensory physiology, vol 2)

Burnett NG, Dallenbach KM (1927) The experience of heat. Am J Psychol 38:418–431

Burton H, Tershima SI, Clark J (1972) Response properties of slowly adapting mechanoreceptors to temperature stimulation in cats. Brain Res 45:401–416

Casey KL (1978) Neural mechanisms of pain. In: Carterette EC, Friedman MP (eds) Handbook of perception, vol VIB, Feeling and hurting. Academic, New York, pp 183–230

Chambers MR, Andres KH, Düring M, Iggo A (1972) The structure and function of the slowly adapting type II mechanoreceptor in hairy skin. Quart J Exp Physiol 57:417–445

Cutolo F (1918) A preliminary study of the psychology of heat. Am J Psychol 29:442

Dallenbach KM (1927) The temperature spots and end-organs. Am J Psychol 39:402–427

Dallenbach KM (1939) Pain: history and present status. Am J Psychol 52:331–347

Dawson WW (1963) The thermal excitation of afferent neurones in the mammalian cornea and iris. In: Herzfeld CM (ed) Temperature – its measurement and control in science and industry, vol 3, part 3. Reinhold, New York, pp 199–210

Dawson WW (1964) Thermal stimulation of experimentally vasoconstricted human skin. Percept Mot Skill 19:775–788

Dennis W (1948) Readings in the history of psychology. Appleton, New York

Dodt E, Zotterman Y (1952a) Mode of action of warm receptors. Acta Physiol Scand 26:345–357

Dodt E, Zotterman Y (1952b) The discharge of specific cold fibres at high temperatures. (The paradoxical cold.) Acta Physiol Scand 26:358–365

Donaldson HH (1885) Research on the temperature sense. Mind 10:399–416

Duclaux R, Kenshalo DR (1972) The temperature sensitivity of the type I slowly adapting mechanoreceptor in cats and monkeys. J Physiol (Lond) 244:647–664

Duclaux R, Kenshalo DR (1973) Cutaneous receptive fields of primate cold fibers. Brain Res 55:437–442

Duclaux R, Kenshalo DR (1980) Response characteristics of cutaneous warm receptors in the monkey. J Neurophysiol 43:1–15

Dykes RW (1975) Coding of steady and transient temperatures by cutaneous "cold" fibres serving the hand of monkeys. Brain Res 98:485–500

Ebbecke U (1917) Über die Temperaturempfindungen in ihrer Abhängigkeit von der Hautdurchblutung und von den Reflexzentren. Pflügers Arch Ges Physiol 169:395–462

Erickson RP (1973) On the intensive aspect of the temperature sense. Brain Res 61:113–118

Erickson RP, Poulos DA (1973) On the qualitative aspect of the temperature sense. Brain Res 61:107–112

Geblewicz E (1940) La sommation spatiale des excitations thermiques. Ann Psychol 39:199

Goldscheider A (1884) Die spezifische Energie der Temperaturnerven. Monatsh Prakt Dermatol 3:198–208

Greenspan J, Kenshalo DR Sr (in press) Spatial summation in thermal sensations of human and monkeys measured by signal detection methods. Somatosensory Res I

Hagbarth K-E, Vallbo AB (1967) Mechanoreceptor activity recorded percutaneously with semi-microelectrodes in human peripheral nerves. Acta Physiol Scand 69:121–122

Hagen E, Knoche H, Sinclair DC, Weddell G (1953) The role of specialized nerve terminals in cutaneous sensibility. Proc R Soc [Biol] 141:279–287

Hardy JD, Oppel TW (1937) Studies in temperature sensation. III. The sensitivity of the body to heat and spatial summation of the end-organ responses. J Clin Invest 16:533–540

Hardy JC, Oppel TW (1938) Studies in temperature sensation. IV. The stimulation of cold by radiation. J Clin Inves 16:771–777

Harrington T, Merzenich MM (1970) Neural coding in the sense of touch, human sensations of skin indentation compared with the responses of slowly adapting mechanoreceptive afferents innervating the hairy skin of monkeys. Exp Brain Res 29:771–777

Hartman CG (1962) Science and the safe period. Williams and Wilkins, Baltimore

Heinbecker P, Bishop GH, O'Leary JO (1933) Pain and touch fibers in peripheral nerves. Arch Neurol Psychiat 29:771–789

Hellon RR, Misra NK (1973) Neurones in the dorsal horn of the rat responding to scrotal temperature changes. J Physiol (Lond) 232:375–388

Hendler E, Hardy JD (1960) Infrared and microwave effects on skin heating and temperature sensation. IRE Trans Med Electron 7:114–152

Hensel H (1950) Temperaturempfindung und intracutane Wärmebewegung. Pflügers Arch Ges Physiol 252:165–215

Hensel H (1952) Physiologie der Thermoreception. Ergeb Physiol 47:166–368

Hensel H (1973) Cutaneous thermoreceptors. In: Iggo A (ed) Handbook of sensory physiology. II. Somatosensory system, ch 2. Springer, New York, pp 79–110

Hensel H (1981) Thermoreception and temperature regulation. Academic, New York

Hensel H, Iggo A (1971) Analysis of cutaneous warm and cold fibers in primates. Pflügers Arch Ges Physiol 329:1–8

Hensel H, Kenshalo DR (1969) Warm receptors in the nasal region of the cat. J Physiol (Lond) 204:99–112

Hensel H, Witt I (1959) Spatial temperature gradient and thermoreceptor stimulation. J Physiol (Lond) 148:180–187

Hensel H, Wurster RD (1970) Static properties of cold receptors in nasal area of cats. J Neurophysiol 33:271–275

Hensel H, Zotterman Y (1951a) The response of the cold receptors to constant cooling. Acta Physiol Scand 22:96–113

Hensel H, Zotterman Y (1951 b) Quantitative Beziehungen zwischen der Entladung einzelner Kältefasern und der Temperatur. Acta Physiol Scand 23:291–319

Hensel H, Zotterman Y (1951 c) The effect of menthol on the thermoreceptors. Acta Physiol Scand 24:27–34

Hensel H, Zotterman Y (1951 d) The response of mechanoreceptors to thermal stimulation. J Physiol (Lond) 115:16–24

Hensel H, Zotterman Y (1951 e) Action potentials of cold fibres and intracutaneous temperature gradient. J Neurophysiol 14:377–385

Hensel H, Andres KH, von Düring M (1974) Structure and function of cold receptors. Pflügers Arch Ges Physiol 352:1–10

Herget CM, Hardy JD (1942) Temperature sensation: spatial summation of heat. Am J Physiol 135:426–429

Herget CM, Granath LP, Hardy JD (1941) Warmth sense in relation to skin area stimulated. Am J Physiol 135:20–26

Hering E (1874) Zur Lehre vom Lichtsinn. Wien Akad Wiss Math-Naturwissenschaftliche. Klasse Sitzungsberichte 72:310–348

Hering E (1877) Grundzüge einer Theorie des Temperatursinnes. Wien Akad Wiss Math-Naturwissenschaftliche. Klass Sitzungsberichte 75:101–135

Hering E (1879) Der Raumsinn und die Bewegungen des Auges. In: Hermann L (ed) Handbuch der Physiologie, vol 3. Vogel, Leipzig, S. 343–601

Iggo A, Muir AR (1969) The structure and function of a slowly adapting touch corpuscle in hairy skin. J Physiol (Lond) 200:764–796

Iggo A, Ogawa H (1977) Correlative physiology and morphological studies of rapidly adapting mechanoreceptors in cat's glabrous skin. J Physiol (Lond) 266:275–296

Jenkins WL (1941 a) Studies in thermal sensitivity. 16. Further evidence on the effects of stimulus temperature. J Exp Psychol 29:413–419

Jenkins WL (1941 b) A new basis for cutaneous temperature sensitivity. Am Inst Physics 6:502–508

Jenkins WL (1951) Somesthesis. In: Stevens SS (ed) Handbook of experimental psychology. Wiley, New York, pp 1172–1190

Jenkins WL, Karr AC (1957) Paradoxical warmth: a sufficient condition for its arousal. Am J Psychol 70:640–641

Johnson KO, Darian-Smith I, LaMotte C (1973) Peripheral neural determinants of temperature discrimination in man. A correlative study of responses to cooling skin. J Neurophysiol 36:347–370

Kenshalo DR (1960) Comparison of thermal sensitivity of the forehead, lip, conjunctiva, and cornea. J Appl Physiol 15:987–991

Kenshalo DR (1964) Temperature sensitivity of furred skin of cats. J Physiol (Lond) 172:439–448

Kenshalo DR (1966) Changes in the cool threshold associated with phases of the menstrual cycle. J Appl Physiol 21:1031–1039

Kenshalo DR (1972) Cutaneous senses. In: Kling JW, Riggs LA (eds) Experimental psychology, vol I. Holt, Rinehart, and Winston, New York, pp 117–168

Kenshalo DR (1976) Correlations of temperature sensitivity in man and monkey: a first approximation. In: Zotterman Y (ed) Sensory functions of the skin in primates. Pergamon, New York, pp 305–330

Kenshalo DR (1978) Biophysics and psychophysics of feeling. In: Carterette E, Friedman MP (eds) Handbook of perception 6 B. Academic, New York, pp 29–74

Kenshalo DR, Bergen DC (1975) A device to measure cutaneous temperature in humans and subhuman species. J Appl Physiol 39:1038–1040

Kenshalo DR, Brearley EA (1970) Electrophysiological measurements of sensitivity of the cat's upper lip to warm and cool stimuli. J Comp Physiol Psychol 70:5–14

Kenshalo DR, Duclaux R (1977) Response characteristics of cutaneous cold receptors in the monkey. J Neurophysiol 40:319–332

Kenshalo DR, Hall EC (1974) Thermal thresholds of the rhesus monkey (*Macaca mulatta*). J Comp Physiol Psychol 86:902–910

Kenshalo DR, Nafe JP (1962) A quantitative theory of feeling. 1960. Psychol Rev 69:17–33

Kenshalo DR, Scott HH Jr (1966) Temporal course of thermal adaptation. Science 151:1095–1096

Kenshalo DR, Nafe JP, Brooks B (1961) Variations in thermal sensitivity. Science 134:104–105

Kenshalo DR, Decker T, Hamilton A (1967a) Comparisons of spatial summation on forehead, forearm, and back produced by radiant and conducted heat. J Comp Physiol Psychol 63:510–515

Kenshalo DR, Duncan DG, Weymark C (1967b) Thresholds for thermal stimulation of the inner thigh, foot pad, and face of cats. J Comp Physiol Psychol 63:133–138

Kenshalo DR, Holmes CE, Wood PB (1968) Warm and cool thresholds as a function of rate of stimulus temperature change. Percept Psychophys 3:81–84

Kenshalo DR, Greenspan J, Rożsa A, Molinari H (1980) Temperature sensitivity in human and non-human primates. In: Anderson D (ed) Physiology past, present, and future: a symposium in honor of Yngve Zotterman. Pergamon, Oxford, pp 87–98

Konietzny F, Hensel H (1979) The neural basis of the sensory quality of warmth. In: Kenshalo D (ed) Sensory functions of the skin of humans. Plenum, New York, pp 241–260

Lele PP, Weddell G (1956) The relationship between neurohistology and corneal sensibility. Brain 79:119–154

Lele PP, Weddell G (1959) Sensory nerves of the cornea and cutaneous sensibility. Exp Neurol 1:334–359

Lele PP, Weddell G, Williams CM (1954) The relationship between heat transfer, skin temperature, and cutaneous sensibility. J Physiol (Lond) 126:206–234

Lipkin M, Hardy JD (1954) Measurement of some thermal properties of human tissues. J Appl Physiol 7:212–217

Locke J (1690) An essay concerning human understanding. Book II, chap VIII, par 21

Maréchaux E, Schäfer K (1949) Über Temperaturempfindungen bei Einwirkung von Temperaturreizen verschiedener Steilheit auf den ganzen Körper. Pflügers Arch Ges Physiol 251:765–784

Marks WB, Dobelle WH, MacNichol EF Jr (1964) Visual pigments of single primate cones. Science 143:1181–1183

Melzack R, Wall PD (1962) On the nature of cutaneous sensory mechanisms. Brain 85:331–356

Molinari HH, Rożsa AJ, Kenshalo DR (1976) Rhesus monkey (Macaca mulatta) cool sensitivity measured by a signal detection method. Percept Psychophys 19:246–251

Molinari HH, Greenspan JD, Kenshalo DR (1977) The effects of rate of temperature change and adapting temperature on thermal sensitivity. Sens Processes 1:354–362

Müller J (1840) Handbuch der Physiologie des Menschen für Vorlesungen, vol 2. Holschen, Coblenz

Nafe JP (1929) A quantitative theory of feeling. J Gen Psychol 2:199–211

Nafe JP (1934) The pressure, pain, and temperature senses. In: Murchison C (ed) Handbook of general experimental psychology, ch 20. Clark University Press, Worchester, pp 1037–1087

Nafe JP (1942) Toward the quantification of psychology. Psychol Rev 49:1–18

Nafe JP, Wagoner KS (1936) II. The sensitivity of the cornea of the eye. J Psychol 2:433–439

Nafe JP, Wagoner KS (1937) The insensitivity of the cornea to heat and pain derived from high temperatures. Am J Psychol 49:631–635

Nafe JP, Wagoner KS (1941b) The nature of sensory adaptation. J Gen Psychol 25:295–321

Nafe JP, Wagoner KS (1941b) The nature of pressure adaptation. J Gen Psychol 25:323–351

Neff WD (1960) Sensory discrimination. In: Fields J, Magoun HW, Hall VE (eds) Handbook of physiology vol 3, Neurophysiology. American Physiological Society, Washington DC, pp 1447–1470

Poggio GF, Mountcastle VB (1963) The functional properties of ventrobasal thalamic neurons studied in unanesthetized monkeys. J Neurophysiol 26:775–806

Poulos DA, Lende RA (1970a) Response of trigeminal ganglion neurons to thermal stimulation of oral-facial regions. II. Steady state response. J Neurophysiol 33:508–517

Poulos DA, Lende RA (1970 b) Response of trigeminal ganglion neurons to thermal stim-
    ulation of oral-facial regions. II. Temperature change response. J Neurophysiol 33:518–
    526
Rice CE, Kenshalo DR (1962) Nociceptive threshold measurements in the cat. J Appl
    Physiol 17:1009–1012
Rożsa AJ, Kenshalo DR (1977) Bilateral spatial summation of cooling symmetrical sites.
    Percept Psychophys 21:455–462
Rożsa A, Molinari HH, Greenspan J, Kenshalo DR Sr (in press) Human and monkey
    thermal sensitivity as a function of skin temperature. Somatosensory Res
Sinclair DC, Weddell G, Zander E (1952) The relationship of cutaneous sensibility to neuro-
    histology in the human pinna. J Anat (Lond) 86:402–411
Starling EH (1930) Principles of human physiology, 5 th edn. Churchill, London
Stevens JC, Marks LE (1971) Spatial summation and the dynamics of warmth sensation.
    Percept Psychophys 9:391–398
Sumino R, Dubner R, Starkman S (1973) Responses of small myelinated "warm" fibers to
    noxious heat applied to the monkey's face. Brain Res 62:260–263
Tapper DN (1965) Stimulus-response relationships in the cutaneous slowly-adapting mech-
    anoreceptors in hairy skin of the cat. Exp Neurol 13:364–385
Vendrik AJH, Vos JJ (1958) Comparison of the stimulation of the warmth sense organ by
    microwave and infrared. J Appl Physiol 13:435–444
Vierordt K (1871) Grundriß der Physiologie des Menschen, 4 th edn. Laupp, Tubingen
von Euler C (1947) Selective responses to thermal stimulation of mammalian nerves. Acta
    Physiol Scand 14:1–75
von Frey M (1895) Beiträge zur Sinnesphysiologie der Haut. III. Ber Sachs Ges (Akad) Wiss
    47:166–184
von Helmholtz H (1860) Handbuch der physiologischen Optik. Voss, Hamburg
von Helmholtz H (1863) Die Lehre von den Tonempfindungen als physiologische Grund-
    lage für die Theorie der Musik. Vieweg, Brunswick
Weber WH (1846) Der Tastsinn und das Gemeingefühl. In: Wagner R (ed) Handwörterbuch
    der Physiologie, vol 3. Vieweg, Braunschweig, S. 481–588
Weddell G (1941 a) Pattern of cutaneous innervation in relation to cutaneous sensibility. J
    Anat 75:346–367
Weddell G (1941 b) The multiple innervation of sensory spots in the skin. J Anat 75:441–446
Weddell G, Pallie W (1954) Observations on the neurohistology of cutaneous blood vessels.
    In: Wolstenholme GEW, Freeman JS (eds) Peripheral circulation in man. Churchill,
    London
Weddell G, Zander E (1950) A critical evaluation of methods used to demonstrate tissue
    neural elements, illustrated by reference to the cornea. J Anat 84:168–195
Weddell G, Zander E (1951) The fragility of non-myelinated nerve fibres. J Anat 85:242–250
Weddell G, Pallie W, Palmer E (1954) The morphology of peripheral nerve terminations in
    the skin. Q J Micro Sci 95:483–501
Weddell G, Palmer E, Pallie W (1955) Nerve endings in mammalian skin. Biol Rev Cam-
    bridge Philos Soc 30:159–195
Wunderli A (1860) Experimentelle Beiträge zur Physiologie des Tastsinnes. Moleschotts
    Untersuch 7:393
Young T (1802) On the theory of light and colours. Phil Tr Roy Soc 92:12
Zander E, Weddell G (1951) Observations on the innervation of the cornea. J Anat 85:68–99

CHAPTER 15

The Sensory Detection of Vibrations

Wolf D. Keidel

A. Introduction

To deal with the systems for perception of vibratory stimuli in man one must look at tactile mechanoreception by means of a special filter: the *dynamic* and *periodic* ways of perceiving the *Umwelt* (surroundings) (Geldard and Sherrick 1966–1981; Keidel 1956).

There is – in contradiction of the view of David Katz – no such special sense as a "sense of vibration;" mechanoreception and perception of nonstatic, nonstationary tactile stimulation (in other words, of a temporally and, in most cases, simultaneously spatially changing stimulatory pattern) together have the function of such a sense, however.

This "sense" involves an even less atavistic and rudimentary type of perception in the case of man, since animals of other species react much more perfectly than we can to transversal displacement of surface waves. Grasshoppers and locusts, for example, sitting on four feet, need close and intimate contact with their world, the grass beneath them.

But man in the course of evolution lifted himself from the ground to walk on two feet, and in order to communicate with his world developed a language, which, being transmitted via the air, was better adapted to his new posture than body waves received from the ground on which he stood. Auditory communication via airborne sound (longitudinal compression waves) made man what he is, the *princeps* (chief) of living animals, the conqueror of the world.

Following this line of thought, it is a miracle that, after many thousands of years of evolutionary habituation to the conditions of their world, the members of the human race still remain sensitive to the other, more primitive type of mechanoperception, which is what I should like to deal with in this chapter.

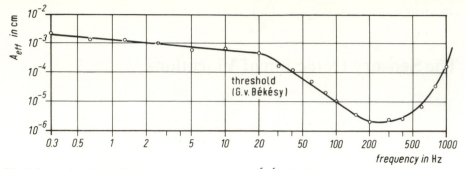

Fig. 1. Intensity threshold curve measured by VON BÉKÉSY (1939 a)

B. First Papers on Vibration (Historical Aspects)

There is a long distance to cover in a backward look with modern eyes of our day's state of the art. As early as in the middle of the nineteenth century, E. H. WEBER (1846) and VALENTIN (1852) in Erlangen (Germany) wrote papers about that topic as VON FREY did in his paper entitled „Physiologische Versuche über das Vibrationsgefühl", summarizing his research, in 1915. One of those early authors (VALENTIN 1847, 1848) had written a textbook on physiology (in German language). Curiously enough, his first article about vibration could be found in the old book's cabinet of the library of the same institute which is now headed by the author. It was this article which actually triggered the author's interest in research in the perception of vibratory stimuli.

One of the two main roots of the interest in vibration is the *clinical observation* that the different qualities of mechanoreception – touch and vibration – can deteriorate differently when measured quantitatively in pathological cases; the one not actually being affected by a disease (e.g., by tabes), the other – quite in contrast – revealing severely raised thresholds. Such observations were made by the Berlin group headed by GOLDSCHEIDER, a well-known Professor of Internal Medicine at the Charité, and triggered the research of a group in Paris under DEJÉRINE (1914). Both institutions had good scientific contact and exchanged young fellows, EGGER joining DEJÉRINE in Paris in 1899, for example.

The second root of interest was more basic research. The sense organs located in the skin gained increasing attention from theoreticians, especially experimental physiologists – mainly VON FREY, working at Würzburg (and Heidelberg). He wrote about quite a few topics in mechanoreception, his main interest being the *Sinnespunkte* (sensory spots) (VON FREY 1894, 1911, 1914, 1915), including the broader question of how those receptors would deal with dynamic – say vibratory – stimulation rather than static pressure or touch.

There have been long and intensive discussions (RUMPF 1889; TREITEL 1897; EGGER 1899; VON FREY 1894; RYDEL and SEIFFER 1903; GOLDSCHEIDER 1904; HERZOG 1906; BING 1910; VON WITTICH 1869; GRANDIS 1902; VALENTIN 1852) as to whether the skin receptors or receptors located around the bones were the mediators of vibratory sensations, and at what frequencies the type of sensation would change from discontinuous single beats to some sort of continuous and specifically vibratory *(schwirrende)* sensations, until finally, above a given upper frequency limit around 1 kHz, the sensation would cease even for very strong stimuli. Another open question at that early stage was whether nerve endings or evolutionarily differentiated corpuscles (MEISSNER'S, MERKEL'S, and others) should be regarded as the transducers for the mechanical (and electrical) stimuli into physiological "excitation" (nerve impulses, conducted signals, etc., in modern nomenclature).

A third root of interest was brought into discussion by experimental psychology, at that time (1923) focused around the laboratory of DAVID KATZ at Rostock, where he was Professor of Philosophy and Pedagogy. Using oscillating forks as sources of stimulation, he claimed the "vibratory sense" to be a special modality in the sense of VON HELMHOLTZ, as distinguished from the concept of VON FREY that vibratory sensation was a modified type of the simple sensation of touch or pressure. KATZ (1923) stood alone with this concept. On the other hand, he started to measure quantitatively the threshold for intensity (displacement of skin microscopically determined) versus frequency of sinusoidal oscillations. The results from the Psychological Institute of Rostock were reported in an article entitled „Über die kleinsten vibratorisch wahrnehmbaren Schwingungen" (On the Smallest Vibrationally Perceivable Oscillations) (KATZ and NOLDT 1925). As minimum displacement at 50 Hz he found 0.3 μm to be the absolute threshold for intensity.

In the USA, at Northwestern University, Evanston, Illinois, GAULT (1927 a–d), KNUDSEN (1928), PEARSON (1928), and GOODFELLOW (1933, 1934) first tried to use the vibratory sensitivity of the human skin to convey speech through the skin. The main activity on vibratory sensation and perception, however, has been concentrated for a long time at the psychological laboratory of the University of Virginia, starting with three consecutive papers by its head, FRANK GELDARD, and his group (GELDARD and VON HALLER-GILMER 1934; VON HALLER-GILMER 1937). In 1935, B. VON HALLER-GILMER, a student of FRANK GELDARD, gave an excellent review of the history of the matter, going back to DUNLAP in 1911. DUNLAP used a set of 11 specially constructed tuning forks, ranging in vibration rate from 420 to 460 Hz, successively applied in pairs to the palmar side of the hand. In his first paper, DUNLAP (1911) reported frequency discriminations as low as 5% (0.2% in audition under optimal conditions). DUNLAP (1913) subsequently reported tactile discrimination of beats and difference tones as distinct and characteristic as auditory beats and difference tones. Here he made use of properly tuned forks of 128 and 256 Hz, mounted in such a way that the two forks were applied simultaneously to the palm.

In 1925 GAULT inaugurated a series of experiments in which he made attempts to enable the deaf to "hear" through the sense of touch. GOLDSTEIN (1926) made similar investigations. KNUDSEN (1928) conducted a study to determine to just what extent the sense of touch is endowed with analytic functions required for hearing speech or music. This investigation was the first to give recognition to the problem of amplitude of the skin's displacement in studying the range of frequency response as mediated through touch. He used an electromagnetic telephone receiver adapted to communicate its vibrations to a pivoted lever. Amplitudes of displacement by the vibration (vacuum tube oscillator) were measured by an optical system like Miller's phonodeik. KAMPIK (1930) performed experiments in which his subjects could often distinguish between noises and musical tones through their fingers. In the same year FESSARD (Institute Marey, Paris) made the first investigations toward a reliable measurement of threshold for intensities of vibration. The frequencies ranged from 15 to 650 Hz. The skin's displacement while receiving vibratory stimuli was recorded by means of a mirror, thus respecting the damping factor of the tissue. In 1932 GRIDLEY performed experiments in the discrimination of short intervals of time by the fingertip and the ear.

ROBERTS (1932) reported experiments on frequency discrimination by the sense of touch. Then GOODFELLOW (1933), applying a revised form of GAULT's Teletactor, studied the sensitivity of the fingertips to vibrations at various frequency levels, ranging from 12 Hz to 3,000 to 4,000 Hz. GOODFELLOW reports perceived frequencies as high as 8,192 Hz. Both FESSARD and KNUDSEN found the "absolute threshold for intensity" in the frequency range of 250–256 Hz. VON HALLER-GIL-MER (1935) refined all those data in GELDARD's laboratory. The absolute intensity threshold at 356 Hz was in the order of 20×10^{-6} cm displacement.

Those threshold studies were continued in parallel at the Institute for Vibration Research in Berlin by SETZEPFAND (1935) and by HUGONY (1935). However, the main effort toward a series of very thorough studies at that time stems from GEORG VON BÉKÉSY, who first worked at Budapest and then went to an industrial laboratory (Siemens) in Berlin. He later emigrated (via Sweden) to the United States. Here, after World War II, he worked for a long period of his life, establishing his world-famous laboratory in the basement of Harvard Memorial Hall in Cambridge, Massachusetts, where together with S. S. Stevens he was senior fellow. He moved to Honolulu, Hawaii shortly before his death in 1973. We shall come back to his work later in this chapter. VON BÉKÉSY's curve for intensity threshold is shown in Fig. 1.

C. Physics of the Skin

One significant difference between small animals and man with respect to the physical parameters of vibratory stimuli is due to the fact that the wavelengths of vibratory stimuli in small animals are long compared to the body size of the entire animal. On the other hand, vibrating sources on the human skin initiate concentric traveling waves along great areas of the body surface. This means that wave velocity and skin impedance influence the displacement and phase which exist simultaneously on different sites of the stimulated skin. Since the neuronal networks by which the mechanoreceptors are excited act together in a highly complex pattern, with alternating facilitatory and inhibitory areas, the integral activation is not a simple function of the traveling waves itself. In addition, convergent and divergent fiber connections play an important role for the physiological encoding processes, so that the situation becomes even more complicated. In contrast, the ear, and specifically the basilar membrane, clearly show a physical frequency dispersion essential for the overall function of the organ of Corti (the *Reizverteilungsorgan* according to OTTO F. RANKE (RANKE 1931, 1950). In the early days of vibratory perception it was highly tempting to look at similar features of vibratory traveling waves. Interesting data on this subject were collected in the late 1940s and 1950s in the laboratory of HENNING VON GIERKE, OESTREICHER, and FRANKE at Wright-Patterson Air Force Base, Dayton, Ohio.

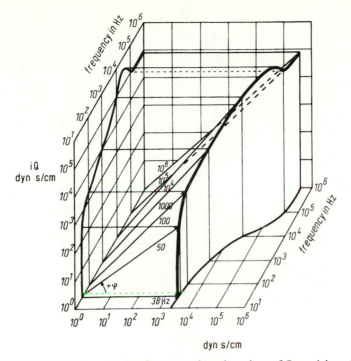

Fig. 2. Mechanical impedance versus frequency based on data of Oestreicher. After KEIDEL (1956)

Perpendicular placements of the human skin, both for quasi-stationary conditions and for dynamic vibrations, cause complex vectors with respect to the deformation of a given partition of the skin. In addition, the human skin under those circumstances can be regarded as consisting of two different layers of tissue, a superficial one (the tegmentum) and a deep layer beneath the epidermis with a high lipid component content. The integral mechanical impedance of the skin is therefore synthesized from two different values – for the skin itself and for the tissue beneath. On the other hand, the forces originated by the indentation of the skin do *not* obey the law of Hooke. In other words, the relation between the indentation and the vectorial force is a nonlinear one (VON GIERKE et al. 1952).

An important special case is bony tissue beneath the skin. The pronounced stiffness of the bones increases the reactance considerably. This explains all the controverseries at the beginning of the history of vibration [VON FREY (1915); GOLDSCHEIDER (1904)] about why vibrations of the skin above bones are perceived so differently from those of skin over fatty tissue. In general, the different body areas yield different mechanical impedances measurable quantitatively by the equations and models developed by the Dayton group in the early 1950s.

The second parameter by which the mechanical impedance is physically influenced in the *frequency* of vibration. Again reliable data have been reported by VON GIERKE (1950) and FRANKE (1951) for a frequency range from 10 Hz to 10 MHz for the human surface (normal skin). These results are demonstrated in Fig. 2

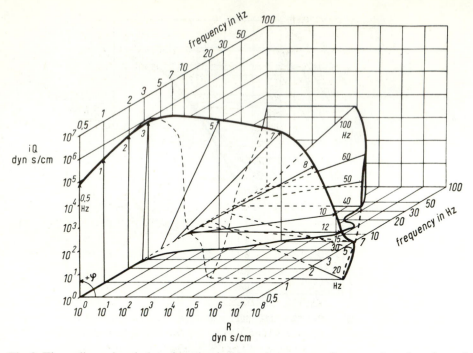

Fig. 3. Three-dimensional plot of mechanical impedance versus frequency based on data of VON BÉKÉSY for frequencies below 100 Hz. After KEIDEL (1956)

(KEIDEL 1956), which is based on the Dayton data. On the other hand, the situation is strikingly different for frequencies below 100 Hz (Fig. 3). The singular point at 3 Hz can be seen clearly. As COERMANN (1953, personal communication) pointed out, this is in clear agreement with the maximal energy transfer for vibrations to the entire body of man at this frequency, e.g., when traveling by car or aircraft.

The measurement of the velocities of the wave propagation began at the same time at two different laboratories: that of the Dayton group and, in the early 1950 s, that of the Erlangen group (KEIDEL 1956). Using stroboscopic light the wave propagation could be photographed. Some of the first pictures were taken by FRANKE (1951) and VON GIERKE et al. (1952). The latter is shown in Fig. 4.

More detailed and systematic studies in respect of the elasticity coefficient of the different tissues underlying the human skin were performed at the Physiological Institute of Erlangen (Germany) between 1949 and 1956 (see KEIDEL 1956).

Using a vibrator energized by an electromagnetic coil at a frequency of 50 Hz and illuminated by stroboscopic light, identical driving forces from a vibrating plate delivered to the skin above three typically different underlying tissues revealed the different waveforms of the traveling vibratory waves. The propagation velocity could be measured quantitatively. Having ascertained the vibratory frequency by recording the wavelength above fatty tissue, above muscle, and above bone in man, it was possible to demonstrate that the lowest frequency was to be found above fat and by far the highest above bone, that above muscle being somewhere between. Thus the time during which a given receptor was exposed to skin

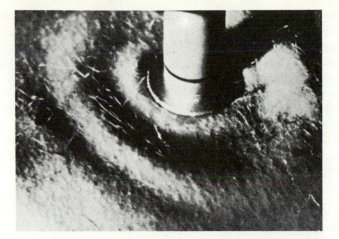

Fig. 4. Stroboscopic photograph of the wave propagation on the leg of a human subject vibrated by a piston at a frequency of 64 Hz. After VON GIERKE et al. (1950, 1952)

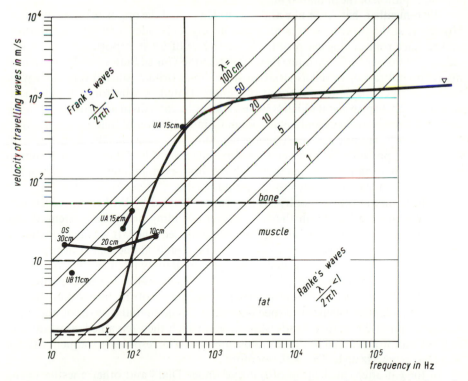

Fig. 5. Frequency dispersion for the wave propagation velocity on the human skin then vibrating at frequencies of between 10 and 100 kHz. The steepest part of the frequency dispersion curves lies between 30 and 500 Hz, just covering the physical vibratory frequencies in man. *Black circles*, after KEIDEL (1956); *crosses*, after FRANKE et al. (1951); *triangles*, after FRUCHT (1953). *UA*, Unterarm; *UB*, Unterbauch; *OS*, Oberschenkel

deformation was shortest at the high propagation velocity on bony subtissue and longest above fat. Most strikingly, the change in the propagation velocity could be recorded when relaxed skeletal muscle was phasically innervated, so increasing its elasticity module. In this case, the wave velocity above the isometrically contracted muscle was enlarged in comparison to the relaxed muscle. Putting all those data together it could be proved that, similarly to the case within the inner ear, the human vibrated skin showed a *clear frequency dispersion* for the physiologically interesting frequency range.

In Fig. 5 a plot of the velocity of the vibratory wave propagation versus vibratory frequency summarizing all the data reveals clearly the *frequency dispersion* for *vibratory skin waves* in man. The frequency ranges from 10 Hz to 100 kHz.

D. Encoding Processes

From the very beginning of the research on vibratory perception in man, there was discussion about the possible existence of specific receptors on the one side and the nonspecific dynamic type of receptor excitation in the encoding processes to vibratory stimulation of the human skin.

We remember that von Frey and David Katz had the opposite interpretation. However, at that time there was only psychophysical evidence in experimentation and no electrophysiological proof. Hence it was of great importance that a few electrophysiologists, for instance Pfaffmann in the United States and Fessard and his group in France, as well as Hoagland in Great Britain, started very early with records of the time pattern of trains of signals elicited by vibratory stimuli. Fitzgerald used displacement of hairs (whiskers) in the cat. All, in accordance with the early research of Adrian and his school in Cambridge, found that the main difference between the static and the dynamic encoding processes was the following one: static touch, pressure and hair bending somehow arouse stochastic trains of signals with different distances between them, while vibratory stimuli up to a certain upper frequency limit lead to synchronized discharges (Fig. 6 b). At MIT in 1957 a group from the communication biophysics laboratory headed by Walter A. Rosenblith made several experiments on the cat whisker encoding processes, systematically changing the two main parameters, intensity and frequency. It was demonstrated that the mammals behave very similarly to the reptiles: I succeeded in recording single-receptor activation indicated by single-unit activity from the dorsocutaneal nerve of the frog (Keidel 1955). As Fig. 6 a shows, a step-like increase in intensity above threshold of such a receptor within a small area of the frog's skin showed the typical adaptive behavior of mechanoreceptors: an initial overshoot and a decrease in impulse rate to a steady state value, which then remained constant and in itself was proportional to the stimulus intensity. The responsive frequency range was from a few Hz up to 300–400, not more.

In the cat after enucleation of one eye under Dial® and other anesthesia the maxillary nerve could be lifted and put on a pair of electrodes. Then the bending of the whiskers in the cat clearly prompted the same behavior as described for the frog (Keidel et al. 1960).

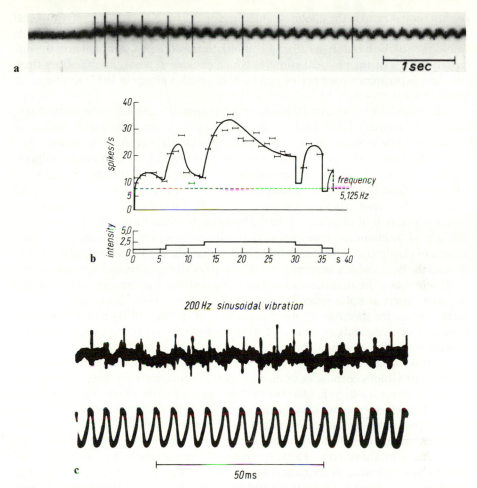

Fig. 6. a Single-fiber record from the frog's dorsocutaneal nerve, showing the typical time course of adaptation; **b** number of spikes versus increasing and decreasing steps of stimulus intensity, showing the initial overshoot, the steady state for the adapted condition, and silent periods within the time course of adaptation; **c** synchronized responses at 200 Hz. After KEIDEL (1955)

This series of experiments revealed that the vibration-sensitive frequency range in the higher animals is extremely comparable to that previously found by means of psychophysical technique in man.

The adaptation time course allows one to separate the static and dynamic intensity functions ranging over not more than 35–50 dB, compared to 130 dB in the auditory system. In other words, the steepness of S.S. Stevens' power functions had to be much steeper (in the order of the exponent n of 0.85 to 1, while in the auditory system it is in the order of 0.3). This holds for the steady state just as for the initial overshoot. The question whether the displacement of the hair itself or its differential ratio is the adequate stimulus for the triggering of the physiological signal running in the maxillary or cutaneous nerve in the frog in the early trials found the solution that it is rather a combination of the proportional and the differential parts of the physical stimulus which decides at what time the fiber fires. All these experiments were performed by Rosenblith's group in 1957 (Keidel et al. 1958, 1960).

Later, in the 1970s at the Physiological Institute in Marburg (Germany), Nier, working at Hensel's laboratory, confirmed these data using the cat's whiskers as site of vibratory stimulation, and obtained very accurately performed results.

Another group of experimenters was able to show that the interosseal Golgi receptors and the Vater Pacinian special mechanoreceptors in man are similarly excitable to those in the cat on which they made their experiments. Again it could be shown that, respecting the physics of the underlying tissues as described in the preceding section of this chapter, in the bony parts of the human body quite a few specialized mechanoreceptors respond to vibratory stimuli. It is the interosseal lamina of elastic and collagenous tissue rather than the highly pain-sensitive "skin" around the bones which are sensitive to this type of dynamic mechanostimulation.

If one tries to fit all those results together it follows that there is not one special receptor. There is not a special sense of vibration as David Katz believed; it is rather the entire spectrum of mechanoreceptors specialized by evolution during hundreds of thousands of years, all with high sensitivity to periodic (vibratory) stimulation by the environment.

So it is not a question of whether one should look to Meissner's, Pacinian's, Merkel's or Golgi's corpuscles when seeking the transducers for the encoding processes for vibratory stimuli. One must rather think in terms of von Frey's conception and my (Keidel 1956) idea that all types of mechanical stimuli can be encoded by all types of mechanosensitive receptors into physiological signals. Periodic vibratory stimuli are as effective on the skin covering a fatty underlying tissue as they are on the skin above bone. However, it is not the skin itself that is sensitive but the mechanoreceptors of the connecting tissues, as we know now. For a thorough coverage of our knowledge on this problem see my chapter in *Contributions to Sensory Physiology*, Vol. 3 (Keidel 1968).

Another point to be touched upon is the difference between the simple mechanoreception of the skin and the advanced one in the auditory system. The upper limit of frequency in the nonspecialized mechanoreceptor systems in animals and in man is defined more or less by the reciprocal of the refractory period of the sensory nerves, a time which is in the order of 1 ms. This means that the highest repetition rate of a synchronized periodic train of nerve impulses elicited by a vibratory stimulation in the skin is limited to a maximum of 1 kHz. Under physiological conditions a maximum of 400 pps is even more likely. That the auditory system is able to convey information of frequencies ranging up to 18 kHz is due to an evolutionary specialization first described by Glen Wever (1949), and labeled the "volley" principle.

If one now looks at the decoding system of this mechanism, the summed up activity gives signals in the order of 10 kHz although a single receptor and its fiber fire only at a rate of 1,000/s maximally. But the matter is even more complicated. We will see that this clear difference between the two systems of mechanoreception plays an important role if one tries to convey complex speech stimuli via the skin or via a severely damaged ear; in other words, in the situation existing for prosthetic cochlear implants. This will be discussed later in this chapter (Sect. G).

E. More Recent Studies on the Psychophysics of the Vibratory System

More recent studies on the psychophysics of vibratory perception have been concentrated in a few laboratories in the United States, one being the laboratory of sensory communication at Syracuse University, headed by Joe Zwislocki, and another, FRANK GELDARD and CARL SHERRICK's laboratory of cutaneous communication at Princeton University.

A series of quite compelling papers has been published from Zwislocki's laboratory, mainly by RONALD T. VERILLO (1965a–c, 1966a–e). He collected data about vibrotactile thresholds on human glabrous and hairy skin. Vibrotactile thresholds on human glabrous skin were determined for short monopolar pulses and for two directions of skin displacement. Positive and negative pulses showed no threshold differences. Neither was any threshold difference obtained when movement into the skin was compared to outward movement of the contactor. Thus the threshold appeared to be independent of the direction of displacement. Absolute thresholds have been measured on the hairy skin of the volar forearm. Some differences could be detected between hairy and glabrous skin. The overall trend, however, for the U-shaped thresholds for both types of skin (hairy and glabrous) was similar: a U-shaped function of frequency with a slope of -12 dB for the lower frequencies and of $+9$ dB for the higher ones (above 220 Hz). Thresholds of vibration decrease in direct proportion to the contactor area with a slope of -3 dB per doubling area.

Another paper from that laboratory dealt with the temporal summation in vibrotactile sensitivity VERILLO (1965b). Here Zwislocki's theory of temporal summation was tested for vibrotactile sensitivity. Vibrotactile thresholds were determined as a function of (mechanical) pulse repetition rate and pulse number for short pulses. Thresholds for various burst durations of sinusoidal signals were also determined. The results indicate that the theory is sufficient to predict vibrotactile thresholds for the temporal patterns used. The earlier findings, which suggested that glabrous skin contains at least two populations of mechanoreceptors, namely Pacinian corpuscles and free nerve endings (in hairy skin surrounding the end and middle part of the hair), were confirmed by using contactors of varying size. When the absolute threshold on the human tongue was compared to that on the hand (VERILLO 1966a–e), the results emphasized the role of the Pacinian corpuscles; the skin of the hand is richly endowed with free nerve endings which may also be sensitive to stimuli eliciting painful sensations at much higher intensity levels. Thus Pacinian corpuscles are specifically sensitive to mechanical vibrations. In another paper, threshold responses to vibratory stimuli have been compared in psychophysical and electrophysiological experiments. There was a striking similarity between the two sets of data. The hypothesis of a duplex mechanism for taction was supported and there was compelling evidence that the Pacinian corpuscle is *the*

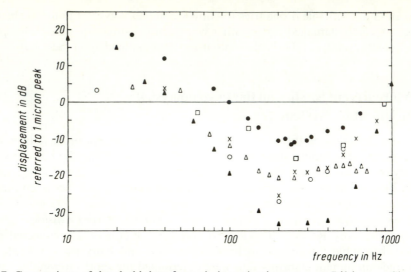

Fig. 7. Comparison of threshold data from six investigations. ▲, von Békésy; ×, Sherrick; □, von Haller-Gilmer; △, Setzepfand; ○, Hugony; ●, Verrillo. After VERRILLO (1962)

neurotransducer of vibrating stimuli. The effect of spatial parameters in the vibrotactile thresholds (1966) was object to another study by VERRILLO (1966 d), with the result that thresholds for vibration decrease in direct proportion to the extent of protrusion by the contactor (which implies the effect of the static pressure exerted on the skin by the contactor). In addition, VERRILLO found an inverse relation between thresholds and contactor area, with a slope of 3 dB per doubling of area. The threshold, however, was unaffected by changes in the gradient and curvation of the displacement of the skin but varied inversely with the number of stimulus pulses presented. An inverse proportionality exists between the threshold and the contactor area. Absolute thresholds for short pulses revealed that cutaneous mechanoreceptors summate energy increments resulting from an increase in repetition rate and in the size of the contactor. Discrepancies between measurements obtained using short pulses and sine waves could be quantitified. Those results are consistent with the hypothesis that a duplex mechanism of mechanoreception exists over most of the body surface. All this later work of VERRILLO (1962) proved the results of his "investigations of some parameters of the cutaneous threshold for vibration."

Here, sensitivity to vibration on the hand was determined as a function of frequency, contactor dimension, contactor configuration, and distance of the contactor from a rigid support. It has been found that each of these parameters affects the threshold in a different way. In the frequency range between 25 and 640 Hz, the absolute threshold as a function of frequency yielded a U-shaped curve, reaching a maximum of sensitivity in the region of 250 Hz (Fig. 7). These findings are thus in good agreement with the very early measurements in the first half of the century, although some refinement of data with regard to the geometric, temporal, and spatial parameters was added to our knowledge by the Syracuse group.

As early as 1953, the Charlottesville-Princeton group published a summarizing paper, "Variables Affecting Sensitivity of the Human Skin to Mechanical Vibration" (SHERRICK 1953). SHERRICK's hypothesis at that time was based on the assumption that the receptors sensitive to mechanical vibration do not respond selectively to frequency, and that either skin or bone tissue possesses mechanical characteristics such that it has a natural period of vibration, with maximum spread of disturbance in the frequency region of 100–300 Hz. The implications of this hypothesis are as follows:

1. If skin tissue does not have a natural period, but body tissue does, the relative sensitivities of regions such as the tongue and finger-tips should differ at various frequencies;

2. The conductivity of the skin should be maximal at the frequency of greatest sensitivity to vibration, and bony tissue should conduct vibration more efficiently than relatively bone-free areas; and

3. The mechanical impedance of tissue should be minimal at the frequency of greatest sensitivity, and the impedance of bony tissue should differ from that of tissue further removed from bone. This is supported by experimental results.

Thus the Virginia group was the first to mention the importance of the mechanical impedance and of the biophysics of the skin in general for the shape of threshold curves and the different threshold in different sites of the body. Some parts of this hypothesis were not borne out by later experimental data: this was the trigger for the Dayton group and the Erlangen group to develop the theory of frequency dispersion of skin waves and to make their influence upon the vibratory perception in man.

Later work of the Virginia group was concerned with comparison of the effects of electrical and of mechanical stimulation of the skin by vibratory stimuli. Interactions resulting from *simultaneous* electrical and mechanical vibratory stimuli have also been described, by JACK A. VERNON (1953). When stimulation was delivered to a common locus of the fingertip, this interaction led to the detection of cutaneous beats and was best produced in the narrow frequency range of about 280–310 Hz. The effect was visible as a decrease in the normal mechanically elicited threshold. Accordingly, when the two phases were presented in phase relation of 180° difference between the two types of stimulus, there was little or no departure from normal thresholds. Furthermore, the evidence showed that electrical stimuli do not stimulate the skin by first producing mechanical movements in the skin.

At the same laboratory, JAMES C. CRAIG matched loudness at a given single locus on the right hand to an increasing number of up to five vibrators on the left hand (CRAIG 1966, 1968; CRAIG and SHERRICK 1969). An increase from one to five vibrators produced a doubling (6 dB) in vibratory loudness. An example of this important result is shown in Fig. 8. Neither loudness level of the components nor distance between the vibrators had any effect on the slope of the overall loudness gross function. Finally, the specific loci stimulated did not appear to have any effect on vibrotactile loudness addition.

Another topic in psychophysics covered by the research of the Charlottesville-Princeton group was the spatial discriminations of vibrotactile patterns (GILSON 1968; CHOLEWIAK 1979; GESCHEIDER 1965). Cholewiak's results made clear that:

1. Cutaneous localization was as accurate for tonal as for noise stimuli;

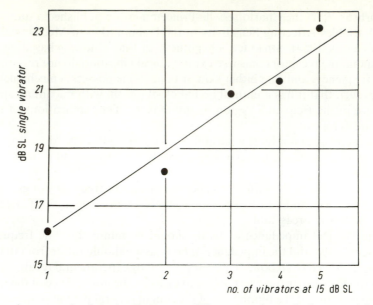

Fig. 8. Loudness match of single vibrators to different numbers of vibrators. After CRAIG (1966) and GELDARD and SHERRICK (1965)

2. Auditory localization was more precise for random noise bursts than for low-frequency tones; and
3. Cutaneous localization of low tones was a great deal more precise than auditory localization of low tones (GILSON 1968).

By means of recently designed compact electromechanical transducers BICE 1961; and GELDARD and SHERRICK 1965 were able to select bodily loci "in as spread out a fashion as possible." The more convenient finger pads, however, "have been used more for cutaneous study than any other region of the body, save for study on cutaneous pain" (VON HALLER-GILMER 1965). Moreover, nearly all attempts at cutaneous communication systems have employed the fingers (GELDARD 1966). For example, the Braille system, the numerous attempts to communicate speech through the skin (GAULT 1927 a–d; WIENER 1948); recent multidimensional skin communication systems (HIRSCH et al. 1964; FOULKE et al. 1966); and various reading devices as reviewed by NYE (1964), have all used the fingers as sites for stimulation. In view of this concentration on the hand, it was considered desirable to compare the discriminability of patterns applied to the fingers with the discriminability of patterns applied to the body. GILSON's experiments, therefore, substituted the fingertips for the ten body loci used by GELDARD and SHERRICK (1965). As a result, a comparison between the original body data and the present data confirmed the earlier data that the fingers make about 25% more errors than the body. The combination of small finger vibrators with application to noncorresponding finger sites can improve discriminability to within the range of that described by GELDARD and SHERRICK for the body (1965). CHOLEWIAK (1979), using 64 contactor vibrotactile matrices computer driven and placed on the thigh, finally succeeded

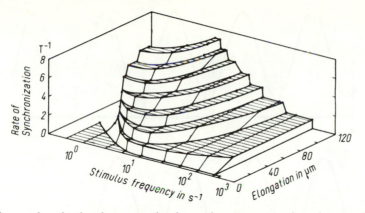

Fig. 9. The synchronization between stimulus and responses reaches plateaus *(shadowed parts of the three-dimensional plot)*. Rate of synchronization means number of spikes per period. The maximal number of responses in a train is seven. *1* in the *ordinate* corresponds to a strict one-to-one synchronization. The *two abscissae* are frequency and intensity of the sinusoidal stimuli. *Elongation* means size of bending of a vibrissa in micrometers. After NIER (1970)

in some refinement of data with regard to the relationships between active elements, their physical intensity, and the overall sensation magnitude of complex spatiotemporal patterns.

F. Electrophysiology 1970–1980

I. Encoding Processes

Apart from some more pioneering papers (e.g., FITZGERALD 1940; KEIDEL 1955–1968; HUNT 1961), the Marburg group (inaugurated by H. Hensel) has been especially active in careful studies of receptor physiology, while other groups concentrated their interest more upon the decoding part of the somesthetic channel. K. NIER at Marburg started a series of papers in 1970 using sinusoidal stimuli on the cat's vibrissae (NIER 1970, 1972, 1977). Suprathreshold sinusoidal stimulation yielded frequency- and phase-locked excitation in the afferent neurons, in full agreement with our own work.

The phase-locking principle is fairly complicated, however. It is dependent (a) on the stimulus frequency, and (b) on intensity (Fig. 9), and it seems that the increasing bending phase of the stimulus is what triggers the neuronal spike in this type of experiment.

NIER (1977) later investigated the neuronal encoding processes for sinusoidal vibrating stimuli on another animal, the catshark (*Scyliorhinus canicula*). The site of stimulation was the placoid squamas on the body surface. A special microvibrator was used for this purpose. In addition to simple sinusoids, rectangular jumps in indentation of single squamas were applied, enabling the observation of responses elicited in single afferent cutaneous fibers.

Summarizing those results in the fish, the Marburg group distinguished two submodal classes of mechanoreceptor, namely push- and pull-sensitive units. They

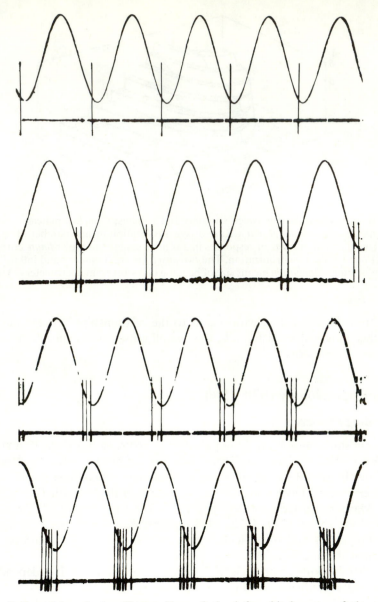

Fig. 10. Pull-sensitive single afferent fiber of the infraorbital nerve of the catshark. Frequency of sinusoidal stimuli, 0.5 Hz; elongation of microvibration of the shark's skin, 80 μm. Triggering of neuronal spikes near maximal pressure on the skin. *Top to bottom,* increasing steady additional pressure. After NIER (1977)

showed no spontaneous activity and could be activated strictly only by pushing or by pulling, especially in the push phase or in the pull phase of a rectangular deformation. Both classes of receptor revealed a differential or, more commonly, a proportional differential behavior and a slow adaptation time course of the neuronal activity.

When stimulated sinusoidally in the low-frequency range at the surface of the skin, a partial or, at higher stimulus intensities, a full synchronization of the afferent pulse pattern with the stimulus periodicity could be observed. The transformation and encoding of the stimulus intensity in single fibers was discontinuous. In the corresponding transformation function for all even pulse rates of the neural activity, plateaus of synchronization appeared. However, in a multifiber preparation a steady continuous transformation function could be obtained, indicating an encoding mechanism which can be regarded as similar to Wever's volley principle in the auditory system. Thus the stimulus intensity was represented in the neuronal pattern by the rate of pulses and the number of activated units; the stimulus frequency was represented by the synchronized pulse rate and the synchronized frequency of pulses within each train or volley.

The frequency functions showed a parallel slope at very low frequencies of the stimuli, then a slowly decreasing slope up to the best frequency between 2–20 Hz. At higher frequencies the frequency function increased very steeply.

The phase versus frequency function resulted in an increasing positive phase lag in the sense of an increasing delay between response and stimulus. At up to 10 Hz, the spikes were elicited roughly in the phase range around the maximum of the exerted pressure at the skin.

Additional static pressure yielded a lower threshold of the synchronization and a positive drift of the frequencies with respect to the synchronization. Furthermore, in this case, the steepness of the transformation functions was considerably increased both for single-fiber and multiple-fiber preparations. Also, the phase lag of triggering of responses was decreased within a given period of sinusoidal stimulation, comparable to the same effect resulting from an increase in stimulus intensity (Fig. 10).

The receptive fields were found to be very variable (areas from 0.5 up to 60 mm², with considerable overlapping. Accordingly, the spatial difference limens (DL) in the perioral region of the sharks could be measured as 8 mm², compared to a mean DL of 28 mm for the dorsolateral skin.

The activity of MOUNTCASTLE's group working at Johns Hopkins in Baltimore has focused on vibration, beginning in 1967 with the cooperation of Kornhuber as guest. In a first paper a comparison was made between the detection thresholds for oscillatory movement of the skin of the human hand and response properties of first-order myelinated mechanoreceptive afferents from the monkey hand, activated by an identical stimulus pattern. Those experiments indicate that flutter vibration is a *dual* form of mechanical sensibility, where the peripheral encoding processes are performed by two different sets of fibers. This statement was proved by counting the number of cutaneous movement detectors ($n=67$) and comparing it with the number of Pacinian corpuscles involved ($n=20$). If one plots the distribution of receptors versus the frequency of sinusoidal vibratory stimulation, then it becomes clear – in complete agreement with VON BÉKÉSY's early psychophysical measurements in man – that below 20 Hz the Pacinian corpuscles cannot account for the vibratory perception (thus explaining the break of the vibratory threshold in man). On the other hand, between 20 Hz and 300 Hz (and probably higher) Pacinian's corpuscles play an important role at least for the skin. This is shown in Table 1. Even for low intensities the neural responses are phase-locked and

Table 1. Percentages of the two populations of afferents which will be locked in phase at stimulus intensities and frequencies at which human perceive flutter vibration (Krause, top row; Pacinian, bottom row). After MOUNTCASTLE et al. (1967)

Afferent population	Frequency (cycles/s)										
	2	5	10	20	40	60	80	100	150	200	300
Cutaneous movement detectors ($n=67$)	10	27	27	34	7	3	0	0	0	0	0
Pacinian corpuscles ($n=20$)	0	0	0	0	10	30	40	25	20	15	10

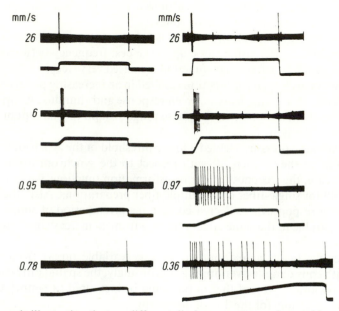

Fig. 11. Records illustrating the two different discharge patterns observed in quickly adapting mechanoreceptive afferents innervating the glabrous skin of the monkey hand. Fibers of the type the records of which are shown to the *left* display classic on–off behavior, and require a minimal rate of skin indentation at discharge threshold. Those of the type illustrated to the *right* continue to discharge so long as movement continues, at least over the range of several seconds tested experimentally. The different discharge patterns are not determined by stimulus intensity, which is here supramaximal for each fiber. *Left:* fiber-innervated receptive field on distal pad of thumb. Stimulus duration 610 ms; total skin indentation 320 μm. Stimulus slopes indicated in mm/s; critical slope was about 0.80 mm/s. *Right:* fiber-innervated receptive field on the thenar eminence. Stimulus duration 780 ms; total skin indentation 850 μm. Fibers isolated for study by microdisection of median nerves. After TALBOT et al. (1968)

frequency-following, although some periods may be omitted for responses of an isolated single afferent fiber in the monkey.

The same group elaborated fundamental discoveries and facts in their next paper (TALBOT et al. 1968). They studied 523 single fibers innervating glabrous skin of the monkey hand. The results obtained appeared to be of a highly complex type: On one side there were fibers of a more or less on–off type when either steady stim-

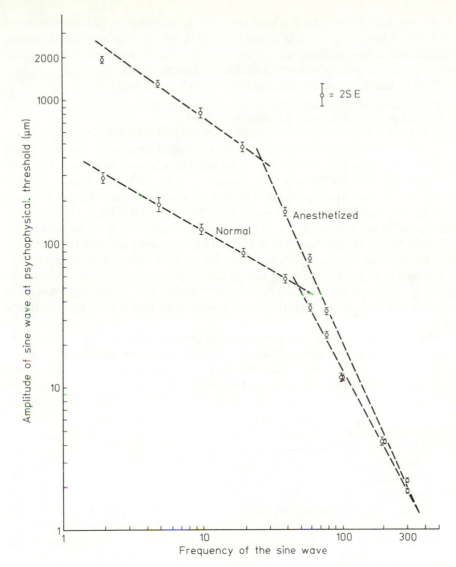

Fig. 12. Relation between the amplitude of a sine wave oscillatory movement of the skin and the human threshold for the perception of movement, at a series of different frequencies. Stimuli delivered to the glabrous skin of the thenar eminence of the hand. Points on the graphs are the means for ten observers. Cutaneous anesthesia by cocaine iontophoresis elevated the thresholds for perception of low-frequency stimuli (2–40 cycles/s) by factors of 5–10; sensitivity to high-frequency oscillation was little affected by skin anesthesia. The *SE* *bars* on the graphs refer to the total dispersion of all observations by all subjects. Dissociation by cutaneous anesthesia of the double-limbed threshold function suggests that the sense of flutter vibration on the hand is served by two sets of primary afferents, one terminating in the glabrous skin, the other in deeper tissues. After TALBOT et al. (1968)

uli or ramp-like stimulation was used (Fig. 11). A second class of fiber responded to a steady stimulus (a constant indentation) with an ongoing burst and to ramps with a slowly adapting firing rate. Thus the entire ensemble under research could be separated into quickly adapting and slowly adapting fibers.

With respect to the receptors the classification was threefold:

1. Superficial receptors located within the skin, adapting quickly;
2. Superficially located receptors, adapting slowly; and
3. Single or small clusters of Pacinian corpuscles located in deep tissues.

A further consideration was the frequency range of sinusoidal stimuli to which the fibers were sensitive. In the case of the quickly adapting movement detectors with fiber diameters (in the median nerve) of 5–12 µm, the best frequencies of their tuning curves were at circa 30 Hz. The slowly adapting fibers showed a steady periodic discharge frequency when modulated by sinusoidal stimuli at between two and ten cycles per second. Those two groups could easily be distinguished under light anesthesia (psychophysically in man). This procedure elevated the threshold for the second group (the slowly adapting fibers) by a factor of 5–10, leaving the first group (the quickly adapting fibers) nearly unaltered (Fig. 12). Finally, the third population, innervating the Pacinian corpuscles, were exquisitely sensitive to oscillating stimuli in the high-frequency range, with best tuning points around 250 Hz.

MOUNTCASTLE'S group also compared the single-fiber studies in monkey with psychophysical measurements of human threshold curves obtained from the corresponding areas of the glabrous skin. It turned out that the quickly adapting fibers covered the low-frequency part of the human threshold curve, while the Pacinian corpuscle fibers revealed tuning curves fitting the high-frequency part of the human threshold curve. Quite correspondingly, in the typical sensation associated with the stimulation by sinusoids starting at very low frequencies and ending at high frequencies, a clear change in the quality and subjective localization was elicited insofar as the low-frequency range originated some sort of flutter vibration rather than ordinary vibration. The flutter vibration could be observed in the frequency range below 40–80 Hz; between 40–80 Hz there was a transient range. Above those frequencies (80–300 Hz) clearer vibratory sensations could be felt, with an optimum sensitivity between 200–300 Hz, in accordance with the findings of all other observers. Moreover, the site of sensation changed too: the lower-frequency range, with a flutter vibration sensation, was felt in the skin itself; the high-frequency range, in contrast, was localized clearly in the deeper tissue, with a sensation of vibratory hum. Therefore, some attempt has been made to establish the distinction of three different groups of afferent fibers which would correspond to force- (indentation-), pressure-, and acceleration-sensitive afferents (JOHNSON et al. 1975, 1980 a, b). Whether those three groups, however, would be identical with the slowly adapting fiber (2–10 Hz), the quickly adapting fiber (best frequency 30 Hz), and the Pacinian (best frequency 250 Hz) groups is still an open question. A summary of the results of this careful study is given in Table 2.

The MOUNTCASTLE group has been able to make guesses as to what type of receptor would feed the three types of afferent with information about the vibratory stimulation of the glabrous skin. They assert that:

Table 2. Mechanoreceptors ending in joint capsules and ligaments and in periosteum and deep tissue. A small proportion of the movement detectors behave differently as slope changes. After TALBOT et al. (1968)

Class	Size (μ)	Peripheral termination	Receptive field	Adaptive properties	Dynamic sensitivity
QA movement detectors	5–12	Dermal ridges of glabrous skin	Small, continuous, graded. Activation by traveling waves limited to 5-mm surround	QA on–off type response to steady stimuli. Require liminal slope for activation	Exquisitely sensitive to oscillating stimuli in low-frequency range. Best tuning points ca. 30 cycles/s
Slowly adapting movement and intensity detectors	5–12	Dermal ridges of glabrous skin	Small, continuous, graded. Precise detectors of variations of intensity	Onset transient a function of slope. Succeeding periodic discharge a function of intensity	Steady periodic discharge frequency modulated by sinusoidal stimuli in 2–10 cycles/s range
Pacinian afferents movement detectors	5–12	Single or small cluster of Pacinian corpuscles, sub-dermal and deep tissues	Point of greatest sensitivity, but field is unlimited. Activated by traveling waves from great distances	QA on–off type response to step stimuli. Require liminal slope for activation	Exquisitely sensitive to oscillating stimuli in the high-frequency range. Best tuning points ca. 250 cycles/s

QA, quickly adapting

1. Meissner's corpuscles are related to the quickly adapting fibers (10–60 Hz).
2. The slowly adapting fibers (2–20 Hz) are served by Merkel's disks, both situated within the skin itself.
3. There is a much smaller number in the underlying tissue, and these are very sensitive to high-frequency components of mechanical stimuli delivered anywhere within a very wide receptive field. They may be entrained to discharge one impulse per cycle by high-frequency (100–400 Hz) mechanical sinusoids, and are therefore thought to terminate peripherally in the Pacinian corpuscles of the subcutaneous and deep tissues.
4. There are afferents which innervate the joint capsules and ligaments, and which are sensitive to the speed and direction of joint movement and to steady joint position.
5. There is a class of afferents terminating in fascia and periosteum which have never been studied in detail. (Afferents from muscle and mechanoreceptive fibers less than 6 μm in diameter are not included in this classification, all other four classes having fiber diameters greater than 6 μm).

II. Cortical Decoding Processes for Vibratory Stimuli

Extensive data on this topic have been collected by MOUNTCASTLE's group. They recorded (MOUNTCASTLE et al. 1969) from the postcentral gyrus from single neuronal units of an unanesthetized monkey on sites where the projection fibers for the hand end mainly across areas 1 and 3. The goal was a comparison between the human capacity to detect oscillatory mechanical stimuli delivered to the glabrous skin of the hand and the pattern of nerve impulses evoked by them in first-order mechanoreceptive afferents. Typical records revealed regularly periodic trains of nerve impulses at the cortical level, corresponding to the appearance of similar trains in certain sets of the driving afferents elicited by sinusoidal stimuli. One example of a record from a single cortical neuron is shown in Fig. 13.

It was concluded that the perception of movement of the skin depends upon the appearance of these trains. It was therefore postulated that discrimination between stimuli of different frequency would depend on a cortical mechanism which "measures" the length of the periods in the input trains (with or without some demultiplicative process occurring in deeper layers of the somesthetic channel).

Earlier studies by the same group suggested that what is commonly regarded as the sense of vibration is (at least) dual in nature (see above). The existence of two sets of primary afferents was considered to underlie these two sensibilities. They are differentially sensitive in the low- and high-frequency ranges, but otherwise show similar dynamic responses. Quickly adapting and Pacinican corpuscle fibers examined in single-fiber studies in the median nerve would be the neurophysiological correlates to the two (psychophysically measurable) sensations, flutter vibration and normal vibration. Now, the results can be classified into neural mechanisms operating in low-frequency flutter sensibility and those operating in high-frequency vibratory sensibility. For the first class, the flutter sensibility, the evidence cited suggests that the glabrous quickly adapting set of cortical neurons receives input from the quickly adapting afferent fibers, which are thought to end in Meissner's corpuscles. A marked degree of specificity of action in the lemniscal component of the somatic afferent system would play a leading role in the periodicity analysis for the low-frequency sensibility. The periodic entrainment of the cortical units cascaded from periphery to cortex. Consequently, a synchronized, periodic discharge in multiunit recordings from first-order fibers *and* cortical

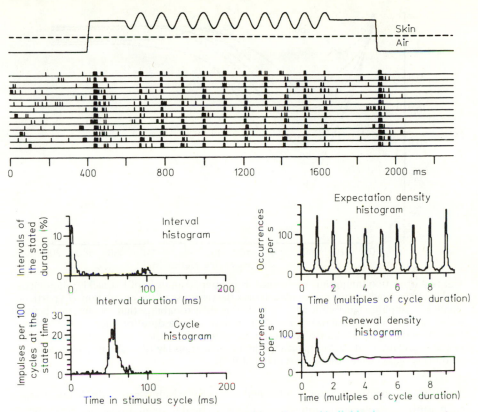

Fig. 13. Composite showing stimulus pattern replicas of several individual responses and examples of the four basic methods of analysis. Stimulus pattern and impulse train replicas share the same time base *(top)*. The stimulus probe is initially in the air above the skin, is moved to indent the skin 560 μm (a fixed value), and then after a 200-ms delay set into sinusoidal movement for a period of 1 s. After a further 300 ms delay the probe is removed from the skin. Typically, this pattern is repeated 16 times at a rate of one presentation each 5 s before the sine wave frequency and/or amplitude is changed. All other parameters are fixed. Transient discharges at onset and removal of the step stimulus are typical of quickly adapting neurons. For the histogram analysis only data collected during actual sinusoidal stimulation are used. Note that the period of the stimulating sine wave is approximately 105 ms. This defines the rightmost meaningful bin in the cycle histogram and has been used as the time mark in the expectation and renewal density histograms in order to emphasize the regularity of the amplitude modulation seen therein. The multiple discharge seen in the impulse train replicas is characteristic of the response to very low frequency sinusoidal stimulation. It obscures the representation of the period of the stimulating sine wave and its subharmonics, which are frequently seen in interval histograms. After MOUNTCASTLE et al. (1969)

neurons suggests a match between the range of frequencies to which the first-order fibers are sensitive and the "band pass" of the serially arranged synaptic transfer, from about 5 Hz to about 100 Hz. The best frequencies of the system appeared to be set at about 30–40 Hz, encoded at the periphery (Fig. 14).

Intensity functions for the quickly adapting cortical neurons differ markedly from those obtained at the periphery. So at 5–6 dB above threshold (best frequency

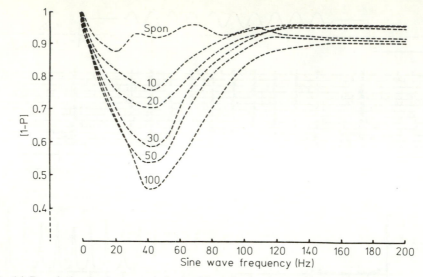

Fig. 14. Population tuning curves obtained from interval analysis of 13 quickly adapting cortical neurons. Each tuning curve characterizes the response of the population to a particular sine wave amplitude as frequency is varied. P is the probability that any interval between nerve impulses of any one member of the population has a duration equal to the period of the sine wave ($\pm 20\%$). *Curves* reveal that at all intensities there is a better representation of the stimulating sine wave frequency when it is near 40 Hz than at frequencies above or below this value. After Mountcastle et al. (1969)

30–40 Hz) a peripheral fiber is entrained perfectly, discharging a single impulse for each stimulus cycle. In the quickly adapting cortical neuron, however, the sequence of events with further increases in stimulus amplitude is a smooth and monotonic increase in the overall frequency of discharge and in the degree of periodicity.

The obvious periodic ordering of discharge pattern therefore seems to be a necessary requirement for the detection of flutter in the glabrous quickly adapting neurons of the postcentral gyrus. It is possible to identify three classes of cortical neuronal element: the thalamocortical fibers; the thin spikes discharged by stellate cells of layer IV and lower layer III; and the regular cortical neurons (largely pyramidal cells). It has been found that the degree of linkage of peripheral fibers, and thus the degree of periodic entrainment, is successively decreased through these three stages. Thus, the change from the abrupt tuning of peripheral fibers to the *gradually* increasing periodicity of the response of central elements to increasing stimulus intensity occurs at the first synapse in the system (namely in the dorsal column nuclei). The depth for quickly adapting cortical neurons is heavily biased toward the middle layers of the cortex.

Similarly important results were obtained by the same group for the neural mechanisms in high-frequency vibratory sensibility (60–400 Hz). This system is driven by the Pacinian afferents. The Pacinian afferent cortical neurons (6% of the postcentral neurons) receive their information from the 9% fibers of the periphery which end up in Pacinian corpuscles. The thalamocortical fibers and the thin spikes of the Pacinian afferent class (areas 1 and 3) can be entrained to periodic discharge over the full range of Pacinian sensitivity (Fig. 15).

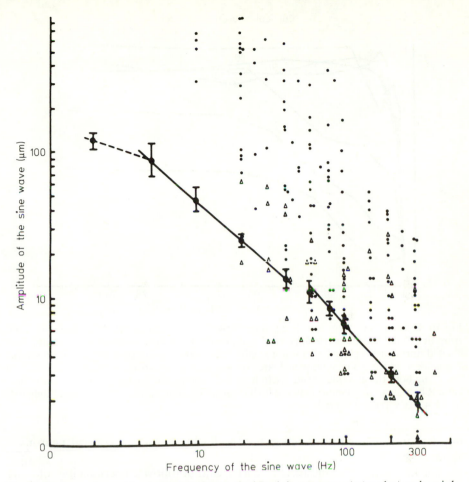

Fig. 15. A comparison of tuning points for cortical Pacinian neurons *(triangles)* and peripheral Pacinian fibers *(dots)*, with the human fingertip frequency–intensity threshold function *(heavy black lines)*. *Each triangle* represents the half-maximal point on an intensity function like those of Fig. 16. *Each dot* represents the lowest stimulus amplitude at which a given peripheral fiber responded with one impulse per stimulus cycle. The fact that the cloud of points (peripheral and cortical) overlaps the high-frequency limb of the psychophysical function, and not the low-frequency limb, supports the contention that high-frequency vibration is a separate sense from low-frequency flutter. After MOUNTCASTLE et al. (1969)

The overall frequency of discharges – in contrast to the intensity function of quickly adapting cortical neurons – rises abruptly to a high plateau at intensities slightly above tuning. Regular cortical neurons of the Pacinian afferent class show a periodic discharge evoked at any stimulus frequency above 100 Hz. The observation that periodic discharges can be elicited in thalamocortical fibers proves that the limiting stage in frequency transmission is at the subsequent intracortical synapses. Up to that level serially linked Pacinian afferent elements can transmit periodic activities up to 300 Hz, indicating a remarkable synaptic security of subcortical pathways leading to the postcentral gyrus. For comparison with the quickly adapt-

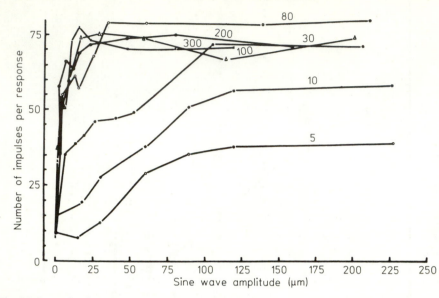

Fig. 16. Intensity functions at several frequencies for a regular cortical cell receiving input from first-order Pacinian afferents. *Each point* marks the average number of nerve impulses elicited during a 1-s period of sinusoidal stimulation at a certain frequency and amplitude. *Points* derived for a single frequency are connected by *lines* labeled with that frequency in Hz. Note both the extreme sensitivity to high frequencies and the fact that response counts cannot be used to distinguish between high frequencies at any given stimulus amplitude. After MOUNTCASTLE et al. (1969)

ing neurons an intensity function for the Pacinian afferent cortical neurons is shown in Fig. 16.

The fact that the unanesthetized cortex cannot follow up periodicities of more than, about, 100 Hz is well known in the physiology of the auditory system. It has also long been known that the auditory nerve activity in a frequency-following type can periodically be driven up to 5 kHz. Nevertheless, some speculations along this line by the group under discussion need more detailed criticism. Of great interest in the connection is the discussion (MOUNTCASTLE et al. 1969) on the neural mechanisms in frequency discrimination for vibratory stimulation of the somesthetic system. Psychophysical data agree that the frequency discrimination capacity in both the quickly acting and the Pacinian-afferent-driven parts is of the same magnitude as the DL for intensity in all sensory modalities, roughly at 10%. GOFF (1967) gave psychophysical data: at middle intensities of stimulation he found for 25 Hz a DL for frequency of 4 Hz (some 18%) and for 200 Hz, 60 Hz (30%) in man. MOUNTCASTLE's comment is:

In the case of frequency discrimination we assume for the purpose of analysis that those sensory events are the observer's estimate of the cycle length of the stimulus, based on his inspection of the periodicities in the postcentral neural discharge. We did find that these two distributions – that of neural events observed experimentally in monkeys and that of behavioural events in man – varied together under two circumstances: changes in frequency and changes in sine-wave amplitude.

Human performance seems to be better, and analyses of the discharges of thalamocortical fibers (rather than cortical neurons themselves) match estimates on humans better than cortical neurons, too. MOUNTCASTLE mentions that his human subjects were conscious of the experimental procedure, while somnolent monkeys were not.

Discrimination in the frequency domain in vibration depends on the Pacinian system. MERZENICH and HARRINGTON (1969) found that there is no decrease in the capacity for frequency discrimination after complete local anesthesia of the glabrous skin, leaving the deep Pacinian corpuscles intact. Two high-frequency stimuli (200 and 250 Hz) engage slightly different populations of cortical neurons because of the differences in mechanical coupling to the tissues and the spatial summation, working for the Pacinian system, not for the quickly acting neurons. This might be quite comparable to the place theory of hearing and to Tunturi's tonotopic principle. Secondly, Pacinian neurons of the second somatic area might possess significantly greater capacity for frequency.

In a later paper, LaMOTTE and MOUNTCASTLE (1975) found DLs for frequencies in the flutter range (around 30 Hz) in the order of 5%–8% (2 Hz) in monkeys' neural responses (primary fibers with Meissner's endings) and of those in trained human subjects. This discussion is indeed of considerable importance for the problems involved in constructing cochlear implants in general.

One more point made by MOUNTCASTLE's group touches the intensity function of *populations* or quickly-acting cortical neurons. Thus the smooth monotonic, negatively accelerating intensity function of glabrous quickly-acting cortical neurons can be explained on the basis of a gradual recruitment of (successively less sensitive) fibers into the population of active first-order fibers, which converge upon such neurons. In addition, a limited spatial as well as this intensive recruitment may provide an explanation of the subjective magnitude function (MOUNTCASTLE et al. 1969).

Finally, in Table 3 (LaMOTTE and MOUNTCASTLE 1975) there is a summary of all the results of MOUNTCASTLE's group concerning the peripheral encoding and cortical decoding mechanisms for certain aspects of the sense of flutter vibration on the basis of comparative behavioral studies in monkeys and in man. The DL for intensity was of the order of 10%, as normal for all sensory modalities; the DL for frequencies was 1.8 Hz for humans and 2.7 Hz for monkeys in the low-frequency range for middle intensities.

Studies on somatosensory-evoked potentials to vibratory stimuli are numerous. We would like mention just two papers of the Kornhuber group in Ulm. In one (JOHNSON et al. 1975), they delivered vibratory stimuli as sinusoids of 250 Hz with 50 and 200 μm indentation to the middle finger knuckle of 15 human subjects. When comparing the cortical evoked potentials and psychophysically obtained magnitude estimations (plotting both functions on a log-log scale following S. S. Stevens) they found that only the large, components of the evoked cortical potentials showed significant correlation to the stimulus intensity. The same was true for ramp indentations (JOHNSON et al. 1980 b). The group stated, however, that it was unlikely that there was a specific correlation between them. It is interesting to mention that ELBERLING et al. (1980) recorded the magnetic field on the human brain with special emphasis upon the auditory evoked potentials. He found a clear

Table 3. Attempt to specify the peripheral and central neural codes thought to be operative in the sense of flutter, for the detection of a mechanical sinusoidal in the frequency range of that submodality in frequency and amplitude discriminations, and in subjective magnitude estimations. Those codes marked with an asterisk are thought to be established with reasonable certainty; those marked with a question mark are considered to be reasonable inferences from the information available. After LaMotte and Mountcastle (1975)

Psychophysical event	Peripheral neural code	Central neural code
Identification: flutter or vibration?	* Place code: which set of peripheral fibers is active	* Place code: which set of cortical neurons shows an increment in activity
Detection of flutter	* Place plus frequency code: appearance of any activity in Meissner afferents	* Place plus frequency code: increment in activity in set of postcentral cortical neurons on which Meissner afferents project
Frequency discrimination	* Place plus temporal order code: appearance of tuned discharges in some small number of Meissner afferents	* Place plus temporal order code: increase above a certain minimal level of cyclic entrainment of activity of that set of postcentral cortical neurons exclusively activated by Meissner afferents
Subjective magnitude estimation	* Place and spatial distribution code: linear increase in size of population of Meissner afferents activated by stimulus	? Place and spatial distribution code: linear growth in size of population of cortical cells in which increments of activity occur
Amplitude discrimination	? Place and spatial distribution code: differences in size of active population of Meissner afferents in two cases discriminated	? Place and spatial distribution code: differences in size of population of cortical cells with incremented activity in two cases

specific correlation in that modality and was able to prove that the site of these potentials was clearly the primary projection areas of the human cortex. This was in contradiction of the conventional galvanic electrical findings, on the basis of which a number of authors asserted the vertex to be the nonspecific origin of auditory evoked potentials. This throws new light upon an article by our group about the specifity of the late components and of the perstimulatory dc shift of the compound evoked potentials in man (Keidel 1970, 1975).

The early deflections of the vibratory evoked responses in man are claimed (Johnson et al. 1975) to be well localized over the contralateral postcentral hand area. The late components resemble the α-rhythm in wavelength and in distribution over both hemispheres, just as the auditory evoked potentials.

Neuronal cortical responses to stimuli delivered to the cat's whiskers have been reported in three papers (Hellweg 1978 a, b; Hellweg et al. 1977) by Creutzfeldt's group in Göttingen. Neurones in the somatosensory cortex of unanesthetized restrained cats were recorded during single trapezoid and repetitive sinusoidal dis-

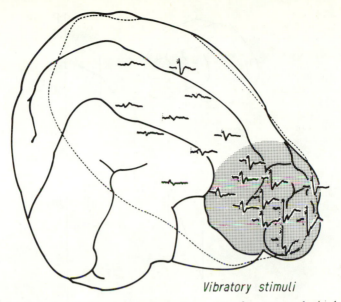

Vibratory stimuli

Fig. 17. Distribution of evoked responses from the cortex of an unanesthetized cat (35 implanted electrodes). Little more than the somesthetic projection areas SI and SII *(cross-hatched area)* are excited by mechanical vibratory stimulation of the cat's paw (burst of 200 Hz). After VON KIETZELL (1971)

placement of single vibrissae. During repetitive mechanical stimulation cortical cells showed adaptive behavior, so that at higher stimulation frequencies the number of cell discharges per stimulus cycle decreased. The one to one ability to follow the repetition of the stimulus was lost between 20 and 60 Hz. On–off type responses to trapezoidal stimuli and typical quickly adapting time functions have been obtained. Similarly, MCINTYRE et al. (1967) in Clayton, Australia recorded cortical responses to impulses from single Pacinian corpuscles in the cat's hind limb.

The *site of cortical projection* for vibratory stimuli elicited from the foot pad of the unanesthetized cat (glabrous skin) has been studied by our group (VON KIET-ZELL 1971) using sinusoidal (and partially rectangular) stimuli ranging between 10 and 1,000 Hz. Particular preference was given to a burst of 200 Hz (trapezoid time course), using 2-ms rise and fall times, the burst lasting for 80 ms. The stimulus site contained high densely packed Pacinian corpuscles in the underlying tissue (GRAY and MATTHEWS 1951). As early as 1940, ADRIAN proved the double representation of that site of the cat's feet in the primary and secondary projection area of the cortex. Averaging technique was used for the evoked corticograms by our group. Repetition rate was 1 per 3 s; 50 and 100 responses were measured. Thirty-five implanted electrodes (V2A steel; 0.2 mm Ø) were positioned epidurally across the cat's head. To avoid auditory evoked potentials the cava tympani were filled. The complete exclusion of the auditory system was controlled by measuring the evoked potentials above the auditory projection areas simultaneously. This procedure proved to be decisive for a concise statement about the cortical distribution across the cat's cortex. The spatial distribution thus obtained is shown in Fig. 17.

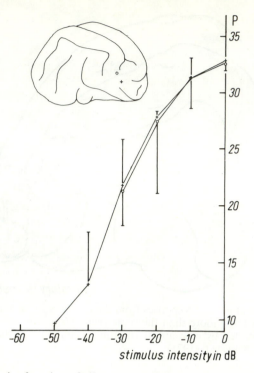

Fig. 18. Typical intensity function of vibratory evoked potential (epidural) from the awake cat. Site of records indicated. *Ordinate,* potential (*P*) N_{30}–P_{60} (linear size). After VON KIET-ZELL (1971)

This work – in contrast to that of other observers – shows clearly the restriction of projection to areas SI and SII in the cat's unanesthetized brain.

The same group studied the cortical intensity functions in the same animals, as shown in Fig. 18. The exponents of Steven's power function were measured carefully and showed a negative acceleration for high intensities only (between 40 and 50 dB). For low intensities (up to 35–40 dB) the mean for *n* of the power functions was between 0.35 and 0.42 ± 0.05 for all 100 intensity functions measured. Individual functions varied considerably inter- and intraindividually when contra- and ipsilateral measurements were compared.

G. Later Research on Vibratese Language

Modern devices for vibratese language are manifold: if one divides them into (a) mechanical, (b) electromechanical, and (c) electrical types (meaning that stimuli of these types are delivered to the skin), then one can describe them as follows.

FRANK GELDARD, the main pioneer of the topic, organized and chaired a very stimulating conference about that goal in Monterey, California, in 1973. Mechanical systems with direct speech mediation began with GAULT's (1926a, b) "speaking tube" and leading to the Teletactor. Vocoder-type systems were inaugurated more theoretically by NORBERT WIENER (1949, 1951) at MIT. GUELKE and HUYSSEN'S

(1959), PICKETT and PICKETT's (1963), KRINGLEBOTN's (1968), and WITCHER and WASHINGTON's (1956) research in that field followed. The use of VON BÉKÉSY's model for the same purpose was brought into discussion by BIBER's (1961) thesis on the work of the Erlangen group (KEIDEL 1961), and was improved by myself (KEIDEL 1968), FINKENZELLER (1973, 1980), and DOLAN et al. (1978).

Pictorial displays started with COLLINS' tactile television system in 1970. Electroftalm was developed by STARKIEWICZ and KULISZEWSKI (1963). Standford Research Institute, California (BLISS et al. 1970), reached best results with the Optacon. This is a direct optical-to-tactile-converting reading aid for the blind, which quantifies an area roughly the size of a letter space into 144 black and white image points (24 rows and 6 columns) and displays the image points on a corresponding array of 144 vibrators. The performance of users depends upon the reading rate, reaching 70% correct alphabetic recognition at 12 words per minute. For 30 words per minute tracking speed, the correct recognition rate drops to less than 50% correct recognition. Final accuracy percentages are above 60%.

Another group of vibratese language procedures used coded languages: Vibratese (GELDARD 1960), Body Braille (GELDARD 1970), Optohapt (GELDARD 1966), Polytap (GELDARD and SHERRICK 1972), air-blast symbols (BLISS et al. 1966), and Visotactor (SMITH and MAUCH 1968) show the eminently productive role in the development of such devices of the Charlottesville-Princeton group of FRANK GELDARD and CARL SHERRICK. Also in this class, braille and its derivatives, finger spelling (BEST 1943), and string writing must be mentioned. The technique of tracking and monitoring uses vibrators and air jets on hands or forehead as information mediator (HILL 1970, 1973; HOWELL 1960; BLISS et al. 1970). Electromechanical devices and an electrostatic "textured" matrix have been used by STRONG and TROXEL (1970) and others.

Electrical application of the stimuli to the skin as a direct speech mediation system has been used by WIENER (1951) and LINDNER (1936) in the Vocoder type of vibratese. Simple dermal electrodes have been applied by LINDNER (1936), DUPONT (1907), and by BREINER (1968). Coded languages expressed by means of direct electrical stimulation have been devised (Katakama by FOULKE and STICHT 1966). International Morse (FOULKE and BRODBECK 1968) and "electrocutaneous Vibratese" (FOULKE et al. 1966) have been introduced. Tracking and monitoring using single multiple electrodes on fingers, arms, legs, or neck have been described by HOFMAN and HEIMSTRA (1972) and by LOEB and HAWKES (1962). Electrical pictorial display has finally been included in the Tactile TV, Electroftalm, and Optacon.

Our own group has published research performed on vibratese languages in several papers and review articles. We gave special attention to the possible application of the basic principles of vibratese to electrical stimulations of the completely deaf ear (besides the application to the skin of the forearm both mechanically and electrically.)

H. The Cochlear Model in Skin Stimulation

If one compares the auditory and the vibrotactile systems as was first done by GEORG VON BÉKÉSY, it can be seen that there are two main differences: the intensity

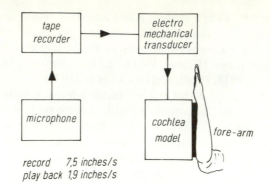

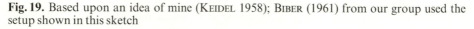

Fig. 19. Based upon an idea of mine (Keidel 1958); Biber (1961) from our group used the setup shown in this sketch

range and the frequency range. While the intensity range for the auditory system is of the order of 130 dB, that for the vibrotactile system is only about 35 dB from threshold to the useful upper limit. The frequency range in the auditory system covers a bandwidth of some 18 kHz for the young subject. The vibrotactile system has its upper frequency limit somewhere between 400–500 Hz. The reason for this difference is clearly that the vibrotactile system is the more primitive one, the auditory system the more sophisticated one. More specialized functional characteristics have been developed by the latter system in the course of evolution. Biber, working at our Institute in 1961, could show that there was a third important difference between the two sensory systems, namely the poor memory of the vibrotactile system compared with the highly developed one of the auditory system. In seeking to feed information into the vibrotactile system in an optimal manner, one should consider these differences.

As I have reported previously (Keidel 1958, 1968), our own approach toward the transmission of maximum information to the skin was based on the following considerations. The hair cells of the inner ear react differently from the receptors of the skin in two respects:

1. The important frequency range for speech received by the ear is 300–3,000 Hz, while vibratory receptors are best stimulated by frequencies in the range of 40–400 Hz.
2. The time for full development of sensation after onset of a stimulus is 0.18 s for the ear and about 1.2 s for the skin.

Furthermore, the auditory system is specialized for great accuracy in frequency discrimination. The DL for auditory frequency discimination is optimally of the order of 0.2%; that for the vibratory system does not fall below 5%–10%. This deficiency on the part of the somesthetic system can be overcome by transforming frequency differences into spatial differences, which are readily discriminated by the somesthetic system. Von Békésy showed how such a transformation might be accomplished. He designed and constructed a tactile model of the inner ear; the model operated in a frequency range that is optimal for vibratory perception. By storing speech on magnetic tape and displaying it eight times more slowly in speed, it should, according to our thinking, also be possible to enlarge the time for vibratory perception by the same factor. Attaching the von Békésy model to the

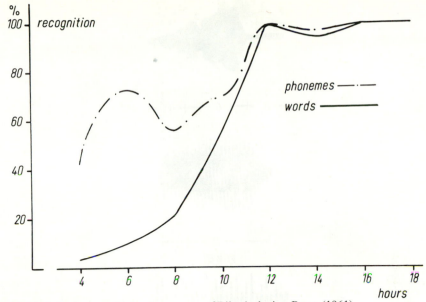

Fig. 20. Training curves obtained by means of Biber's device. BIBER (1961)

forearm of a human subject, BIBER (1961) trained people at our laboratory to recognize three types of monosyllabic words. The three types differed in terms of
frequency range: very low, middle, and very high. In addition, BIBER slowed down
the speed of the type between recording and playback not only by a ratio of 1:8,
but also by other ratios, such as 1:4 and 1:2. Considering the loss of transmitted
information due to poor tactile memory, and also considering the fact that physically, the information processing should be best at a ratio of 1:8, it becomes clear
that somewhere between 1:1 and 1:8 the best performance should be reached by
our technique of producing vibratese language. The optimal ratio was found experimentally by BIBER to be 1:4. His setup is shown in Fig. 19. After this fact was
established, training was continued only at the ratio of 1:4, using endless tape loops
with known syllables and, later, words made up of the three different frequency
bands, as described above. By means of this technique, it was possible in 18 hours
to train inexperienced people to recognize 83% of unknown words correctly
through the skin, and after 32 hours training, practically 100% correct answers
were given to unknown words. Examples of the learning curves are shown in Fig.
20. It is obvious that the advantage of this technique is the adequate type of stimulation in combination with the utilization of the cutaneous neural network structure of the skin.

On the other hand, this technique contains serious disadvantages, which must
be discussed. It is well known that the different modalities of the human sensory
systems as a whole usually act together. For any type of information transmission
– not only for speech transfer systems – the brain uses a combination of visual,
auditory, tactile, gustatory, and olfactory stimuli simultaneously to recognize a
given change in environmental conditions. This can be performed well only when

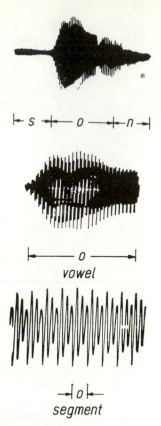

Fig. 21. Time course of speech signal for the word "son." The vowel "o" is dilated in time to show the redundancy in speech. After KUSCH (1971)

identical timing for the different sensory modalities is used. Our technique, however, is not compatible with this demand, since the speed of tactile information transfer used is four times slower than the speed of information transfer in the other sensory modalities. This makes lipreading or simultaneous use of visual speech techniques impossible. For a pilot in an aircraft, relatively slow vibrotactile information would clearly confuse the even more important incoming information from visual and auditory signals. This statement was clearly emphasized by experiments which we performed on deaf people during the 1960s.

Working with VON BÉKÉSY's cochlea model in real time, therefore, we looked for possibilities of transformation in the frequency domain, while avoiding a change in the time domain. While doing so, we found a very interesting similar problem in the auditory system.

KUSCH (1971) described a new method of improving voice quality in an atmosphere containing helium by technologically performing a similar task; by namely, transforming speech frequencies to lower bands in real time. He summarizes his work as follows:

At great depths beneath the surface of the ocean only a helium atmosphere can be used for respiration. Since such an atmosphere has a considerably increased velocity of sound the

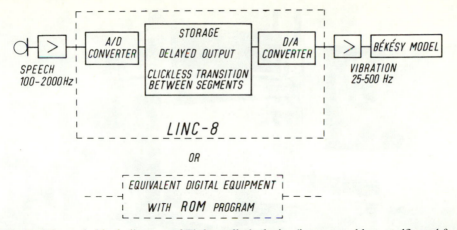

Fig. 22. Schematic block diagram of Finkenzeller's device (inaugurated by myself) used for our new type of vibratese language on the basis of von Békésy's cochlea model. The frequencies are transformed in a ratio of 4:1 by means of a special computer program. The vibratory frequencies thus obtained from spoken words in the auditory frequency range are fed into VON BÉKÉSY's model in real time. KEIDEL (1974)

spoken words become unintelligible. An on-line method is proposed which processes the spoken information in such a way that intelligibility is reestablished. The method makes use of the fact that a sound is characterized by a segment which is repeated several times. Each second segment is selected by means of a computer and dilated in time. The output waveform is the sequence of the dilated segments. A prototype apparatus converts speech disturbed by the helium atmosphere in an intelligible form.

KUSCH's discovery that speech, like most daily life information, is highly redundant can obviously be used to effect the frequency transformation needed for vibrotactile application. In Fig. 21 this redundancy for a spoken sound is shown for the phoneme "o". Our modification of his device described above is demonstrated schematically in Fig. 22.

If one tries to generalize this concept to all kinds of repetitive complex time patterns by which, for special purposes, the skin might be stimulated, one should look for some small computer program which would enable one to feed any type of information to the VON BÉKÉSY model. The sole restriction would be the condition that the time pattern with which the model is fed must contain considerable redundancy, a condition which, however, is obviously fulfilled for human speech, the most complex time pattern we know. It thus seems possible to use the general idea of this special program for nearly all types of vibrotactile signal: sinusoids, trains of pulses, etc.

Now what have been the experimental results? I shall confine myself to FINKENZELLER's work done at our laboratory during recent years. He used our LINC-8 computer in combination with the VON BÉKÉSY model in the way shown in Fig. 23, using a program which he developed, named FRQ. The result, shown as the output to the vibrator, is demonstrated for a single sinusoidal tone of 500 Hz. This tone is then reduced to 124 Hz. The original frequency range (100–2,000 Hz) is thus reduced automatically to 25–500 Hz for the VON BÉKÉSY model. Thus far the realization of the basic idea – transfer of frequencies in a ratio of 4:1 in real time – seems

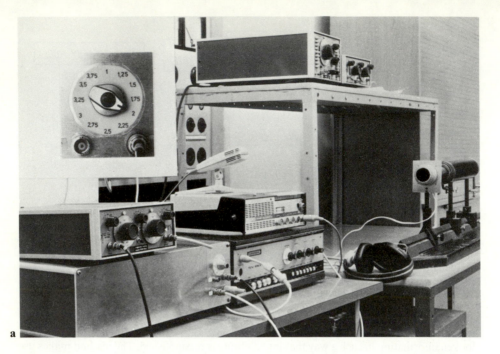

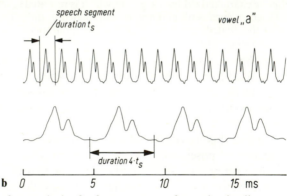

Fig. 23. a Setup for our device for frequency transformation in vibratese. *Left top,* the switch for setting the rate of frequency transformation can be seen. *Below,* the microcomputer used. *Right in the background* the von Békésy model is located. For details see KEIDEL (1981). Setup and program developed by FINKENZELLER 1980. **b** Frequency transformation of the vowel "a" by a factor of 4:1 using the setup shown in Fig. 23 a. The information typical for the given vowel "a" remains in the lower-frequency range in the real time domain. After KEIDEL (1974) and FINKENZELLER (1980)

to be relatively easy. In addition, this technique can be used for any type of very complex stimulus, as in speech. This is shown in Fig. 24 for typical vowels and consonants.

However, there was one difficulty which had to be eliminated. The time series at the output of the system consists of equal time divisions which have been combined sequentially by the computer. This sequence of 50/s was felt very clearly by

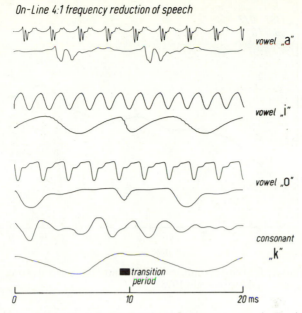

Fig. 24. Application of the setup shown in Fig. 23 to human speech. Typical examples for the vowels "a," "i," and "o" and for the consonant "k" are shown. *Each upper trace* represents the original language, *each lower trace*, the output to VON BÉKÉSY's model. KEIDEL (1974)

the VON BÉKÉSY model. Such unwanted periodicity was very disturbing to the perception of the actual information to be transmitted as a signal via the skin. Since for complex patterns phase-locking – the easiest solution – could not be applied for general purpose use, a special part of the final program allowed a smooth transition period between each two segments. This program, therefore, fortunately works for all input frequencies between 100 and 2,000 Hz and their combinations, so that in the final version of the program no unwanted periodicity at all can be felt at the forearm. The reason for this is that the absolute time of the transition period is too brief to be felt by the skin. This new system for the use of VON BÉKÉSY's model for information transfer through the skin is now under investigation. The preliminary results are very promising because: (a) it now works in real time; (b) tactile memory is not overloaded; and (c) vibrotactile information can be combined with that from other sensory modalities simultaneously without any interference with the timing (in contrast to the case with the BIBER-type application of the model).

A completely different approach is at present being developed, however. FIN-KENZELLER has built an electronic model of the basilar membrane, which will be reported elsewhere. This model was originally conceived for the audio frequency range; it was to be used in combination with an additional model imitating the neuronal network of both the auditory and vibrotactile systems simply by changing the frequency parameter and the type of interconnection between the outputs of the artificial basilar membrane and the first-order neuronal layer.

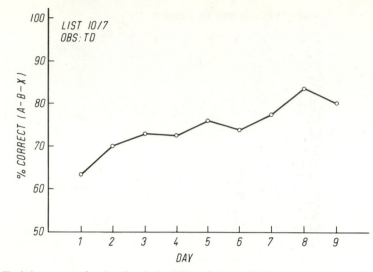

Fig. 25. Training curves for the discriminability of monosyllabic words perceived in real time via the von Békésy model. Dolan et al. (1978)

Compatibility with the physiological frequency dispersion of the hydrodynamics of the inner ear is evident. Up to 64 outputs of the model can be used simultaneously in conjunction with 64 separate vibrators when the frequency parameter is changed to that of vibratory stimuli (25–500 Hz). Thus spatial discrimination is preprocessed by the model as in the ear, and will be improved (a) by some electronic network simulating lateral inhibition of the receptors, and (b) by the natural network of the skin of the forearm, which in turn enlarges the gradient between every two sites of vibratory stimulation. Therefore, using this device, the performance of the von Békésy model in its ability to transform temporal into spatial distributions is considerably improved electronically. On the other hand, the temporal pattern of the input stimuli is fully available, as in audition for periodicity hearing.

Data obtained in 1978 and published in 1979 (Dolan et al. 1978) used the frequency transformation technique up to a ratio of 1:4. During the experiments single monosyllabic words, stored either in a computer or on magnetic tape, were transformed and presented to the observer via the vibrotactile transducer (the von Békésy model). The observer sat inside a soundproof chamber with his arm resting on the ramp of the model (in order to eliminate acoustic artifacts) while noise was presented through headphones during the course of each data-collecting session.

The first experiment, the results of which are indicated in Fig. 25, involved the use of an A-B-X paradigm to measure the discriminability of monosyllabic words. As a reminder, the A-B-X paradigm involves the presentation of three words on each trial–word A, word B, and word X. Word X is a repeat of either A or B, and the observer's task is to determine whether word X was A or B. The stimuli were words randomly selected from the W-22 list of 200 monosyllabic words published by Hirsh (1952). The words were not normalized in any manner and were paired in a random fashion from trial to trial. The only feedback provided the observer was the percentage of correct estimates at the end of every 50 trials. Each data point indicates the overall percentage of correct estimates each day: 250 trials were run daily. As indicated, performance generally improved during the 9 days summarized on the slide. An analysis of the data, however, suggested that some of the pairings were easily discriminated even in the first few days, while other pairings remained difficult even after 9 days. I should add, after reading a paper by PICKETT and PICKETT (1963), that the word X was not simply a recording of word A or B, but a fresh utterance of the word. PICKETT and PICKETT found a significant difference in discrimination scores depending on whether single or fresh utterance was employed.

After the initial training on the A-B-X paradigm, a series of experiments was conducted to determine the dynamic range of the tactile system, using the same device and the spectral content utilized in the discriminations. The results of these experiments were similar to those that have already been reported – the dynamic range was approximately 40 dB and only very low frequencies were used.

The advantage of the frequency transformation procedure is obvious, since in contrast to BIBER's use of the VON BÉKÉSY model the spoken words can now be fed into the skin in *real time,* while the older technique could be performed only with a considerable time expansion by a factor of at least 4. Now the training curves reach nearly 90% correct answers, as they did with BIBER's technique, but the real time presentation allows additional application of spoken word information by means of other sensory modalities, such as visual lipreading. The main disadvantage, however, is the problem that consonants do not have the same degree of redundancy as vowels do, so that information is lost by the frequency transformation procedure (DOLAN et al. 1978).

At the present time, therefore, the Erlangen group is working on a multichannel tactual display utilizing a set of vibrators (piezoelectric ceramics) in which each element conducts information from different spectral regions. Further, artificial means of increasing the discriminability are being considered. For example, it may be possible to add acoustic information to the waveforms to be perceived, improving the perception of the consonants.

I. Similarities Between Skin Sensation and Hearing

The idea of comparing vibration and hearing systematically to gain better understanding of the auditory system stems from the Nobel prizewinner GEORG VON BÉKÉSY. His own research began very early, simultaneously with his research and experimentation on the auditory system. However, he placed more and more emphasis on this part of his research as he gained more experience in general. His classic work in this field gained topical interest in connection with the efforts in the 1960s to try to build "artificial ears" or "cochlear implants" for completely deaf people and for the severely hearing-impaired. With the improvement of electronic techniques, especially the miniaturization of computers from space technology, it becomes possible to construct small devices to be surgically implanted near man's cochlea. These prostheses were able to preprocess information for the remainder of the auditory channel.

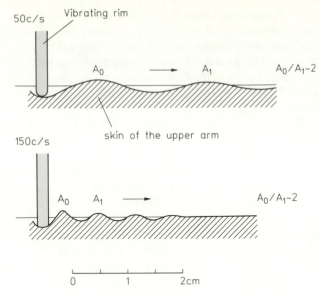

Fig. 26. Traveling waves at the surface of the skin elicited by the vibrating rim indicated in the drawing at frequencies of 50 Hz *(top)* and at 150 Hz *(bottom)*. The ratio of the maxima of dislocation A_0/A_1 following each other can be observed to be in the order of 2. VON BÉKÉSY (1955)

When the cochlea is degenerate, the neuronal pathway of audition and the somesthetics of vibration prove to have very similar capabilities, even for stimuli as complex as those necessary for conveying speech signals to the decoding systems of the human brain.

VON BÉKÉSY himself was mainly concerned with four subtopics:
1. The principle of lateral inhibition, inherent in all sensory modalities;
2. Interactions between intensity and frequency of vibratory stimuli and their effect on perceived pitch;
3. The problem of how, by including the neuronal part of the vibratory system, the human brain is able to measure the degree of synchrony and periodicity of neuronal signals to the projection areas of the brain; and
4. Similarities between the traveling waves in the cochlea and those in the skin.

Since his work now is of a classic type, this cannot be the place to describe all his manifold and ingenious experiments in detail. The interested reader is referred to the original literature. Numerous papers were published, mainly in the Journal of the Acoustical Society of America *(JASA)* and in psychological journals, and two monographs, *Experiments in Hearing* VON BÉKÉSY (1960) and *Sensory Inhibition* VON BÉKÉSY (1967). I will restrict myself to just one typical example of each of the four mentioned subtopics of his interest in this field. Actually, VON BÉKÉSY (1959c) wrote a review article on exactly this topic, "Similarities Between Hearing and Skin Sensation."

In Fig. 26 one example of each of the two types of traveling wave, here for the skin, is shown for two frequencies, for sinusoidal vibrations of 50 and 150 Hz. The type of traveling wave running along the basilar membrane in the cochlea is well known and needs no explanation, since its equation as a Bessel function is now well

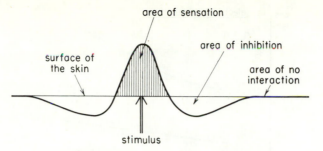

Fig. 27. The area of sensation originated by a vibratory stimulus is surrounded by a ring-like concentric area of inhibition. VON BÉKÉSY (1959 b)

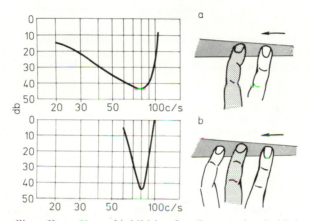

Fig. 28 a, b. Funnelling effect of lateral inhibition for vibratory thresholds in man compared for the two cases **a** when two fingers and **b** when three fingers touch a vibrating rim. Vibratory thresholds are measured psychophysically. VON BÉKÉSY (1961 c)

established. Neural funneling, originating in the principle of lateral inhibition, is demonstrated for the skin in Figs. 27 and 28.

The underlying idea is a convergence–divergence type of fiber connection between the successive relay stations, both for the somesthetic (WERNER and MOUNT-CASTLE 1965) and the auditory channels. This network is similar in principle to that within the retina of the eye, which has been long known to be due to the horizontal cell layer situated within it. The so-called physiological contrast in the eye is thus clearly comparable to the process of funneling, both in the auditory system and in the somesthetic channel.

Finally, the observation presented in Fig. 29 touches on the last subtopic above. Curves of equal pitch sensation can be obtained by matching frequency and intensity to identical pitch sensations elicited by mechanical vibrations on the human skin. Thus, for example, the same pitch can be elicited by a sinusoidal stimulus 10 dB above threshold at 100 Hz, or by another stimulus 40 dB above threshold and at a frequency of 135 Hz.

This gave rise to profound questions about the underlying neurophysiological pitch detection abilities of the decoding systems of the brain. When a given number

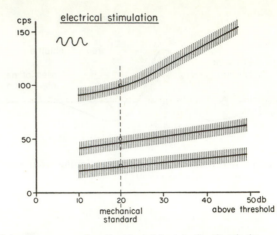

Fig. 29. Match of the frequency of a vibratory (electrical) stimulation and its intensity. The *three curves* describe curves of equal pitch sensation. Thus, for example, a stimulus of 20 dB at 100 Hz is felt equally to a stimulus of 40 dB at 135 Hz. VON BÉKÉSY (1957b)

of signals reaches, say, the cortical area SI, running through the described complex network of neuronal connections between all relay nuclei, then a given large number of spikes can be originated by a high intensity of more or less random time course; or it can be originated by more or less periodic trains of signals, with sections of high and low pulse density within the corresponding time course. Two types of sensation, pitch, and magnitude, are thus conveyed by one type of signal only. The decisive and essential information for the brain stems only from the degree of the synchronization of the signals to the periodicity of the stimulus. This is true for both systems, the skin and the ear. Things are even more complex, since there exists a spatial distribution too, and therefore temporal and spatial interactions take place until finally the time course of the signals within an ensemble of neurons at cortical level is made up by the entire sensory channel.

Although only a few examples of VON BÉKÉSY's work[1] could be discussed here in detail, they may be able to prove the great importance of this type of research for a better understanding of the more primitive type of mechanoreception, vibration, and for techniques of feeding auditory speech signals into the remainder of the auditory channel (in the case of a complete loss of hair cells or auditory nerve fibers in severely hearing-impaired patients).

---

1 These and similar experiments by VON BÉKÉSY gave rise to quite a lot of experiments by other scientists, especially the Princeton group. All those experiments led to FRANK GELDARD's (1982) important discovery of the "rabbit phenomenon." FRANK GELDARD writes in his abstract of that review: When temporally restricted and spatially separated stimuli excite the skin, systematic mislocations of some magnitude are likely to occur. This phenomenon, sensory saltation, is reviewed from its discovery to the present. Experiments designed to reveal the general characteristics of saltation, its distribution over the integument, and the possible underlying neural mechanisms responsible for it are described. Close analogs in vision and audition are shown to exist. Finally, directions for research needed in the future are indicated

References

Names containing *von* are alphabetized in this list under *v*

Adrian ED (1926) The impulses produced by sensory nerve-endings, part I. J Physiol (Lond) 61:49–72

Adrian ED (1940) Double representation of the feet in the sensory cortex of the cat. J Physiol (Lond) 98:16P

Best H (1943) Deafness and the deaf in the United States. MacMillan, New York

Biber KW (1961) Ein neues Verfahren zur Sprachkommunikation über die menschliche Haut. Dissertation, Universität Erlangen

Bice RC (1961) Electromechanical transducer for vibrotactile stimulation. Rev Sci Instrum 32:856–857

Bing R (1910) Über Vibrationsgefühl und Skelettsensibilität. Korresp Bl Schweiz Ärzte 1:2–9

Bliss JC, Crane HD, Mansfield PK, Townsend JT (1966) Information available in brief tactile presentations. Percept Psychophys 1:273–283

Bliss JC, Katcher MH, Rogers CH, Shepard RP (1970) Optical-to-tactile image conversion for the blind. IEEE Trans MMS 11:58–65

Breiner HL (1968) Versuch einer elektrokutanen Sprachvermittlung. Z Exp Angew Psychol 15:1–48

Cholewiak RW (1979) Spatial factors in the perceived intensity of vibrotactile patterns. Sens Processes 3:141–156

Coermann RR (1962) The mechanical impedance of the human body in sitting and standing position at low frequencies. Hum Factors 4:227–253

Collins CC (1970) Tactile television-mechanical and electrical image projection. IEEE Trans MMS 11:65–71

Craig JC (1966) Vibrotactile loudness addition. Percept Psychophys 1:185–190

Craig JC (1968) Vibrotactile spatial summation. Percept Psychophys 4:351–354

Craig JC, Sherrick CE (1969) The role of skin coupling in the determination of vibrotactile spatial summation. Percept Psychophys 6:97–101

Déjerine J (1914) Sémiologie des affections du système nerveux. Citation from: Echlin FA, Fessard A (eds) (1938) Synchronized impulse discharges from receptors in the deep tissues in response to vibrating stimulus. J Physiol 93:312–334

Dolan TR, Finkenzeller P, Keidel WD (1978) Vibrotactile encoding of speech signals. J Acoust Soc Am 63:80

Dunlap K (1911) Palmesthetic difference sensibility for rate. Am J Physiol 29:108–114

Dunlap K (1913) Palmesthetic beats and difference tones. Science 37:532–535

DuPont M (1907) Dur des courants alternatifs de périodes variées correspondant à des sons musicaux et dout les périodes des mêmes rapports que les sons; effects physiologiques de ces courants alternatifs musicaux rythmés. C R Seances Acid Sci [III] 144:336–337

Egger M (1899) De la sensibilité ossense. Journal de Physiolog et de Pathol génerale I a, 511–520

Elberling C, Bak C, Kofoed B, Lebech J, Saermark K (1980) Magnetic auditory responses from the human brain. Scand Audiol 9:185–190

Fessard A (1937) Quelques suggestions apportées par la physiologie au problème du sens vibratoire. Année Psychol 38:22

Finkenzeller P (1973) Hypothese zur Schallcodierung des Innenohres. Habilitationsschrift, Universität Erlangen

Finkenzeller P (1980) Auditory prostheses – a challenge for neurophysiology. Audiology 19:176–187

Fitzgerald O (1940) Discharges from the sensory organs of the cat's vibrissae and the modification in their activity by ions. J Physiol (Lond) 98:163–178

Foulke E, Brodbeck AA Jr (1968) Transmission of Morse code by electrocutaneous stimulation. Psychol Rec 18:617–622

Foulke E, Sticht TG (1966) The transmission of the katakana syllabary by electrical signals applied to the skin. Psychologia 9:207–209

Foulke E, Coates G, Alluisi EA (1966) Decoding of electrocutaneous signals: effects of dimensionality on rates of information transmission. Percept Mot Skills 23:295–302

Franke EK (1951) Mechanical impedance measurements of the human body surface, AF technical report no 6469. United States Air Force, Wright Air Development Center, Wright-Patterson Air Force Base, Dayton, Ohio

Franke EK, von Gierke H, Oestreicher HL, von Wittern WW (1951) The propagation of surface waves over the human body, AF technical report no 6464. United States Air Force, Wright Air Development Center, Wright-Patterson Air Force Base, Dayton, Ohio

Frucht AH (1953) Die Schallgeschwindigkeit im menschlichen und tierischen Gewebe. Naturwiss 39:491–492

Gault RH (1926a) Control experiments in the relation to identification of speech sounds by aid of tactual cues. J Abnorm Soc Psychol 21

Gault RH (1926b) Touch as substitute for hearing in the interpretation and control of speech. Arch Otolaryngol 3:121–135

Gault RH (1927a) Hearing through the sense organs of touch and vibration. J Franklin Inst 204:329–358

Gault RH (1927b) Fingers instead of ears. Welfare Magazine

Gault RH (1927c) On the upper limit of vibrational frequency that can be recognized by touch. Science 65:403–404

Gault RH (1927d) On the identification of certain vowel and consonantal elements in words by their tactual qualities and by their visual qualities as seen by the lip-reader. J Abnorm Soc Psychol 22

Gault RH, Goodfellow LD (1933) Eliminating hearing in experiments on tactual reception of speech. J Gen Psychol 9:223–234

Geldard FA (1960) Some neglected possibilities of communication. Science 131:1583–1588

Geldard FA (1966) Cutaneous coding of optical signals: the Optohapt. Percept Psychophys 1:377–381

Geldard FA (1970) Vision, audition, and beyond. In: Neff WD (ed) Contributions to sensory physiology, vol 4. Academic, New York, pp 1–17

Geldard FA (1982) Saltation in somesthesis. Psychol Bull 92:136–175

Geldard FA, von Haller Gilmer B (1934) A method for investigating the sensitivity of the skin to mechanical vibration. J Gen Psychol 11:301–310

Geldard FA, Sherrick CE (1965) Multiple cutaneous stimulation: the discrimination of vibratory patterns. J Acoust Soc Am 37:797–801

Geldard FA, Sherrick CE (1966–1981) Princeton cutaneous research project. Reports no 5–37, University of Princeton, Princeton

Gescheider GA (1965) Cutaneous sound localization. J Exp Psychol 70:617–625

Gilson RD (1968) Some factors affecting the spatial discrimination of vibrotactile patterns. Percept Psychophys 3:131–136

Gilson RD (1969) Vibrotactile masking: some spatial and temporal aspects. Percept Psychophys 5:176–180

Goff GD (1967) Differential discrimination of frequency of cutaneous mechanical vibration. Journal of Experimental Psychology 74:294–299

Goldscheider A (1904) Über das Vibrationsgefühl. Berl Klin Wochenschr 14:353–356

Goldstein M (1926) Practical demonstrations of modern pedagogic methods in training the deaf child. Laryngoscope 36:31–42

Goodfellow LD (1933) Sensitivity of finger tips to tactile stimulation. J Franklin Inst 216:387–392

Goodfellow LD (1934) The sensitivity of various areas of the body to vibratory stimuli. J Gen Psychol 11:435

Grandis V (1902) Sur la perception des impressions tactiles. Arch Ital Biol 37:96–116

Gray JAB, Matthews PBC (1951) Adaptation of Pacinian corpuscle. J Physiol (Lond) 114:454

Gridley PF (1932) The discrimination of short intervals of time by finger tip and by ear. Am J Psychol 44:18–43

Guelke RW, Huyssen RMJ (1959) Development of apparatus for the analysis of sound by the sense of touch. J Acoust Soc Am 31:799–809

Hellweg FC (1978 a) Complex functional properties of cortical whisker cells. In: Brazier MAB, Petsche H (eds) Architectonics of the cerebral cortex. Raven, New York, pp 385–391

Hellweg FC (1978 b) Responses of cells in the somatosensory cortex of unanaesthetized cats after sinusoidal displacements of single vibrissae. J Comp Physiol 125:29–35

Hellweg FC, Schultz W, Creutzfeldt OD (1977) Extracellular and intracellular recordings from cat's cortical whisker projection area: thalamocortical response transformation. J Neurophysiol 40:463–479

Herzog F (1906) Über das Vibrationsgefühl. Dtsch Z Nervenheilk 31:96–107

Hill JW (1970) A describing function analysis of tracking performance using two tactile displays. IEEE Trans MMS 11:92–101

Hill JW (1973) Limited field of view in reading letter shapes with the fingers. In: Geldard F (ed) Cutaneous communication systems and devices. Psychonomic Society, Austin

Hirsch J, Shafer JH, Eitan A (1964) Experiments in tactile communication. 6th Ann. Aviat. Astronaut., Tel Aviv and Haifa, 410–468

Hirsh IJ (1952 a) Certain temporal factors in audition. Science 116:523

Hirsh IJ (1952 b) The measurement of hearing. McGraw-Hill, New York

Hoagland H (1935) Pacemakers in relation to aspects of behaviour. MacMillan, New York

Hofman MA, Heimstra NW (1972) Tracking performance with visual, auditory, and electrocutaneous displays. Hum Factors 14:131–138

Howell WC (1960) On the potential of tactile displays: an interpretation of recent findings. In: Hawkes GR (ed) Symposium on cutaneous sensitivity, USAMRI rep no 424, pp 103–113

Hugony A (1935) Über die Empfindung von Schwingungen mittels des Tastsinns. Z Biol 96:548–553

Hunt CC (1961) On the nature of vibration receptors in the hind limb of the cat. J Physiol (Lond) 155:175–186

Johnson D, Jürgens R, Kongehl G, Kornhuber HH (1975) Somatosensory-evoked potentials and magnitude of perception. Exp Brain Res 22:331–334

Johnson D, Jürgens R, Kornhuber HH (1980 a) Somatosensory-evoked potentials and perception of skin velocity. Arch Psychiatr Nervenkr 228:95–100

Johnson D, Jürgens R, Kornhuber HH (1980 b) Somatosensory-evoked potentials and vibration. Arch Psychiatr Nervenkr 228:101–107

Kampik A (1930) Experimentelle Untersuchungen über die praktische Leistungsfähigkeit der Vibrationsempfindung. Arch Psychol 76:3

Katz D (1923) Über die Natur des Vibrationssinns. M M W 70:706–708

Katz D, Noldt F (1925–1926) Über die kleinsten vibratorisch wahrnehmbaren Schwingungen. Z Psychol 99:104–109

Keidel WD (1955) Aktionspotentiale des N. dorsocutaneus bei niederfrequenter Vibration der Froschrückenhaut. Pflügers Arch 260:416–436

Keidel WD (1956) Vibrationsreception. Der Erschütterungssinn des Menschen. Erlanger Forsch Reihe B2

Keidel WD (1958) Note on a new system for vibratory communication. Percept Mot Skills 8:250

Keidel WD (1961) Grundprinzipien der akustischen und taktilen Informationsverarbeitung. Ergeb Biol 25:213–246

Keidel WD (1968) Electrophysiology of vibratory perception. In: Neff WD (ed) Contributions to sensory physiology, vol 3. Academic, New York

Keidel WD (1970) Speaking as a neurophysiologist: what do we really know about the human cortical averaged potential after all? Ist International symposium of the ERA group, Freiburg, 1–4 April 1970

Keidel WD (1974) The cochlear model in skin stimulation. In: Geldard F (ed) Conference on vibrotactile communication. Psychonomic Society, Austin

Keidel WD (1975) Simultaneous computation of ECG, early response and ERA. International ERA study group, Biennial symposium, London, 28–30 July 1975

Keidel WD (1981) Physiological background of hearing prostheses. In: Syka J, Aitkin L (eds) Neuronal mechanisms of hearing. Plenum, New York

Keidel WD, Keidel UO, Kiang NYS, Frishkopf L (1958) Time course of adaptation of evoked response from the cat's somesthetic and auditory system. Q Prog Rep Res Lab Electron MIT 48:121

Keidel WD, Keidel UO, Kiang NYS (1960) Peripheral and cortical responses to mechanical stimulation of the cat's vibrissae. Arch Int Physiol Biochim 68:241–262

Knudsen VO (1928) Hearing with the sense of touch. J Gen Psychol 1:320–352

Kringlebotn M (1968) Experiments with some visual and vibrotactile aids for the deaf. Am Ann Deaf 113:311–317

Kusch H (1971) Ein neues Verfahren zur Verbesserung der Sprache in Heliumatmosphäre. Acustica 25:42–46

LaMotte RH, Mountcastle VB (1975) Capacities of humans and monkeys to discriminate between vibratory stimuli of different frequency and amplitude: a correlation between neural events and psychophysical measurements. J Neurophysiol 38:539–559

Lindner R (1936/1938) Physiologische Grundlagen zum elektrischen Sprachetasten und ihre Anwendung auf den Taubstummenunterricht. Z Sinnesphysiol 67:114–144

Loeb M, Hawkes GR (1962) Detection of differences in duration of acoustic and electrical cutaneous stimuli in a vigilance task. J Psychol 54:101–111

McIntyre AK, Holman ME, Veale JL (1967) Cortical responses to impulses from single Pacinian corpuscles in the cat's hind limb. Exp Brain Res 4:243–255

Merzenich MM, Harrington T (1969) The sense of flutter-vibration evoked by stimulation of the hairy skin of primates: comparison of human sensory capacity with the response of mechanoreceptive afferents innervating the hairy skin of monkeys. Exp Brain Res 9:236–260

Mountcastle VB, Powell TPS (1959) Neural mechanisms subserving cutaneous sensibility, with special reference to the role of afferent inhibition in sensory perception and discrimination. Bull John Hopkins Hosp 105:201–232

Mountcastle VB, Talbot WH, Kornhuber HH (1966) The neural transformation of mechanical stimuli delivered to the monkey's hand. In: de Reuck AVS, Knight S (eds) Touch, heat, and pain (a Ciba Foundation symposium). Churchill, London

Mountcastle VB, Talbot WH, Darian-Smith I, Kornhuber HH (1967) Neural basis of the sense of flutter-vibration. Science 155:597–600

Mountcastle VB, Talbot WH, Sakata H, Hyvärinen J (1969) Cortical neuronal mechanisms in flutter-vibration studied in unanesthetized monkeys. Neuronal periodicity and frequency discrimination. J Neurophysiol 32:452–484

Nier K (1970) Transformationscharakteristik von Vibrissenreceptoren bei sinusförmiger Reiz-Zeitfunktion. Dissertation, University of Marburg/Lahn

Nier K (1972) Phasenfrequenzgang neuraler Impulsmuster von Vibrissenrezeptoren. Pflügers Arch 334:357–366

Nier K (1977) Neurale Afferenz cutaner Mechano- und Thermoreceptoren bei Selachiern. Dissertation, University of Marburg/Lahn

Nier K, Hensel H, Bromm B (1976) Differential thermosensitivity and electric prepolarization of the ampullae of Lorenzini. Pflügers Arch 363:181–185

Nye PW (1964) Reading aids for blind people – a survey of progress with the technological and human problems. Med Electron Biol Enging 2:247–264

Pearson GHJ (1928) Effect of age on vibratory sensibility. Arch Neurol 20:482

Pfaffmann C (1939) Afferent impulses from the teeth due to pressure and noxious stimulation. J Physiol (Lond) 97:207–219

Pickett JM, Pickett BH (1963) Communication of speech sounds by a tactual Vocoder. J Speech Hear Res 6:207–222

Ranke OF (1931) Die Gleichrichter-Resonanztheorie. Habilitationsschrift. J.F. Lehmann, München

Ranke OF (1950) Theory of operation of the cochlea. J Acoust Soc Am 22:772–777

Roberts WH (1932) A two-dimensional analysis of the discrimination of differences in the frequency of vibrations by means of the sense of touch. J Franklin Inst 213:283–310

Rumpf HTM (1889) Über einen Fall von Syringomyelie nebst Beiträgen zur Untersuchung der Sensibilität. II. Neurol Centralblatt 8:222–230

Rydel, Seiffer (1903) Untersuchungen über das Vibrationsgefühl oder die sogenannte „Knochensensibilität" (Pallästhesie). Arch Psychol 37:488

Setzepfand W (1935) Zur Frequenzabhängigkeit der Vibrationsempfindung des Menschen. Z Biol 96:236–240

Sherrick CE Jr (1953) Variables affecting sensitivity of the human skin to mechanical vibration. J Exp Psychol 45:273–282

Smith GC, Mauch HA (1968) The development of a reading machine for the blind. Summary report VA prosthetic and sensory aids service

Starkiewicz W, Kuliszewski T (1963) Active energy reading systems: the 80-channel Electroftalm. In: Clark LL (ed) Proceedings of international congress technology Blindness, vol I. American Foundation for the Blind, New York, pp 157–166

Strong RM, Troxel DE (1970) An electrotactile display. IEEE Trans MMS 11:72–79

Talbot WH, Darian-Smith I, Kornhuber HH, Mountcastle VB (1968) The sense of flutter-vibration: comparison of the human capacity with response patterns of mechanoreceptive afferents from the monkey hand. J Neurophysiol 31:301–334

Treitel L (1897) Über das Vibrationsgefühl der Haut. Arch Psychiatr Nervenkr 29:633–640

Valentin G (1847) Lehrbuch der Physiologie des Menschen, Bd. 1 und Bd. 2. F. Viehweg & Sohn, Braunschweig

Valentin G (1848) Lehrbuch der Physiologie des Menschen. Bd. 2. 2. Abhandlung. F. Viehweg & Sohn, Braunschweig

Valentin G (1852) Über die Dauer der Tasteindrücke. Arch Physiol Heilkunde 11:438–587

Vernon JA (1953) Cutaneous interaction resulting from simultaneous electrical and mechanical vibratory stimulation. J Exp Psychol 45:283–287

Verrillo RT (1962) Investigation of some parameters of the cutaneous threshold for vibration. J Acoust Soc Am 34:1768–1773

Verrillo RT (1965a) The effect of number of pulses on vibrotactile thresholds. Psychon Sci 3:73–74

Verrillo RT (1965b) Temporal summation in vibrotactile sensitivity. J Acoust Soc Am 37:843–846

Verrillo RT (1965c) Vibrotactile threshold and pulse polarity. Psychon Sci 3:171

Verrillo RT (1966a) Specificity of a cutaneous receptor. Percept Psychophys 1:149–153

Verrillo RT (1966b) Vibrotactile sensitivity and the frequency response of the Pacinian corpuscle. Psychon Sci 4:135–136

Verrillo RT (1966c) Taction thresholds for short pulses. Psychon Sci 4:409–410

Verrillo RT (1966d) Effect of spatial parameters on the vibrotactile threshold. J Exp Psychol 71:570–575

Verrillo RT (1966e) Vibrotactile thresholds for hairy skin. J Exp Psychol 72:47–50

von Békésy G (1939a) Über die Vibrationsempfindung. Akust Z 4:315–334

von Békésy G (1939b) Über die Empfindlichkeit des stehenden und sitzenden Menschen gegen sinusförmige Erschütterungen. Akust Z 4:360–369

von Békésy G (1955) Human skin perception of traveling waves similar to those on the cochlea. J Acoust Soc Am 27:830–841

von Békésy G (1957a) Sensations on the skin similar to directional hearing, beats, and harmonics of the ear. J Acoust Soc Am 29:489–501

von Békésy G (1957b) Neural volleys and the similarity between some sensations produced by tones and by skin vibrations. J Acoust Soc Am 29:1059–1069

von Békésy G (1959a) Synchronism of neural discharges and their demultiplication in pitch perception of the skin and in hearing. J Acoust Soc Am 31:338–349

von Békésy G (1959b) Neural funneling along the skin and between the inner and outer hair cells of the cochlea. J Acoust Soc Am 31:1236–1249

von Békésy G (1959c) Similarities between hearing and skin sensations. Psychol Rev 66:1–22

von Békésy G (1960) Experiments in hearing. McGraw-Hill, New York

von Békésy G (1961a) Pitch sensation and its relation to the periodicity of the stimulus. Hearing and skin vibrations. J Acoust Soc Am 33:341–348 von Békésy G (1961 b) Concerning the fundamental component of periodic pulse patterns and modulated vibrations observed on the cochlear model with nerve supply. J Acoust Soc Am 33:888–896

von Békésy G (1961 c) Über die Gleichartigkeit einiger nervöser Prozesse beim Hören und Vibrationssinn. Proceedings of the 3rd international congress for acoustic. Elsevier, Amsterdam, pp 13–20

von Békésy G (1967) Sensory inhibition. Princeton University Press, Princeton

von Frey M (1894) Beiträge zur Physiologie des Schmerzsinns. Berichte Königlich Sächsischer Gesellschaft der Wissenschaften, Leipzig, 46:283–296

von Frey M (1911) Die Wirkung gleichzeitiger Druckempfindungen aufeinander. Z Biol 56:574

von Frey M (1914) Beobachtungen an Hautflächen mit geschädigter Innervation. Z Biol 63:335–376

von Frey M (1915) Physiologische Versuche über das Vibrationsgefühl. Z Biol 65:417–427

von Frey M (1926) Die Tangoreceptoren des Menschen. In: Bethe A, Bergmann GV, Embden G, Ellinger A (Hrsg.) Rezeptionsorgane I. Springer, Berlin (Handbuch der normalen und pathologischen Physiologie, XI)

von Gierke HE (1950) Measurement of the acoustic impedance and the acoustic absorption coefficient of the surface of the human body. AF Technical Report no 6010. United States Air Force, Wright Air Development Center, Wright-Patterson Air Force Base, Dayton, Ohio

von Gierke HE, Oestreicher HL, Franke EK, Parrack HO, von Wittern WW (1952) Physics of vibrations in living tissues. J Appl Physiol 4:886–900

von Haller-Gilmer B (1935) The measurement of the sensitivity of the skin to mechanical vibration. J Gen Psychol 13:42–61

von Haller-Gilmer B (1937) The relation of vibratory sensitivity to pressure. J Exp Psychol 21:456–463

von Haller-Gilmer B (1965) Some problems in cutaneous communications research. Report no 6, U.S. Public Health Service Grant, Project HBO 2020, Carnegie Institute of Technology, May 1965

von Helmholtz H (1909) Handbuch der physiologischen Optik, 3rd edn. Voss, Leipzig

von Kietzell HR (1971) Vibratorisch evozierte Hirnrindenpotentiale bei der wachen Katze. Dissertation, University of Erlangen

von Wittich W (1869) Bemerkungen zu Preyers Abhandlung über die Grenzen des Empfindungsvermögens und Willens. Pflügers Arch 2:329

Weber EH (1846) Der Tastsinn und das Gemeingefühl. In: Wagner (Hrsg.) Wörterbuch der Physiologie, Bd. 3. Vieweg, Braunschweig

Werner G, Mountcastle VB (1965) Neural activity in mechanoreceptive cutaneous afferents: stimulus-response relations, Weber functions, and information transmission. J Neurophysiol 28:359–397

Wever EG (1949) Theory of hearing. Wiley, New York

Wiener N (1948) Cybernetics. Wiley, New York

Wiener N (1949) Sound communication with the deaf. Philos Sci 16:260–262

Wiener N (1951) Problems of sensory prosthesis. Am Math Soc Bull 57:27–35

Witcher CM, Washington L (1956) Vocatac (sensory replacement project). Q Prog Rep Res Lab Electron MIT January:133–137, July:66–68, October:118–121

CHAPTER 16

Fifty Years of Vestibular Science

OTTO LOWENSTEIN

A. Introduction

This chapter on the foundations of vestibular science will focus attention on the historical and technological factors which have operated in the advance of the subject during the past five decennia.

Parts 1 and 2 of Vol. 6 of the *Handbook of Sensory Physiology* (KORNHUBER 1974a, b) deal with the present state of knowledge concerning form and function of the vestibular system, and it will therefore be not only economical but also reasonable to use their contents as the basis of fact and theory for the treatment of the subject here. This applies especially to the wealth of illustrations enshrined in these volumes. Constant reference to these will not only avoid duplication, but will also serve the purpose of directing the reader's attention to the chapters illustrated by them.

History is made by Man, and a historical treatment of a subject will have to highlight the role played in the subject's advance by individual protagonists, and in this respect, the treatment of the subject will differ from the customary approach found in a handbook.

The individual scientific mind's merit in many cases is to have served in "seed-ing" the crystallization of problems dissolved in the sea of circumstance and in act-ing as a catalyst for the efforts of others. Progress is, of course, equally dependent on the utilization of new research tools becoming available through technical ad-vances in other fields of scientific activity. In such cases the individual innovator's contribution is to have perceived the potentialities offered by them.

In this context a parenthetic reference to educational policy suggests itself. The instances of the pathfinding value of such "opportunism" (in the good sense of the word) are so numerous, especially in the biological sciences, as to make the demand for a wide-ranging comprehensive scientific education a most compelling one. Ear-ly specialization on the secondary school level and, equally, on the level of aca-demic undergraduate courses, is apt to restrict the chances of the "one great step forward" event in creative science.

To return to our introductory delineation of approach. The five decennia (1930–1980) of vestibular research to be scrutinized for specifically pathfinding dis-coveries and insights are not a continuum. They are punctuated by the Second World War, and it will be seen that, on the one hand, the war brought a hiatus in the momentum gained in the study of sensory systems after the introduction of the high-gain electronic amplifier and associated recording devices, whilst on the other hand, enhancing the development of techniques made possible by a rapid advance in the design and general availability of the electron microscope, which literally open-ed up new vistas for the understanding of the functional morphology of sense or-gans (and not least of the end organs of the inner ear on an ultrastructural level).

The rapid progress made in computer design, also catalysed by the demands of the war, and the spectacular increase in the availability of laboratory computers to be used in computer-controlled experiments and data evaluation, is another hallmark characterizing the last three decennia under review.

An account of the achievements of the first 100 years of vestibular research (1824–1924) will be sketched out here by way of introduction to the historical sur-vey of progress made during the period from the early 1930s to the present. That period itself may then be subdivided into four phases of research activity governed by the advent of the new technologies, which facilitated breakthroughs in research methods and the attack on unsolved problems.

B. The First 100 Years

On 15 November 1824, Flourens transected a horizontal semicircular canal in the pigeon and discovered the now well-known deficiencies in orientation following upon such an operation on the vestibular organ (FLOURENS 1842). This epoch-making experiment ushered in the first 100-year-long period of exploration of ves-tibular function characterized by the almost exclusive use of the method of oper-ative elimination of the organ in parts or as a whole; this was followed by a descrip-tion of "deficiency phenomena" *(Ausfallserscheinungen)* in the control of posture and movements by the experimental animal, their comparison to pathological states in man and their imputed relationship to morbid changes in the inner ear.

The achievements of this period are exhaustively reviewed in the relevant chapters by Kolmer, Fischer, MAGNUS and DE KLEIJN, GRAHE, Rohrer and Masuda in BETHE'S (1926) *Handbuch der normalen und pathologischen Physiologie* Vol. 11/1. These reviews deal with the morphology of the vestibular organ, its function in nonmammalian and mammalian organisms (including man) and investigations into the physics of the semicircular canals and otolith organs. The reviews demonstrate that, after a very slow start, vestibular science gained momentum in the last quarter of the nineteenth century with the work of MACH (1875), BREUER (1889, 1891), CRUM-BROWN (1873), and EWALD (1892).

Fortunately, the experimental investigation of this period extended over the whole of the vertebrate phylum (with important cross-references to relevant work on invertebrate statoreceptors) instead of being confined to a few standard animals used in medical physiology for the elucidation of "clinically important" aspects of vestibular function not accessible to direct observation and experimentation in man. In fact vestibular science was, and still is, in the field of sensory science as a whole, the least encumbered by psychophysical "prejudice," a fact that is to be ascribed largely to the poor representation of vestibular inputs in the above-cerebellar brain centres. In other words, the output from vestibular end organs, like that from myotatic receptors, does not impressively contribute to human conscious experience, unless when functionally disturbed or incongruous in range and configuration with phylogenetically fixed "normal" stimulation patterns.

A concise overview of the state of theory and knowledge in the vestibular field at the end of the first quarter of the present century was given by myself in a review entitled "The Equilibrium Function of the Vertebrate Labyrinth" (LOWENSTEIN 1936). This represents a summing-up of achievements at the very end of the period of vestibular research. These were based chiefly on the method of operative elimination complemented by experiments with natural and artificial stimulation applied to the exposed vestibular organ as a whole or in parts.

It may be useful here to quote the Summary of this review article in full. Naturally some of the statements are now in need of modification in the light of work in the subsequent periods of vestibular research, and attention will be drawn to them at the end of this quotation.

1. The vertebrate labyrinth can be divided into a pars superior, consisting of the utriculus and the semicircular canals, and a pars inferior, consisting of the sacculus and its various appendages.

2. Only the pars superior is concerned with the maintenance of muscle tone and with reflex reactions to gravity and to linear and angular accelerations. This has been demonstrated for fishes, amphibia, and mammals, and, although the evidence is not completely satisfactory, it probably holds for reptiles and birds as well.

The pars inferior takes no part in any of these functions (again with the above reservation as to reptiles and birds), but, even in those vertebrates which lack the organ of Corti, is concerned with sound reception.

Breuer's theory of the localisation of the non-acoustic function of the labyrinth has thus been shown to be erroneous.

3. Attempts have been made, by eliminating separately the various endings to discover which of the receptor endings of the pars superior are involved in each of its functions. The results obtained are not entirely consistent. Production of the static reflexes and of the reflexes to centrifugal force and fast linear acceleration is in all probability the main function of the otolith organ (utriculus). It appears, however, that the assumption that the otolith organ is purely static in function is incorrect, for it has been shown that the utriculus can be involved in dynamic responses to rotations.

The main function of the semicircular canals is the release of the dynamic reflexes. It has, however, been claimed that the vertical canals take part in the production of static reflexes as well.

Both the utriculi and the semicircular canals are involved in the maintenance of muscle tone.

4. In the discussion of the general conclusions as to the function of the utriculi and of the semicircular canals it is shown that one of the important functional differences between the two receptors consists in their different reaction time, which may be due to the difference in their auxiliary structures and to a different pattern of their nervous connection with the effector organs.

Here are some critical comments on the above. Both the sacculus and the lagena have meanwhile been shown in certain vertebrate types to function as receptors for gravitational and innertial stimuli, notably in the elasmobranch fishes (LOWENSTEIN and ROBERTS 1949) and in amphibians (MacNAUGHTON and McNALLY 1946), whereas there is some evidence for the participation of the utriculus in low-frequency sound reception in herring-type fishes (DENTON and BLAXTER 1976) and of its intrinsic vibration sensitivity in the elasmobranch labyrinth (LOWENSTEIN and ROBERTS 1951). The quoted comment on Breuer's theory of functional localization is, therefore, invalid *sensu stricto*.

It is quite clear that at the time of the publication of BETHE's (1926) *Handbuch* and the above quoted review (1936), the method of operative elimination, etc. had made its maximum contribution to the functional analysis of the vestibular system. The scene was set for a new methodological approach to the wealth of outstanding problems concerning basic functional mechanisms.

It may be appropriate here to enumerate some of these open problems in order to highlight the significance of the methodological advance made in what may be called the second period in the history of vestibular science, which is to be the starting point of the historical survey for the purposes of this book.

The asymmetries in eye position and body posture observed after unilateral elimination of vestibular receptors pointed to a lasting and continuously ongoing "tonic" action by the remaining intact organ. The idea of the labyrinth as an important source of tonic innervation, not only for the muscles of the effector organs involved in the control of posture and movement, but also for the body musculature in general, stemmed from EWALD's (1892) concept of the "tonus labyrinth." The gradual compensatory recovery from such asymmetries, as well as their reappearance after the subsequent elimination of the remaining intact labyrinth, suggested the additional involvement of central nervous tonus sources. However, the question of the mechanism of peripheral tonus generation by vestibular receptors had remained an open problem.

Another unresolved problem concerned the mode of function of the semicircular canals in response to oppositely directed angular accelerations. The question, as formulated at the time, was whether semicircular canals should be considered to be unidirectional or bidirectional receptors for angular accelerations in the plane of their optimal sensitivity (LOWENSTEIN 1932, 1937).

BREUER (1889, 1891) and EWALD (1892) had been in favour of bidirectionality, but recognized one direction as dominant in sensitivity over the opposite one. This had been suggested by the results of elimination experiments in fishes, birds, and mammals. Results of experiments on amphibian and reptilian labyrinths, however, pointed to exclusive unidirectionality of canal receptors, with ampulla-trailing (horizontal canal) or, alternatively, ampulla-leading (vertical canals) being the only effective rotational directions (MCNALLY and TAIT 1925; TRENDELENBURG and KÜHN 1908).

A third fundamentally important and hotly debated question concerning stimulus transduction in the labyrinth referred to the otolith organs and centered around the nature of the adequate primary stimulus. Was it a change in pressure or in traction of the otolith or otoconial mass on the underlying sense endings (QUIX 1924; MYGIND 1948; MAGNUS and DE KLEIJN 1926), or their shearing displacement tangentially to the surface of the sensory epithelium (BREUER 1889, 1891)? Here again majority opinion tended to support Breuer's shearing hypothesis, which was to find strong support later in the results of von Holst's behavioural experiments on fishes (in which he studied the balance between responses controlled by vision on the one hand and by vestibular mechanisms on the other). Here the measurement of the contribution by vestibular directional component pointed quite unequivocally to a tangential action of the otolith organ (VON HOLST 1950).

C. The Electrophysiological Era

I. Exploration of Basic Function

The year 1926 is memorable for the publication by Adrian and collaborators of the first four of six epoch-making papers that described the recording of nerve impulses in sensory nerves by means of an electronic valve amplifier at first coupled to a capillary electrometer and consequently to a mechanical oscillograph, de signed by B. H. C. Matthews at Cambridge (ADRIAN and ZOTTERMAN 1926a–c; ADRIAN and ECKHARD 1926; ADRIAN 1930, 1947). This method supplanted the laborious use of the fickle string galvanometer in the measurement of neuro-electric events. The rapid response, especially of the mechanical oscillograph (to be displaced later by the distortion-free high-intensity cathode-ray oscillograph) made possible for the first time in the history of neurophysiology the analysis of fast electrical events (action potentials). These were found in single sensory nerve fibres and receptor organs.

In the vestibular field the following "calendar entries" may convey an idea of the magnitude and importance of the initial harvest by means of this new technique in terms of discoveries fundamental to our knowledge of intrinsic receptor mechanisms. At the same time we shall see how the technique opened the way to the solution of the outstanding problems outlined above as left unsolved at the end of the first century of vestibular research.

1926: ADRIAN and ZOTTERMAN (1926a) in their first account of oscillographic recordings from single fibres of sensory nerves of the frog's myotatic system meet resting activity in the overtly unstimulated afferent pathway, and discuss its obscure origin and functional significance.

1934: ASHCROFT and HALLPIKE record impulses from the saccular branch of the eighth nerve in the frog in response to substrate-conducted vibration, and postulate an auditory function for the sacculus. Their work represents the first application of the oscillographic technique to the vestibular system.

1936: Ross publishes an account of recordings from the eighth nerve of the frog, in which he describes a variety of responses both to movement and position, including also the occurrence of resting activity in the absence of overt stimulation. In the critical assessment of his findings he rightly refrains from making definitive postulates on the origin within the vestibular organ of the various responses, and leaves open the question as to whether the resting activity is an artefact and, if not, what its functional significance migth be.

1936: LOWENSTEIN and SAND publish a first account of an oscillographic analysis of the response from an isolated branch of the eighth nerve innervating the horizontal semicircular canal in the dogfish labyrinth. The records are taken from the visually identified nerve branch in the surviving spinal fish by means of a forceps electrode inserted through an opening in the posterior wall of the exposed orbit. A number of active fibres make contact with the electrode and a multifibre response is registered. The adequate stimulus is supplied by the rotation of a large hand-operated turntable carrying a screening cage in which the whole fish is mounted in air, its gills being continuously irrigated with sea-water. Mercury slip-rings carry the impulse response and the action signal monitoring the turntable movement to the three-stage high-gain amplifier and mechanical oscillograph with paper-film camera as designed by Matthews.

The results of this study not only confirm the existence of a significant level of resting activity, but demonstrate that in this case the resting activity is an integral part of the response mechanism in so far as it forms the basis for the bidirectionality of the canal receptors. Its increase on ampulla-trailing and its decrease on ampulla-leading angular acceleration of the horizontal semicircular canal enables the organ to signal two oppositely directed rotatory stimuli to the vestibular centre by the increase and decrease above and below a basic level of "spontaneous" impulse activity.

At the same time, the continuous outflow from the vestibular end organ of impulse activity even in the absence of stimulation furnishes evidence for the correctness of the assumption that the labyrinth is an important source of background tonus, at least in the effector musculature associated with it, if not in the whole of the body. Finally, units showing such resting activity may be assumed to be practically "thresholdless" when adequately stimulated.

These first steps in the qualitative exploration of fundamental vestibular function were for obvious technical reasons confined to the study of the horizontal semicircular canal. The bulky live fish and the necessity of gill irrigation did not lend itself to the exploration of responses to rotational stimuli in the planes of the vertical canals, and the heavy turntable and large screen cage could not be made to furnish quantitatively controlled angular accelerations.

Sand's previous experience in experiments on the lateral line organs in surviving isolated preparations of the rostral part of the head of the ray, *Raja clavata* (SAND 1937), suggested the use of the isolated head of this elasmobranch fish for further experimentation. In fact, it emerged that the responses from such a preparation did not significantly differ from those obtained from whole live spinal dogfish, and that typical responses could be obtained from such preparations for at least 2 h after the isolation of the head.

This change of tactics opened up the way to a survey of the responses recorded from the nerve branches innervating individual ampullae from all three semicircular canals. Furthermore, a falling-weight-operated drive to a small turntable facilitated an analysis of the responses from single-fibre units in the nerve from the horizontal canal to quantitatively controlled angular accelerations and decelerations. The recording technique, too, was greatly improved by the use of a cathode-ray oscillograph and a push–pull amplifier with a high signal-to-noise ratio. The responses recorded from the vertical canals yielded confirmation of the notion that they differ from the horizontal canal in responding with increased activity to ampulla-leading and with decreased activity to ampulla-trailing acceleration, as postulated earlier on the grounds of studies of compensatory eye movements.

A scheme of the integrated collaboration of the three pairs of corresponding canals in the two labyrinths was postulated in terms of their control over the activities of individual eye muscles involved in such compensatory eye movements accompanying angular movements of the head in space (LOWENSTEIN and SAND 1940a).

Recordings in which the pick-up electrode makes effective contact with more than one fibre in a nerve branch (multifibre recordings) are adequate for such qualitative investigations. Attempts at gaining information on quantitative stimulus–response relationships can only be successful if the pick-up is restricted to effective contact of the electrode with a single nerve fibre (single-unit recording). When this was achieved, accurate quantification of the angular acceleration stimulus produced evidence for a linear relationship over an extended range of stimulus intensities between angular acceleration and the rate of change in discharge frequency, as well as an approximation to a response threshold of $3°/s^2$ for the horizontal canal. It could also be demonstrated that the effective stimulus for a canal is angular acceleration, whereas during prolonged rotation at constant speed the impulse activity from canal-controlled units reverts to the resting level within 20–30 s.

The way was now open for an interpretation in physical terms of the mechanical properties of the cupula-endolymph system, to account for the observed time relations of compensatory effector responses such as the tonic deviations and pre- and post-rotational nystagmus of the eyes (LOWENSTEIN and SAND 1940b).

The outbreak of the Second World War put a stop to these joint experiments, which were carried out in the Laboratory of the Marine Biological Association of the United Kingdom at Plymouth. With the death of Alec Sand before the end of the war, a most fruitful collaboration came to an untimely end. An appraisal of historical and personal aspects of this collaboration has been published under the title "Biographical Notes on the Early Electrophysiological Exploration of Vestibular Function" (LOWENSTEIN 1975; see Appendix to this chapter).

A most important confirmation of the basic pattern of canal-controlled impulse activity was furnished by ADRIAN (1943) in his recordings from the cat vestibular system. Responses picked up from what appeared to be axons of first-order canal-controlled neurons in the root of the vestibular nerve in the medulla showed the same bidirectionality against a background of resting activity as described by myself and Sand (LOWENSTEIN and SAND 1940a, b).

Like Ross (1936) in his work on the frog, Adrian found gravity-dependent responses and believed them to be derived chiefly from the sacculus, whereas he attributed certain responses to linear acceleration in the horizontal plane to the utriculus. In this he followed the interpretation of the functional mechanisms of otolith organs as given by MAGNUS (1924). This interpretation is not compatible with the now generally accepted shearing hypothesis of BREUER (1889, 1891), and Adrian's tentative localization of the origins of the observed responses can no longer be considered valid. Nevertheless, this first electrophysiological study of mammalian vestibular function, carried out successfully despite the inaccessibility of the vestibular nerve in the higher vertebrates, represents a historical landmark in the field of vestibular physiology.

A further confirmation of the findings on the fish semicircular canals was published by LEDOUX (1949), who recorded impulse activity from the eighth nerve in the isolated head of the frog, and found identical response characteristics demonstrating bidirectionality based on a modulation of resting activity in the amphibian semicircular canals for which a unidirectional response mode had been postulated (MCNALLY and TAIT 1925).

In addition, Ledoux drew attention for the first time to a sensitivity of canal receptors to positional (gravity-controlled) stimuli. This finding, however, being out of keeping with the theoretical concept of basic canal mechanics, appeared at the time to be a possible consequence of the surgical interference with the system rather than a demonstration of an aspect of normal canal function.

By the beginning of the era under consideration here, many of the standard clinical test procedures in the investigation of vestibular pathology had been well established. They were extensively reviewed by GRAHE (1926). Outstanding contributions to the problems of vertigo and of spontaneous or enforced nystagmus were made with new and redirected vigour at the beginning of the present century under the impact of the recognition of the role of the vestibular portion of the inner ear in the control of posture and movement. The investigations of BÁRÁNY (1907) by means of the caloric test method and by means of the rotating chair (Bárány chair), as well as the development of various methods of observation of eye nystagmus in patients suffering from vertigo, characterize the clinical research of this period into the normal and pathological physiology of the vestibular system in man, as carried out at a number of research centres in Europe.

The observation and measurement of nystagmus, having proved to be an important if not indispensable diagnostic aid in clinical otology and neurology, was, and still is a subject for intensive research, and was later to be furthered by the introduction of electronic methods of recording.

Despite the fact that Bárány is reputed to have thought that in man the vestibular organ may be in a state of functional regression, with posture and movement being largely controlled by vision and by the kinesthetic and myotatic sensory systems, his work early in this century made a pathfinding contribution to the study of optic nystagmus by the method of caloric stimulation of the canal system. The theoretical aspects of this work were investigated by DOHLMAN (1925). He was able to demonstrate conclusively that the caloric stimulus acts via thermomechanical endolymph displacement rather than by directly affecting the nerve endings of the receptors. He also elaborated an optical technique of nystagmography for the quantitative evaluation of some of the important nystagmus parameters.

The strong interaction between vestibular and optokinetic eye reflexes made it imperative to exclude visual orientation in test procedures. Palpation of the bulbi through closed eyelids during tests carried out with the rotating chair were one means of studying eye responses of purely vestibular origin, and the introduction of specially designed, strongly convex, illuminated spectacles served this purpose (FRENZEL 1925), although a serious disturbance in the configuration of the vestibular eye response by light as such, despite the absence of visible landmarks, was pointed out by OHM (1926).

It is evident from what has just been said that perhaps (even more than in other fields of sensory science) clinical study of the receptor organ's function, or rather dysfunction, provided a potent driving force for the initiation and diversification of research effort. Although the contributions of clinical research to the advance in vestibular physiology will obviously find their proper place in our story, especially when they provide important signposts on the forward path to knowledge, an account of the history of clinical methodology in the service of diagnosis and treatment of inner ear disease is outside the scope of this chapter and the competence of its author.

Among the pressing tasks awaiting the vestibular physiologist after the war was a further clarification of the mode of functioning of the otolith-controlled end organs of the labyrinth. The response analysis, based on the separate elimination of parts of the frog labyrinth by the sectioning of individually identified nerve branches carried out by MCNALLY and TAIT (1925), had posed important questions as to the integration of function between the otoconia-bearing maculae of the utriculus, sacculus, and lagena. This challenge had been taken up by ROSS (1936), and here it is incumbent on the historian to set out his contribution to progress in some detail, as this will be seen to have clearly delineated the existing problems and encouraged later electrophysiological attack on them. Attention is drawn to the evaluation of Ross's work on p. 102 of Vol. 6/1 of the *Handbook of Sensory Physiology* (LOWENSTEIN 1974a). Consultation of Ross's original paper reveals the work as that of an experimenter of high skill and, above all, of meticulously critical realism. Recording impulse responses of mixed origin from portions of the eighth nerve, he demonstrated a number of fundamental characteristics of gravity-sensitive end organs innervated by the anterior and posterior rami of the nerve. He clearly realized that the utriculus responds to tilts of the head about more than one axis, and found two types of gravity-related response in pick-ups from the ramus posterior. He also confirmed the existence of vibration receptors innervated by the posterior ramus, first described by ASHCROFT and HALLPIKE (1934) and attributed to the sacculus. An outstanding aspect of the quality of Ross's work is the way in which he abstained from any attempt to go beyond the confines of direct evidence furnished by his experiments in his suggestions as to the specific localization of origin of the recorded response. By this critical recognition of the limitations of his techniques he made an invaluable pioneering contribution to the formulation of questions concerning the nature and functional range of otolith organs.

The overriding necessity of an unequivocal identification of the origin of nerve fibres for the analysis of responses to rotational and static displacement of the head in space led to the post-war continuation of electrophysiological work on the isolated elasmobranch labyrinth, from which unit responses can be recorded from individual nerve twigs where they emerge from the directly identified sensory epithelia (LOWENSTEIN and ROBERTS 1949, 1951). The results of this work are reviewed in the above-quoted contribution to Vol. 6/1 of the *Handbook of Sensory Physiology,* which incorporates the illustrations referred to below. It will be useful in the context of our present scrutiny of the foundations on which our field of sensory science rests to single out from this work specific points of historical interest.

It must be said that it is, here as always, hazardous to make findings obtained in experiments on a given species of organism the basis for generalizations claiming validity even for relatively closely related species, let alone for representatives of other taxa within the vertebrate subkingdom. The labyrinth of a comparatively primitive fish, such as an elasmobranch, serves a specific range of functions satisfying the organism's requirements and potentialities within its specific environment. Nevertheless, we may expect the sensory equipment of such an animal to furnish the basis for evolutionary and adaptive elaboration of function in higher forms of differing modes of life. The organ may thus be thought to represent a "basic blueprint" modifiable in the light of emerging functional demands. It is clear, therefore, that some of the functional characteristics of the various vestibular end organs revealed by the elasmobranch labyrinth may either have relevance for all vertebrates or represent adaptations to aquatic or even specifically elasmobranch existence.

The aspect of otolith-controlled receptor function which is likely to have universal validity for all vertebrate labyrinths is, in contrast to that of the semicircular canal receptors, the lack of directional uniformity. The otolith organs share with the canals a range of adaptation to constant levels of stimulation. This, in turn, is responsible for the characterization of two extreme types of units within the family of receptors for gravitational stimuli and linear accelerations in general. They are separated into two classes, albeit with transitional types between them: the maximally static receptors (position sensors); and the dynamic units, which respond to changes in head position, but adapt relatively rapidly to the resting level of activity characteristic for the normal head position (irrespective of the spatial orientation of the point of arrest of the tilting movement, which this type of receptor unit is incapable of signalling). There are also individual differences within the population of otolith-controlled receptor units with respect to the spatial angle covered by their response range. The example illustrated in Fig. 15, p. 103, Vol. 6/1 of the *Handbook of Sensory Physiology* (LOWENSTEIN 1974 a) shows a case of a 360° range of coverage by one unit, although it obviously incorporates two ranges of ambiguity (i.e. between side-down and upside-down and side-up and normal), for which the frequency readings are indistinguishable. There exist within the receptor population types of units covering restricted ranges of tilt angle, being insensitive to considerable portions of the 360° spatial angle (range fractionation).

In considering the results of the elasmobranch experiments from the point of view of distribution within the labyrinth of responses to the various types of stimulus, such as vibration or displacement from or return to the normal position, we are faced with the problem of deciding what are specific elasmobranch characteristics and what are features of general validity. That the sensory epithelia of both the utriculus and the sacculus were found to incorporate, besides gravity-sensitive areas, others that were exclusively vibration-sensitive may apply basically to all vertebrate labyrinths, although the manner of their distribution may vary among vertebrate types. What the study presently discussed has established is that the otolith-controlled end organs of the vertebrate labyrinth are capable of functioning as vibration receptors, as well as receptors for linear acceleration (including gravity-dependent stimuli). The salient feature of the work on elasmobranches is the certainty in the localization of the origin of the recorded responses.

II. Experimental Tests of Functional Equations

A scrutiny of the literature on sensory science published in the 1950s shows a general preoccupation of sensory physiologists with cutaneous, kinesthetic, and myotatic mechanisms and audition within the sphere of mechanoreception, and above all with vision. Fundamental vestibular research (apart from work relevant to clinical otology) during that decennium might be described as having "withdrawn in preparation for a new assault," as if awaiting the advent of new technical weaponry. However, important progress was made in the theoretical field. The work of the Utrecht school under Van Egmond (VAN EGMOND et al. 1949), based on STEINHAUSEN's (1931, 1933) concept of the torsion pendulum model of semicircular canal function, resulted in the formulation of equations for the time course of the mechanical events during the displacement of the cupula of the canal caused by angular acceleration of the head.

This phase of theoretical research into vestibular function has been summarized by GUEDRY (1974) in his chapter on the psychophysics of vestibular sensation in Vol. 6/2 of the *Handbook*. Here we are interested in how some pathfinding insights into vestibular mechanics were gained at the time.

In a paper of fundamental importance, VAN EGMOND et al. (1949) describe the behaviour of the cupula during constant angular acceleration by the equation:

$$x \simeq a\tau_1\tau_2 \left(1 - e^{\frac{-t}{\tau_1}}\right), \tag{1}$$

where $x=$ the assumed cupula deflection and $a=$ the acceleration; τ_1 denotes the "long" time constant represented by the quotient Π/Δ or the ratio of the viscous to the elastic term, and τ_2 represented by the quotient θ/π or the ratio of the inertial to the viscous term in the torsior pendulum equation:

$$\ddot{x} + \frac{\Pi}{\theta}\dot{x} + \frac{\Delta}{\theta}x = 0, \tag{2}$$

where $\ddot{x}$, $\dot{x}$ are the second and first derivatives of the cupula deflection from rest x.

For measuring the time course of the decay of excitation (or inhibition) of the canal response towards the condition existing at rest, the mechanical impulse caused by the sudden arrest of a constant-velocity rotation of the head in the plane of the canal was chosen. Tests for threshold by registration of the so-called sensation cupulogram from maximum deflection at sudden arrest yielded by the equation:

$$x = x_{max} e^{\frac{-t}{\tau_1}}. \tag{3}$$

The actual values derived from these cupulogram measurements for time constants and threshold have been the subject of a good deal of subsequent research and revision, but the method of measurement has retained its usefulness.

A second method of arriving at quantitative estimates of these functional parameters is based on the investigation of responses measured in the frequency domain by the application to the system of sinusoidal oscillations on a torsion swing. This method was pioneered by GROEN and JONKEES (1948), following no doubt the very early application of this principle by MACH (1875) in his search for a threshold of sensation of turning. Chosing a frequency range between 0.6 and 1.3 rad/s, assumed to be near the natural frequency of the canal system, Groen and Jonkees showed that the sensation was a function of the rotational velocity. The output–input ratio plotted in the form of a Bode plot demonstrated that this ratio is constant over a certain range of frequencies, including the natural frequency. The so-called phase angle plotted against frequency is given by the relationship:

$$\varphi = \frac{\pi}{2} - \tan^{-1}\omega_f\tau_1 - \tan^{-1}\omega_f\tau_2 \tag{4}$$

where ω_f is the cycle frequency and τ_1 the long time constant. The natural frequency of the system is indicated by the steady-state range characterized by $\varphi = 0$.

At this point in the exploration of the validity of the torsion pendulum model of canal function it became obvious that direct measurements of the time course of the afferent impulse activity recorded from a canal receptor unit would furnish an important check on the results gained from subjective tests on the human observer.

For this purpose the isolated surviving elasmobranch labyrinth offered yet again the ideal test preparation. Unit responses could be obtained from nerve strands innervating the horizontal canal. These responses were exclusively afferent, as all possible sources of feedback were severed by the removal of the brain. Such units would function normally for extended periods of time and would make possible the application to the labyrinth of lengthy stimulation routines; these routines consisted of mechanical impulses produced by sudden arrest of constant-velocity rotation of a turntable driven by a motor geared down to the required speeds, or of sinusoidal oscillations of a platform suspended from wires the adjustable effective length of which controlled the circle frequency. All movements were monitored photo-electrically by means of a slotted disc mounted coaxially with the platform, the signals being recorded on the paper film in conjuction with the nerve impulses trains. This work was again carried out at the Marine Biological Laboratory at Plymouth by myself in collaboration with J.J. Groen and A.J.H. Vendrik (GROEN et al. 1952).

From a historical point of view it may be of interest to present-day electrophysiologists to recall the effort called for in the acquisition of quantitative data of this kind at that time. The nerve impulses displayed on the screen of a cathode-ray oscillograph were recorded together with the monitored stimulus parameters by means of a camera on 61-m reels of paper film, the suitability of the output from the preparation being assessed by means of a monitor speaker. After the processing and drying of the film, the recorded impulse frequencies had to be laboriously analysed by measuring the interspike distances and correlated with the action signals and the signals indicating the film velocity. The resulting tables of figures then had to be plotted in the manner called for, either in the form of decay curves or of phase angles against circle frequencies (Bode plots). The data so obtained had to be entered in the appropriate equations and subjected to evaluation. Three investigators were thus kept busy often into the small hours of the morning if the biological preparation of a set of afferent canal units had been successfully achieved. All this may be compared with the present-day use of magnetic tape and a computer delivering impulse interval or impulse frequency histograms on call, as well as the desired graphics, with the additional possibility of automatic stimulus application and control. It may in a way be considered a morale-boosting fact that the operating skills necessary in producing physiological preparations have, as yet, not been automated!

The results of this work showed that the torsion pendulum model of canal function was, in fact, within limits applicable to the peripheral organ. The parameters obtained for the horizontal canal of the ray (*Raja clavata*) by the two different modes of stimulation were found to tally well. Average values for Δ/θ and Π/θ were computed from swing frequencies significantly higher and lower than the natural frequency of the canal, and were averaged at 1.0 s^{-2} and 36 s^{-1} respectively. The measurements of the responses to mechanical impulse stimuli yielded similar values for Π/θ. The internal diameter of the horizontal canal of *Raja* being 0.068 cm, the density of the endolymph (ϱ) being estimated at 1.0 g cm^{-3} and the viscosity (η) at 0.010 cgs units yielded a value of 35 s^{-1} for Π/θ, using the relationship:

$$\frac{\Pi}{\theta} = \frac{8\eta}{2\varrho r^2}. \tag{5}$$

The following differential equation was, therefore, suggested as a description of the mechanical behaviour of the cupula-endolymph system of *Raja*:

$$\ddot{\varkappa} + 35\,\dot{\varkappa} + \varkappa = 0. \tag{6}$$

How this equation compares with similar ones proposed for the human vestibular organ on the basis of cupulometric and nystagmographic measurements was critically discussed at a later date by MAYNE (1974), and compared to data by VAN EGMOND et al. (1949) and by NIVEN and HIXON (1961), as well as to the early computations of SCHMALTZ (1932). MAYNE (1974, p. 505) gives a Bode plot of the canal response in Fig. 2, in which the transition of lead to lag relative to velocity lies at the cycle frequency $\omega_f = 0.5 \text{ Hz} (3.14 \text{ rad s}^{-1})$, the gain being flat over the approximate range 0.05–2 Hz $(0.3–12.6 \text{ rad s}^{-1})$.

It must not be overlooked in this context that internal radius of the horizontal canal of *Raja* is over twice that given for this canal in man (JONES and SPELLS 1963), a fact which would make the elasmobranch value of 35 for *Raja* and that of 16 given by Niven and Hixon for man approximately equivalent, emphasizing the lower frequency response of the canal in fish (MAYNE 1974).

In 1949 DE VRIES attempted to arrive at an estimate of the absolute threshold of vestibular receptors to compare it with those found in other sense organs. He observed otolith displacements by tilts using X-ray photography, and estimated maximum displacements to be of the order of 0.0006 cm/dyn. A similar estimate was arrived at by Vilstrup and Vilstrup (1952). In a study of the minimum perceptible angular acceleration in man, De Vries reached the conclusion that the absolute threshold lay within the order of magnitude of molecular heat motion. He also studied vestibular microphonics and recognized the frequency doubling by the microphonic response so characteristic of the lateral line receptors. A rationale for this phenomenon emerged much later from ultrastructural data. Vilstrup and Vilstrup's investigations on elasmobranches yielded much valuable information on the morphology of their labyrinth, and exploratory work on the reaction of elasmobranchs to sound involving a procedure of conditioning led them to the conclusion that sharks can hear and that apart from the skin and the lateral line, the pars inferior, especially the sacculus, was involved in the reception of sonic stimuli.

Both De Vries and T. Vilstrup showed great promise and pioneering spirit in their early contributions to vestibular science. De Vries's untimely death and T. Vilstrup's switch to an exclusive pursuance of clinical practice cut short some very promising work.

This appears to be the proper place to recall in more detail the work of Von Holst and collaborators on the mode of functioning of otolith organs, which contributed so significantly to the consolidation of Breuer's shearing hypothesis of otolith action. Von Holst (1950) made use of what is known as the "dorsal light reflex," which makes fish (and other aquatic organisms) attempt under lateral illumination to orient the sagittal plane of their body in line with the direction of incident light; their final orientation is in the direction of the resultant between the "force vectors" of light and gravity. When the g vector was varied by centrifugation and the intensity and direction of the light stimulus were kept constant, it was found that the orientation of the sagittal plane of the fish was a function of the changing g vector times the sine of the angle of deviation from the normal or from the light-related angle. It could be seen, therefore, that the otolith-controlled component of orientation is caused by otolith displacement tangentially to the sensory epithelium, whereas a mechanism dependent on changes in pressure or traction would have involved a cosine relationship. Thus an ingeniously designed behavioural experimental procedure has made a decisive contribution to the solution of an important but, until then, highly controversial physiological problem. The whole field of work was critically reviewed later by one of von Holst's closest collaborators (Schöne 1959). It is only fair, however, to refer in this context to the early work of perhaps the strongest advocates of the rival pressure-traction hypothesis, namely Quix (1924), Werner (1929), and above all Mygind (1948).

III. Exploration of Biophysical Mechanisms

During the decennium at present scrutinized we witness an intensification of the interest in the nature and molecular composition of the endolymph and perilymph fluids of the mammalian ear with the work by Smith et al. (1954), Citron et al. (1956), and Rauch and Koestlin (1958). Similar analytical work on lower vertebrates was carried out by Ledoux (1949) on the frog, and by Vilstrup et al. (1954)

and later MURRAY and POTTS (1961) on elasmobranches (see also PETERSON et al. 1978).

The most important feature of this work was the finding that the potassium and sodium contents of the endolymph bathing the apical aspect of the hair cells has, at least in the mammalian labyrinth, an ionic composition resembling that of the cell interior – i.e. a high potassium and a low sodium concentration, whereas the perilymph to which the basal synaptic region of the sensory epithelia is exposed shows, inversely, the high sodium and low potassium levels characteristic of intercellular fluids (see LOWENSTEIN 1974 a, p. 87, Table 1).

As we now know, the two intralabyrinthine media are separated by a system of intercellular tight junctions between hair cells and supporting cells, which are considered to form an ion-tight seal separating these two fluid environments of the hair cells.

The recognition of the nature of the ionic environment of the hair cell had important repercussions in the study of the processes involved in the mechano-electric transduction and signal generation in the vestibular organ. TRINCKER'S measurements of the dc potentials in the semicircular canal system of the guinea pig showed how the ionic composition of the endolymph and the difference in dc potential between endolymph and perilymph enter into the interpretation of signal transduction (TRINCKER and PARTSCH 1959).

In agreement with the results of work on the mammalian cochlea (VON BÉKÉSY 1951; TASAKI and SPYROPOULOS 1959) were Trincker's first findings on the relationship between vestibular dc potentials and stimulus transformation (TRINCKER and PARTSCH 1959). The pursuance of this problem by this author continued well into the early 1960s, but it may suffice here to quote as an additional reference his treatment of the matter in his all-embracing review, "Physiologie des Gleichgewichtsorgans" (TRINCKER 1965). Trincker measured potential changes between the lumen of the semicircular canal ampulla of the guinea pig close to the crista and the perilymphatic space during adequate stimulation by means of manometrically controlled cupula displacements. Pressure and suction, moving the cupula in opposite directions, yielded oppositely directed changes in the resting dc potential proportional to the degree of cupula deviation. Utriculopetal displacement in the horizontal canal resulted in a depolarization (increased negativity), utriculofugal displacement in hyperpolarization (increased positivity), with the reverse changes being found in the vertical canals.

It is interesting in the context of the then existing controversy among clinicians concerning the validity of the so-called second law of Ewald, dealing with the inequality of the reflex effect of oppositely directed canal stimulation, that Trincker found in his mammalian preparation that the magnitude of depolarization was almost always significantly larger than the corresponding hyperpolarization.

The importance attached to this question of asymmetry versus symmetry, especially in the field of clinical diagnostics, can be gauged by the fact that an International Symposium on Problems of Otoneurology at Basel in 1960 had this as its chief theme of discussion, with contributions by C.S. HALLPIKE (1960), G.F. DOHLMAN (1960a), A. LEDOUX (1960), R. MITTERMAIER (1960), J.J. GROEN (1960), A.M. DI GIORGIO (1960), J.D. HOOD (1960), and A. MONTADON (1960). The cases for and against rejection of Ewald's second law were argued on clinical and on fundamental grounds, but no unanimous conclusion was reached. However, it was fairly generally accepted that within a limited range of stimulus intensities, the peripheral organ may, especially in mammals, generate symmetrically equal excitatory and inhibitory responses, whereas electrophysiological studies revealed that over an extended range of stimulus intensities the total excitatory response may be significantly preponderant over the associated inhibitory one. This applies especially to canal responses in the lower vertebrates. Reflex responses observed in amphibians and reptiles after unilateral labyrinth loss had earlier on led to the conclusion that, far from effecting symmetrically strong bidirectional responses, the semicircular canals were to be assumed to respond exclusively unidirectionally, namely in the excitatory direction only (McNALLY and TAIT 1933; MAIN 1931; TRENDELENBURG and KÜHN 1908). This appears to point to a difference in central nervous utilization of the inherently bidirectional canal responses in squatting animals enjoying a mechanically stable equilibrium (terrestrial amphibia and reptiles).

The graphic representation of dc potential changes is given by TRINCKER (1965) in conjunction with the discharge frequencies from three units of the horizontal semicircular canal of the guinea pig, and shows an impressive parallelism between the dc changes during manometrically controlled cupula deflections and the changes in discharge frequency recorded from the canal nerve after sudden arrests of constant-velocity rotations in the excitatory and inhibitory directions. Two units exhibiting resting activity show almost symmetrical excitatory increases and inhibitory decreases of discharge frequency from the resting level. The third unit displayed was silent at rest and showed, therefore, only a unilaterally excitatory response.

As will be seen later, such spontaneously silent units are present in the sensory epithelia of canal cristae in considerable numbers, and are bound to contribute quite substantially to asymmetry in end organ response as postulated by Ewald's second law. As they are now known to have a higher threshold, but also a higher sensitivity, their presence will make itself felt, particularly at relatively high stimulus intensities. We shall return to this aspect of end organ function in a different context.

When dealing with the earlier theories relating to the ionic composition of the vestibular fluids and the resulting resting dc potential between endolymph and perilymph, and with the assumptions concerning the mechano-electric transduction process in the hair cell, it has to be kept in mind that the leading exploratory ideas were developed for the cochlea. This topic is discussed in the chapter by Davis in this volume. His original work on the guinea pig cochlea led him to conceive the fundamental theory of cochlear action associated with his name (DAVIS 1960, 1965). He developed his ideas with close reference to the work of VON BÉKÉSY (1952, 1953) on cochlear resting potentials and microphonics, and on the travelling wave model concept.

It may suffice here to enumerate those principles which, mutatis mutandis, have also been thought to apply to the transduction process in vestibular sense endings.

Davis, concerning himself with the final step in the transduction mechanism, believed that the electric events around and in the hair cells may excite the afferent nerve endings either directly or with the mediation of a chemical transmitter. The central point of this theory is that the dc potentials and their stimulus-dependent fluctuations form an essential link in transduction, although Davis pointed out at the time that there existed no absolute proof for this contention.

The intracellular resting potential of − 50 to − 80 mV in the cochlear hair cells, as all intracellular potentials in tissue cells, is dependent for its maintenance on ion-separating mechanisms, so-called ion-pumps, which derive their energy from oxidative metabolic processes, and are therefore sensitive to anoxia and antimetabolic poisons. In the search for the possible way by which the mechanical stimulus to the apical part of the hair cell would lead to a fluctuation in the intracellular potential, Davis proposed for the cochlea the intervention of a so-called endocochlear potential measurable between the endolymph of the cochlear duct (scala media) and a reference point in the perilymph of the scala tympani or scala vestibuli. This positive potential is associated with the high potassium and low sodium concentrations in the endolymph maintained by the metabolic activity of the stria vascularis tissue (TASAKI and SPYROPOULOS 1959). Davis suggested that this endocochlear potential represents the electromotive force of a battery, which acts as a source for a current flowing through the hair cells proportional in strength to changes in their resistance brought about by the mechanical deformation (displacement) of the hair processes by the action of the travelling wave created by sound in the scala media. Davis postulated in addition that the intracellular potential of the hair cell drives yet another battery in series with the first. Its potential fluctuations (cochlear microphonics) act as receptor potentials responsible in turn for the depolarization of the dendritic membranes of the afferent first-order neurons generating the all-or-nothing impulses in the afferent axon. The possible intervention of a chemical transmitter process was here envisaged.

Davis recognized that the endocochlear potential may be a unique feature not paralleled by similarly large potentials between the endolymphatic and perilymphatic spaces of the vestibular apparatus, for which, therefore, no corresponding "first battery" mechanisms could be postulated. This is likely to be so in spite of the fact that, at least in the mammals, but also to a lesser degree in lower vertebrates, the concentrations of potassium and sodium ions in the endolymph resemble the intracellular concentrations to such an extent that no large enough working gradient appears to exist for these ions across the hair cell membrane apically above the level of the tight junctions between hair cells and supporting cells (reticular membrane). The basal part of the hair cell soma, however, is bathed by intercellular fluid and perilymph, which characteristically have low potassium and high sodium content. Here, i.e. in the region of the synaptic endings of afferent and efferent nerves, exist the extra- to intracellular gradients necessary for depolarization and hyperpolarization. We shall have to return to these aspects of hair cell biophysics and physiology when dealing with the problems of transduction in the light of present-day research.

D. The Electron Microscopic Study of Vestibular Ultrastructure

In 1956 WERSÄLL gave the first comprehensive account of the ultrastructure of the hair cell and of other components of the sensory epithelium of the crista of the semicircular canal of the guinea pig as revealed by the electron microscope. This study yielded evidence of a dimorphism of the hair cell, which Wersäll described by the now universally accepted designation as type I and II. This was later found to be valid for the labyrinth of reptiles, birds, and mammals, but not for the lower vertebrates, the hair cells of which conform in appearance and innervation to Wersäll's type II.

The essential features of the two types may be summarized as follows (Wersäll and Bagger-Sjöbäck 1974, p. 124, Fig. 30). Type I cells are flask-shaped and the near-spherical part of their soma is enveloped by a chalice-shaped end formation of the dendritic part of the afferent first-order neuron. This makes synaptic contact with the hair cell membrane where membrane features and intracellular synaptic bars, with their assembly of vesicles, display all the characteristics of chemical transmission sites. Typical efferent nerve endings make contact with the outside of the chalice membrane and are, therefore, postsynaptically situated with respect of the afferent pathway.

The innervation of the cylindrical type II hair cells is different. Here, both the afferent and the efferent endings are of approximately equal shape and size and make contact with the hair cell membrane directly, their characteristic synaptic structures being discretely distributed over the basal part of the cell soma.

There is little difference in the structure and arrangement of the hair processes at the apical end of the two types of hair cell. A kinocilium rooted in a basal body shows the 9–2 longitudinal filamental structure characteristic of motile cilia, and is accompanied by an array of macrovilli (stereocilia), the length of which decreases with increasing distance from the kinocilium. These stereocilia are anchored by tapering root formations in a so-called cuticular plate composed of densely packed granules and situated immediately below the plasma membrane. So-called tight junctions are situated near the apical end of the hair cells and separate them from the adjoining supporting cells.

Wersäll's findings immediately suggested to me the possibility of investigating the directional aspects of hair cell stimulation in a vestibular organ, the directional responses of which had been demonstrated with absolute certainty by single-unit electrophysiological analysis. Such a case was presented by the results of the work on the horizontal semicircular canal of the elasmobranch fish *Raja clavata* (Lowenstein and Sand 1940a, b; Groen et al. 1952). A collaboration was arranged between Wersäll and myself at the Plymouth Laboratory, aimed at the mapping of the distribution and orientation of the hair cells within the sensory epithelia of the canal cristae, and also within the maculae of the otolith organs in the utriculus, sacculus, and lagena of the ray labyrinth. So far as the canal cristae are concerned, the opportunity offered itself to define the functional polarization of the hair cells in the light of the directionally uniform responses of given canals to angular accelerations. The results of the electron microscopic survey justified these expectations insofar as in all canal cristae the hair cells were found to be deployed so that the kinocilia pointed uniformly in the same direction on both slopes of the crista. In the horizontal canal, all the kinocilia pointed away from the canal end of the ampulla towards the opening into the utriculus, whereas in the vertical canals they were found to face the canal, pointing away from the utriculus. It was thus clearly demonstrated, in correlation with the electrophysiological results, that a displacement of the hair bundle towards the kinocilium produced an excitatory effect, and a displacement in the opposite direction produced an inhibitory effect on the discharge activity generated by the hair cell, and that the hair cell was, in fact, functionally polarized in a plane going through the kinocilium and the so-called basal foot of its root structure and the centre of the stereocilial array (LOWENSTEIN et al. 1964). At the same time, the long-accepted difference between the horizontal and the vertical canals in their responses to ampullopetal and ampullofugal endolymph displacement was elucidated as a consequence of hair cell orientation. GROEN (1960) proposed a simple embryological explanation for the apparent oppositeness of hair cell arrangement as between the anterior vertical and the horizontal canal, pointing out that the two adjacent sensory epithelia develop from a common placode, extending symmetrically across the opening of the ampulla into the utricular cavity.

The hair cell maps of the otoconia-bearing maculae were found to be more complex (LOWENSTEIN 1974a, p. 91, Fig. 10). Once the functional polarization of the hair cell was accepted as a guide-line for the directional sensitivity of canal cristae and the various regions within maculae, hair cell maps were obtained from representatives of all vertebrate classes, as well as for the mammalian cochlea, both by means of transmission and by scanning electron microscopy (see ADES and ENGSTRÖM 1972; WERSÄLL and BAGGER-SJÖBÄCK 1974; and H. Engström's chapter in this volume).

The theoretical implications of the established hair cell polarization range far and wide, as will be seen in connection with the acoustic function of the otolith organs in animals without cochlea.

It is beyond the scope of this chapter to attend to the cochlear hair cells in any detail. However, it is relevant to add in connection with what follows that both the inner and the outer hair cells of the adult organ of Corti lack a kinocilium, although its basal body remains extant. An assessment of the functional role of this organelle must take this fact into account in theoretical considerations concerning the nature of the mechano-electric transduction process in all hair-cell-bearing vertebrate sense endings.

E. The Search for the Mechanisms of Mechano-Electric Transduction

We have now entered the decade of the 1960s, and a survey of the advances in vestibular science in that decade shows that the newly won insights into the ultrastructure and the deployment of the hair cell in the various end organs gave a new impetus to research and theorizing concerning the mechanical and mechano-electric processing of the adequate rotatory, translatory, and gravity-dependent stimuli to which vestibular end organs respond.

The jelly-like covering structures (cupulae and otolith membranes, the latter weighted by calcareous otoliths or otoconia, as well as unweighted in certain regions) are the first target for the mechanical inertial or specific gravity-controlled forces resulting from adequate stimulation of the vestibular end organs.

The final unit response to adequate mechanical stimulation can be of two kinds. In afferent axons, which carry an ongoing resting discharge, it manifests itself as a modulation of the discharge frequency up or down, the frequency envelope being a function of the force and direction of the mechanical stimulus. The resulting afferent message is, however, not necessarily a strict stimulus analogue. The shape of the response curve, when recorded in the time domain, is linear with the stimulus only over a restricted intensity range. When recorded in the frequency domain, it provides evidence for the operation of adaptive processes besides that for the underlying response parameters derived from the mechanical properties (elasticity, viscosity) of the hair processes and the surrounding medium, namely the endolymph and covering structures. Recorded in the frequency domain (sinusoidal stimulation), the responses from spontaneously active units show similar non-linearities, the theoretical evaluation of which will be attended to in the context of more recent analytical work.

Apart from the units exhibiting a resting discharge, the effect of adaptation is, of course, most evident in the so-called phasic units described above as spontaneously silent. They act as unidirectional receptors, responding only to stimuli in the excitatory direction. They have a relatively high threshold, and a higher sensitivity in terms of impulses per unit acceleration. Their rapid adaptation even to stimuli of relatively short duration yields extremely non-linear response curves. In records taken from multiunit preparations of the afferent nerve, the admixture of the response of such units is responsible for impressive response asymmetries resembling those found in the study of whole-organism responses such as nystagmus and subjective sensation.

The search for the mechanisms governing the functional links between the displacement of the covering structures and the final impulse response recorded from the afferent first-order axon has, to the present day, not yielded a satisfactorily complete story. In the early 1960 s it was still taken as axiomatic that the hair bundles of the sensory cells are extensively ensheathed in the gelatinous cupulae and otolith membranes, and that these two components of the transduction apparatus are therefore mechanically closely coupled. The time course of the observed displacements of the covering structures and that of the enclosed hair processes were considered to be to all intents and purposes identical, except for a possibility of "slippage" caused by overstimulation. For the purpose of this historical account we retain this model concept, although it may no longer be wholly acceptable.

The time course of hair displacement was considered to be fully governed by the mechanical effects of the viscous and elastic properties of cupulae, otolith membranes and surrounding endolymph. The mechanical differential equations describing the response behaviour of canal and otolith organs (cf. pp. 523–525) rested on this assumption. The next step in the transformation of the mechanical stimulus offered considerable interpretative difficulties. It raised the question as to which of the components of the sensory hair bundle was the actual link between mechanical displacement and the physicochemical changes in the hair cell membrane leading to its depolarization or hyperpolarization. The first model concept suggested involved the kinocilium. This organelle, having all the structural characteristics of a motile cilium as found in many types of organism and tissue, was considered to be capable of functioning "in reverse." This means that instead of undergoing a mechanical deformation during active ciliary beat (a process believed to be controlled by changes in the electrical state in or around the basal apparatus), the vestibular kinocilium was thought to transform passive deformation into an electric event in or near its basal apparatus. This would then, in turn, be responsible for changes in the polarization of the hair cell membrane in its vicinity (GRAY and PUMPHREY 1958). The hypothesis just outlined had, however, a serious flaw, in so far as a kinocilium is absent in fully developed hair cells of the cochlea. The kinocilial basal apparatus persists, but the apical hair bundle both in the inner and the outer hair cells consists of characteristically patterned arrays of stereocilia only. As it is generally assumed that the cochlear hair cells serve as mechano-electric transducers in a manner similar to those of the vestibular organ and those of the lateral line of aquatic vertebrates, the kinociliar hair process at least could not be considered to be a necessary link in transduction. The question of the functional role of the basal apparatus was left open. The possibility must here be considered that the kinocilium – if not involved in transduction – may be a centre of organization responsible for hair cell development and maintenance. The story of the possible role of kinocilia in mechano-electric transduction does, however, not end here. The fact that, in the analogous hair cells found in the statodynamic receptor organs of the molluscs among the invertebrates, the arrays of apical hair processes are composed exclusively of typical kinocilia (MARKL 1974), presents us in our search for a functional generalization with a situation in which the cochlear hair cell appears very much as an outsider.

Naturally, the stereocilia, with their characteristic arrangements in orderly array patterns covering much of the apical aspect of hair cells, their lengths sloping away in a gradient from the kinocilial pole of the cell, suggested themselves as an alternative means of transfer of the mechanical stimulus to the cell membrane. Their association firm rooting in with, and the dense cuticular plate suggested the possibility that their joint displacement may either directly (by a concomitant displacement of the cuticular plate within the cytoplasm) initiate the depolarization or hyperpolarization of the hair cell membrane in a region below the tight junctions of the reticular membrane, or indirectly act on the closely adjoining basal apparatus of the kinocilium with similar effect. In this connection, it may be of interest to recall that the hair cell of the lamprey (among the cyclostomes) was found to contain a striated organelle intervening between the base of the cuticular plate and the basal parts of the soma in the vicinity of the afferent synaptic bars and vesicles (LOWENSTEIN and OSBORNE 1964; LOWENSTEIN 1974a, p. 85, Fig. 8). It would have been reasonable to consider this structure to be a possible direct intracellular link between the cuticular plate and the synaptic loci, if similar organelles had been generally found in hair cells. However, the search for them has, until recently, been unsuccessful.

An entirely different way in which the stereocilia might be involved in mechano-electric transduction was suggested by DOHLMAN (1960b) and TRINCKER (1965). The stereocilia present an impressive surface enlargement of the apical hair cell membrane, having a surface area approximately 20 times that of the rest of the cell. Their deformation cannot, however, be directly associated with the usual mechanism of excitation of their covering membrane. They are bathed in endolymph, the ionic composition of which resembles that of the cell interior and appears to preclude at least the operation of a potassium-sodium mechanism of change in membrane potential. As an alternative to this, CHRISTIANSEN (1964) and TRINCKER (1965) drew attention to the fact that the hair processes are coated with a layer of acid mucopolysaccharide, which intervenes between them and the covering cupula of otolith membrane. Such mucopolysaccharides, and especially their potassium salts, are demonstrated reversibly to generate so-called displacement potentials in response to mechanical deformation. An ion-impermeable stereocilial membrane in conjunction with its mucopolysaccharide coating suggested the model concept of an electrolyte capacitor effect acting as a trigger for polarity changes in membrane regions below the reticular membrane, where the cell membrane is exposed to perilymph of an ionic composition favouring a potassium-sodium mechanism. TRINCKER (1965) points to the observation of stimulus-synchronous vestibular microphonics up to 120 kHz which occur in the semicircular canal ampulla (described by TRINCKER and PARTSCH 1959) as possibly generated at the apical hair cell surface. This might then be assumed to act as an ion-condenser microphone. The high potassium content of the endolymph might thus find a reasonable interpretation as a necessary condition for a mucopolysaccharide-based mechanism.

The presence of synaptic structures characteristic for chemical transmission had removed the possibility of direct electrical stimulus transmission from the field of theoretical considerations. The membrane of the dendritic processes of the afferent first-order neuron was considered to conform to the type of electrically inexcitable electrogenic membrane (GRUNDFEST 1966), being subjected to the action of chemical transmitter substance only. It was therefore assumed that experimental electrical stimulation of the hair cell system, as carried out by myself (LOWENSTEIN 1955), affected the presynaptic hair cell membrane controlling the transfer of transmitter substance, increasing it by ascending and decreasing it by descending galvanic current routed through the afferent nerve. These experiments with galvanic polarization showed not only that the responses to adequate stimulation of a semicircular canal could be qualitatively mimicked by this procedure, but also that it produced responses both in the time and in the frequency domain, showing many of the quantitative features concerning time course and adaptation which were usually attributed to the mechanical behaviour of the cupula–endolymph system, yet in circumstances in which no displacement of cupula or endolymph is likely to occur. The question therefore presented itself as to whether the mechanical processes which formed the premises for the classic differential equations describing vestibular receptor behaviour were really directly responsible for the above-mentioned response parameters.

There is, indeed, now reason to believe that a special so-called encoder mechanism associated with the afferent terminals at the hair cell may be responsible for the different dynamic properties observed in the peripheral afferent semicircular canal (and also otolith-controlled) units (PRECHT et al. 1971).

Among the topics of vestibular science attracting the special attention of theoreticians and experimenters throughout this decade, two deserve close scrutiny. The first is concerned with the neuroanatomy and mode of functioning of the efferent pathways connecting the vestibular centres with the individual vestibular end organs; the second relates to the analysis of the vestibulo-ocular reflexes, the architecture of their neurological foundations and the diagnostic aspects, both fundamental and clinical, of their manifestation in experiment and disease. Both topics have been extensively reviewed in the *Handbook of Sensory Physiology,* the first by GACEC (1974) and PRECHT (1974a, b), the second by COHEN (1974); the neuro-anatomical basis for both topics were dealt with by BRODAL (1974).

F. The Efferent System

The identification by electron microscopy of the efferent endings at the vestibular hair cells (WERSÄLL 1956) established the fact that the vestibular periphery was subject to central control. The search for the origin of this control and the specific pathways serving it yielded the following information (for comprehensive review see PRECHT 1974a).

After the first demonstration of efferent neurons in the auditory system by RAS-MUSSEN (1946, 1953), GACEC (1960, 1967) investigated the efferent system associated with the vestibular end organs, and in a study of the system in the kitten (GACEC and LYON 1974) described the vestibular efferent pathway as converging with the cochlear efferents at the vestibular root of the eighth nerve. In the vestibular nerve the efferent fibres are assembled compactly into bundles, taking up a central position within the dorsal aspect of the nerve. They then split up on their way to the ganglion of Scarpa to reach the various vestibular end organs. As the fibres are small in diameter (2–3 µm), the cells of origin were expected to be small also. In fact, RASMUSSEN (1946) found the cell bodies from which the crossed cochlear fibres originate to be small multipolar cells situated dorsomedially to the superior olivary nucleus. The fibres stain in a way characteristic of the cholinergic system and can therefore be traced by the acetylcholine method (DOHLMAN et al. 1958; HILDING and WERSÄLL 1962; IRELAND and FARKASHIDI 1961).

In short, the control mechanisms originate chiefly in the vestibular nuclei and in the cerebellum, with a possible additional involvement, either directly or indirectly, of the reticular formation. Basically, it appears most reasonable to interpret efferent action as inhibitory in the form of a negative feedback to the periphery, triggered and controlled by the afferent signal. However, the possibility that at least some of the efferents may be excitatory, either immediately or via disinhibition somewhere along the pathway, cannot be ruled out. Such feed-forward action would have to be experimentally and rigorously demonstrated before it could be accepted as part of the efferent mechanism. Otherwise, one may be led to the development of theoretical constructs which, although rationally possible, are epicyclically capable of yielding any desired explanation. Such rational procedures are rather devoid of concrete usefulness.

Nevertheless, the very existence of an efferent control system suggests a variety of plausible scenarios. The simplest one is the negative feedback mechanism directly affecting the degree of afferent synaptic transmission from hair cell to first-order afferent neuron. GROEN et al. (1952) developed the model concept of a biasing process capable of shifting the "working point" of a canal unit along its S-shaped "characteristic" and so controlling the linearity and mode of output from such a unit.

The second possible mode of utilization of sensory efferents has been suggested by the work of RUSSELL (1968, 1971) on the lateral line of *Xenopus,* in which an efferent modulation of the activity in lateral line afferents was demonstrated to occur whenever the ventral column motor pool was being activated in the context of locomotory (swimming) activity of the limbs. The rationale for this type of efferent action suggested by Russell was the neutralization of signals monitoring and localizing delicate changes in water displacements in the vicinity of the animal when swimming activity produces massive disturbances in the surrounding water mass. This could be interpreted as a means of preventing a swamping of the central analyser with meaningless information and also possibly preventing an overload of the peripheral synaptic system.

A similar functional interpretation was suggested by KLINKE (1970) and KLINKE and GALLEY (1971) in work on the goldfish, where even in the immobilized animal (Flaxedil) exposed to a rotating visual environment which would normally elicit a locomotory persuit response, the afferent discharge from the vestibular receptors was inhibited during the period of optokinetic stimulation. It may appear that we are dealing here with the effect of an unexecuted motor command, which could be ascribed to a manifestation of a centrally stored enregistration of this motor command described as "efference copy" by VON HOLST (1950).

This type of functional role of sensory efference may be of quite common occurrence when automatic reflex responses to environmental stimulus situations are being overruled by voluntary action, e.g. as found in the neutralization of righting reflexes during voluntary positional change.

Finally, there is a recent claim (BIENHOLD and FLOHR 1980) that the cholinergic efferent system associated with vestibular centers plays a role in the compensation of the effects of unilateral loss of vestibular function. Its apparent influence on the activity level of the vestibular nuclei on the damaged side can be abolished by the systemic or intracysternal application of anticholinesterases. This decompensatory action of substances like eserine, isofluorophate, E 600 and E 605 in the unilaterally delabyrinthized frog point to a role played by cholinergic synapses in the development and maintenance of compensation.

G. Centres and Effectors

The account of the work on the significance of efferent control of vestibular function just rendered shows that the problems investigated in the 1960s are still under very active investigation at present. It therefore appears impracticable to separate the last two decades of our history.

I. Vestibular Centres

The characteristics of the complex vestibular nuclei in mammals have been summed up by BRODAL (1974) so succinctly that a near-verbal quotation from that summary can serve our purpose better than any paraphrase. Brodal deals in turn with the four principal nuclei, i.e. superior, lateral, medial, and descending (or inferior).

[1.] The superior vestibular nucleus appears to be particularly closely related to the oculomotor apparatus and to serve the mediation of vestibular and cerebellar influences on these nuclei ... The vestibular influences appear to come mainly from the cristae. Possible relations of the superior nucleus with the spinal cord can only be indirect. The superior nucleus on one side must be functionally linked with its fellow on the other side.

[2.] The lateral vestibular nucleus appears to be of primary importance as a station in pathways mediating cerebellar influences on the spinal cord. The pathways ... all appear to be somatotopically organized and are presumably essential in the production of somatotopically organized effects on the spinal motor apparatus elicitable from the cerebellar vermis. The preponderant contribution of primary vestibular afferents from the utriculus to the nucleus, the restriction of these fibres to the forelimb region and the contribution of small as well as large cells of the vestibulo-spinal tract are features of functional interest. There are indications of relative functional independence of the nuclei on both sides.

[3.] The medial vestibular nucleus appears to be organized in a less specific manner than the superior and lateral nuclei. Like the superior nucleus the medial appears to have its main task in the orderly transmission of impulses from the cristae to the motor nuclei of the ocular nerves. Its projection to the cervical cord suggests that the nucleus may be of functional importance for the integration of movements of the eyes and the neck.

[4.] The descending nucleus in many respects resembles the medial, but it appears scarcely to be concerned with vestibular influences on the ocular muscles. It must be subjected to a differentiated cerebellar control, and has ample possibilities for cooperation with the contralateral descending nucleus.

There follows a summing up of findings with respect to smaller cell groups of the vestibular nuclear complex, including the interstitial nucleus of the vestibular nerve, which receives primary vestibular fibres and may be the only group

... which receives afferents from all five receptor regions of the vestibular apparatus, although the presence of fibres from the maculae is disputed. Cerebellar connections appear to be absent. The nucleus may be particularly related to vestibular influences on the movements of the eyes.

II. Central Processing

The functional aspects of the localization of processing of primary afferents from canals and otolith organs have been reviewed by PRECHT (1974 b).

The methods used in this functional analysis are:

1. The recording at canal- and otolith-controlled sites in the complex of vestibular nuclei of responses to adequate stimulation by angular acceleration as well as by lateral and fore-and-aft tilting;

2. The exploration and localization as well as the time relationships of responses by electrical stimulation of the peripheral organ and the first-order afferents and by the study of field potentials in the nuclear sites (PRECHT and SHIMAZU 1965). The most thoroughly investigated end organ is, of course, for technical reasons the horizontal canal. Here the four *response types* as classified by DUENSING and SCHAEFER (1958) have been fully confirmed.

Type I is represented by the typical primary afferent response from the horizontal canal, consisting of an increase in the frequency of the resting activity on ipsilateral and a decrease on contralateral angular acceleration. *Type II* is reversely characterized by an inhibition of the resting activity on ipsilateral and excitation on contralateral angular acceleration. *Type III* is characterized by excitation on both ipsilateral and contralateral angular acceleration. *Type IV* is inhibited on both ipsilateral and contralateral angular acceleration.

Type II, III, and IV responses are confined to pick-ups from sites in the vestibular nuclei, and are never obtained in open-loop recordings from primary afferents. They are evidently the result of various patterns of convergence of activities from disparate peripheral sources and from intranuclear interaction.

The resting discharge so characteristic of the activity of first-order canal-controlled afferents is also found in the associated second-order neurons in the vestibular nuclei.

The existence of a tonic and a phasic type of response could be demonstrated at nuclear sites (DUENSING and SCHAEFER 1958; SHIMAZU and PRECHT 1965; PRECHT et al. 1971). Tonic units have a pronounced resting activity, low threshold and little or no adaptation to continued stimulation. Phasic (kinetic) units are silent at rest, have a relatively high threshold but a considerably larger gain, and adapt fairly rapidly. It may be recalled that it is generally believed that these two response types originate in hair cells of different topographic location (i.e. the tonic units are associated with hair cells lying on the slopes of the crista and innervated by nerve fibres of moderate diameter, whereas the phasically responding cells are believed to be situated at or near the apical aspect of the crista). They are innervated by large-diameter fibres. In the higher vertebrates these hair cells could be Wersäll's type II and type I respectively, whereas in the lower vertebrates both response types derive from cells morphologically of Wersäll's type II conformation.

The existence of tonic and phasic receptors both in the canal cristae and in the otolith maculae raises the question of the functional significance of such a dualism. The difference between the two types in sensitivity (threshold) and in adaptive behaviour suggests a search for the response parameters in the various effector systems. So far as optic nystagmus is concerned, this is, of course, associated with a turning sensation, and as PRECHT (1975) points out, the tonic units with their low threshold may be responsible for the overall sensitivity of the system, whereas the phasic (kinetic) units with their high threshold could cope with high stimulus intensities of short duration. An association of these peripheral response types with nystagmus on the one hand and turning sensation on the other could be associated with the control by these two different types of afferent. The afternystagmus after a sudden stop of constant-velocity rotation lasts longer than the associated turning sensation, and the cross-over of the cupulograms based on these two is reminiscent of similar differences in the slopes of response curves from tonic and peripheral phasic units. PRECHT et al. (1969) report having obtained supporting evidence for this assumed association in experiments in which they recorded the activity in the abducent nucleus of the cat.

The rapid and far-reaching adaptation found in first-order afferents from phasic receptors has so far not been found in second-order neurons of higher vertebrates, in contrast to the case in the frog, for example, where such adaptation of second-order neurons has indeed been observed (PRECHT et al. 1971; RICHTER and PRECHT 1972).

The synaptology, too, of phasic and tonic peripheral receptors appears to be different. Whereas electrical stimulation of the eighth nerve produces short-latency responses from units identified as phasic, the tonic units appear to be generally linked polysynaptically with the second-order neuron pools (PRECHT and SHIMAZU 1965).

III. Vestibulo-Ocular Interaction

The fact that one of the most, if not the most, overtly important sets of effector organs under vestibular control are the extrinsic eye muscles has been recognized right from the beginning of the exploration of labyrinthine reflexes. An exhaustive coverage of the relevant literature is given by COHEN (1974). The late 1950s and the 1960s saw methodological advances in the registration of eye movements and poses, which, fostered by the increasing need for a refined analysis of optic nystagmus, above all for clinical purposes, focussed research interest on the mechanism of vestibulo-ocular interaction, including the exploration of the central nervous circuitry subserving it.

Horizontal eye movements in response to active and passive rotation of the head about its vertical (z) axis manifest themselves in the simplest case as a compensatory movement of the eyeball in a direction opposite to that of the head under the control of the internal and external (anterior and posterior) straight eye muscles. They are effective in maintaining over a certain range a stationary image of the environment on the retina. Their compensatory range is limited, however, and when the active or passive rotation continues beyond that limit, the eye is reset to its central position by a rapid saccadic return movement. Farther displacement of the head elicits a repeat of this sequence of eye movements. A succession of such eye responses is known by the term "nystagmus." When passive head rotation is abruptly stopped, a so-called post-rotatory nystagmus (afternystagmus) is observed, with slow and rapid phases beating in a direction opposite to those of the per-rotatory nystagmus, i.e. with the slow phase in, and the saccade against, the direction of the preceding rotation. This type of nystagmus is of vestibular origin and is observed in the dark, i.e. in the absence of visual fixation. In the light the per-rotatory nystagmus is reinforced by the simultaneous operation of a so-called optokinetic image, which stabilizes movement of the eye interrupted by saccadic return towards the center of the central position in the orbit (optokinetic nystagmus). Cessation of the movement is followed by an optokinetic afternystagmus in the opposite directions.

The optokinetic eye movements can be observed in organisms without functioning vestibular organs. Rotations of the head about other axes elicit rotary and vertical nystagmus and nystagmus in vectorially intermediate directions. It has been held that all three pairs of semicircular canals are concerned in the control of nystagmus responses of vestibular origin. The central nervous circuitry involving the vestibular and oculomotor nuclei in the medulla is still the object of intensive research.

The circumstance that the eye musculature, being one of the principal vestibular effector organs, forms an essential element in the control of the receptive activity of the eye raises the study of vestibulo-ocular interaction to a level of fundamental importance which makes it understandable that it has commanded the attention of several prominent research groups all over the world. The analysis of this interaction – apart from the physiology of the peripheral sense organs – necessarily extends to the study of the central nervous circuitry forming its morphological and physiological substrate.

The general conclusions as presented by COHEN (1974) and HENN et al. (1980) point to the following insights into the complexities of reciprocal collaboration of the two sensory systems. The interaction manifests itself in a reinforcement of the compensatory eye movements or in their suppression, as the case may be. One of the first authors to draw attention to the latter was OHM (1926), who investigated the influence of vision on vestibular per- and post-rotatory nystagmus. More recently, the participation of the vestibular organ in the shaping of the optokinetic nystagmus and afternystagmus has been investigated by Cohen and co-workers, who found that the vestibular afternystagmus could be completely abolished by the adjustment of relative optokinetic and vestibular stimulation (COHEN et al. 1973). Pure visually induced sensation of self-movement (circular vection) has been found to be dominant in so far as the actually moving stimulating scene tends to be experienced as a stationary background against which the body is felt to be moving. The central nervous system, therefore, interprets the event as of vestibular origin. This can be demonstrated in recordings from second-order vestibular neurons whose activity can be shown to be modulated by visual stimulation.

The involvement of the cerebellum appears likely (MAEKAWA and SIMPSON 1972; ITO et al. 1974). The reverse influence of the vestibular system on the visual one has been less well explored (COHEN 1974). Of course, there are other systems that influence the levels of activity in the vestibular centers. Foremost among them, neck receptors and somatic proprioceptors more generally, as well as integumental mechanoreceptors, all contribute to the final integrated control of body posture and movement. The experimental isolation of any given single contributing modality is, therefore, by no means easy.

More specifically in the vestibular realm, eye reflexes are under the control of both the semicircular canals and the otolith organs. The study of these effector responses dates back to the earliest epochs of vestibular research, and they were explored qualitatively just at the beginning of the period under review here by LORENTE DE NÓ (1931).

The method of recording the responses of the various eye muscles to electrical stimulation of first-order vestibular afferents and second-order neurons in vestibular nuclei has revealed short-latency pathways, whereas the existence of multisynaptic pathways responsible for compensatory eye movements was demonstrated by LORENTE DE NÓ (1933), SZENTÁGOTHAI (1950, 1964) and by the work of Precht and co-workers, who showed the role of cerebellar structures in the control of eye responses of vestibular origin (PRECHT 1972, 1974b). Other workers who have made substantial contributions to this field of research are Shimazu and Susuki (for references see COHEN 1974).

It appears that our knowledge of otolith-controlled eye responses (counter-rolling and static eye deviations) is as yet rather patchy (SZENTÁGOTHAI 1964; FLUUR and MELLSTRÖM 1970a, 1971; SUSUKI et al. 1969). The study of counter-rolling of the eyes in response to head-tilting movement and maintained tilts has shown that its compensatory effect is rather limited (not more than 10% of the total angular displacement of the retina). An open problem concerns the possible participation of the sacculus as well as the utriculus in these responses (FLUUR and MELLSTRÖM 1970b, 1971).

The mapping of the central nervous pathways involved in eye movement control and in vestibulo-ocular interaction has now entered a new methodological era with the introduction of the use of substances such as horseradish peroxidase, which are transported along individual axons after injection into or near the neurons of origin, and are therefore capable of tracing individual pathways within and between central nuclei and between them and peripheral receptor elements. This method promises not only to demonstrate hitherto unknown pathways but also to supplement the results of previous laborious and time-consuming studies by means of retrograde degeneration, for example, apart from the classic staining methods (Nissl, Golgi, thionine and others) described by BRODAL and POMPEIANO (1957, 1958), BRODAL et al. (1962), and BRODAL (1974).

H. Vestibular Problems in the "Spacious Present"

We have now reached a point in our account of the development of vestibular science where it becomes clear that the rendering of history is changing into story-telling. This is to say we are coming up against the fact that – as historians quite rightly avow – it is impossible to treat the present historically. The present can, of course, be surprisingly extended in time. This is governed in the realm of science by the protracted continuity in the pursuance of problems by individual or by whole schools extending over much of the lifetime of the individual or over a period of unchanging composition and programme of a school or research group.

Topics foremost under consideration at present concern one or the other aspect of stimulus transduction, be it mechanical, biophysical, biochemical or neurological. A detailed report on recent work dealing with such topics lies outside the scope of this historical survey. However, it may be desirable to draw the reader's attention to the relevant literature under the various headings.

In the mechanical and biophysical fields the emphasis is on the role of the cupula of the semicircular canal ampulla (DOHLMAN 1971, 1980; HILLMAN 1972; OMAN and YOUNG 1972; MCLAREN and HILLMAN 1976; FLOCK et al. 1977; MCLAREN and HILLMAN 1979; OMAN et al., to be published). The mode of functioning of otolyth organs is dealt with by HUDSPETH and JACOBS (1979), HUDSPETH et al. (1980), FLOCK et al. (1977, 1981), and MACARTHEY et al. (1980).

The microchemical interest centers chiefly on the role of Ca^+ (SAND 1975) in the transduction process (see also TRINCKER 1965). An important element in the stimulus–response relationship is peripheral adaptation. This has been elucidated by the work of GOLDBERG and FERNANDEZ (1971 a, b) for the various types of receptor element (WERSÄLL and BAGGER-SJÖBÄCK 1974), and the sites of the adaptive response regulation have been discussed by SAND (1975) and LOWENSTEIN (1981).

Systems-analytic and neurological work relating to transduction based on the earlier torsion pendulum hypothesis of semicircular canal function (STEINHAUSEN 1931, 1933; SCHMALTZ 1925, 1932; DOHLMAN 1935; VAN EGMOND et al. 1949; GROEN et al. 1952) has yielded formulations which strongly suggest imperfections and oversimplifications in the earlier functional models (GOLDBERG and FERNANDEZ 1971 a, b; YOUNG 1969; YOUNG and OMAN 1968, 1969; MAYNE 1974). Otolith-controlled responses have so far lent themselves less to such treatment (LOWENSTEIN and SAUNDERS 1975).

The advent of space travel has highlighted problems arising from space-sickness, which is probably triggered by mismatches of information from the semicircular canals and the eyes with that from the otolith organs, which are specifically affected by exposure to the reduction or absence of gravitational stimuli in orbital flight. There are recent reviews of this subject by Graybiel (1968), Guedry (1968), Money (1970), Mayne (1974), Melvill Jones (1974), and Reason and Brand (1975), and a report of experimental work with an animal preparation in orbital flight by Bracchi et al. (1975); see also the papers by Kellog and Graybiel (1967), Graybiel et al. (1974), Vinnikov (1974), and Benson (1974).

Vestibulo-ocular interaction in normal and disturbed situations are at present under intensive scrutiny by a number of research groups and a full account of this work is given by Cohen (1981).

The acoustic function of the vestibular organ largely restricted to lower aquatic vertebrates has been left unreviewed here. However, there follow some references to some early papers and to recent review articles on this important aspect of vestibular science, the detailed treatment of which would be more advantageously rendered in an article on bioacoustics or hearing: Ashcroft and Hallpike (1934); von Frisch (1936); Lowenstein and Roberts (1951); Tavolga (1971); Lowenstein (1971); Kleerekoper and Chagnon (1954); Enger (1968); Popper and Fay (1973); Blaxter and Tytler (1978).

J. Postscript

During a lifetime of work in the field of vestibular science I have had the good fortune to enjoy the collaboration of the late A. Sand, the late J. J. Groen, and of J. Wersäll, as well as of my research assistants T. D. M. Roberts and R. D. Saunders. The story of the early pioneering on the electrophysiology of the elasmobranch labyrinth carried out in collaboration with Alec Sand has been told in a biographical manner, published under the title "Biographical Notes on the Early Electrophysiological Exploration of Vestibular Function" in the *Canadian Journal of Otolaryngology* (Lowenstein 1974 b) and reprinted in the *Journal of Comparative Biochemistry and Physiology* (Lowenstein 1975).

K. Appendix: Biographical Notes[1]

It all started in the Professor's room in the Zoology Department in Munich in 1933. At that time I had just lost a research assistantship held under the auspices of the *Notgemeinschaft der Deutschen Wissenschaften* because the National Socialist Government would not allow grants of this or any kind to be held by anybody who could not prove that he was of pure Aryan descent. However, Karl von Frisch, my teacher and *Doktorvater* (doctor father), had told me when my grant dried up that he wanted me to continue my work in the Department on the labyrinth of tench and pike – a continuation of my work on the minnow labyrinth (Lowenstein 1932), which had earned me my doctorate. He said he had a private fund available

---

1 Quoted from an article first published in the *Canadian Journal of Otolaryngology* in 1974

from which he could continue to let me have my monthly cheque, which was to be collected from his office. It was only much later that I realized that these monthly cheques orginated in his private purse!

It must have been on one of those occasions that, after a survey of the fate of various unsuccessful attempts to place me in one or the other laboratory abroad, he asked me what I would do research-wise, if I was successful in finding a place and research facilities. I answered by extolling to him the exciting possibilities in sensory physiology opened up by Adrian's electrophysiological method, and said I would try to apply this technique to the analysis of the function of individual parts of the labyrinth.

I still remember the frown on von Frisch's brow and the terse comment heralded by it: "So you want to put all this gadgetry between yourself and the animal?" This remark was not entirely unexpected. Although he had put me in charge of the care of the physical apparatus in the Department, and had charged me with the duty of advising research workers intending to use it, he was suspicious of young biologists becoming enmeshed in such methods for their own sake and in danger of losing sight of the biological aspects of their problem.

When I left Germany in 1933 to work as a displaced scholar in the Zoology Department of the University of Birmingham (England), a chance meeting with Alec Sand at the Plymouth Marine Laboratory opened up the possibility of a joint electrophysiological analysis of the impulse responses to rotary and postural stimuli in specific branches of the vestibular nerve in elasmobranch fishes.

After a preliminary anatomical exploration of the eighth nerve and its individual branches had indicated the marginal feasibility of such a project, Sand and I arranged for a period of joint work at the Plymouth laboratory. Most promising technically, and also very important theoretically, was to attempt a recording of the impulse responses from the horizontal ampulla of the dogfish to rotational stimuli in the horizontal plane.

Our theoretical expectations were based on my hypothesis (LOWENSTEIN 1932, 1937) that a semicircular canal ought to be able to signal bidirectional information, and also on Sand's experience with sensory units of the lateral line, where he had found side by side two types of unit responding with an increase of the resting discharge to perfusion of the canal in one direction and with a decrease to perfusion in the opposite direction, each individual unit, however, was excited and inhibited respectively by perfusion in opposite directions (SAND 1937).

It is not surprising, therefore, that we were somewhat disapointed to find that angular acceleration of the turntable in one direction (counter-clockwise for the left labyrinth) invariably produced an increase, and clockwise rotation a decrease in the frequency of the resting discharge in units of the horizontal canal. This meant that there were no receptor endings in a given ampulla that could respond by excitation to contralateral angular acceleration. Only ipsilateral acceleration could produce such a "positive" response in a horizontal canal. Translated into terms of the immediate physical stimulus, this meant that only ampullopetal endolymph displacement resulted in a positive response.

Did this, then, mean that my hypothesis of a bidirectional canal response was wrong? It gradually dawned on us that this was not the case. After all, we did obtain reliably repeatable effects by rotating in opposite directions – an excitatory increase in the resting activity in response to ipsilateral and an equally striking "inhibitory decrease or even complete abolition of the resting activity in response to contralateral angular acceleration." The simple postulate that the central nervous relay stations were capable of recognizing and processing both an increase and a decrease in a pre-existing peripheral activity sufficed to establish the bidirectionality of the semicircular canal receptor (Lowenstein and Sand 1936).

What is more, we suddenly saw a rationale behind the resting activity, allotting to it the specific function of serving as a background for bidirectional modulation of a peripheral signal, apart from its obvious importance as a constant source of labyrinthine tonus. In fact, it was the more complex arrangement in the lateral line end organs that demanded an explanation in terms of functional "advantage."

The expedition to Plymouth had, after all, been crowned with success. Not only had we demonstrated to ourselves that electrophysiological work on the elasmobranch labyrinth was possible, we had also produced the first direct evidence for the modus operandi of vestibular end organs. Twenty-eight years later, it was my good fortune to be able to demonstrate in collaboration with Osborne and Wersäll how the bidirectionality has its base in the ultrastructural polarization of the vestibular hair cell and its topographic deployment within the various sensory epithelia of the labyrinth.

Before proceeding to describe the next joint step in the electrophysiological analysis of vestibular function, I feel it might be of interest to provide a memory picture of the personality of Alec Sand, especially as his tragic early death at the end of the Second World War prevented so many contemporary sensory physiologists from enjoying the pleasure and privilege of meeting face to face this man of outstanding personal and scientific qualities.

Sand was born in 1901 in Warsaw. In 1907 his parents moved to England, where he received a grammar school education with an emphasis on arts subjects. His teachers remember him as an exceptionally bright boy, of short stature but with a splendid physique, a good sportsman and very gifted artistically, especially as a pianist.

After a year at Reading University, he went to the University of British Columbia to study dairy science. With a degree in agriculture he took up farming, but felt this gave him insufficient intellectual outlets. He therefore went to McGill to read for an MSc in Bacteriology. It was at McGill that he met Lancelot Hogben, who persuaded him to accept a lectureship in zoology when he was appointed to the Chair of that department at Cape Town University. Sand accepted that offer in preference to a fellowship at Yale. When Hogben left Cape Town, Sand worked with T. A. Stephenson until 1933, when he obtained leave of absence to work for the Cambridge PhD under James Gray. And thus we met.

Sand impressed me not only by his wide-ranging interests, which covered all branches of science, quite apart from his wide specialist knowledge of comparative physiology, but also by his enlightened outlook on life and his unobtrusive but ever-present awareness of cultural values. He was five years my senior, but for all I knew we belonged to the same generation, and there was always an implicit mutual understanding between us on all things that mattered.

There was a sombre strain in his make-up which I attributed to his Russian heritage, but this was amply compensated by his wonderful sense of humour and wit. He could be rather despondent at times when things went wrong with an experiment, but soon recovered his sense of enterprise, in which he was helped not only by his skill and ingenuity in the planning and carrying out of experiments but also by his sheer craftsmanship and talent for improvization. If one adds to this his penetrating critical faculties and his gift for lucid writing, one can imagine how fortunate I felt myself to have found such a congenial workmate, willing at all times to enter into an exchange of ideas and a frictionless division of labour which is the hallmark of a successful scientific collaboration.

When war broke out, he was the first member of the staff of the Plymouth Laboratory to volunteer for active service in the Navy, a step which was for him not only a matter of duty to his country, but a means of settling a score with a regime which he considered to menace the only acceptable way of life, to say nothing of the misdeeds perpetrated against his fellow-Jews, an aspect of the times which occasionally made him despair of the future fate of *Homo sapiens* and of the possibility of the advent of a humanist global society.

When I said goodbye to him at the end of our joint labours on the work about to be described, which coincided with the outbreak of the war, we made plans for a continuation of our collaboration after its end, not knowing that this end would be so distant, and that he was not destined ever again to work at Plymouth. His untimely death in 1945, when we both believed that a new joint venture was just around the corner, deprived the scientific world of a physiologist of the highest promise and me of a man whose friendship I had learned to treasure.

The new approach that enabled us to analyse the response of all three semicircular canals was based on our realization that reliably repeatable responses had been obtained in spinal dogfish that failed to recover at the end of an experimental session. This, together with Sand's experience with work on isolated preparations of the lateralis organs in the ray, encouraged us to develop the technique of the isolated labyrinth (LOWENSTEIN and SAND 1936). It soon became clear that on dimensional grounds and from the point of view of better accessibility, the ray labyrinth was more suitable than that of the dogfish. The gain in experimental convenience was, of course, very considerable. We were able to dispense with the large unwieldy turntable, and instead of having to cope with a whole fish under artificial respiration we were now dealing with the isolated brain case, which gave access from all sides for the pick-up from the nerves of all three ampullae. The result was the proposal of a schema for the integrated collaboration of the three canals during angular accelerations about the three main body axes, and its relation to the known eye muscle reflexes occurring in response to these rotational stimuli.

However, the responses recorded were massive responses from multifibre pick-ups that did not allow rigorously quantitative analysis of the stimulus–response relationships. Moreover, the pictures obtainable with the mechanical oscillograph lacked the clarity obtainable by means of the cathode-ray oscillograph, which was coming into use at that time.

Before we proceeded to our next subject (LOWENSTEIN and SAND 1940 a, b), Sand had the good fortune to benefit from the advice and help of the American physiologist Otto Schmitt (at A. V. Hill's laboratory in London) for the building of a sophisticated balanced high-gain amplifier system and cathode-ray oscillograph with a performance which was then years ahead of its time.

When we resumed work, we felt that we should aim at a single-unit pick-up, and this was achieved by the introduction of a forceps electrode instead of the looped silver wire used up till then. Furthermore, the aim at a quantitative treatment of the responses made necessary the quantification of the acceleratory stimulus. This was achieved by the design of a falling-weight drive to the turntable and the installation of a photo-electric signalling system incorporating a precision-cut slotted disc for the interception of the light beam. In all these developments Sand's practical ingenuity played a leading part.

The result was the fitting of the impulse responses from the horizontal semicircular canal to the physical properties of the cupula, as described by STEINHAUSEN (1933), as a basis for the time relations of rotatory and post-rotatory nystagmus described in our paper, the completion of which coincided with the outbreak of the war (LOWENSTEIN and SAND 1940a, b).

References

Names containing *von* are alphabetized in this list under *v*

Ades HW, Engström H (1972) Inner ear studies. Acta Otolaryngol [Suppl] (Stockh) 301:3–75
Adrian ED (1930) The mechanism of the sense organs. Physiol Rev 10:336–374
Adrian ED (1943) Discharges from vestibular receptors in the cat. J Physiol (Lond) 101:389–407
Adrian ED (1947) The physical background of perception. Clarendon, Oxford
Adrian ED, Eckhard R (1926) Impulses in the optic nerve. J Physiol (Lond) 62:23–24P
Adrian ED, Zotterman I (1926a) The impulses produced by sensory nerve endings. I. J Physiol (Lond) 61:49–72
Adrian ED, Zotterman I (1926b) The impulses produced by sensory nerve endings. II. The responses of a single end-organ. J Physiol (Lond) 61:151–171
Adrian ED, Zotterman I (1926c) Impulses from a single sensory end-organ. J Physiol (Lond) 61:8
Ashcroft DW, Hallpike CS (1934) On the function of the saccule. J Laryngol Otol 49:450–460
Bárány R (1907) Physiologie und Pathologie des Bogengangsapparates beim Menschen. Deutike, Wien
Bethe A (ed) Handbuch der normalen und pathologischen Physiologie. Springer, Berlin
Benson AJ (1974) Modification of the response to angular accelerations by linear accelerations. In: Kornhuber HH (ed) Vestibular system pt 2 psychophysics, applied aspects and general interpretations. Springer, Berlin Heidelberg New York, pp 281–360
Bienhold H, Flohr H (1980) Role of cholinergic synapse in vestibular compensation. Brain Res 195:476–478
Blaxter JHS, Tytler P (1978) Physiology and function of the swimbladder. Adv Comp Physiol Biochem 7:311–367
Bracchi F, Gualtierotti T, Morabito A, Rocca E (1975) Multiday recordings from primary neurons of the statoreceptors of the labyrinth of the bullfrog. Acta Otolaryngol [Suppl] (Stockh) 334:1–27
Breuer J (1889) Neue Versuche an den Ohrbogengängen. Pflügers Arch 44:134–152
Breuer J (1891) Über die Funktion der Otolithen-Apparate. Pflügers Arch 48:195–306
Brodal A (1974) Anatomy of the vestibular nuclei and their connections. In: Kornhuber HH (ed) Vestibular system, pt 1 basic mechanisms. Springer, Berlin Heidelberg New York, pp 239–352 (Handbook of sensory physiology, vol 6/1)
Brodal A, Pompeiano O (1957) The vestibular nuclei in the cat. J Anat 91:438–454

Brodal A, Pompeiano O (1958) The origin of ascending fibres of the longitudinal fasciculus from the vestibular nuclei. An experimental study in the cat. Acta Morphol Neerl Scand 1:306–328

Brodal A, Pompeiano O, Walberg F (1962) The vestibular nuclei and their connections, anatomy, and functional correlation. Oliver and Boyd, Edinburgh

Christiansen JA (1964) On hyalouronate molecules in the labyrinth as mechano-electric transducers and as molecular motors acting as resonators. Acta Otolaryngol (Stockh) 57:33–49

Citron LD, Exley D, Hallpike CS (1956) Formation, circulation, and chemical properties of the labyrinthine fluids. Br Med Bull 12:101–104

Cohen B (1974) The vestibulo-ocular reflex arc. In: Kornhuber HH (ed) Vestibular system, pt 1 basic mechanisms. Springer, Berlin Heidelberg New York, pp 477–540 (Handbook of sensory physiology, vol 6/1

Cohen B, Uemura T, Takemori S (1973) Effects of labyrinthectomy on optokinetic nystagmus (OKN) and optokinetic after nystagmus (OKAN). Equil Res 3:80–93

Cohen B (ed) (1981) Vestibular and oculomotor physiology. International meeting of the Bárány society. Ann New York Acad Sci Vol 374

Crum-Brown A (1873) On the sense of rotation and the anatomy and physiology of the semicircular canals of the internal ear. J Anat 8:327–331

Davis H, Eldredge DH (1959) An interpretation of the mechanical detector action of the cochlea. Ann Otol Rhinolaryngol 68:665–674

Davis H (1960) Mechanism of excitation of auditory nerve impulses. In: Rasmussen GL, Windle WF (eds) Neural mechanisms of the auditory and vestibular systems. Thomas, Springfield

Davis H (1965) A model for transducer action in the cochlea. Cold Spring Harbor Symp Quant Biol 30:181–190

Denton EJ, Blaxter JHS (1976) The mechanical relationships between the clupeid swim bladder, inner ear, and lateral line. J Mar Biol Assoc UK 56:787–807

De Vries H (1949) The minimum perceptible angular acceleration. Acta Otolaryngol (Stockh) 37:218–229

Di Giorgio AM (1960) La seconde loi d'Ewald est-elle justifiée? Acta Otolaryngol [Suppl] (Stockh) 159:47–49

Dohlman GF (1925) Physiokalische und physiologische Studien zur Theorie des kalorischen Nystagmus. Acta Otolaryngol [Suppl] (Stockh) 5:1–196

Dohlman GF (1935) Some practical and theoretical points in labyrinthology. Proc R Soc Med 50:779–790

Dohlman GF (1960a) On the case for repeal of Ewald's second law. Acta Otolaryngol [Suppl] (Stockh) 159:15–24

Dohlman GF (1960b) Some aspects of the mechanism of vestibular hair cell stimulation. Confin Neurol 20:169

Dohlman GF (1971) The attachment of the cupulae, otolith, and tectorial membranes to the sensory cell areas. Acta Otolaryngol (Stockh) 71:89–105

Dohlmann GF (1980) Critical review of the concept of cupula function. Acta Otolaryngol [Suppl] (Stockh) 376:1–30

Dohlman GF, Farkashidi J, Salomm F (1958) Centrifugal nerve fibres to the sensory epithelium of the vestibular labyrinth. J Laryngol Otol 78:784

Duensing F, Schaefer KP (1958) Die Aktivität einzelner Neurone im Bereich der Vestibularis-Kerne bei Horizontalbeschleunigungen unter besonderer Berücksichtigung des vestibularen Nystagmus. Arch Psychiat Nervenkr 198:225–252

Enger PS (1968) Hearing in fish. In: De Reuck AVS, Knight S (eds) Hearing mechanisms in vertebrates. Churchill, London, pp 4–17

Ewald JR (1892) Physiologische Untersuchungen über das Endorgan des Nervus octovus. Bergmann, Wiesbaden

Fernandez C, Goldberg JM (1971) Physiology of peripheral neurons innervating the semicircular canals of the squirrel monkey. II. The response to sinusoidal stimulation and dynamics of the peripheral vestibular system. J Neurophysiol 34:661–675

Flock Å, Flock B, Murray E (1977) Studies on the sensory hairs of receptor cells in the inner ear. Acta Otolaryngol (Stockh) 83:85–91

Flock Å, Cheung HC, Flock B, Utter G (1981) Three sets of actin filaments in sensory cells of the inner ear. Identification and functional orientation determined by gel electrophoresis, immunofluorescence, and electronmicroscopy. J Neurocytol 10:133–147

Flourens P (1842) Recherches expérimentales sur les propriétés et les fonctions du système nerveux dans les animaux vertébrés, 2 nd edn. Crevot, Paris

Fluur E, Mellström A (1970 a) Utricular stimulation and oculomotor reactions. Laryngoscope 80:1701–1712

Fluur E, Mellström A (1970 b) Saccular stimulation and oculomotor reactions. Laryngoscope 80:1713–1721

Fluur E, Mellström A (1971) The otolith organs and their influence on oculomotor movements. Exp Neurol 30:139–147

Frenzel H (1925) Nystagmusbeobachtung während der Drehung. Z Hals Nasen Ohrenheilk 12:637

Gacek RR (1960) Efferent component of the vestibular nerve. In: Rasmussen GL, Windle WF (eds) Neural mechanisms of the auditory and vestibular systems. Thomas, Springfield

Gacek RR (1967) Anatomical evidence for an efferent vestibular pathway. Third symposium on the role of the vestibular organs in space exploration. Naval Aerospace Medical Institute, Pensacola, Florida

Gacek RR (1974) Morphological aspects of the efferent vestibular system. In: Kornhuber HH (ed) Vestibular system, pt 1 basic mechanisms. Springer, Berlin Heidelberg New York, pp 213–220 (Handbook of sensory physiology, vol 6/1)

Gacek RR, Lyon M (1974) The localization of vestibular efferent neurons in the kitten with horseradish peroxidase. Acta Otolaryngol (Stockh) 77:92–101

Goldberg JM, Fernandez C (1971 a) Physiology of peripheral neurons innervating semicircular canals of the squirrel monkey. I. Resting discharge and response to constant angular accelerations. J Neurophysiol 34:635–660

Goldberg JM, Fernandez C (1971 b) Physiology of peripheral neurons innervating semicircular canals in the squirrel monkey. III. Variations among units in their discharge properties. J Neurophysiol 34:676–684

Grahe K (1926) Die Funktion des Bogengangsapparates und der Statolithen beim Menschen. In: Bethe A (ed) Handbuch der normalen und pathologischen Physiologie, vol 11. Springer, Berlin, S. 909

Gray EG, Pumphrey RJ (1958) Ultrastructure of the insect ear. Nature 181:618

Graybiel A (1968) Structural elements in the concept of motion sickness. NAMI-1055:1–39

Graybiel A, Miller EF II, Homick JL (1974) Experiment M131: human vestibular function. In: Graybiel A (ed) NASA Tech Memo X-58154 Lyndon B. Johnson Space Center 1:169–198

Groen JJ (1960) On the repeal of Ewald's second law. Acta Otolaryngol [Suppl] (Stockh) 159:42–46

Groen JJ, Jonkees LBW (1948) The turning test with small regulable stimuli. IV. The cupulogram obtained by subject angle estimation. J Laryngol Otol 62:236–240

Groen JJ, Lowenstein O, Vendrik AJH (1952) The mechanical analysis of the responses from the end-organs of the horizontal semicircular canal in the isolated elasmobranch labyrinth. J Physiol (Lond) 117:329–346

Grundfest H (1966) Comparative electrobiology of excitable membranes. Adv Comp Physiol Biochem 2:1–116

Guedry FE Jr (1968) Conflicting sensory orientation cues as a factor in motion sickness. NASA Spec Publ 187:45–51

Guedry FE Jr (1974) Psychophysics of vestibular sensation. In: Kornhuber HH (ed) Vestibular system, pt 2 psychophysics. Springer, Berlin Heidelberg New York, pp 3–154 (Handbook of sensory physiology, vol 6/2)

Hallpike CS (1960) On the case for repeal of Ewald's second law: some introductory remarks. Acta Otolaryngol [Suppl] (Stockh) 159:7–14

Henn V, Cohen B, Young LR (1980) Visual-vestibular interactions in motion perception and the generation of nystagmus. Neuros Res Program Bull 18:459–651

Hilding DA, Wersäll J (1962) Cholinesterase and its relation to the nerve endings in the inner ear. Acta Otolaryngol (Stockh) 55:205–217

Hillman DE (1972) Observations on morphological features and mechanical properties of the peripheral vestibular receptor system in the frog. Brain Res 37:69–75

Hillman DE, McLaren JW (1979) Displacement configuration of semicircular canal ampullae. Neuroscience 4:1989–2000

Hood JD (1960) The neuro-physiological significance of cupular adaptation and its bearing upon Ewald's second law. Acta Otolaryngol [Suppl] (Stockh) 159:50–55

Hudspeth AJ, Jacobs R (1979) Stereocilia mediate transduction in vertebrate hair cells. Proc Nat Acad Sci USA 76:1506–1509

Hudspeth AG, Shotwell SL, Jacobs R (1980) Directional sensitivity of individual vertebrate hair cells to controlled deflection of their hair bundles. Cohen B (ed) Conf vest oculomotor physiol. International Meeting of the Bárány Society, New York. Academy of Sciences Press, New York

Ireland P, Farkashidi J (1961) Studies on the efferent innervation of the vestibular end organs. Ann Otolaryngol Chir Cervicofac 70:490–503

Ito M, Shida T, Yagi N, Yamamoto M (1974) Visual influence on rabbit horizontal vestibulo-ocular reflex presumably effected via the cerebellar flocculus. Brain Res 65:170–174

Jones GM, Spells KE (1963) A theoretical and comparative study of the functional dependence of the semicircular canal upon its physical dimensions. Proc R Soc Lond B 157:403–419

Kellog RS, Graybiel A (1967) Lack of response to thermal stimulation of the semicircular canals in the weightless phase of parabolic flight. Aerospace Med 38:487–490

Kleerekoper H, Chagnon EC (1954) Hearing in fish, with special reference to *Semotilus atromaculatus atromaculatus* (Mitchill). J Fisheries Res Board Can 11:130–152

Klinke R (1970) Efferent influence on the vestibular organ during active movements of the body. Pflügers Arch 318:325–332

Klinke R, Galley N (1971) Efferent innervation of vestibular and auditory receptors. Physiol Rev 54:315–357

Kornhuber HH (ed) (1974a) Vestibular system, pt 1 basic mechanisms. Springer, Berlin Heidelberg New York (Handbook of sensory physiology, vol 6/1)

Kornhuber HH (ed) (1974b) Vestibular system, pt 2 psychophysics. Springer, Berlin Heidelberg New York (Handbook of sensory physiology, vol 6/2)

Kornhuber HH (1974c) History of vestibular research. In: Kornhuber HH (ed) Vestibular system, pt 1 basic mechanisms. Springer, Berlin Heidelberg New York, p 14 (Handbook of sensory physiology, vol 6/1)

Ledoux A (1949) Activité électrique des nerfs des canaux semi-circulaires du saccule et de l'utricule chez la grenouille. Acta Otorhinolaryngol Belg 3:335–349

Ledoux A (1960) Contribution à la discussion sur la validité de la seconde loi d'Ewald. (Arguments tirés de l'étude electrophysiologique du canal semi-circulaire.) Acta Otolaryngol [Suppl] (Stockh) 159:15–24

Lorente de Nó R (1931) Ausgewählte Kapitel aus der vergleichenden Physiologie des Labyrinthes. Die Augenmuskelreflexe beim Kaninchen und ihre Grundlagen. Ergebn Physiol 32:73–242

Lorente de Nó R (1933) Vestibulo-ocular reflex arc. Arch Neurol Psychiat 30:245–291

Lowenstein O (1932) Experimentelle Untersuchungen über den Gleichgewichtssinn der Elritze (*Phoxinus laevis*). Z Vergl Physiol 17:806–854

Lowenstein O (1936) The equilibrium function of the vertebrate labyrinth. Biol Rev 11:113–145

Lowenstein O (1937) The tonic function of the horizontal semicircular canals in fishes. J Exp Biol 14:473–482

Lowenstein O (1955) The effect of galvanic polarization on the impulse discharge from sense endings in the isolated labyrinth of the thornback ray (*Raja clavata*). J Physiol (Lond) 127:104–117

Lowenstein O (1971) The labyrinth. In: Hoar WS, Randall DJ (eds) Fish physiology, vol 5. Academic, New York, pp 207–240

Lowenstein O (1974a) Comparative morphology and physiology. In: Kornhuber HH (ed) Vestibular system, pt 1 basic mechanisms. Springer, Berlin Heidelberg New York, pp 75–120 (Handbook of sensory physiology, vol 6/1)

Lowenstein O (1974 b) Biographical notes on the early electrophysiological exploration of vestibular function. Can J Otolaryngol 3:254–261

Lowenstein O (1975) Biographical notes on the early electrophysiological exploration of vestibular function. Comp Biochem Physiol 51:1–5

Lowenstein O (1981) The origin and functional significance of the resting activity and peripheral adaptation in the vestibular system. In: Gualtierotti T (ed) The vestibular system: function and morphology. Springer, Berlin Heidelberg New York, pp 317–328

Lowenstein O, Osborne MP (1964) Ultrastructure of sensory hair-cells in the labyrinth of the ammocoete larva of the lamprey, *Lampetra fluviatilis*. Nature 204:197–198

Lowenstein O, Roberts TDM (1949) The equilibrium function of the otolith organs of the thornback ray (*Raja clavata*). J Physiol (Lond) 110:392–415

Lowenstein O, Roberts TDM (1951) The localization and analysis of the responses to vibration from the isolated elasmobranch labyrinth. A contribution to the problem of the evolution of hearing in the vertebrates. J Physiol (Lond) 114:471–489

Lowenstein O, Sand A (1936) The activity of the horizontal semicircular canal of the dogfish, *Scyllium canicula*. J Exp Biol 13:416–428

Lowenstein O, Sand A (1940a) The individual and integrated activity of the semicircular canals of the elasmobranch labyrinth. J Physiol (Lond) 99:89–101

Lowenstein O, Sand A (1940b) The mechanism of the semicircular canal. A study of the responses of single-fibre preparations to angular accelerations and rotation at constant speed. Proc R Soc Lond B 129:256–275

Lowenstein O, Saunders RD (1975) Otolith-controlled responses from the first-order neurons of the labyrinth of the bullfrog (*Rana catesbiana*) to changes in linear acceleration. Proc R Soc Lond B 191:475–505

Lowenstein O, Osborne MP, Wersäll J (1964) Structure and innervation of the sensory epithelia of the labyrinth in the thornback ray (*Raja clavata*). Proc R Soc Lond B 160:1–12

Mach E (1875) Grundlinien der Lehre von den Bewegungsempfindungen. Engelmann, Leipzig

Macartney JC, Comis SD, Pickles JO (1980) Is myosin in the cochlea a basis for active motility? Nature 288:491–492

MacNaughton IPJ, McNally WJ (1946) Some experiments which indicate that the frog's lagena has an equilibrium function. J Laryngol Otol 61:204–214

Maekawa K, Simpson JI (1972) Climbing fiber activation of Purkinje cells in the flocculus by impulses transferred through the visual pathway. Brain Res 35:245–251

Magnus R (1924) Körperstellung. Springer, Berlin

Magnus R, de Kleijn A (1926) Funktion des Bogengangs- und Otolithenapparates bei Säugern. In: Bethe A (ed) Handbuch der normalen und pathologischen Physiologie, vol 11. Springer, Berlin, pp 868–908

Main RJ (1931) Stereotropism and geotropism of the salamander, *Triturus torosus*. Physiol Zool 4:409

Malcolm R, Mellvill Jones G (1970) A quantitative study of vestibular adaptation in humans. Acta Otolaryngol (Stockh) 70:126–135

Markl H (1974) The perception of gravity and of angular acceleration in invertebrates. In: Kornhuber HH (ed) Vestibular system, pt 1 basic mechanisms. Springer, Berlin Heidelberg New York, pp 17–74 (Handbook of sensory physiology, vol 6/1)

Mayne R (1974) A systems concept of the vestibular organs. In: Kornhuber HH (ed) Vestibular system, pt 2 psychophysics. Springer, Berlin Heidelberg New York, pp 493–580 (Handbook of sensory physiology, vol 6/2)

Mayne R, Belanger F (1966) The function and operating principles of otolith organs. III. Interpretation of single-fibre or few-fibre recordings. Goodyear Aerospace Corp, Rep. GERA 1113

McLaren JW, Hillman DE (1976) Configuration of the cupula during endolymph pressure changes. Abstracts of the 6th annual meeting of the society of neuroscientists, Toronto, p 1060

McLaren JW, Hillman DE (1979) Displacement of semicircular canal cupula during sinusoidal rotation. Neuroscience 4:2001–2008

McNally WJ, Tait J (1925) Ablation experiments on the labyrinth of the frog. Am J Physiol 75:155–179

McNally WJ, Tait J (1933) Some results of section of particular nerve branches to the ampullae of the four vertical semicircular canals of the frog. Q J Exp Physiol 23:147–196

Melvill Jones G (1974) Adaptive neurobiology in space flight. Proc Skylab Life Sci Symp NASA TMX-58154 11:847–859

Mittermaier R (1960) Zur Gültigkeit des zweiten Ewaldschen Gesetzes beim Menschen. Acta Otolaryngol [Suppl] (Stockh) 159:35–41

Money KE (1970) Motion sickness. Physiol Rev 50:1–39

Montandon A (1960) Discussion au sujet de la seconde loi d'Ewald. Acta Otolaryngol [Suppl] (Stockh) 159:56–59

Murray RW, Potts WTW (1961) The composition of the endolymph, perilymph and other body fluids of elasmobranchs. Comp Biochem Physiol 2:65–75

Mygind GH (1948) Static function of the labyrinth. Attempt at a synthesis. Acta Otolaryngol [Suppl] (Stockh) 70:1–114

Niven GI, Hixon WC (1961) Frequency response of human semicircular canals. I. Steady-state ocular nystagmus response to high level sinusoidal angular rotations. In: Graybiel A (ed) NSAM-459. Naval School of Aviation Medicine, Pensacola

Ohm J (1926) Über den Einfluß des Sehens auf den vestibulären Drehnystagmus. Z Hals Nasen Ohrenheilk 16:521–540

Oman CM, Young LR (1972) The physiological range of pressure difference and cupula deflections in the human semicircular canal: theoretical considerations. Acta Otolaryngol (Stockh) 74:324–331

Oman CM, Frishkopf LS, Goldstein MH (to be published) Cupula motion in the semicircular canal of the skate *Raja erinacea:* an experimental investigation. Acta Otolaryngol (Stockh)

Peterson SK, Frishkopf LS, Lechène C, Oman CM (1978) Element composition of inner ear lymphs in cats, lizards, and skates, determined by electrode probe microanalysis of liquid samples. J Comp Physiol 126:1–14

Popper AN, Fay RR (1973) Sound detection and processing by teleost fishes: a critical review. J Acoust Soc Am 53:1515–1529

Precht W (1972) Vestibular and cerebellar control of oculomotor functions. Bibl Ophthalmol (Basel) 82:71–88

Precht W (1974a) Physiological aspects of the efferent vestibular system. In: Kornhuber HH (ed) Vestibular system, pt 1 basic mechanisms. Springer, Berlin Heidelberg New York, pp 221–236 (Handbook of sensory physiology, vol 6/1)

Precht W (1974b) The physiology of the vestibular nuclei. In: Kornhuber HH (ed) Vestibular system, pt 1 basic mechanisms. Springer, Berlin Heidelberg New York, pp 353–416 (Handbook of sensory physiology, vol 6/1)

Precht W (1975) Vestibular system M.T.B. In: Guyton AC, Hunt CC (eds) International review of sciences, neurophysiology physiology series 1 vol 3. Butterworth, London, pp 82–149

Precht W, Shimazu H (1965) Functional connections of tonic and kinetic vestibular neurones with primary vestibular afferents. J Neurophysiol 28:1014–1028

Precht W, Richter A, Grippo J (1969) Responses of neurons in cat's abducent nuclei to horizontal angular acceleration. Pflügers Arch 309:285–309

Precht W, Llinas R, Clarke M (1971) Physiological responses of frog vestibular fibres to horizontal angular rotation. Exp Brain Res 13:378–407

Quix FM (1924) Die Otolithenfunktion in der Otologie. Z Hals Nasen Ohrenheilk 8:516

Rasmussen GL (1946) The olivary peduncle and other fiber projections of the olivary complex. J Comp Neurol 84:141

Rasmussen GL (1953) Further observations of the afferent cochlear bundle. J Comp Neurol 99:61

Rauch S, Köstlin A (1958) Aspects chimiques de l'endolymphe et de la periphymphe. Pract Oto-Rhino-Laryngol 20:287–291

Reason JT, Brand JJ (1975) Motion sickness. Academic, London

Richter A, Precht W (1972) Responses of frog vestibular neurons to physiological stimulation of the labyrinth. Pflügers Arch [Suppl] 335:79

Ross DA (1936) Electrical studies on the frog's labyrinth. J Physiol (Lond) 86:117–146

Russel IJ (1968) The influence of efferent fibres on a receptor. Nature 219:177–178

Russel IJ (1971) The role of the lateral-line efferent system in *Xenopus laevis*. J Exp Biol 54:621–641

Sand A (1937) The mechanism of the lateral line. Proc R Soc Lond B 123:477–495

Sand O (1975) Effects of different ionic environments on the mechano-sensitivity of lateral line organs in the mudpuppy. J Comp Physiol 102:27–42

Sand O, Ozawa S, Hagiwara S (1975) Electrical and mechanical stimulation of brain cells in the mudpuppy. J Comp Physiol 102:13–26

Schmaltz G (1925) Versuche zu einer Theorie des Erregungsvorganges im Ohrlabyrinth. Pflügers Arch 207:125–128

Schmaltz G (1932) The physical phenomena occurring in the semicircular canals during rotary and thermic stimulation. Proc R Soc Med 25:360–381

Schöne H (1959) Die Lageorientierung mit Statolithenorganen und Augen. Ergebn Biol 21:161–209

Shimazu H, Precht W (1965) Tonic and kinetic responses of cat's vestibular neurons to horizontal angular acceleration. J Neurophysiol 28:991–1013

Smith CA, Lowry OH, Wu ML (1954) The electrolytes of the labyrinthine fluids. Laryngoscope 64:141–153

Steinhausen W (1931) Über den Nachweis der Bewegung der Cupula in der intakten Bogengangsampulle des Labyrinthes bei der natürlichen rotatorischen und calorischen Reizung. Pflügers Arch 228:322–328

Steinhausen W (1933) Über die Beobachtung der Cupula in den Bogengangsampullen des Labyrinthes des lebenden Hechtes. Pflügers Arch 232:500–512

Suzuki J, Tokumasu K, Goto K (1969) Eye movements from single ultricular nerve stimulation in the cat. Acta Otolaryngol (Stockh) 68:350–362

Szentagothai J (1950) The elementary vestibulo-ocular reflex arc. J Neurophysiol 13:395–407

Szentágothai J (1964) Pathways and synaptic articulation patterns connecting vestibular receptors and oculomotor nuclei. In: Bender MB (ed) The oculomotor system. Hoeber Medical Division, Harper and Row, New York, pp 205–223

Tasaki I, Spyropoulos CS (1959) Stria vascularis as source of endocochlear potential. J Neurophysiol 22:149–155

Tasaki I, Davis H, Eldredge DH (1954) Exploration of cochlear potentials in guinea pig with a microelectrode. J Acoust Soc Am 26:765

Tavolga WN (1971) Sound production and detection. In: Hoar WS, Randall DJ (eds) Fish physiology, vol V. Academic, New York, pp 135–205

Trendelenburg W, Kühn A (1908) Vergleichende Untersuchungen zur Physiologie des Ohrlabyrinthes der Reptilien. Arch Anat Physiol [Suppl] 160–188

Trincker D (1965) Physiologie des Gleichgewichtsorgans. In: Berendes J, Link R, Zöllner ZF (eds) Handbuch der Hals-, Nasen- und Ohrenheilkunde, vol 3/1. Thieme, Stuttgart, pp 311–361

Trincker D, Partsch CJ (1959) The AC potentials (microphonics) from the vestibular apparatus. Ann Otol Rhinol Laryngol 68:153–158

Van Egmond AAJ, Groen JJ, Jonkees LBW (1949) The mechanics of the semicircular canal. J Physiol (Lond) 110:1–17

Vilstrup G, Vilstrup T (1952) Does the utricular otolithic membrane move on postural changes of the head? Ann Otol Rhinol Laryngol 61:189–197

Vilstrup T, Jensen CE, Koefoed J (1954) Reports on the chemical composition of the fluids of the labyrinth. Ann Otolaryngol Chir Cervicofac 63:157–163

Vinnikov YAA (1974) Sensory reception, cytology, molecular mechanisms, and evolution. Springer, Berlin Heidelberg New York

von Békésy G (1951) DC potentials and energy balance of the cochlear partition. J Acoust Soc Am 22:576–582

von Békésy G (1952) DC resting potentials inside the cochlear partition. J Acoust Soc Am 24:72–76 von Békésy G (1953) Description of some mechanical properties of the organ of Corti. J Acoust Soc Am 25:786–790

von Békésy G (1960) Experiments in hearing. McGraw-Hill, New York

von Frisch K (1936) Über den Gehörsinn der Fische. Biol Rev 11:210–246

von Holst E (1950) Die Arbeitsweise des Statolithenapparates bei Fischen. Z Vergl Physiol 32:60–120

Werner CF (1929) Über die Erregungsvorgänge im Labyrinth. Verh Dtsch Zool Ges 1929:99–104

Wersäll J (1956) Studies on the structures and innervation of the sensory epithelium of the cristae ampullares in the guinea pig. Acta Otolaryngol [Suppl] (Stockh) 126:1–85

Wersäll J, Bagger-Sjöbäck D (1974) Morphology of the vestibular sense organ. In: Kornhuber HH (ed) Vestibular system, pt 1 basic mechanisms. Springer, Berlin Heidelberg New York, pp 123 (Handbook of sensory physiology, vol 6/1)

Young LR (1969) The current status of vestibular system models. Automata 5:369–383

Young LR, Meiry YL (1967) A revised dynamic otolithic model, NASA Spec Publ 152:363–366

Young LR, Oman CM (1968) A model for vestibular adaptation to horizontal rotation. 4th Symposium on the role of the vestibular organs in space exploration. NASA Spec Publ 187:363–380

Young LR, Oman CM (1969) A model of vestibular adaptation to horizontal rotations. Aerospace Med 40:1076–1080

Author Index

Page numbers in *italics* refer to the references

Subject Index

Handbook of Sensory Physiology
Volumes I–IX

Volume I
Principles of Receptor Physiology

Editor: W.R.Loewenstein
1971. 262 figures. XII, 600 pages
ISBN 3-540-05144-9

From the Reviews: "This will undoubtedly become the authoritative treatise on sensory physiology…"
American Reference Books Annual

Volume II
Somatosensory System

Editor: A.Iggo
1973. 240 figures. XI, 851 pages ISBN 3-540-05941-5

From the Reviews: "…supported by excellent illustrations, including some crucial anatomical diagrams with added color… This volume should stand for years as a standard reference work…"
BioScience

Volume III

Part 1:
Enteroceptors

Editor: E.Neil
1972. 91 figures. VIII, 233 pages
ISBN 3-540-05523-1

Part 2:
Muscle Receptors

Editor: C.C.Hunt
1974. 128 figures. VIII, 310 pages
ISBN 3-540-06891-0

Part 3:
Electroreceptors and Other Specialized Receptors in Lower Vertebrates

Editor: A.Fessard
1974. 118 figures. VIII, 333 pages
ISBN 3-540-06872-4

Volume IV
Chemical Senses

Editor: L.M.Beidler

Part 1:
Olfaction

1971. 212 figures. VIII, 518 pages
ISBN 3-540-05291-7

Part 2:
Taste

1971. 176 figures. VIII, 410 pages
ISBN 3-540-05501-0

Volume V
Auditory System

Editors: W.D.Keidel and W.D.Neff

Part 1:
Anatomy, Physiology (Ear)

1974. 305 figures. VIII, 736 pages
ISBN 3-540-06676-4

Part 2:
Physiology (CNS), Behavioral Studies, Psychoacoustics

1975. 12 tables, 209 figures. VII, 526 pages
ISBN 3-540-07000-1

Part 3:
Clinical and Special Topics

1976. 343 figures. VII, 811 pages ISBN 3-540-07129-6

From the Reviews: "…attention to clarity and detail characterizes the entire book. For the audiological research worker or the serious student wishing a compilation of auditory physiology, this book is invaluable." *Journal of the American Medical Association*

Volume VI
Vestibular System

Editor: H.H.Kornhuber

Part 1:
Basic Mechanisms

1974. 251 figures. VIII, 676 pages
ISBN 3-540-06889-9

Part 2:
Psychophysics, Applied Aspects and General Interpretations

1974. 198 figures. VIII, 680 pages
ISBN 3-540-06864-3

Springer-Verlag
Berlin
Heidelberg
New York
Tokyo

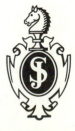

Springer-Verlag
Berlin
Heidelberg
New York
Tokyo

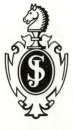